PHLEBOTOMY

Exam Review

THIRD EDITION

PHLEBOTOMY

Exam Review

THIRD EDITION

Ruth E. McCall, BS, MT(ASCP)
Retired Phlebotomy Program and Clinical Laboratory
Assistant Program Director
Central New Mexico Community College
Albuquerque, New Mexico

Cathee M. Tankersley, BS, MT(ASCP), CLS (NCA)
Retired Phlebotomy Program Director
Faculty Emeritus
Phoenix College
Phoenix, Arizona

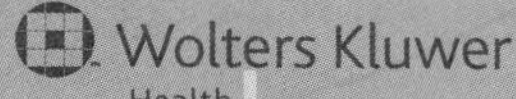

Lippincott Williams & Wilkins
Philadelphia • Baltimore • New York • London
Buenos Aires • Hong Kong • Sydney • Tokyo

Acquisitions Editor: Barrett Koger
Managing Editor: Michael Marino
Marketing Manager: Nancy Bradshaw
Associate Production Manager: Kevin P. Johnson
Creative Director: Doug Smock
Compositor: International Typesetting and Composition

Third Edition

Lippincott Williams & Wilkins, a Wolters Kluwer business.

351 West Camden Street
Baltimore, MD 21201

530 Walnut Street
Philadelphia, PA 19106

Printed in the United States

9 8 7 6 5 4 3 2 1

Library of Congress Cataloging-in-Publication Data

McCall, Ruth E.
Phlebotomy exam review/Ruth E. McCall, Cathee M. Tankersley.—3rd ed.
p. ; cm.
Includes bibliographical references and index.
ISBN-13: 978-0-7817-7855-8
ISBN-10: 0-7817-7855-7
1. Phlebotomy—Examinations, questions, etc. I. Tankersley, Cathee M. II. Title.
[DNLM: 1. Phlebotomy—Examination Questions. WB 18.2 M4777p 2008]
RB45.15.M332 2008
616.07'561—dc22

2007037827

DISCLAIMER

To all of the thousands of students who have graced our classrooms in the past and made our teaching careers so worthwhile. Thank you.

Ruth E. McCall
Cathee M. Tankersley

PREFACE

The demand for phlebotomists and other allied health workers who perform phlebotomy to demonstrate competency through national certification has increased in light of recent federal safety requirements and healthcare accrediting agency requirements for quality assurance. In addition, some states, such as California, require national certification by an approved certification agency as a condition of obtaining licensure.

Phlebotomy Exam Review, 3rd edition, continues the tradition of the second edition by providing a comprehensive review of current phlebotomy theory and offers an ideal way to study for phlebotomy licensing or national certification exams. It also makes an excellent study guide for students taking formal phlebotomy training programs.

Answering the questions in this review provides you with an opportunity to test your knowledge and application of current phlebotomy theory. Theory questions address recent federal safety standards, Clinical and Laboratory Standards Institute (CLSI) guidelines, and the National Accrediting Agency for Clinical Laboratory Sciences (NAACLS) phlebotomist competencies when applicable. Questions are standard multiple-choice, like those used on national exams, with choices that often test your critical thinking abilities.

The question section of the book follows the same chapter sequence as that of the companion textbook, *Phlebotomy Essentials,* 4th edition, by the same authors. This format makes it an ideal chapter-by-chapter study reference when used in conjunction with the textbook in phlebotomy training programs.

Outstanding unique features include:

- An expanded table of contents that corresponds to the companion textbook, *Phlebotomy Essentials,* 4th edition
- Current information on the various exams, including names and contact information for eight organizations that offer phlebotomy certification exams
- A pretest and pretest analysis to help you evaluate your knowledge and application of current phlebotomy theory
- A process for creating your very own study plan and way to track your study hours
- A section on study and test-taking skills to help ensure success on the exam
- Overview and study tips pertinent to each chapter
- Preparation tips for test-taking for ESL students
- 1,383 multiple-choice questions with correct answers, each answer having a detailed explanation of why it is correct
- Question choices that are concise, to lessen the chance of confusion, and similar in length, to enhance validity of results by minimizing guessing based on length
- Two comprehensive mock exams, one traditional (pencil and paper) and one computer-based on CD

This book is designed to help you succeed by providing the information and tools you need to help you pass any national exam you might choose to take. We have incorporated years of test-writing experience and major revisions to make this latest exam review book a stimulating learning experience. It is not intended to replace formal education in phlebotomy theory, nor is there any guarantee that using this exam review will ensure passage of any certification or licensing exam.

The authors wish to express their gratitude to all who assisted and supported this effort, with special thanks to Pat DeVere, Mimi Roush, and Jack Nida.

RUTH E. MCCALL
CATHEE M. TANKERSLEY

CONTENTS

PHLEBOTOMY

Exam Review

THIRD EDITION

Guide to Certification Success

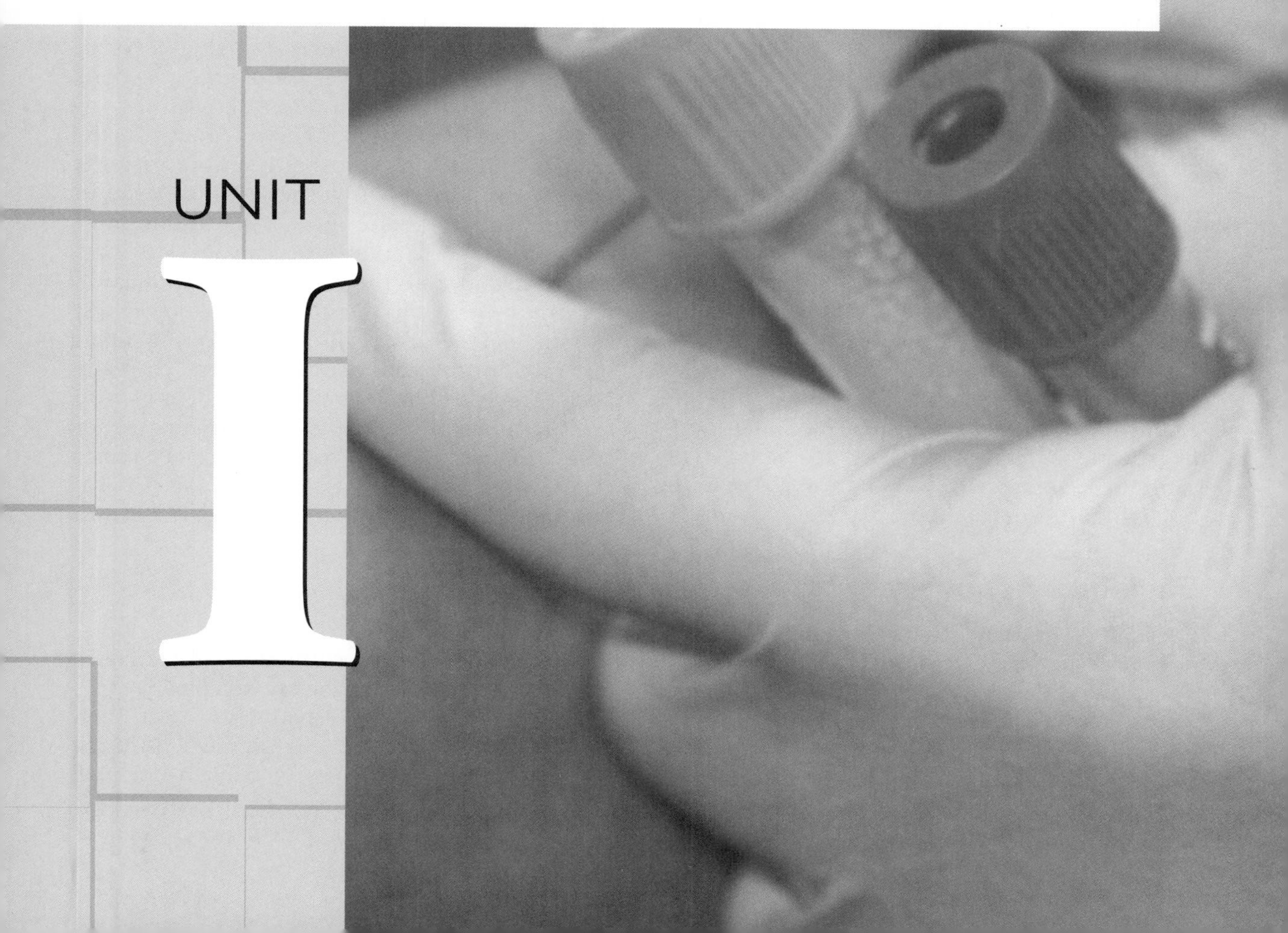

UNIT I

THE CERTIFICATION PROCESS

Certification

Certification is a process in which a national nongovernmental organization recognizes the competence of an individual in a particular profession or discipline. In today's healthcare climate, recognition through certification is becoming more popular because of the need for healthcare professionals to show evidence of proficiency in many different areas of practice. Most laboratory errors occur in the preanalytical phase, so it is essential that all healthcare workers who collect blood specimens prove their competence in an effort to ensure quality patient care. In addition, national certification in phlebotomy is required by many institutions to address federal safety and QA requirements and to meet licensing requirements in some states.

Credentials

Proof of certification is provided by credentials awarded to candidates who have met the educational or experiential requirements of a certifying organization and have successfully passed the organization's certification exam. Certification credentials provide evidence that the individual has mastered fundamental competencies in the profession. Certification credentials indicate competence at the time of the exam, and recertification is a mechanism used to demonstrate continued competence either through re-exam or continuing education.

Eligibility Requirements

Eligibility requirements for obtaining certification vary according to the certifying organization; however, most certifying organizations recognize several eligibility routes. Eligibility routes typically include graduation from an approved educational program, other specific education requirements, or work experience. Requirements to maintain or renew certification also vary, from no requirements (meaning once certified, always certified) to submitting proof of a minimum number of hours of continuing education and payment of a renewal fee.

Exam Format

Although some certification exams are still traditional hard copy exams taken with pencil and paper, many exams are computer-based. Computer-based testing (CBT) is the equivalent of a paper test that is administered by computer and has the advantage of faster scoring. One example of a computer-based exam is the National Credentialing Agency (NCA) phlebotomy certification exam.

Some exams may involve computer adaptive testing (CAT). When a question is answered correctly on a CAT exam, the very next question comes from a somewhat higher level of difficulty. The difficulty level of the questions presented to the examinee continues to increase until a question is answered incorrectly. At that time, a question that is a little easier is presented. Consequently, the test is tailored to the individual's ability level. CAT testing attempts to establish an appropriate level of performance and stops the test once the candidate's performance is determined to be at the highest sustainable level. Because CAT scoring takes into account which questions were correctly answered as well as how many, candidates who answer more difficult questions obtain higher scores than those who correctly answer easier questions. The American Society for Clinical Pathology (ASCP) phlebotomy certification exam is a CAT exam.

Exam Content

Regardless of the format, currently available exams are based on similar versions of accepted competencies for entry-level phlebotomists. Most often these competencies are determined through job/task analysis surveys. The National Accrediting Agency for Clinical Laboratory Sciences (NAACLS) outlines competencies for phlebotomy programs approved by their organization. Outlines reflecting exam content and references used in developing questions are available from most certifying organizations and are usually sent automatically to applicants. Exam questions typically are based on standards for venipuncture, skin puncture, and other phlebotomy procedures developed by the Clinical and Laboratory Standards Institute (CLSI). The number of questions varies from 80 to 250, depending on the offering agency. Some exams have a practical component. Examples are the American Certification Agency (ACA) and American Medical Technologists (AMT) phlebotomy certification exams.

Choosing an Exam

Once you have decided to become certified, your next job is to decide which organization's exam you would like to take. Currently, at least eight organizations offer certification in phlebotomy. All of these organizations have exam sites throughout the United States. Several of them also offer exams in United States territories, such as Puerto Rico, and in other countries such as Canada.

Generally speaking, employers do not favor any single certifying organization, but applicants may find that one exam better suits their needs than another. In addition, requirements vary by organization, so your choice may be limited depending on your ability to meet the eligibility requirements for the particular exam you choose. Table I-1 (Phlebotomy Certification Organizations) has information that can help you decide which exam or exams you might be interested in taking. To find out if you are eligible for the exam of your choice, go to the agency's website listed in the table. Websites have applications you can download, and in some cases you can even apply online.

Application Deadlines

Application deadlines for exams offered during a particular period vary according to organization policies. Applications can generally be submitted at any time throughout the year but will typically apply to the exam offering that corresponds with the deadline closest to the date that the application is received. Applications can be submitted by mail or online, depending on the organization.

Knowing What to Study

You have decided to become nationally certified. This is a worthy goal, but now where to start? Just what should be studied and how much time should it take? The pretest and pretest analysis that follow can help point out what subjects you need to study and how much time you will need to devote to each of those subjects.

THE PRETEST AND PRETEST ANALYSIS

The pretest and pretest analysis help you determine your strengths and weaknesses in three major categories of phlebotomy: specimen collection and handling, quality assurance, and general knowledge. For study purposes, the categories have been divided into 23 subject areas. The pretest contains questions for each area.

The Pretest

This test is simply to indicate the subject areas in which you will need to study. Consequently, when you sit down to take it, do not rush and do not time yourself. Answer each question by writing the answer on a separate piece of paper. This allows you to retake the test as many times as you like. After taking the pretest found in Unit IV, perform the pretest analysis, which will show you how much time to devote to each of the subject areas.

The Pretest Analysis

The pretest analysis, which takes approximately 45 to 50 minutes, shows you which topics are in need of additional study time and

Table I-1 Phlebotomy Certification Organizations

Organization	Address	Website	Contact Person
American Certification Agency (ACA)	P.O. Box 58 Osceola, IN 46561	acacert.com	Shirley Evans Carole Mullins
American Medical Technologists (AMT)	10700 West Higgins Road, Suite 150 Rosemont, IL 60018	amt1.com	Geri Mulcahy Chris Damon Dr. James Fidler
American Society of Clinical Pathology (ASCP)	33 West Monroe Street, Suite 1600 Chicago, IL 60603	ascp.org	Iris McLemore
American Society of Phlebotomy Technicians (ASPT)	P.O. Box 1831 Hickory, NC 28603	aspt.org	Helen Maxwell
National Credentialing Agency for Laboratory Personnel (NCA)	P.O. Box 15945-289 Lenexa, KS 66285	nca-info.org	Sheila O'Neal Deborah Grooms
National Center for Competency Testing (NCCT)	7007 College Blvd., Suite 700 Overland Park, KS 66211	ncctinc.com	Stan Adams Bruce Brackett Nancy Graham
National Healthcareer Association (NHA)	7 Ridgedale Avenue, Suite 203 Cedar Knolls, NJ 07927	nhanow.com	Jon S. Brandt Ruth Glickman
National Phlebotomy Association (NPA)	1901 Brightseat Road Landover, MD 20785	nationalphlebotomy.org	Altonese Reese

how much time should be allotted for each. You will find that time invested here saves you time in the long run. It is a three-step process, and when it is completed you will know minimum recommended study times for each subject and major category and a recommended total review time. The process involves filling out Tables I-2 and I-3. Copies of the tables have been provided in the back of the book so that you can perform the analysis more than once if you desire. You can also make additional copies of the tables.

Step 1

Each answer on the pretest has been assigned to a subject area that corresponds to 1 of 23 subjects listed in Table I-2. When you have finished the pretest, go back and check each question. Put a check mark in the box provided by the question

Telephone	E-mail	Fax	Testing Period	Testing Site
574-277-4538	info@acacert.com	574-277-4624	Contact office	Contact office
800-275-1268 847-823-5169	RPT@amt1.com geri.mulcahy@amt1.com	847-823-0458	Self-scheduled; open all year	More than 200 test centers throughout the United States
312-541-4999	bor@ascp.org	312-541-4998	Jan.–Mar. April–June July–Sept. Oct.–Nov.	More than 200 test centers throughout the United States
828-294-0078	office@aspt.org	828-327-2969	Contact office for times	Contact office for sites
913-895-4613	soneal@goamp.com nca-info@goamp.com	913-895-4652	5 days/week 52 weeks/year No application deadline	150+ nationally located assessment centers with international testing locations available as well
800-875-4404	stan@ncctinc.com nancy@ncctinc.com	913-498-1243	Contact office	Contact office for nearest test site
800-499-9092 973-605-1881	info@nhanow.com drglickman@nhanow.com	973-644-4797	Every day	More than 1,000 national and international sites
866-329-9108	naltphle@aol.com	301-386-4203	As scheduled	Where requested

if the answer was incorrect or if you were unsure and it required a significant amount of time to decide on the answer.

Now review the pretest again and count the total boxes checked for each subject area. Write this number in the corresponding box in Table I-2. For example, if you have three answers checked for Anatomy and Physiology, you would put a 3 in that box. Put a "happy face" in the subject box if there are no check marks for that subject.

Step 2

When you have reviewed all of the questions on the pretest and have filled in all of the boxes in Table I-2, you can estimate your study time in the following way:

- 0–1 in a topic box implies reasonable knowledge of that particular topic and a recommended study time of a minimum of 1.0 hour. For every topic box that has a 0–1, place a "1"

Table I-2 Exam Topics and Study Hours by Topic

General Knowledge 26%	Specimen Collection 60%	Quality Assurance 14%
Healthcare System ☐ Recommended study time__ hr.	Patient Considerations ☐ Recommended study time__ hr.	Regulatory Agencies ☐ Recommended study time__ hr.
Communication ☐ Recommended study time__ hr.	Equipment ☐ Recommended study time__ hr.	Preanalytical Considerations ☐ Recommended study time__ hr.
Professionalism ☐ Recommended study time__ hr.	Venipuncture ☐ Recommended study time__ hr.	The Law and Ethics ☐ Recommended study time__ hr.
Infection Control ☐ Recommended study time__ hr.	Capillary ☐ Recommended study time__ hr.	Professional Standards ☐ Recommended study time__ hr.
Safety ☐ Recommended study time__ hr.	Arterial ☐ Recommended study time__ hr.	
Anatomy & Physiology ☐ Recommended study time__ hr.	Handling ☐ Recommended study time__ hr.	
Circulatory System ☐ Recommended study time__ hr.	Processing ☐ Recommended study time__ hr.	
Terminology ☐ Recommended study time__ hr.	Transporting ☐ Recommended study time__ hr.	
Tests & Disorders ☐ Recommended study time__ hr.	Specimen Types ☐ Recommended study time__ hr.	
	POCT ☐ Recommended study time__ hr.	

in the corresponding blank for recommended study time.

- 2 in a topic box implies partial knowledge of that particular topic and a recommended study time of a minimum of 2.0 hours. For every topic box that has a 2, place a "2" in the corresponding blank for recommended study time.
- 3 in a topic box implies limited knowledge of that particular topic and a recommended study time of a minimum of 3.0 hours. For every topic box that has a 3, place a "3" in the corresponding blank for recommended study time.

Table I-3 Summary of Study Hours

Study Item	Hours
Pretest Suggested Study Hours	
Additional study hours added for Specimen Collection and Handling which is >50% of the test questions on all exams	4
Timed mock exam (computer or written) and final prep hours	4
Total suggested minimum study hours	

Step 3

Add up all of the recommended study hours in Table I-2 and write that total number in the appropriate blank in Table I-3. Add up all hours in Table I-3 and write that number in the "total suggested minimum study hours" blank.

Your pretest analysis is now complete. The results reveal your subject area strengths and weaknesses and provide a recommended minimum study time for each subject. In Table I-3, Summary of Study Hours, you will see that the total review time includes suggested study hours for mock exams and final preparation hours. This summary has been tested and tried and shows good results when followed.

STUDYING AND TEST-TAKING TIPS

Regardless of the type of test you are preparing for, you can use numerous techniques to study and review effectively and improve your test-taking ability. The following information is designed to help you develop a study plan, control the study and test-taking environment, and learn key ways to retain information while studying. The desired result is to be able to effectively express your knowledge of a subject while taking a test.

Strategies for ESL Students

Studying for a national exam can be a challenge. It can be an even greater challenge if English is not your primary language. The following strategies are meant to help ESL (English as a Second Language) students meet that challenge.

- Fluency in English is obviously a plus when taking a national exam. If you have difficulty reading or speaking English, consider taking the Combined English Language Skills Assessment (CELSA) tests for non-English speakers. These tests, which are available at most community colleges, identify your level of English. Several Internet sites offer online English skills assessment tools and other resources for ESL students.
- Most exam agencies ask for proof of high school graduation or the equivalent as one of the requirements to sit for the exam. If your English skills are not at the level of a high school graduate, you may have a hard time passing a national exam and should consider taking an ESL course at a local community college or other school.
- Purchase or borrow an ESL dictionary (to help you with unfamiliar terms) and an ESL medical terminology book (to help you learn how to identify the meanings of basic elements of medical terms). Make flash cards for terms you need to work on.
- Most questions and choices in this exam review are short and concise to lessen confusion. However, you may still encounter problems understanding a question or choice. If so, focus on the words or parts of the question you do understand to lead you in the right direction when trying to figure it out. If it still doesn't make sense, work backwards by studying the explanation of the correct choice to see if that helps. Practicing this technique with the exam review questions will help prepare you to tackle difficult questions on the certification exam.
- The saying "two heads are better than one" is quite often true. Try to find a study partner whose native language is English or an ESL individual who is already fluent in English. Choose someone who is motivated and organized and who will encourage and inspire you to do your best.
- Wait to sign up for an exam until you are confident of your abilities. There is a big advantage to studying the material at your leisure without an exam deadline fast approaching. Use the studying and test-taking tips that follow, and you will be well on your way to a successful certification experience.

Preparing to Study

Cultivate a Positive Attitude

The adage, "You can do anything if you set your mind to it," makes a lot of sense. Those who think they can succeed at something and have a plan to achieve it are usually successful. Those who think they will fail usually do. If your goal is to pass a national certification exam, tell yourself that you can pass it and visualize being successful. Your belief that you will be able to successfully pass the exam actually helps you achieve that goal. In addition, your attitude plays an important role in determining how you approach preparation for the exam and ultimately how well you do on the actual exam. A positive attitude during the study process will result in more effective studying and increase learning and retention. Bringing a positive attitude to the test will help relieve the stress associated with the testing process and leave your mind free to think logically and make you a more successful test-taker.

Plan to Study

A key element of effective studying is the ability to manage your study or review time. Plan to study. Develop a routine by establishing a particular time and place to study. Committing yourself to a regular routine eliminates the continual need to decide when and where to study. This keeps you in control and helps eliminate procrastination.

Establish a Consistent Study Setting

Choose a site that is compatible with study activities, such as a desk or table. Make sure the site is comfortable and has adequate lighting to minimize eyestrain and fatigue. Resist the temptation to get too comfortable, however. Avoid beds or couches, where you may become too relaxed and fall asleep.

Limit Distractions and Commitments

Select a place to study where you are less likely to be disturbed by family members, roommates, pets, TV, phones, and other distractions.

- Do not answer the phone. If you do not have an answering machine, consider unplugging the phone. Turn off your cell phone or at least the ring tone.
- Put a "Do Not Disturb" sign on the door.
- Do not disrupt your study schedule unless it is really important. Learn to say "no."

When to Study

Study When You Are Rested

You are more alert when you are rested. Do not study when you are already physically or emotionally tired, and never study to the point of exhaustion. Studies have shown that getting a good night's sleep soon after learning information helps retention, so avoid the temptation to stay up until the wee hours of the morning, especially on the day of the exam.

Follow Your Daily Biorhythm

If possible, study during a time of day when you are most alert and efficient. For example, if you are a morning person, try to arrange study time in the morning.

How to Study

Have a Review Strategy

Decide in advance how you will review the material and allow adequate time to accomplish everything you want to do. Use whatever method works best for you. Effective study strategies include reviewing your notes, textbook, and study questions and taking practice tests or mock exams.

Consider Forming a Study Group

Set aside some time to study with other students or peers who are also preparing to take the same exam. Members of study groups tend to motivate each other. Members can also share study tips and techniques that work well for them. Socializing and conversations unrelated to the topic at hand are distracting and reduce actual study time. Agree ahead of time that you will limit socializing and other distractions to within the first few minutes of arriving and after the allotted study time is over.

Establish a Realistic Study Schedule

Avoid resorting to marathon study sessions. Short 1- to 3-hour study sessions on a regular basis are usually more beneficial than occasional long, drawn-out sessions.

Use Time Effectively

Copy information that needs to be memorized into a small notebook or on note cards and carry them with you. That way you can study small amounts while waiting in line, riding the bus, or waiting for appointments. Note cards can also be taped on mirrors or cupboards,for quick reviews in between other chores or activities.

Take Breaks

Do not forget the old saying, "All work and no play makes Jack a dull boy." You by no means want to be "dull" on test day. Schedule breaks into your allotted study time. The ideal break should be short enough to relieve stress but not so extended that you lose focus, interest, or rhythm.

Watch the Time

Keep track of the time and do not waste it. If you get frustrated or your attention starts to wander, take a break.

Study What Is Appropriate

Try not to study more than necessary. Do not repeatedly go over material you already know. Review it every so often to make certain you still remember it, but do not spend a great deal of time on it. For example, it would be a waste of time to read the textbook or your class notes over and over. A more effective method would be to review your notes and refer to the textbook to clarify concepts or information you have forgotten or do not completely understand.

Study Difficult Topics First

Although the pretest has given you an idea of what subjects you need to study and a recommended amount of study time for each subject, you still have to decide the order in which to study them. It is usually advantageous to study difficult or boring concepts or topics first while your mind is clear. Trying to master a difficult topic at the end of your allotted study time can result in frustration because of a reduced ability to concentrate.

Don't Try to Study Everything At Once

Think about the answer to the joke, "How do you eat an elephant?" Answer: "One bite at a time!" Divide extensive topics into smaller portions.

Use the Exam Review Effectively

Once you feel that you are familiar with the material, try to answer the questions in the exam review. Refer to the textbook for information if you cannot answer a question or still need to clarify material after you read the explanation for the correct answer.

Take the Sample Exams

When you feel you have a good grasp of the material and have answered the review questions, take the sample exams. Again, refer to the text or class notes when you cannot answer a question. Never attempt to memorize questions and answers. The intent of the study questions and sample exams is to help you identify areas in which your knowledge is weak. In addition, because many exams are computer-based, taking the sample computer exam will help you feel more comfortable taking computer exams in the future.

How to Improve Your Thinking Skills

Multiple-choice questions usually cover six commonly recognized thinking levels. From lowest to highest they are memory, comprehension, application, analysis, synthesis, and evaluation. When studying for multiple-choice tests, many students mistakenly spend their study time learning at the lowest level, memorizing facts without understanding how to analyze and apply the information. Learning how to identify the various thinking levels and using the skills associated with them as you study should help to enhance your knowledge of the subject and help you be a successful test-taker.

Memory Skills

Memory questions require the lowest level of thinking and involve the ability to recall specific information such as terminology, structures, classifications, facts, or concepts. Information of this type is most commonly memorized using techniques involving constant repetition. Examples of memorization techniques include reciting information aloud, listing information, and using flash cards. Information learned this way is committed to short-term memory and may be forgotten unless reinforced using other study methods or practical application.

The following are ways to assist in the memorization of information and enhance recall.

ABCS

Associating information with letters of the alphabet is an effective means of recalling information. Each letter of the alphabet acts as a cue or hint to recall information. You can make up your own ABCs to remember information and use established ones such as the following: the ABCs of cardiopulmonary resuscitation are A = airway, open the airway; B = breathing, perform rescue breathing; and C = circulation, initiate chest compressions.

ACRONYMS

Another helpful technique used to recall information is the use of acronyms, or words formed by the first letter of a series of statements or facts. Each letter of the word jogs the memory to recall previously learned information. An example is the acronym RACE, used to remember action to take in the event of a fire: R = rescue, A = alarm, C = confine, E = extinguish.

ACROSTICS

Acrostics are catchy phrases or jingles in which the first letter of each word helps you to remember certain information. An example is the jingle used to help remember the order of draw for the evacuated tube method of venipuncture: Stop light red, stay put, green light, go. S = sterile collections such as blood culture bottles or tubes, L = light blue top tubes, R = red top tubes, S = serum separator tubes (SSTs), P = plasma separator tubes (PSTs), G = green top tubes, L = lavender top tubes, G = gray top tubes.

IMAGING

Forming a mental picture associated with the information is another technique used to recall information. For example, one way to remember that a lipemic specimen is caused by fatty substances in the blood that make the serum appear cloudy or milky-looking is to visualize a fat, white cloud when thinking about or saying the term "lipemic."

Comprehension Skills

Comprehension questions test your ability to understand information. To answer comprehension questions, you not only must recall information but also be able to understand the significance of the information. Comprehension questions test your ability to interpret information to draw conclusions or determine consequences, effects, or implications. A good way to enhance comprehension of material is to ask yourself, "What is the significance of this information—how or why is this information useful?" Again, using the term "lipemic" as an example, once we know what the term lipemic means and what a lipemic specimen looks like, we can now ask ourselves, "What is the significance of a lipemic specimen? Why or how is this information useful?" One answer is that a lipemic specimen is a clue that the patient was not fasting. This is significant if the test was ordered fasting. Lipemia also interferes with the testing process for some chemistry tests. Now we not only can recall facts but are also learning to comprehend the significance of these facts.

Application Skills

Application questions test your ability to use information. Answering application questions requires that you not only remember and comprehend information but are also able to relate that information to a real-life situation. Again, using the example of the term "lipemic," an application question might be: "When processing a specimen for a fasting glucose test, you notice that the specimen is lipemic. What does this tell you about the specimen?" Thought process: Lipemia can occur after eating fatty foods. If the specimen is lipemic, the patient must have eaten recently, which means the specimen is probably not a fasting specimen.

Analysis Skills

Analysis questions test your ability to analyze or evaluate information. Analysis questions often require you to evaluate several options to reach an answer. You must be able to recognize differences and determine the significance of several choices before arriving at your answer.

Example: Which of the following specimens would most likely be rejected for testing? A:

a. lipemic specimen for glucose testing.
b. platelet count drawn in an EDTA tube.
c. routine UA in an unsterile container.
d. potassium specimen that is hemolyzed.

The following is a typical thought process used to analyze the choices for the question above and determine the correct answer:

a. A lipemic specimen is an indication that the patient was not fasting, but it does not say it was a fasting glucose. In addition, a few people have lipemic serum for other reasons, so the specimen would not necessarily be rejected.
b. A platelet count *should* be collected in EDTA, so it would not be rejected for that reason.
c. A urine C&S *must* be collected in a sterile container, but a routine UA *does not have to be,* so an unsterile container would not cause it to be rejected.
d. Hemolysis liberates potassium from the red blood cells. That means a hemolyzed potassium specimen would most likely be rejected. The correct answer is "d."

How to Answer Multiple-Choice Questions

- For written exams, jot down memory aids in the margins if you are allowed.
- Read the question carefully.
- Do not assume information that is not given.
- Eliminate choices that are clearly incorrect.
- Answer the easy questions first.
- Do not spend a great deal of time on questions you cannot answer.
- If you do not know the answer, skip the question and come back later. Information in other questions may remind you of the correct answer. If you still do not know the answer, try to make an educated guess.
- Do not change answers without a good reason. Your first guess is usually your best unless other questions remind you of the correct response.

TIPS FOR TEST DAY

- Get a good night's sleep before the test. The more rested you are, the more you will be able to think clearly and do your best on the test.
- Collect the items that you must bring to the test, such as identification and test documents, ID, calculator, and pencils ahead of time so that you will not be scrambling to find them at the last minute.
- Wear comfortable clothes to the exam. Dress in layers so that you can adapt in case the room is too cold or too warm.
- Know your test site. If the test is in a location with which you are unfamiliar, drive by the testing site a day or two before the exam. If possible, travel during the same time of day as when you will be traveling to take the actual test. Allow yourself extra travel time the day

of the test in case there are unexpected delays.

- Arrive early for the test. That way you can get yourself situated and mentally prepared. You also have the opportunity to situate yourself in a location that is comfortable for you and suits your needs, rather than having to choose quickly from the seats that are left.
- Listen carefully while test directions are given. Ask for clarification from the proctor if you do not understand something.
- Try to relax. Change positions, or pause to take a deep breath and stretch now and then.

OVERCOMING TEST ANXIETY

Keep in mind that some anxiety or tension before an exam is normal, although excessive anxiety is not. Being well prepared is an excellent way to keep anxiety levels low. Having familiarity with the material builds confidence. The more familiar you are with the material, the more confident you will be. The more confident you are, the better you will do on the exam. Confidence in your ability and a positive attitude about your chances of success go a long way toward relieving stress or anxiety about the testing process. So prepare yourself well, approach the exam with confidence, banish negative thoughts, and visualize success.

Exam Review

UNIT

II

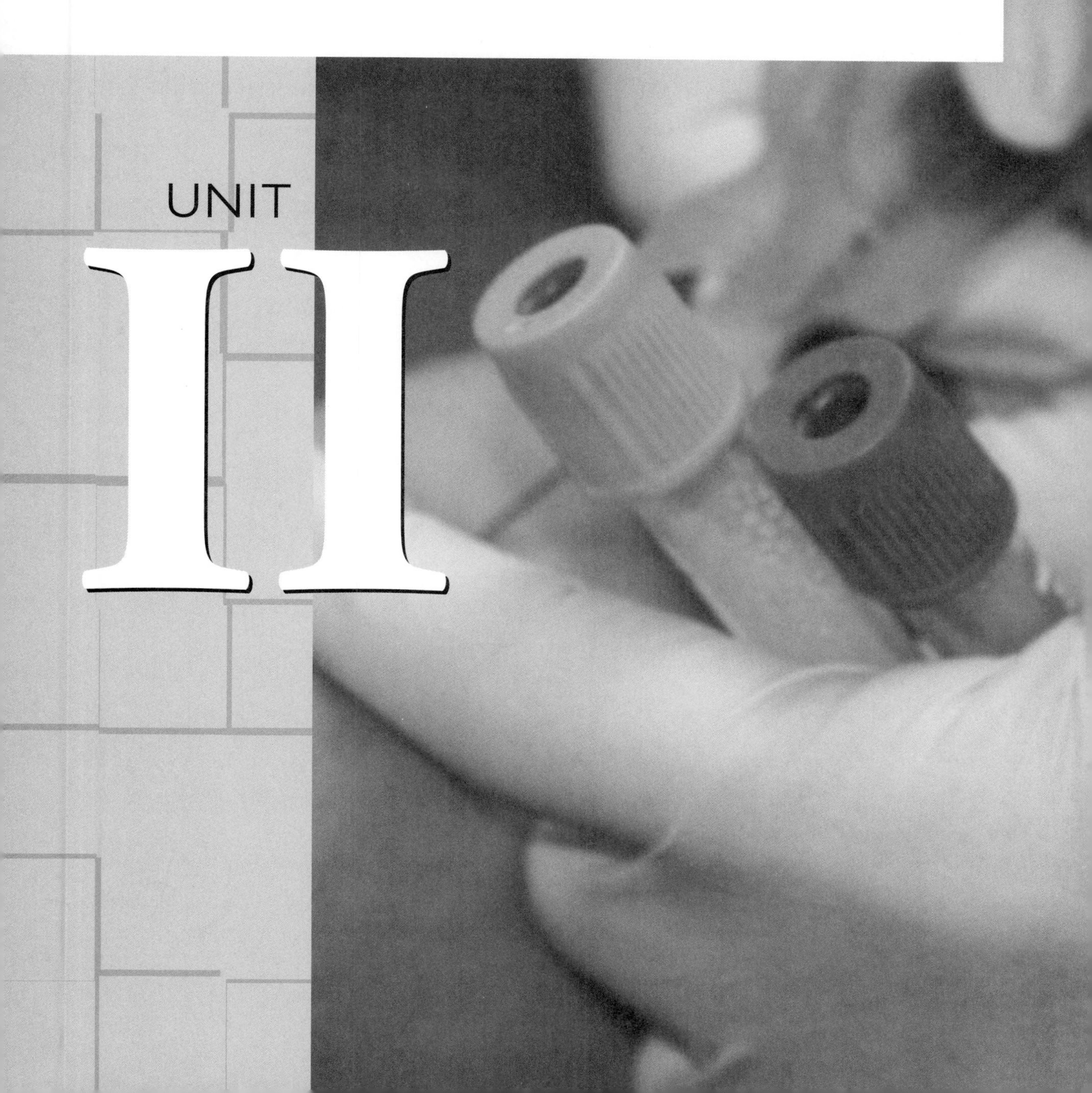

CHAPTER 1

PHLEBOTOMY: PAST AND PRESENT AND THE HEALTHCARE SETTING

study tip

Questions in this chapter test the ability to describe the evolution of phlebotomy practice and equipment into the role the phlebotomist plays in healthcare today, including traits that form the professional image of phlebotomists, organizations that support professional recognition of phlebotomists, and the basic elements of communication. Questions also test the ability to describe the healthcare delivery system, including healthcare settings and financing, and to identify and describe medical specialties, hospital and clinical laboratory departments, and related personnel.

overview

This chapter deals with the integrated healthcare delivery system, focusing on the clinical laboratory that provides physicians with some of medicine's most powerful diagnostic tests. As key players in the delivery of healthcare, phlebotomists must be familiar with the healthcare system and understand their role in healthcare delivery.

This chapter assesses knowledge of phlebotomy from its historical beginnings to the present-day role of the phlebotomist, with a special emphasis on the clinical laboratory. An understanding of phlebotomy from a historical perspective helps phlebotomists appreciate the significance of this role.

REVIEW QUESTIONS

Choose the BEST answer.

1. All of the following infectious disease services are offered through regional Public Health Services agencies EXCEPT:
   a. education.
   b. monitoring.
   c. screening.
   d. treatment.

2. This is an abbreviation for an independent group of hospitals and physicians that offers services to employers at a discounted rate in exchange for a steady supply of patients.
   a. CPT
   b. DRG
   c. PHS
   d. PPO

3. The abbreviation for the current coding system for physician billing is called:
   a. CPT.
   b. DRGs.
   c. PPO.
   d. PPS.

4. This is an abbreviation for large organizations that contract with local providers to establish a complete network of services.
   a. APC
   b. MCO
   c. PHS
   d. PPS

5. A nationally endorsed principle ensuring that patients and their families understand their rights and responsibilities while in a healthcare facility comes from:
   a. federal HIPAA regulations.
   b. prepaid healthcare plans.
   c. Protected Health Information.
   d. the Patient Care Partnership.

6. Managed Care Organizations control costs by all of the following ways EXCEPT:
   a. encouraging healthy lifestyles.
   b. detecting risk factors early.
   c. limiting patient enrollment.
   d. offering patient education.

7. The term used to describe a holistic, coordinated system of healthcare services is:
   a. continuum of care
   b. entitlement program
   c. health insurance plan
   d. public health services

8. This is the abbreviation for a classification system implemented in 2000 that is used to determine payment to hospitals for outpatient services.
   a. APC
   b. DRGs
   c. ICD-9
   d. PPS

Use Figure 1-1 (Example of Hospital Organizational Chart on page 17) to answer the following 5 questions:

9. Which Director, Chief Officer, or Vice President would have the administrative responsibility for ancillary testing, such as magnetic resonance (MR) scans?
   a. Sr. Director Performance Excellence
   b. VP Clinical & Support Services
   c. VP/Chief Nursing Officer
   d. VP & Chief Medical Officer

10. Who has the responsibility for control of hospital-induced infections in the healthcare facility?
    a. Sr. Director Performance Excellence
    b. VP Clinical & Support Services
    c. VP/Chief Nursing Officer
    d. VP & Chief Medical Officer

11. Who is responsible for the physicians who practice in the hospital?
    a. Sr. Director Performance Excellence
    b. VP Clinical & Support Services
    c. VP/Chief Nursing Officer
    d. VP & Chief Medical Officer

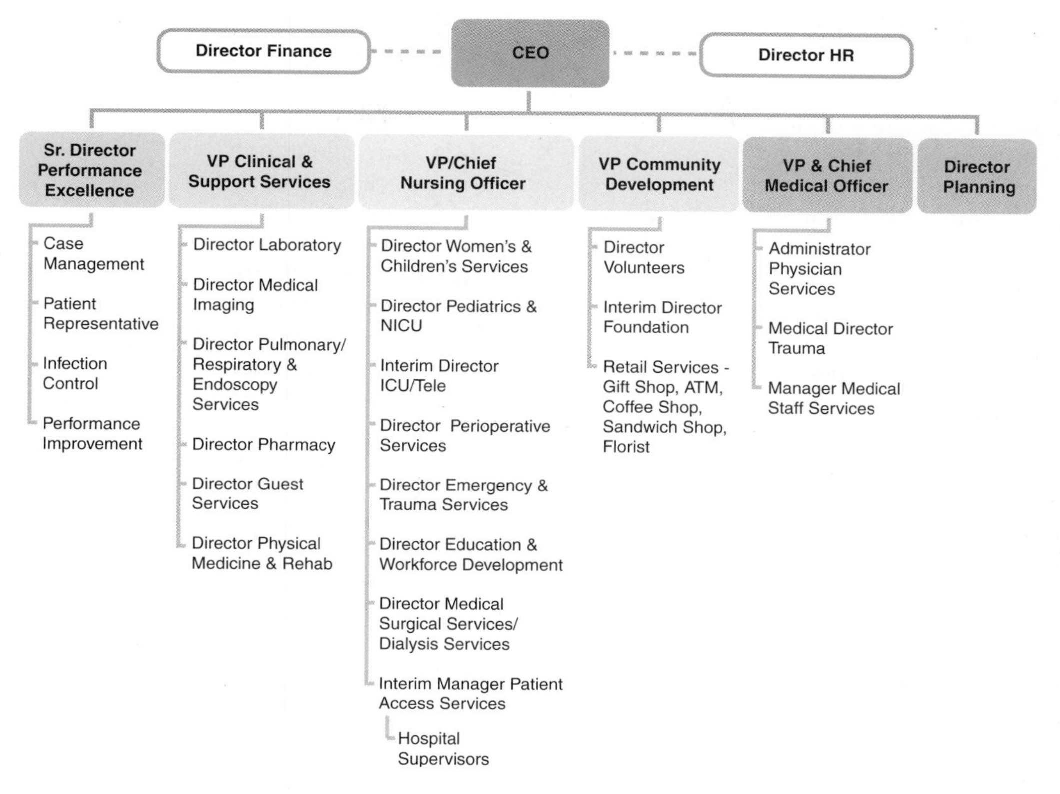

FIGURE 1-1 Example of a hospital organizational chart.

12. Which Director, Chief Officer, or Vice President has the administrative responsibility for outpatient medical services?
    a. Sr. Director Performance Excellence
    b. VP Clinical & Support Services
    c. VP/Chief Nursing Officer
    d. VP & Chief Medical Officer

13. Which Director, Chief Officer, or Vice President has the responsibility for quality performance and patient satisfaction?
    a. Sr. Director Performance Excellence
    b. VP Clinical & Support Services
    c. VP/Chief Nursing Officer
    d. VP & Chief Medical Officer

14. Which phlebotomist's duty involves TB and Cocci testing?
    a. collect routine venous specimens
    b. perform electrocardiography
    c. perform point-of-care testing
    d. prepare specimens for transport

15. Which phlebotomist's duty does *not* involve telephone etiquette?
    a. comply with instituted procedures
    b. maintain patient confidentiality
    c. perform quality control checks
    d. promote good public relations

16. Which of the following is an agency that certifies phlebotomists?
    a. ASCP
    b. CLIAC
    c. CLSI
    d. NAACLS

17. The primary duty of a phlebotomist is to:
 a. accession all specimens.
 b. collect blood specimens.
 c. document the workload.
 d. perform skin tests.

18. Promoting good public relations is a part of the phlebotomist's role for all of the following reasons EXCEPT:
 a. a phlebotomist is a representative of the laboratory.
 b. good public relations promotes harmonious relationships.
 c. patients equate experiences with overall caliber of care received.
 d. skilled public relations can cover up inexperience and insecurity.

19. *Primum non nocere* comes from the Hippocratic Oath and means:
 a. do first things first.
 b. first do no harm.
 c. quality is foremost.
 d. ready to serve.

20. Which of the following is an example of good work ethics?
 a. assertiveness
 b. noncommunicative behavior
 c. dependability
 d. indifference toward others

21. Phlebotomy is used as a therapeutic treatment for:
 a. diabetes.
 b. hypothyroidism.
 c. phlebitis.
 d. polycythemia.

22. All of the following are reasons for a phlebotomist to participate in continuing education programs EXCEPT:
 a. eliminate annual evaluations.
 b. learn new skills and techniques.
 c. renew licensure or certification.
 d. stay current in the latest procedures.

23. The term "phlebotomy" is derived from Greek words that, literally translated, mean to:
 a. cut a vein.
 b. draw blood.
 c. stick a vein.
 d. withdraw blood.

24. One of a phlebotomist's duties is to:
 a. assist with inserting IV cannulas.
 b. help nurses with direct patient care.
 c. inform patients of their test results.
 d. perform lab computer operations.

25. What are the credentials of an NCA-certified phlebotomist?
 a. CLPlb
 b. CPT
 c. PBT
 d. RPT

26. Which of the following ancient bloodletting instruments has a counterpart in a modern-day bleeding device?
 a. bleeding bowl
 b. cup
 c. fleam
 d. syringe

27. Proof of participation in a workshop to upgrade skills required by some agencies to renew certification is called:
 a. accreditation verification.
 b. continuing education units.
 c. essentials confirmation.
 d. reciprocity substantiation.

28. While staying in a healthcare facility, one patient expectation as listed in *The Patient Care Partnership* brochure is the right to:
 a. a 1:1 patient-to-nurse ratio.
 b. a quiet, private room.
 c. help with billing claims.
 d. information on roommates.

29. Personal "zone of comfort" is a radius of:
    a. 1–18 inches.
    b. $1\frac{1}{2}$–4 feet.
    c. 4–12 feet.
    d. over 12 feet.

30. All of the following are examples of barriers to effective communication EXCEPT the patient:
    a. does not speak English.
    b. is a very young child.
    c. is emotionally upset.
    d. is a mature male HCW.

31. Which of the following is an example of a confirming response to a patient?
    a. "I am on a tight schedule right now."
    b. "I do not know what you mean."
    c. "I have no idea how long it will take."
    d. "I understand how you must be feeling."

32. Which of the following is an example of negative kinesics?
    a. eye contact
    b. frowning
    c. good grooming
    d. smiling

33. Which one of the following projects a professional image for a phlebotomist?
    a. closed-toe, conservative shoes
    b. long hair that is not tied back
    c. natural-looking artificial nails
    d. very strong-smelling cologne

34. All of the following are good ways to earn a patient's trust EXCEPT:
    a. act knowledgeably.
    b. convey sincerity.
    c. dismiss patient fears.
    d. look professional.

35. Which one of the following represents improper telephone protocol?
    a. answer the phone promptly
    b. clarify and record information
    c. hang up on hostile individuals
    d. restate information received

36. Proxemics is the study of an individual's:
    a. body language.
    b. concept of space.
    c. facial expressions.
    d. verbal communication.

37. Elements of good communication in healthcare involve all of the following EXCEPT:
    a. accepting the patient as a unique individual who has special needs.
    b. allowing patients to feel a sense of control by expressing their wishes.
    c. disguising the truth to the patient with statements like "this won't hurt".
    d. listening thoughtfully and patiently while patients vent their emotions.

38. The best way to handle a "difficult" or "bad" patient is to:
    a. help the patient to feel in control of the situation.
    b. leave the room without collecting the specimen.
    c. speak firmly to maintain charge of the situation.
    d. threaten to report the patient to his or her doctor.

39. Which of the following is an example of proxemics?
    a. eye contact
    b. facial expression
    c. personal contact
    d. personal hygiene

40. Which of the following situations allows patients to feel in control?
    a. agreeing with patients that it is their right to refuse a blood draw
    b. informing patients that you are going to collect a blood sample
    c. insisting that patients cooperate and let you draw needed samples
    d. telling patients they are not to eat or drink anything during a test

41. What is the average speaking rate of a normal adult?
a. 75–100 words per minute
b. 125–150 words per minute
c. 250–350 words per minute
d. 500–600 words per minute

42. Another term for outpatient care is:
a. ambulatory care.
b. nonambulatory care.
c. nursing home care.
d. rehabilitation care.

43. Which laboratory department performs tests to identify abnormalities of the blood and blood-forming tissues?
a. chemistry
b. hematology
c. microbiology
d. urinalysis

44. Which department is responsible for administering a patient's oxygen therapy?
a. cardiodiagnostics
b. electroencephalography
c. physical therapy
d. respiratory therapy

45. Which of the following tests would be performed in surgical pathology?
a. compatibility testing
b. enzyme immunoassay
c. frozen section
d. triglycerides

46. The phlebotomist is asked to collect a specimen from a patient in the nephrology department. A patient in this department is most likely being treated for a disorder of the:
a. joints.
b. kidneys.
c. lungs.
d. nose.

47. The phlebotomy supervisor asked a phlebotomist to collect a specimen in the otorhinolaryngology department. The phlebotomist proceeded to go to the department that provides treatment for:
a. bone and joint disorders.
b. ear, nose, and throat disorders.
c. eye problems or diseases.
d. skin problems and diseases.

48. Which of the following tests is performed in the coagulation department?
a. BUN
b. CBC
c. glucose
d. PT

49. Which medical specialty treats patients with tumors?
a. geriatrics
b. oncology
c. ophthalmology
d. orthopedics

50. The medical specialty that treats skeletal system disorders is:
a. gastroenterology.
b. neurology.
c. orthopedics.
d. pediatrics.

51. The specialty of this physician is the treatment of newborns.
a. gerontologist
b. neonatologist
c. obstetrician
d. pediatrician

52. Another name for blood bank is:
a. immunohematology.
b. immunology.
c. microbiology.
d. serology.

53. All of the following are hematology tests EXCEPT:
a. glycosylated hemoglobin.
b. hematocrit.
c. platelet count.
d. reticulocyte count.

54. All of the following departments typically play a role in cerebrospinal fluid (CSF) analysis EXCEPT:
    a. chemistry.
    b. hematology.
    c. immunohematology.
    d. microbiology.

55. With which other hospital department would the laboratory coordinate therapeutic drug monitoring?
    a. nuclear medicine
    b. pharmacy
    c. physical therapy
    d. radiology

56. Which department processes and stains tissue samples for microscopic analysis?
    a. chemistry
    b. coagulation
    c. histology
    d. microbiology

57. All of the following personnel are required to have a college degree or equivalent EXCEPT:
    a. clinical laboratory scientist.
    b. medical technician.
    c. medical technologist.
    d. phlebotomist.

58. An appendectomy performed in a free-standing ambulatory surgical center is an example of:
    a. managed care.
    b. primary care.
    c. secondary care.
    d. tertiary care.

59. Which department performs blood cultures?
    a. hematology
    b. microbiology
    c. serology
    d. urinalysis

60. Electrolyte testing includes:
    a. bilirubin and creatinine.
    b. BUN and cholesterol.
    c. glucose and uric acid.
    d. sodium and potassium.

61. Which hospital department performs diagnostic tests and monitors therapy of patients with heart problems?
    a. ECG
    b. EEG
    c. ER
    d. ICU

62. Basic metabolic panels (BMPs) are performed in which department?
    a. chemistry
    b. hematology
    c. histology
    d. microbiology

63. Which laboratory department performs chromosome studies?
    a. chemistry
    b. coagulation
    c. cytogenetics
    d. hematology

64. A Pap smear is examined for the presence of cancer cells in this department.
    a. cytology
    b. hematology
    c. histology
    d. microbiology

65. The prepaid group healthcare organizations in which members pay flat fees for defined services are called:
    a. DRGs.
    b. HMOs.
    c. ICDs.
    d. SNFs.

66. The term used to describe sophisticated and highly complex medical care is:
    a. managed care.
    b. primary care.
    c. secondary care.
    d. tertiary care.

67. A patient in labor would normally be admitted to which of the following medical specialty departments?
a. cardiology
b. geriatrics
c. obstetrics
d. pediatrics

68. A primary physician is considered the patient's gatekeeper in this type of managed care plan.
a. HMO
b. IDS
c. MCO
d. PPO

69. Toxicology is often a part of which of the following laboratory departments?
a. chemistry
b. coagulation
c. hematology
d. urinalysis

70. This individual is a physician who is a specialist in diagnosing disease from laboratory findings.
a. administrative technologist
b. laboratory director
c. medical technologist
d. pathologist

71. Which of the following is a hematology test?
a. BMP
b. C&S
c. CBC
d. CSF

72. The department that analyzes arterial blood gases and tests lung capacity is:
a. cardiodiagnostics.
b. electroneurodiagnostics.
c. pharmacy.
d. respiratory therapy.

73. Which department performs CEA testing?
a. chemistry
b. hematology
c. microbiology
d. urinalysis

74. Which department performs radiographic procedures and other imaging techniques to aid in diagnosis?
a. occupational therapy
b. pharmacy
c. radiology
d. respiratory therapy

75. Which of the following is an example of an inpatient care facility?
a. day-surgery facility
b. dentist's office
c. major hospital
d. physician's office

76. Which of the following would most likely be performed in the serology department?
a. BUN
b. CBC
c. PTT
d. RPR

77. Which of the following laboratory personnel has the same qualification as a medical technologist?
a. CLS
b. CLT
c. MLT
d. pathologist

78. Which department would perform a hemogram?
a. chemistry
b. hematology
c. immunohematology
d. immunology

79. This department examines specimens microscopically for the presence of crystals, casts, bacteria, and blood cells.
a. chemistry
b. hematology
c. microbiology
d. urinalysis

80. This hospital department provides therapy to restore patient mobility.
  a. cardiodiagnostics
  b. physical therapy
  c. radiology
  d. respiratory therapy

81. Brain wave mapping and evoked potential are performed by which department?
  a. ECG
  b. EEG
  c. OT
  d. RT

82. All medical laboratories are regulated by:
  a. AMT.
  b. CLIA'88.
  c. HIPAA.
  d. PHS.

83. This is the abbreviation for a relatively new category of multiskilled personnel who work as part of the nursing team, performing nursing and phlebotomy duties.
  a. ADN
  b. CNA
  c. EMT
  d. PCT

84. Which laboratory worker has a bachelor's degree, or equivalent, in medical technology?
  a. CLS
  b. CLT
  c. MLT
  d. PBT

85. Which of the following laboratory personnel has an associate's degree, or equivalent?
  a. CLS
  b. CLT
  c. MT
  d. PBT

86. A specimen for ova and parasite testing would be sent to which department?
  a. chemistry
  b. coagulation
  c. microbiology
  d. urinalysis

87. The test to identify an organism and determine an appropriate antibiotic for treatment is called a:
  a. compatibility screen.
  b. culture and sensitivity.
  c. microscopic analysis.
  d. radioimmunoassay.

88. A glucose test would be performed in which department?
  a. chemistry
  b. hematology
  c. microbiology
  d. radioimmunoassay

89. Which medical specialty treats patients with blood disorders?
  a. dermatology
  b. hematology
  c. internal medicine
  d. urology

90. All of the following services are offered by local public health agencies EXCEPT:
  a. Healthcare worker licensing.
  b. Immunization and vaccination.
  c. Screening for diabetes.
  d. Venereal disease clinics.

91. Which department performs C&S tests?
  a. blood bank
  b. chemistry
  c. immunology
  d. microbiology

92. Blood typing and compatibility testing are performed in this department.
  a. blood bank
  b. chemistry
  c. coagulation
  d. hematology

93. A sample for fibrin degradation products (FDP) testing would be sent to which of the following departments?
a. blood bank
b. chemistry
c. coagulation
d. microbiology

94. Which immunology test detects streptococcus infection?
a. ASO
b. monospot
c. RA
d. RPR

95. This is a federal program that provides medical care for the indigent.
a. homecare services
b. Medicaid
c. Medicare
d. Workers' compensation

96. Which department performs chemical screening tests on urine specimens?
a. coagulation
b. hematology
c. microbiology
d. urinalysis

97. Which department would perform an erythrocyte sedimentation rate (ESR)?
a. chemistry
b. hematology
c. immunology
d. microbiology

98. Diagnosis and treatment of diseases characterized by joint inflammation is part of which medical specialty?
a. dermatology
b. gastroenterology
c. internal medicine
d. rheumatology

99. Which phlebotomist's duty, if not complied with, has a penalty of possible fines or jail time?
a. maintain patient confidentiality
b. participate in continuing education
c. perform quality control checks
d. promote good public relations

100. All of the following factors are considered critical in understanding a diverse population's healthcare needs EXCEPT their:
a. approach to health and illness.
b. family living environment.
c. level of education attained.
d. traditions related to healing.

101. According to CLIA'88, the following is true:
a. A CLIA certificate is only required for hospitals.
b. All laboratories must follow the same standards.
c. Personnel standards are not included in the law.
d. Physician's laboratories are exempt from CLIA.

102. Which of the following specimens would be analyzed in the anatomical pathology area?
a. biopsy tissue
b. cerebrospinal fluid
c. synovial fluid
d. urine

103. Reference laboratories are viable because they offer all of the following EXCEPT:
a. a fast turnaround time.
b. more accurate results.
c. reduced test costs.
d. specialized analysis.

104. The physician is considered the gatekeeper in this category of care.
a. acute care
b. primary care
c. secondary care
d. tertiary care

105. The AMT, ASCP, and NCA are agencies that:
    a. accredit phlebotomy programs.
    b. certify laboratory professionals.
    c. license allied health professionals.
    d. monitor communicable diseases.

106. A phlebotomist is told to take procedure shortcuts to save time when collecting specimens during morning sweeps. She disagrees and chooses to follow the rules. Which professional characteristic is she exhibiting?
    a. compassion
    b. diplomacy
    c. integrity
    d. motivation

107. Which of the following is the name or abbreviation of the federal law that established standards for the electronic exchange of patient information?
    a. CLIA
    b. HIPAA
    c. Medicare
    d. OSHA

108. Which of the following actions by a phlebotomist does not encourage good verbal communication?
    a. active listening
    b. giving feedback
    c. noting nonverbals
    d. using pat clichés

109. A phlebotomist who appears knowledgeable, honest, and sincere is creating in the patient a sense of:
    a. control.
    b. dependency.
    c. empathy.
    d. trust.

110. All of the following are part of the homebound services offered to meet the needs of patients who have extended care after being discharged from the hospital EXCEPT:
    a. minor surgery.
    b. phlebotomy.
    c. physical therapy.
    d. respiratory therapy.

ANSWERS AND EXPLANATIONS

1. Answer: d

   Why: Public Health Services, one of the principal units under the Department of Health and Human Services, have agencies at local and state levels. These agencies are constantly monitoring, screening, protecting, and educating the public about defense against infectious diseases that might spread among the populace. The agencies do not get involved in treatment for infectious diseases.

   Review: Yes ☐ No ☑

2. Answer: d

   Why: Preferred provider organizations (PPOs) are independent groups of physicians or hospitals that negotiate contracts with employers for healthcare services at discounted rates in exchange for a guaranteed number of patients.

   Review: Yes ☐ No ☐

3. Answer: a

   Why: The current procedural terminology (CPT) codes were originally developed in the 1960s by the AMA to provide terminology and coding systems for physician billing.

   Review: Yes ☐ No ☐

4. Answer: b

   Why: Managed Care Organizations (MCOs) evolved from prepaid healthcare plans such as Health Maintenance Organizations (HMOs) and PPOs. MCOs contract with healthcare facilities and physicians to establish a complete network of services. They reimburse providers on the basis of enrollees served. These organizations strive to have the right care from the right provider at the right time for all patients and that way reduce the total cost of care.

   Review: Yes ☐ No ☐

5. Answer: d

   Why: The Patient Care Partnership (Box 1-1) is an easy-to-read brochure that replaces the American Hospital Association (AHA) Patient Bill of Rights and serves as an accepted statement of principle that encourages and guides healthcare institutions to put into writing what a patient can expect during his or her hospital stay. It is designed to help patients understand their rights and responsibilities while being treated in a particular healthcare facility.

   Review: Yes ☐ No ☐

Box 1-1 The Patient Care Partnership

What to expect during your hospital stay

- High-quality hospital care
- A clean and safe environment
- Involvement in your care
- Protection of your privacy
- Help when leaving the hospital
- Help with your billing claims

For more details see AHA website at www.aha.org/aha/resource

6. Answer: c

   Why: Managed care is a generic term for a payment system that manages costs and quality by encouraging healthy lifestyles, detecting risk factors, and offering patient education. This payment system encourages patient enrollment rather than limits it.

   Review: Yes ☐ No ☐

7. Answer: a

   Why: healthcare organizations are reorganizing, merging, and integrating healthcare delivery to form a continuum of care. A continuum of care offers a coordinated system of healthcare from birth to death and has evolved because of increased pressure to contain costs and improve quality.

   Review: Yes ☐ No ☐

8. Answer: a
   Why: The Ambulatory Patient Classification (APC) method was implemented in 2000 for hospitals to use in determining payment for outpatient services. Diagnosis-Related Groups (DRGs) and the *International Classification of Diseases,* Ninth Revision (ICD-9), which were being used at that time, were designed for inpatient services only.
   Review: Yes ☐ No ☐

9. Answer: b
   Why: According to the organizational chart (Figure 1-1), the Director of Medical Imaging where magnetic resonance (MR) scans are performed reports to the Vice President for Clinical & Support Services.
   Review: Yes ☐ No ☐

10. Answer: a
    Why: Infection Control is responsible for controlling nosocomial, or hospital-acquired, infections. This department is listed under the Senior Director of Performance Excellence on the organizational chart (Figure 1-1).
    Review: Yes ☐ No ☐

11. Answer: d
    Why: According to the organizational chart (Figure 1-1), the Administrator of Physician Services reports to the Vice President and Chief Medical Officer.
    Review: Yes ☐ No ☐

12. Answer: c
    Why: The Director of Medical & Surgical Services/Dialysis Services who oversees outpatient services reports to the Vice President and Chief Nursing Officer (see Figure 1-1).
    Review: Yes ☐ No ☐

13. Answer: a
    Why: The Directors of Performance Improvement and Patient Representatives who oversee many areas of quality assurance report to the Senior Director of Performance Excellence (see Figure 1-1).
    Review: Yes ☐ No ☐

14. Answer: c
    Why: One phlebotomist duty (See Box 1-2) is to collect and perform point-of-care testing

Box 1-2 Duties and Responsibilities of a Phlebotomist

- Prepare patients for collection procedures associated with laboratory samples
- Collect routine skin puncture and venous specimens for testing as required
- Prepare specimens for transport to ensure stability of sample
- Maintain patient confidentiality
- Perform quality control checks while carrying out clerical, clinical, and technical duties
- Transport specimens to the laboratory
- Comply with all procedures instituted in the procedure manual
- Promote good public relations with patients and hospital personnel
- Assist in collecting and documenting monthly workload and recording data
- Maintain safe working conditions
- Perform laboratory computer operations
- Participate in continuing education programs
- Collect and perform point-of-care testing (POCT)
- Perform quality control checks on POCT instruments
- Perform skin tests
- Process specimens and perform basic laboratory tests
- Collect urine drug screen specimens
- Perform electrocardiography
- Perform front office duties, current procedural terminology (CPT) coding, and paperwork

(POCT). This means that at some types of healthcare facilities the phlebotomist may perform TB and Cocci skin testing.

Review: Yes ☐ No ☐

15. Answer: c

Why: A phlebotomist should know laboratory procedures and policies and refer to them when answering callers' questions. A phlebotomist who uses proper telephone etiquette promotes good public relations with patients and hospital personnel. A phlebotomist who uses proper telephone etiquette in the laboratory would never leave the phone line open so that conversations can be heard by someone on hold, which would compromise patient confidentiality. Although telephone etiquette is an excellent example of good communication, it is not considered a quality control check.

Review: Yes ☐ No ☐

16. Answer: a

Why: The American Society of Clinical Pathologists (ASCP) is one of several national organizations that certify phlebotomists. Certification is a process that indicates the completion of defined academic and training requirements and the attainment of a satisfactory score on a national exam. The Clinical Laboratory Improvement Advisory Committee (CLIAC) provides scientific and technical advice and guidance regarding the need for, and the nature of, revisions to CLIA standards. The Clinical and Laboratory Standards Institute (CLSI) and the National Accrediting Agency for Clinical Laboratory Sciences (NAACLS) play a role in setting standards of care for healthcare professionals, including phlebotomists.

Review: Yes ☐ No ☐

17. Answer: b

Why: Many duties fall under the role of a phlebotomist, but the primary one is to collect high-quality blood specimens.

Review: Yes ☐ No ☐

18. Answer: d

Why: Positive public relations promote goodwill and harmonious relationships with employees and patients. Because the phlebotomist is an unofficial "public relations officer," everything the phlebotomist does reflects on the whole facility. The phlebotomist is often the only real contact patients have with the laboratory. In many cases, patients equate encounters with phlebotomists with the caliber of care they receive while in the hospital. Being skilled at good public relations does not cover up for inexperience and insecurity, however.

Review: Yes ☐ No ☐

19. Answer: b

Why: The primary objective in any healthcare professional's code of ethics must always be the patient's welfare, "first, do no harm," which is the translation for *primum non nocere* from the Hippocratic Oath taken by physicians about to enter practice.

Review: Yes ☐ No ☐

20. Answer: c

Why: Having good work ethics includes being dependable. A person with good work ethics can be relied on to be there when scheduled or when needed. Dependability shows a determination to "hang in there" no matter what.

Review: Yes ☐ No ☐

21. Answer: d

Why: Polycythemia is a condition caused by overproduction of red blood cells, and therapy includes removing some of the blood to bring levels into the normal range.

Review: Yes ☐ No ☐

22. Answer: a

Why: Continuing education for a healthcare professional is important for maintaining competency in all areas. It is necessary to remain current in the increasingly complex field of healthcare in order to maintain a high quality of care and avoid litigation. By staying current, a phlebotomist can maintain his or her certification through continuing education or by periodically retaking the certification exam. What continuing education does *not* do is eliminate the need for annual evaluations. This valuable tool tells the phlebotomist what additional continuing education he or she might need.

Review: Yes ☐ No ☐

23. Answer: a
    Why: The word phlebotomy comes from the Greek words "phlebos," meaning vein, and "tome," meaning incision, and literally translated means to make an incision in (or cut) a vein.

    Review: Yes ☐ No ☐

24. Answer: d
    Why: With the advent of multiskilling in healthcare, phlebotomists' duties are expanding; however, assisting with the insertion of IV cannulas, helping nurses perform direct patient care, or informing patients of their test results is not normally within a phlebotomist's scope of practice. A big part of a phlebotomist's duties is using the laboratory computer system to access requests and confirm collection.

    Review: Yes ☐ No ☐

25. Answer: a
    Why: Each certifying agency awards a designated title and initials to phlebotomists who successfully pass the national exam. The National Credentialing Agency (NCA) has chosen the initials CLPlb to designate the title of Clinical Laboratory Phlebotomist.

    Review: Yes ☐ No ☐

26. Answer: c
    Why: Today's lancet is the modern-day counterpart of the fleam. A typical fleam (Figure 1-2) had a wide double-edged blade at a right angle to the handle and was used to slice a vein. A special suction device called a cup was placed on the skin to draw blood to the surface before making an incision. The specimen was collected in a "bleeding bowl."

    Review: Yes ☐ No ☐

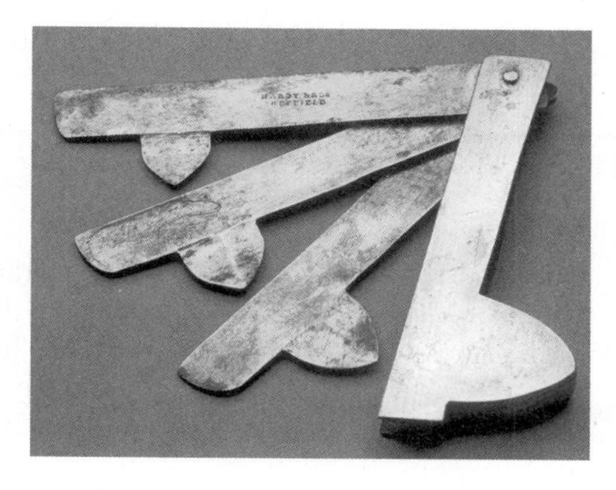

FIGURE 1-2 Typical fleams. (Courtesy Robert Kravetz, MD, Chairman, Archives Committee, American College of Gastroenterology.)

27. Answer: b
    Why: Several organizations sponsor workshops and seminars to enable phlebotomists and other healthcare workers to earn credit required to renew their licenses or certification. Credits indicated on certificates that are awarded on completion of these events are called continuing education units (CEUs). Copies of the certificates can be sent to certifying agencies as "proof of continuing education."

    Review: Yes ☐ No ☐

28. Answer: c
    Why: *The Patient Care Partnership* brochure replaces the AHA Patient's Bill of Rights and is designed to help patients understand their expectations during a hospital stay. One of the expectations is the right to receive help concerning billing issues if required.

    Review: Yes ☐ No ☐

Table 1-1 Territorial Zones and Corresponding Radii

Territorial Zone	Zone Radius
Intimate	1 to 18 inches
Personal	$1\frac{1}{2}$ to 4 feet
Social	4 to 12 feet
Public	More than 12 feet

29. Answer: b
Why: Every individual is surrounded by an invisible bubble of personal territory in which he or she feels most safe. This invisible bubble is known as a zone of comfort. The "zone of comfort" varies with each individual depending largely on how well an intruder into the zone is known and other circumstances surrounding the intrusion. Personal zone of comfort is typically recognized as $1\frac{1}{2}$–4 feet (See Table 1-1).
Review: Yes ☐ No ☐

30. Answer: d
Why: Language, age, and emotions all can be barriers to communication (Figure 1-3) that require special communication techniques for effective exchange of information to occur. In the case of a mature, male healthcare worker (HCW), communication should be without many obstacles because as a practitioner in the healthcare system he understands the process and knows what to expect.
Review: Yes ☐ No ☐

31. Answer: d
Why: Confirming responses help a patient feel recognized as an individual and not a number. "I understand how you must be feeling" is a response that communicates an effort on your part to view the patient as an individual and empathize with his or her situation.
Review: Yes ☐ No ☐

32. Answer: b
Why: Kinesics is the study of nonverbal communication, or body language. Frowning is an example of negative kinesics, or body language. Eye contact, good grooming, and smiling all are examples of positive body language. Examples of nonverbal facial cues are shown in Figure 1-4.
Review: Yes ☐ No ☐

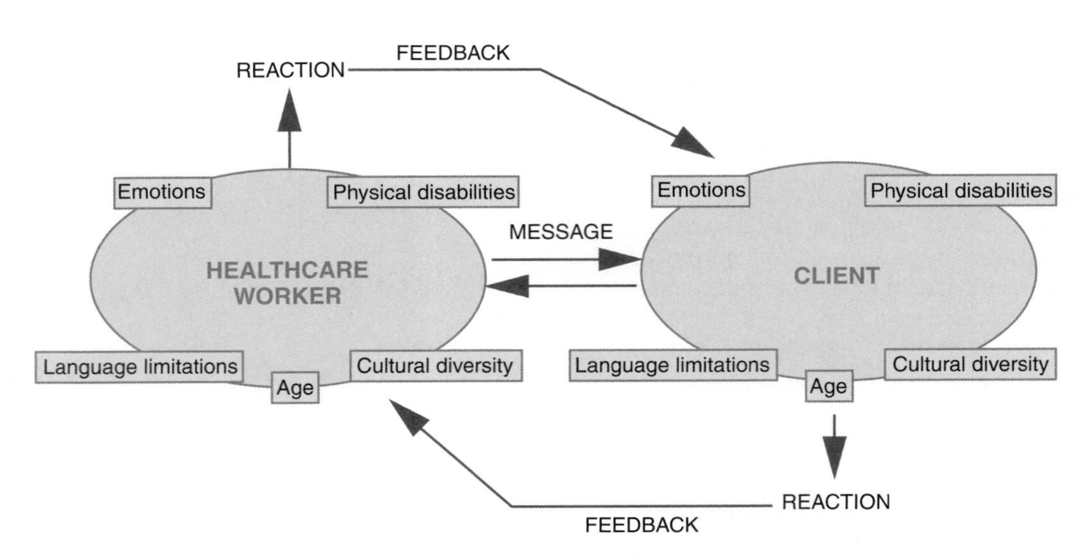

FIGURE 1-3 Verbal communication feedback loop.

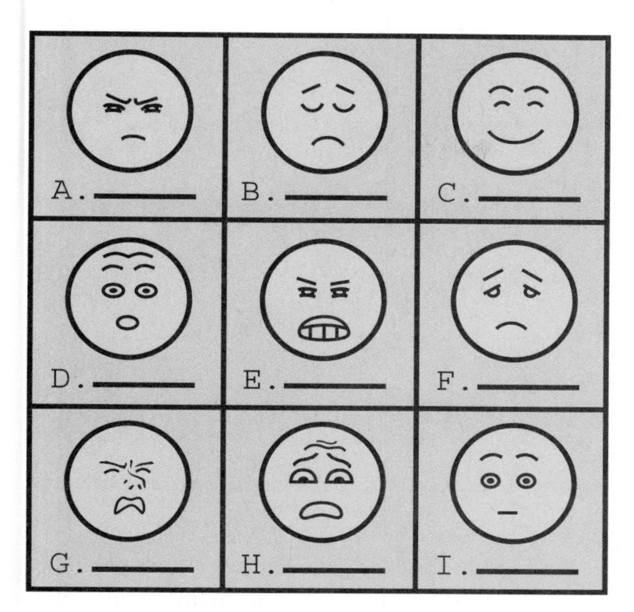

FIGURE 1-4 Nonverbal facial cues. Can you match the sketches with the correct effects? (1) happy, (2) sad, (3) surprise, (4) fear, (5) anger, (6) disgust.

Answers: A-5, B-2, C-1, D-3, E-5, F-2, G-6, H-4, I-3.

33. Answer: a
Why: A neat, clean appearance plays a big part in presenting a professional image. A clean, pressed laboratory coat; closed-toe, conservative shoes; short, clean fingernails (artificial nails not allowed); and long hair pulled back contribute to presenting a professional image. Wearing strong cologne is offensive to some people, especially those who are ill or allergic to perfume, and may interfere with their perceiving the individual who wears it as being professional.
Review: Yes ☐ No ☐

34. Answer: c
Why: Acting knowledgeably, conveying sincerity, and presenting a professional appearance all are part of portraying a professional image that earns a patient's confidence or trust. Dismissing a patient's fears makes the phlebotomist seem insensitive to the situation and the patient's needs and undermines the patient's confidence in the care received.
Review: Yes ☐ No ☐

35. Answer: c
Why: Proper telephone protocol involves answering the phone promptly and restating what has been said to clarify information received before recording it. Callers who are upset and hostile should be handled carefully. Validating a hostile caller's feelings will often diffuse the situation and allow the issue to be addressed. Never hang up on any caller.
Review: Yes ☐ No ☐

36. Answer: b
Why: Proxemics is the study of an individual's concept and use of space. To better relate to the patient in a healthcare setting, it is important to understand this subtle part of nonverbal communication.
Review: Yes ☐ No ☐

37. Answer: c
Why: Trust, as defined in a healthcare setting, is the unquestioning belief by a patient that health professionals are knowledgeable, sincere, and honest. When the statement of a phlebotomist proves to be wrong (even if it seems like a harmless reassurance such as "this won't hurt"), the patient's trust in the phlebotomist is undermined.
Review: Yes ☐ No ☐

38. Answer: a
Why: A hospital is one of the few places where an individual gives up control over most of the personal tasks he or she normally performs. Because of this loss of control, the patient may respond by getting angry and is then characterized as a "difficult" or "bad" patient. The best approach is to help the patient feel in control of the situation.
Review: Yes ☐ No ☐

39. Answer: c
Why: Proxemics is the study of an individual's concept and use of space. It involves four categories of naturally occurring territorial zones (Table 1-1), referred to as zones of comfort, that are very obvious in human interaction. Personal contact involves one of these zones. Entering a patient's personal zone is often necessary in a healthcare setting, and if this is not carefully handled, the patient may feel threatened, insecure, or out of control.
Review: Yes ☐ No ☐

40. Answer: a
Why: Feeling in control is essential to a patient's well-being. Informing, insisting, and telling all are actions that may cause the patient to feel as if he or she has no control over the situation. Allowing the patient the right to either agree to or refuse a procedure allows the patient to exercise control over the situation and generally makes for a more agreeable patient.
Review: Yes ☐ No ☐

41. Answer: b
Why: The average speaking rate of an adult is 125–150 words per minute. Because the average person absorbs verbal messages at 500–600 words per minute (which is approximately four times the speaking rate), the listener must make an effort to stay actively involved in what the speaker is saying to communicate effectively.
Review: Yes ☐ No ☐

42. Answer: a
Why: The term "outpatient care" is synonymous with "ambulatory care." Ambulatory, or outpatient, care is offered to those who are able to come to the facility for care and go home the same day. Nonambulatory care is found in tertiary facilities, where patients must stay over one or more nights. Nursing home or rehabilitation care is considered nonambulatory for the reasons stated above.
Review: Yes ☐ No ☐

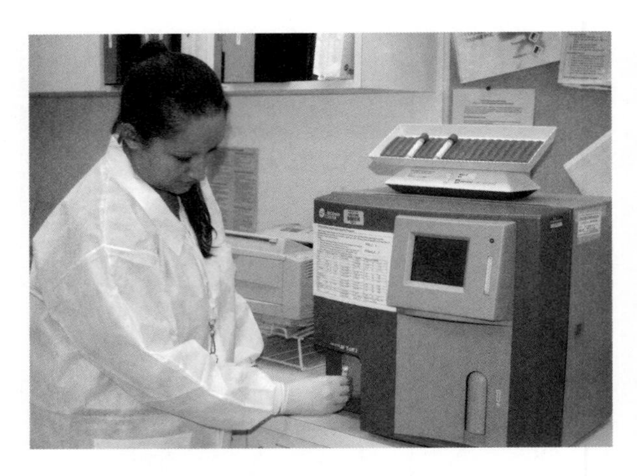

FIGURE 1-5 Coulter A^c Tdiff2 automated hematology analyzer.

43. Answer: b
Why: The hematology department identifies abnormalities of the blood by analyzing whole blood specimens in automated analyzers (see Figure 1-5).
Review: Yes ☐ No ☐

44. Answer: d
Why: Respiratory means relating to respiration or the act of breathing, which provides lungs with oxygen. The respiratory therapy department is responsible for administering oxygen therapy to patients with respiratory disorders.
Review: Yes ☐ No ☐

45. Answer: c
Why: A frozen section is a test performed by a pathologist in the surgical pathology department. Tissue removed during surgery is quickly frozen, and a thin slice of the specimen is microscopically examined for abnormalities while the patient is still under anesthesia. Results of the frozen section analysis determine what further action is to be taken by the surgeon.
Review: Yes ☐ No ☐

46. Answer: b
Why: Nephrology is the study of the kidneys. A patient being treated in the nephrology

department is most likely being treated for a disorder associated with the kidneys.

Review: Yes ☐ No ☐

47. Answer: b

Why: "Oto" means ear, "rhino" means nose, and the "larynx" is a structure in the throat. The otorhinolaryngology department treats disorders of the ear, nose, and throat. Skin disorders are treated in the dermatology department. Eye problems are treated in the ophthalmology department, and bone and joint disorders are treated in the orthopedics department.

Review: Yes ☐ No ☐

48. Answer: d

Why: A prothrombin time (protime, or PT) is performed in the coagulation department. It is most commonly performed to monitor the effects of anticoagulant drugs such as coumarin on the coagulation process. Blood urea nitrogen (BUN) and glucose tests are performed in the chemistry department. A complete blood count (CBC) is performed in the hematology department.

Review: Yes ☐ No ☐

49. Answer: b

Why: The word "onco" means tumor, and the suffix "ology" denotes the study of. The term "oncology" is used to describe the medical specialty that treats patients who have tumors. Geriatrics is the branch of medicine that deals with problems of aging. Ophthalmology deals with eye disorders, and orthopedics deals with musculoskeletal system disorders.

Review: Yes ☐ No ☐

50. Answer: c

Why: The term "orthopedics" is used to describe the medical specialty that treats disorders of the musculoskeletal system. Gastroenterology is the specialty that treats disorders of the digestive tract and related structures; neurology is the specialty that treats disorders of the brain, spinal cord, and nerves; and pediatrics is the specialty that treats children from birth to adolescence.

Review: Yes ☐ No ☐

51. Answer: b

Why: A neonate is a newborn up to the age of 1 month. A neonatologist is a physician who specializes in the study, treatment, and care of newborns. A gerontologist specializes in disorders related to aging; an obstetrician/gynecologist specializes in pregnancy, childbirth, and treatment of disorders of the reproductive system; and a pediatrician treats children from birth to adolescence.

Review: Yes ☐ No ☐

52. Answer: a

Why: The blood bank department is sometimes called immunohematology. Immunology is another name for the serology department. An earlier name for the microbiology department was bacteriology.

Review: Yes ☐ No ☐

53. Answer: a

Why: Glycohemoglobin is a short way of saying glycosylated hemoglobin, which is a chemistry test. Glycosylated hemoglobin is formed when glucose and hemoglobin combine, and it is tested to evaluate long-term glucose control. The most common glycosylated hemoglobin is hemoglobin A_1.

Review: Yes ☐ No ☐

54. Answer: c

Why: Cerebrospinal fluid (CSF) analysis involves several different departments. Chemistry tests performed on CSF include glucose and protein analysis. Cell counts on CSF are performed in the hematology department, and culture and sensitivity testing on CSF is performed in the microbiology department. In addition, syphilis testing may be performed on CSF in the serology/immunology department. There is no reason for this fluid to be tested in the immunohematology department because this department's major responsibility it is to prepare blood products to be used for patient transfusions.

Review: Yes ☐ No ☐

55. Answer: b

Why: Therapeutic drug monitoring is a team effort and requires cooperation between nursing, pharmacy, and the laboratory for quality results.

Review: Yes ☐ No ☐

56. Answer: c

Why: The histology department prepares tissue samples for microscopic exam by a pathologist.

Review: Yes ☐ No ☐

57. Answer: d

Why: A phlebotomist is not required to have a college degree and may not even be required to show any type of certification or proof of training to practice. A few states require licensing of phlebotomists, and many employers require their phlebotomists to be nationally certified. To become nationally certified, a phlebotomist must have a high school diploma or GED and have completed a formal, structured phlebotomy program or have a minimum of 1 year of full-time experience as a phlebotomist. A clinical laboratory scientist (CLS) and a medical technologist (MT) are normally required to have a minimum of a bachelor's degree in medical technology or chemical or biological science. A medical laboratory technician (MLT) is normally required to have a minimum of an associate's degree or equivalent.

Review: Yes ☐ No ☐

58. Answer: c

Why: Secondary care involves care by specialists in a particular area of healthcare. An appendectomy performed in an ambulatory surgical center is an example of secondary care. Managed care is a system of healthcare delivery and financing that involves primary, secondary, and tertiary care. Primary care entails initial consultation and treatment by a family physician or other caregiver. Tertiary care implies highly complex or specialized services delivered primarily in inpatient facilities to patients who stay overnight.

Review: Yes ☐ No ☐

59. Answer: b

Why: Blood cultures are performed in the microbiology department and are blood specimens collected in special nutrient substance or media designed to encourage the growth of microorganisms that might be present in a patient's bloodstream. The process is often automated using a special system such as the BactALERT 3D (Figure1-6).

Review: Yes ☐ No ☐

60. Answer: d

Why: Sodium and potassium are both electrolytes. They can be ordered as individual

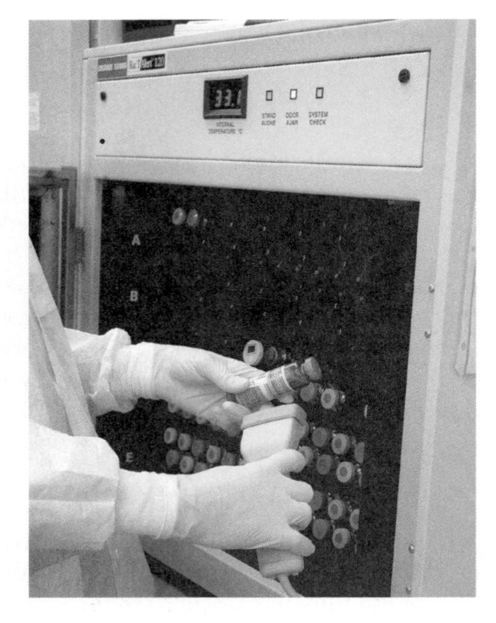

FIGURE 1-6 Microbiologist reviews blood cultures processed by the BactALERT 3D microbiology system.

tests or as part of an electrolyte panel that includes sodium, potassium, chloride, and bicarbonate (commonly measured as carbon dioxide [CO_2]. Bilirubin, blood urea nitrogen (BUN), creatinine, cholesterol, glucose, and uric acid are tests that are performed in the chemistry department and are ordered to check the status of various organs or body systems.

Review: Yes ☐ No ☐

61. Answer: a
Why: ECG (also called EKG) is used as an abbreviation for both the cardiodiagnostic department and the most common test performed by this department, an electrocardiogram. EEG is an abbreviation used for both the electroneurodiagnostic technology (ENT) department—also called the electroencephalography (EEG) department—and its most common test, the electroencephalogram. The emergency room (ER, or emergency department) initially deals with emergency situations involving all types of patients, not just patients with heart problems. ICU stands for intensive care unit, which delivers specialized care for critically ill patients.
Review: Yes ☐ No ☐

62. Answer: a
Why: Basic metabolic panel (BMP) is a term used for one of the Health care Financing Administration (HCFA)-approved disease and organ-specific panels that evaluate the functioning of various body systems. It includes glucose, blood urea nitrogen (BUN), creatinine, sodium, potassium, chloride, carbon dioxide (CO_2), and calcium. These tests can all be performed on an automated analyzer (see Figure 1-7) in the chemistry department.
Review: Yes ☐ No ☐

63. Answer: c
Why: The cytogenetics department performs chromosome studies; however, not all laboratories have a cytogenetics department, in which case these studies are sent to a reference laboratory.
Review: Yes ☐ No ☐

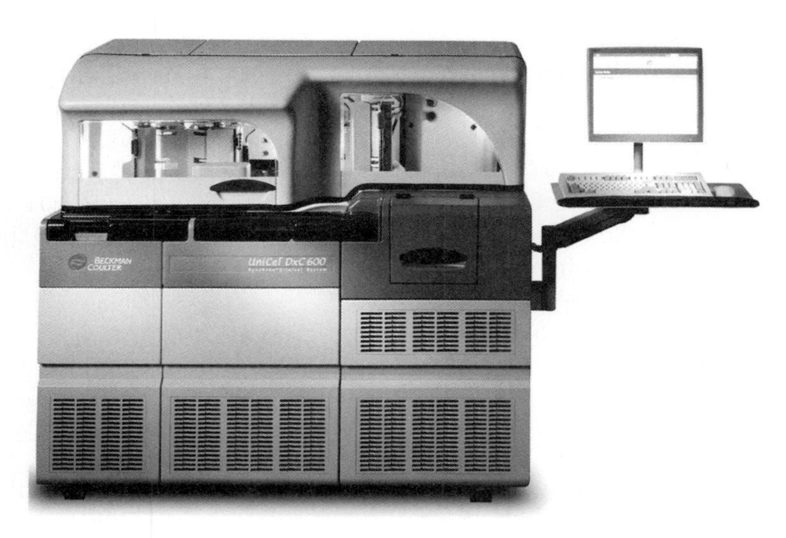

FIGURE 1-7 Unicel ® DXC 600 Synchron ® Clinical System (Courtesy of Beckman Coulter, Inc., 2007)

64. Answer: a
Why: Cytology is the study of the formation, structure, and function of cells. The cells in body fluids and tissues are analyzed in the cytology department to detect signs of cancer. The Pap smear test is named after a cytology staining technique used to detect cancerous cells in specimens obtained from the cervix in the vagina.
Review: Yes ☐ No ☐

65. Answer: b
Why: An HMO charges members a flat fee for a complete package of healthcare services. The fee is normally paid by the member on a monthly basis and is paid regardless of whether the services are used. An additional fee, called a copayment, is charged at the time services are used. The amount of the copayment depends on the type of service chosen.
Review: Yes ☐ No ☐

66. Answer: d
Why: There are three basic levels of care offered in the United States: primary (basic) care through the physician, secondary (specialist) care offered on an outpatient basis, and tertiary (highly sophisticated and complex) care requiring a stay in an inpatient facility.
Review: Yes ☐ No ☐

67. Answer: c
Why: Obstetrics is the medical specialty that includes treating women throughout pregnancy and childbirth. This specialty also treats disorders of the female reproductive system and menopause.
Review: Yes ☐ No ☐

68. Answer: a
Why: A primary care physician is one of the most important concepts in "managed care." HMOs, PPOs, and MCOs are all labels for managed care payment systems. Only in HMOs does the physician truly serve as a gatekeeper because directives to other physicians and services must be accompanied by his request or referral. This type of coordination reduces the time and cost of care. Integrated healthcare delivery systems (IDSs) were developed to coordinate a holistic approach to healthcare performed by many medical facilities and physicians.
Review: Yes ☐ No ☐

69. Answer: a
Why: Toxicology is a subsection of the chemistry department. Toxicology tests determine the presence of poisons or toxic substances in blood or urine specimens.
Review: Yes ☐ No ☐

70. Answer: d
Why: A pathologist is a physician who specializes in diagnosing disease from abnormal changes detected in blood, body fluid, and tissue specimens.
Review: Yes ☐ No ☐

71. Answer: c
Why: A complete blood count (CBC) is the most common test performed in the hematology department. Culture & sensitivity (C&S) testing is performed in the microbiology department. Cerebrospinal fluid (CSF) is analyzed in several different departments. A BMP is a disease and organ-specific diagnostic panel that is performed in the automated chemistry area of the laboratory.
Review: Yes ☐ No ☐

72. Answer: d
Why: The respiratory therapy department diagnoses, treats, and manages patient lung deficiencies, tests capacity of the lungs, and administers oxygen therapy. This department may also analyze arterial blood gas (ABG) specimens, although ABGs are sometimes performed in the clinical laboratory.
Review: Yes ☐ No ☐

73. Answer: a
Why: Carcinoembryonic antigen (CEA) is a substance released during malignant tumor growth and is classified as a "tumor marker." It was first associated with cancer of the colon. Because CEA levels increase in other types of cancer and some nonmalignant conditions, it is no longer considered specific for colon cancer. Monitoring CEA levels is, however, considered a useful tool in the treatment and management of certain cancers. CEA tests are performed in the chemistry department.
Review: Yes ☐ No ☐

74. Answer: c
Why: X-ray procedures and other imaging techniques are functions of the radiology department. The occupational therapy department assists mentally, physically, or emotionally disabled patients in maintaining daily living skills. The pharmacy prepares and dispenses drugs, provides advice on selection and side effects of drugs, and helps coordinate therapeutic drug monitoring. The respiratory therapy department aids in the diagnosis, treatment, and management of lung deficiencies.
Review: Yes ☐ No ☐

75. Answer: c
Why: There are two main types of healthcare facilities: inpatient and outpatient. An inpatient facility is designed for patients who stay overnight. A hospital is primarily an inpatient facility. Outpatient facilities are places where patients receive treatment and go home the same day. Physician and dentist offices and day-surgery centers are examples of outpatient facilities.
Review: Yes ☐ No ☐

76. Answer: d
Why: Rapid plasma reagin (RPR) is a common serology test used in the diagnosis of syphilis. BUN is a chemistry test; CBC, a hematology test; and PTT, a coagulation test.
Review: Yes ☐ No ☐

77. Answer: a
Why: Both the medical technologist (MT) and the clinical laboratory scientist (CLS) have the same qualifications, including a bachelor's degree in medical technology or a chemical or biological science. The title depends on which national certification exam was chosen and passed. A clinical laboratory technician (CLT) and medical laboratory technician (MLT) are both required to have a minimum of a 2-year associate's degree or equivalent. A pathologist is a physician with a specialty in laboratory diagnosis.
Review: Yes ☐ No ☐

78. Answer: b
Why: A hemogram is a hematology test. It is the name given to the graph or printed results of complete blood cell count (CBC) on an automated blood cell counter. It generally includes the major components of a CBC except a manual differential.
Review: Yes ☐ No ☐

79. Answer: d
Why: The urinalysis department performs urinalysis testing, a routine exam of urine that includes a microscopic exam of urine sediment for the presence of blood cells, bacteria, crystals, and other substances.
Review: Yes ☐ No ☐

80. Answer: b
Why: The physical therapy department provides many types of assistance to patients who have physical handicaps, including therapy to restore mobility. The cardiodiagnostics department provides diagnosis, monitoring, and therapy for patients with cardiovascular problems. The radiology department diagnoses medical conditions using x-rays and

other imaging techniques. The respiratory therapy department provides testing, therapy, and monitoring of patients with respiratory disorders.

Review: Yes ☐ No ☐

81. Answer: b
Why: The electroencephalography (EEG) or electroneurodiagnostic technology (ENT) department performs evoked potential testing to determine muscle function and brain wave mapping to diagnose and monitor neurologic disorders. ECG (formerly EKG) is the abbreviation used for an electrocardiogram and also the cardiodiagnostic department where electrocardiograms are performed. The occupational therapy (OT) department assists mentally, physically, or emotionally disabled patients in maintaining daily living skills. The respiratory therapy (RT) department provides testing, therapy, and monitoring of patients with respiratory disease.
Review: Yes ☐ No ☐

82. Answer: b.
Why: Clinical Laboratory Improvement Amendments of 1988 (CLIA'88) mandate that all laboratories must be regulated using the same standards regardless of the location, type, or size. American Medical Technologists (AMT) is a certification agency for allied health professionals. Public Health Services (PHS) agencies function at local and state level to provide services for the entire population of the region. The Health Insurance Portability and Accountability Act (HIPAA) is a bill that established standards for electronic data exchange, including coding systems.
Review: Yes ☐ No ☐

83. Answer: d
Why: A patient care technician (PCT) is a certified nursing assistant (CNA) with additional specialized patient care skills and phlebotomy skills. An ADN is an associate's degree nurse. An emergency medical technician (EMT) is also a multiskilled person, but one who functions at an emergency level only.
Review: Yes ☐ No ☐

84. Answer: a
Why: A clinical laboratory scientist (CLS) and a medical technologist (MT) are required to have a bachelor's degree in medical technology or a chemical or biological science. A clinical laboratory technician (CLT) and a medical laboratory technician (MLT) normally have an associate's degree from a 2-year college or equivalent, or certification from a military or proprietary (private) college. A phlebotomist certified through the ASCP Board of Registry is called a phlebotomy technician (PBT) and has a high school diploma or GED at a minimum.
Review: Yes ☐ No ☐

85. Answer: b
Why: A clinical laboratory technician (CLT) and a medical laboratory technician (MLT) normally have an associate's degree from a 2-year college or equivalent, or certification from a military or proprietary (private) college. A clinical laboratory scientist (CLS) and a medical technologist (MT) are required to have a bachelor's degree in medical technology or a chemical or biological science. A phlebotomist may not be required to have any formal education or certification. Phlebotomy Technician (PBT) is the title awarded to those who successfully pass the ASCP phlebotomy certification exam. To apply for certification, a phlebotomist is typically required to have a high school diploma or GED at a minimum.
Review: Yes ☐ No ☐

86. Answer: c
Why: A subsection of the microbiology department is parasitology, where stool specimens are carefully examined for the presence of parasites or their eggs (ova).
Review: Yes ☐ No ☐

87. Answer: b
Why: The process used to identify microorganisms and determine the appropriate antibiotic for treatment is called culture and sensitivity (C&S) testing.
Review: Yes ☐ No ☐

88. Answer: a
Why: The chemistry department performs tests to evaluate certain analytes such as glucose that are dissolved in the blood. Glucose levels are evaluated to diagnose or monitor diabetes.
Review: Yes ☐ No ☐

89. Answer: b
Why: The word root "hem" means blood, and the suffix "logy" denotes the study of. Hematology is the medical specialty that treats patients with blood disorders. Dermatology is the medical specialty that treats skin disorders. Internal medicine treats disorders of the internal organs and general medical conditions. Urology treats disorders of the urinary tract and male reproductive organs.
Review: Yes ☐ No ☐

90. Answer: a
Why: Public health agencies take care of large-scale healthcare problems at the federal, state, and local levels. Their designated services are to be used by the entire population of an area and include diabetes screening, immunization and vaccination programs, and venereal disease screening clinics. Licensure of personnel is not part of public health service responsibilities.
Review: Yes ☐ No ☐

91. Answer: d
Why: Culture and sensitivity (C&S) testing is performed in the microbiology department.
Review: Yes ☐ No ☐

92. Answer: a
Why: Blood typing and compatibility testing are performed in the blood bank department, which is sometimes called immunohematology.
Review: Yes ☐ No ☐

93. Answer: c
Why: Fibrin Degradation Products (FDP), also called fibrin split products (FSP), are the end-products of the breakdown of fibrin formed during the coagulation process. The test is performed in the coagulation department and is most commonly ordered to diagnose disseminated intravascular coagulation (DIC).
Review: Yes ☐ No ☐

94. Answer: a
Why: The antistreptolysin O (ASO) test is performed to demonstrate the presence of antibodies formed in response to an infection from streptococcus bacteria. A monospot test detects mononucleosis. RA is a rheumatoid arthritis test, and rapid plasma reagin (RPR) is a syphilis test.
Review: Yes ☐ No ☐

95. Answer: b
Why: Medicaid is a state-based, federal program that provides medical care for the poor (indigent). Medicare, a federal program, provides medical care to patients age 65 and older. Workers' Compensation (workers' comp for short) provides benefits to individuals who have been injured on the job. Homecare services that provide medical care to patients in their homes may be federal or state-based programs.
Review: Yes ☐ No ☐

96. Answer: d
Why: The urinalysis department performs chemical screening tests on urine specimens as part of a urinalysis test. Chemical screening involves dipping a special strip (dipstick) impregnated with chemical reagents into the

urine and interpreting color reactions that take place on the strip.

Review: Yes ☐ No ☐

97. Answer: b

Why: An erythrocyte sedimentation rate (ESR) is a whole blood test that is performed in the hematology department.

Review: Yes ☐ No ☐

98. Answer: d

Why: The medical specialty of rheumatology is involved in the diagnosis and treatment of diseases characterized by joint inflammation. Dermatology involves the treatment of skin disorders. Gastroenterology involves the treatment of disorders of the digestive tract and related structures. Internal medicine involves the treatment of disorders of the internal organs and general medical conditions.

Review: Yes ☐ No ☐

99. Answer: a

Why: The Health Insurance Portability and Accountability Act (HIPAA) established national standards for protecting patient health information. Maintaining patient confidentiality is a major concern, and all healthcare workers must sign a confidentiality and nondisclosure agreement affirming that they understand HIPAA and will keep all patient information confidential. Penalties for HIPAA violations include disciplinary action, fines, and possible jail time.

Review: Yes ☐ No ☐

100. Answer: c

Why: Critical factors in the provision of healthcare services that meet the needs of diverse populations include understanding the beliefs and values that shape their approach to health and illness, the family's living environment, and their customs and traditions that relate to health and healing. Education level attained plays a role but is not considered one of the critical factors.

Review: Yes ☐ No ☐

101. Answer: b

Why: CLIA'88 mandates that all laboratories that test human specimens must be regulated using the same standard measurement regardless of the location, type, or size. Personnel qualifications for each of the test complexity type labs *are* stated in the regulations.

Review: Yes ☐ No ☐

102. Answer: a

Why: Biopsy tissue is analyzed by a physician in the anatomical pathology area (Box 1-3). All others fluids listed above will be processed and analyzed in the clinical area of the laboratory.

Review: Yes ☐ No ☐

Box 1-3 Two Major Divisions in the Clinical Laboratory

Clinical analysis areas	Anatomical and surgical pathology
Specimen processing, hematology, chemistry, microbiology, blood bank/immunohematology, immunology/serology, and urinalysis testing	Tissue analysis, cytologic exam, surgical biopsy, frozen sections, and performance of autopsies

103. Answer: b
Why: Reference laboratories are large, independent facilities that receive specimens from many different areas. They provide specialized testing that is not cost-effective in smaller labs and they offer fast turnaround time (TAT). The high volume of tests they perform allows them to reduce costs but does not necessarily mean they have more accurate results than in any other laboratory facility.
Review: Yes ☐ No ☐

104. Answer: b
Why: The primary care physician fills the role of gatekeeper and serves as the patient's advocate to advise and coordinate services for each individual, including advising the patient on care offered through secondary and tertiary sources.
Review: Yes ☐ No ☐

105. Answer: b
Why: American Medical Technologists (AMT), American Society of Clinical Pathologists (ASCP), and the National Credentialing Agency (NCA) are among the agencies that offer certification for all levels of laboratory professionals. Licensure of healthcare and allied health professionals is the responsibility of the states that have passed licensure laws. Phlebotomy programs are accredited by the National Accrediting Agency for Clinical Laboratory Sciences (NAACLS). State and local Public Health Services (PHS) monitor communicable diseases.
Review: Yes ☐ No ☐

106. Answer: c
Why: Professional standards of integrity and honesty require a person to do what is right regardless of the circumstances.
Review: Yes ☐ No ☐

107. Answer: b
Why: The Health Information Portability and Accountability Act (HIPAA) is a federal law that was enacted to more closely secure protected health information (PHI) and regulate patient privacy. The law established national standards for the electronic exchange of PHI.
Review: Yes ☐ No ☐

108. Answer: d
Why: Using clichés or overused expressions is not a form of good communication because they could be misunderstood, especially by those who have language limitations. Using clichés often indicates that the speaker is not using active listening.
Review: Yes ☐ No ☐

109. Answer: d
Why: A very important professional characteristic that a phlebotomist should exhibit is that of being trustworthy. Patients appear comfortable and relaxed when interacting with a sincere, honest, and knowledgeable phlebotomist they feel they can trust.
Review: Yes ☐ No ☐

110. Answer: a
Why: Many homebound older adults require respiratory therapy, nursing care, and physical therapy, as well as laboratory specimens to be collected, where they reside, either in their homes or in long-term care facilities. Several different agencies employ nurses, physical and respiratory therapists, and phlebotomists for this purpose. So far, minor surgery is not a service that is offered to the homebound.
Review: Yes ☐ No ☐

CHAPTER 2

QUALITY ASSURANCE AND LEGAL ISSUES

study tip

Questions in this chapter address quality assurance (QA) and legal issues in healthcare. QA questions test the ability to identify agencies that accredit or establish standards for healthcare facilities, clinical laboratories, clinical laboratory procedures, and clinical laboratory education. They also address the ability to define QA and QA-related terminology, name areas of phlebotomy subject to quality assessment, identify various QA documents, and describe the risk management process. Legal issue questions test the ability to identify civil actions based on tort, define legal terminology, identify and define the various types of patient consent, and describe the litigation process.

overview

This chapter assesses knowledge of quality assurance (QA) and legal issues in healthcare, including the relationship of both to the practice of phlebotomy. Consumer awareness has increased lawsuits in all areas of society. This is especially true in the healthcare industry. Consequently, it is essential for phlebotomists to recognize the importance of following QA guidelines and understand the legal implications of not doing so.

REVIEW QUESTIONS

Choose the BEST answer.

1. Legal actions in which the alleged injured party sues for monetary damages are:
   a. civil action.
   b. criminal action.
   c. malpractice.
   d. vicarious liability.

2. Significant gaps in the quality of testing practices in physicians' offices resulted in the recent development of:
   a. competencies.
   b. good laboratory practices.
   c. quality indicators.
   d. threshold values.

3. The level of care that a person of ordinary intelligence and good sense would exercise under the given circumstances is the definition of:
   a. due care.
   b. quality care.
   c. quality essentials.
   d. standard of care.

4. Deceitful practice or false portrayal of facts either by words or by conduct is the definition of:
   a. battery.
   b. discovery.
   c. fraud.
   d. negligence.

5. Quality improvement involves all of the following EXCEPT:
   a. being directly accountable to the customer.
   b. being required and administered by OSHA.
   c. identifying situations that pose risks to employees.
   d. minimizing circumstances that jeopardize patient care.

6. Quality System Essentials (QSEs) are:
   a. accompanied by quality indicators that monitor workflow.
   b. guidelines for reporting quality assessment incidents.
   c. preanalytical factors that affect the quality of the sample.
   d. threshold values for all measurable aspects of care.

7. All of the following are responsibilities of the Center for Medicare and Medicaid Services (CMS) EXCEPT:
   a. administering of Medicare programs.
   b. managing of federal healthcare programs.
   c. overseeing administration of CLIA '88.
   d. providing healthcare worker insurance.

8. A process in which one party questions another under oath while a court reporter records every word is:
   a. civil action.
   b. deposition.
   c. discovery.
   d. tort.

9. Which one of the following is *not* found in the Procedure Manual?
   a. corrective action
   b. purpose of procedure
   c. required equipment
   d. revision dates

10. An internal process focused on identifying and minimizing situations that pose danger to patients and employees is:
    a. facilitywide risk management.
    b. performance improvement plan.
    c. sentinel (early warning) events.
    d. the delta check procedure.

11. CLIA categorizes certificates for laboratories according to:
    a. complexity of testing.
    b. personnel qualifications.
    c. quality control standards.
    d. size of the laboratory.

12. CLIA laboratories that perform high-complexity testing:
    a. are funded by the federal government.
    b. are subjected to routine inspections.
    c. must hire PhDs to be supervisors.
    d. must renew their certificate annually.

13. The Joint Commission's Sentinel Event QI program policy is designed to do all of the following EXCEPT to:
    a. demonstrate flexibility in setting QC measures.
    b. identify unfavorable events for immediate investigation.
    c. improve the safety of patients in health-care institutions.
    d. prevent unfavorable events from happening again.

14. If a sentinel event occurs, the healthcare organization is required to do all of the following EXCEPT:
    a. monitor improvements to see if they are effective.
    b. perform a thorough analysis of the root cause.
    c. put into practice improvements to reduce risk.
    d. send a complete report to the Joint Commission.

15. A clinical laboratory "path of workflow" is:
    a. defined as the steps necessary to deliver a product or service.
    b. made up of preanalytical, analytical, and postanalytical processes.
    c. monitored throughout the process by quality indicators.
    d. overseen by the hospital administrator through periodic reports.

16. Guides used to monitor all aspects of patient care are called:
    a. QA indicators.
    b. QI core measurements.
    c. Quality System Essentials.
    d. thresholds values.

17. What is the abbreviation for an agency that has an approval process for phlebotomy programs?
    a. CLIA '88
    b. CLSI
    c. NAACLS
    d. NCA

18. A very busy phlebotomist misidentifies the patient when collecting a specimen for transfusion preparation. The possible misdiagnosis of blood type could cause the patient's death. If the phlebotomist's action results in injury, this wrongful act is called:
    a. assault.
    b. battery.
    c. fraud.
    d. negligence.

19. The abbreviation for the federal regulations that established quality standards for all laboratories that test human specimens is:
    a. BBP Standard.
    b. CLIA '88.
    c. HazCom.
    d. OSHA.

20. The abbreviation for a national agency that sets standards for phlebotomy procedures is:
    a. ASCP.
    b. CLSI.
    c. NAACLS.
    d. NCA.

21. Which of the following is *not* an area of phlebotomy subject to quality control (QC) procedures?
    a. patient identification
    b. patient IV adjustment
    c. phlebotomy technique
    d. specimen labeling

22. A laboratory technician asked a phlebotomist to recollect a specimen on a patient. When the phlebotomist asked

what was wrong with the specimen, the technician replied, "The specimen was OK, but the results were inconsistent." How would the laboratory technician have decided that the results were questionable? The results did not:
a. compare with previous results after a delta check.
b. match results of patients with the same diagnosis.
c. measure up to the results on the control specimens.
d. relate well to other patients tested at the same time.

23. Which organization provides voluntary laboratory inspections and proficiency testing?
a. ASCP
b. CAP
c. CLSI
d. OSHA

24. QC protocols prohibit use of outdated evacuated tubes for all of the following reasons EXCEPT:
a. additives that prevent clotting may no longer function as required.
b. specimens collected in these tubes may yield erroneous results.
c. stoppers may have shrunk, allowing specimen leakage if inverted.
d. tubes may not fill completely, changing additive to sample ratios.

25. The Joint Commission:
a. accredits healthcare organizations.
b. approves phlebotomy programs.
c. certifies laboratory personnel.
d. develops phlebotomy standards.

26. All of the following are examples of quality control measures EXCEPT:
a. checking expiration dates of evacuated tubes.
b. documenting maintenance on centrifuge.
c. logging hours on your time sheet daily.
d. recording refrigerator temperature daily.

27. When the threshold value of a QA clinical indicator is exceeded and a problem is identified:
a. a corrective action plan is implemented.
b. an incident report must be filed.
c. patient specimens must always be redrawn.
d. the patient's physician must be notified.

28. Which of the following does *not* represent a QA procedure?
a. checking needles for blunt tips and barbs
b. following strict specimen-labeling requirements
c. keeping a record of employee sick leave
d. recording results of refrigerator temperature checks

29. Which preanalytical factor that can affect validity of test results is not always under the phlebotomist's control?
a. patient identification
b. patient preparation
c. specimen collection
d. specimen handling

30. Which of the following contains a chronologic record of a patient's care?
a. delta check
b. medical record
c. specimen label
d. user manual

31. A phlebotomist redirects the needle several times in a failed venipuncture attempt before switching to the other arm and obtaining the blood sample. The patient later complains of pain in the antecubital area where the phlebotomist was unsuccessful. What claim can be made against the phlebotomist?
a. assault
b. fraud

c. negligence
d. res ipsa loquitur

32. A specimen was mislabeled on the floor by the same phlebotomist for the second time. You, as the phlebotomist's supervisor, are required to fill out a Performance Improvement Plan. Which of the following is the only information that would *not* be included?
a. explanation of the deficiency
b. description of the consequence
c. detailed corrective action plan
d. suggestion for new guidelines

33. An example of a QA indicator is:
a. all phlebotomists will follow standard precautions guidelines.
b. laboratory personnel will not wear lab coats when on break.
c. no eating, drinking, or smoking is allowed in lab work areas.
d. the contamination rate for BCs will not exceed the national rate.

34. What laboratory document describes in detail the steps to follow for specimen collection?
a. OSHA safety manual
b. policy guidelines
c. procedure manual
d. quality control manual

35. Drawing a patient's blood without his or her permission can result in a charge of:
a. assault and battery.
b. breach of confidentiality.
c. malpractice.
d. negligence.

36. The term "tort" means a:
a. criminal action.
b. monetary award.
c. personal injury.
d. wrongful act.

37. All of the following are steps in the risk management process EXCEPT:
a. breach of confidentiality.
b. education of employees.
c. identification of risk.
d. treatment of risk.

38. Which of the following would not violate a patient's right to confidentiality?
a. indicating the nature of a patient's disease on the door
b. keeping a list of HIV-positive patients posted in the laboratory
c. posting a patient's lab results on a board in his or her room
d. sharing information on a "difficult draw" with a coworker

39. Unauthorized release of confidential patient information is called:
a. a type of negligence.
b. failure to use due care.
c. invasion of privacy.
d. violation of discovery.

40. Civil actions involve:
a. legal proceedings between private parties.
b. offenses that can lead to imprisonment.
c. regulations established by governments.
d. violent crimes against the state or nation.

41. Malpractice is a claim of:
a. breach of confidentiality.
b. improper treatment.
c. invasion of privacy.
d. res ipsa loquitur.

42. All of the following are examples of negligence EXCEPT when the phlebotomist:
a. does not return a bedrail to the upright position.
b. fails to report significant changes in a patient's condition.
c. forgets to put a needle in the sharps container.
d. is unable to obtain a specimen from a combative patient.

43. A patient is told that she must remain still during blood collection or she will be restrained. Which tort is involved in this example?
    a. assault
    b. battery
    c. fraud
    d. malpractice

44. A patient agrees to undergo treatment after the method, risks, and consequences are explained to him. This is an example of:
    a. implied consent.
    b. informed consent.
    c. respondent superior.
    d. standard of care.

45. The period within which an injured party may file a lawsuit is known as:
    a. binding arbitration.
    b. litigation process.
    c. statute of limitations.
    d. tort interval.

46. The definition of a minor is anyone:
    a. who is not self-supporting.
    b. who is not the age of majority.
    c. younger than 18 years of age.
    d. younger than 21 years of age.

47. Performing one's duties in the same manner as any other reasonable and prudent person with the same experience and training is referred to as:
    a. risk management.
    b. the standard of care.
    c. the statute of limitations.
    d. vicarious liability.

48. Doing something that a reasonable and prudent person *would not* do, or failing to do something that a reasonable and prudent person *would* do is:
    a. battery.
    b. discovery.
    c. fraud.
    d. negligence.

49. A phlebotomist explains to an inpatient that he has come to collect a blood specimen. The patient extends his arm and pushes up his sleeve. This is an example of:
    a. expressed consent.
    b. implied consent.
    c. informed consent.
    d. refusal of consent.

50. A 12-year-old inpatient who refused to have his blood collected was restrained by a healthcare worker while the phlebotomist collected the specimen. This is an example of:
    a. assault and battery.
    b. implied consent.
    c. malpractice.
    d. negligence.

51. The standard of care used in phlebotomy malpractice cases is often based on guidelines from this organization.
    a. CAP
    b. CLSI
    c. OSHA
    d. NAACLS

52. Which one of the following actions points to negligence?
    a. causing harm as a result of a violation of duty
    b. documenting an unusual happening during a draw
    c. informing the patient of his laboratory test results
    d. watching for implied consent from the patient

53. The process of gathering information by taking statements and interrogating parties involved in a lawsuit is called:
    a. collaboration.
    b. deposition.
    c. discovery.
    d. litigation.

54. The "standard of care" in the practice of phlebotomy is influenced by which of the following organizations?
    a. Environmental Protection Agency
    b. Food and Drug Administration
    c. Health Insurance Privacy Act
    d. The Joint Commission

55. A lawsuit is filed against the phlebotomist after a patient claimed an injury occurred during a venipuncture. In litigation proceedings the phlebotomist is the:
    a. client.
    b. defendant.
    c. plaintiff.
    d. prosecutor.

Use Fig. 2-1 (Microbiology Quality Assessment Form) to answer questions 56–59.

HOSPITAL & HEALTH CENTER
QUALITY ASSESSMENT AND IMPROVEMENT TRACKING
CONFIDENTIAL A.R.S. 36-445 et. seq.

STANDARD OF CARE/SERVICE:

IMPORTANT ASPECT OF CARE/SERVICE:
LABORATORY SERVICES
COLLECTION/TRANSPORT

SIGNATURES:

DIRECTOR

MEDICAL DIRECTOR

VICE PRESIDENT/ADMINISTRATOR

DEPARTMENTS:
DATA SOURCE(S):
METHODOLOGY: [X] RETROSPECTIVE [ ] CONCURRENT
TYPE: [ ] STRUCTURE [ ] PROCESS [X] OUTCOME
PERSON RESPONSIBLE FOR:
- DATA COLLECTION:
- DATA ORGANIZATION:
- ACTION PLAN:
- FOLLOW-UP:

DATE MONITORING BEGAN: 1990
TIME PERIOD THIS MONITOR: 2ND QUARTER 2006
MONITOR DISCONTINUED BECAUSE:
FOLLOW-UP:

INDICATORS	THLD	ACT	PREV	CRITICAL ANALYSIS/EVALUATION	ACTION PLAN
Blood Culture contamination rate will not exceed 3%				**Population: All patients** **All monthly indicators were under threshold, 3%**	**Share results and analysis with Lab staff and ER staff.**
APR - # of Draws: 713 **# Contaminated: 13**	**3.00%**	**1.8%**	**1.2%**	**% Contamination from draws other than Line draws, by unit:**	
MAY - # of Draws: 710 **# Contaminated: 23**	**3.00%**	**2.8%**	**2.3%**	**APR: ER = 4.7% Lab = 0.7%** **MAY: ER = 11.5% Lab = 1.0%** **JUN: ER = 8.6% Lab = 1.1%**	
JUN - # of Draws: 702 **# Contaminated: 17**	**3.00%**	**2.4%**	**1.9%**	**ER was over threshold for each month of quarter.**	
Total for 1st Quarter - **# of Draws: 2125** **# Contaminated: 50**	**3.00%**	**2.4%**	**1.9%**		

FIGURE 2-1 Microbiology quality assessment form. (Courtesy John C. Lincoln Hospital & Health Center.)

56. This quality assessment and tracking tool shows the number of contaminated blood cultures to be highest in what month?
    a. April
    b. May
    c. June
    d. September

57. Which hospital department's blood culture collections exceeded the threshold for each month of the quarter?
    a. emergency room
    b. laboratory
    c. outpatient services
    d. radiology

58. The use of this microbiology quality assessment form for tracking and evaluating blood cultures began in what year?
    a. 1985
    b. 1990
    c. 2000
    d. 2004

59. In which month did the laboratory blood culture collections actually exceed 3% contamination?
    a. the month of April
    b. the month of May
    c. the month of June
    d. none of the above

Use Fig. 2-2 (a page from a nursing services manual) to answer questions 60–62.

60. Which test specimen has to be centrifuged and separated and have the plasma frozen immediately?
    a. antithrombin activity
    b. APTT
    c. aspergillus serology
    d. AST

61. Which test collection time is dependent on the time the patient's coagulation therapy was given?
    a. antithrombin activity
    b. APTT
    c. aspergillus serology
    d. AST

62. Which of the following tests must be collected after a discard tube is drawn?
    a. antithrombin activity
    b. APTT
    c. aspergillus serology
    d. AST

TEST PROCEDURE:	**ANTI THROMBIN III ACTIVITY – PLASMA ACTIVITY**
TEST MNEMONIC:	**AT3**
BILLING NUMBER:	3000070
MANNER OF COLLECTION:	Drawn by Lab
SPECIMEN REQUIRED:	Citrated plasma, 1 Blue Top with Black Insert of 2 Blue Top with White Insert
SPECIAL INSTRUCTIONS:	2, 1 ml citrated plasma aliquots place in plastic tubes. Centrifuge, separate, and freeze plasma immediately.
PATIENT PREPARATION:	None
AVAILABILITY:	At all times
ROUTINE TURN-AROUND TIME:	Dependent on Reference Laboratory's testing schedule
STAT TURN-AROUND TIME:	N/A
LIMITATIONS:	None
NORMAL RANGE:	See Reference Laboratory Report

TEST PROCEDURE:	**APTT**
TEST MNEMONIC:	**APTT (ALSO SEE PTT)**
BILLING NUMBER:	3000030
MANNER OF COLLECTION:	Drawn by Lab
SPECIMEN REQUIRED:	Citrated plasma, Blue Top Tube
SPECIAL INSTRUCTIONS:	If the patient is on heparin, APTT's should be timed so that the blood is not drawn immediately after the dose is given. Draw a red tube before drawing the blue top tube. TESTING CANNOT BE PERFORMED ON OVERFILLED OR UNDERFILLED BLUE TOP TUBES. CORRECT BLOOD VOLUME IN BLUE TOP TUBE IS CRITICAL.
PATIENT PREPARATION:	None
AVAILABILITY:	At all times
ROUTINE TURN-AROUND TIME:	1–2 Hours
STAT TURN-AROUND TIME:	60 Minutes
LIMITATIONS:	None
NORMAL RANGE:	Normal Range: 21.5 – 34.0 seconds

TEST PROCEDURE:	**ARSENIC, URINE**
TEST MNEMONIC:	**ARSENUR**
BILLING NUMBER:	
MANNER OF COLLECTION:	Urine collected by nurse
SPECIMEN REQUIRED:	Random urine
SPECIAL INSTRUCTIONS:	10 ml random urine in acid-washed container, refrigerate
PATIENT PREPARATION:	None
AVAILABILITY:	At all times
ROUTINE TURN-AROUND TIME:	Dependent on Reference Laboratory's testing schedule
STAT TURN-AROUND TIME:	N/A
LIMITATIONS:	None
NORMAL RANGE:	See Reference Laboratory Report

TEST PROCEDURE:	**ASPERGILLUS SEROLOGY**
TEST MNEMONIC:	**ASPTER**
BILLING NUMBER:	3020090
MANNER OF COLLECTION:	Drawn by Lab
SPECIMEN REQUIRED:	1 Red Top Tube
SPECIAL INSTRUCTIONS:	Refrigerate 1 ml serum
PATIENT PREPARATION:	None
AVAILABILITY:	At all times
ROUTINE TURN-AROUND TIME:	Dependent on Reference Laboratory's testing schedule
STAT TURN-AROUND TIME:	N/A
LIMITATIONS:	None
NORMAL RANGE:	See Reference Laboratory Report

TEST PROCEDURE:	**AST (SGOT)**
TEST MNEMONIC:	**AST**
BILLING NUMBER:	3011070
MANNER OF COLLECTION:	Drawn by Lab
SPECIMEN REQUIRED:	Plasma or Serum, 1 Green Top, Red Top, or SST Tube
SPECIAL INSTRUCTIONS:	None
PATIENT PREPARATION:	None
AVAILABILITY:	At all times
ROUTINE TURN-AROUND TIME:	4 Hours
STAT TURN-AROUND TIME:	60 Minutes
LIMITATIONS:	None
NORMAL RANGE:	15–37 U/L

FIGURE 2-2 Page from a nursing services manual. (Courtesy John C. Lincoln Hospital & Health Center.)

ANSWERS AND EXPLANATIONS

1. Answer: a
   Why: Civil lawsuits are concerned with actions between private parties, such as individuals or organizations, and constitute the bulk of the legal actions dealt with in healthcare. Criminal action deals with felonies and misdemeanors. Malpractice, a type of negligence, would fall under a civil action. Vicarious liability is a liability imposed by law on one person for acts committed by another.
   Review: Yes ☐ No ☐

2. Answer: b
   Why: Good Laboratory Practices (GLPs), as seen in Box 2.1, are 10 QA recommendations developed by the Clinical Laboratory Improvement Advisory Committee (CLIAC) for Certificate of Waiver (COW) labs because of problems with the quality of their testing practices. These GLPs emphasize quality assurance when collecting and performing blood work using waived testing kits.
   Review: Yes ☐ No ☐

3. Answer: a
   Why: Due care is a level of care that is expected to be exercised by a person of ordinary intelligence and good sense under the given circumstances. The standard of care is the level of skill and care that is expected to be performed to provide due care. Quality essentials and quality care are simply phrases that might be used in healthcare organizations when discussing QA processes.
   Review: Yes ☐ No ☐

4. Answer: c
   Why: Fraud is a deliberate deception carried out for unlawful gain and is in the form of a deceitful practice or false portrayal of facts, either by words or by conduct. Battery is defined as intentional harmful or offensive touching of or use of force on a person without consent or legal justification. Negligence is failure to exercise due care. If any of these torts make it to court, a formal discovery will occur, which involves taking depositions and interrogating parties involved.
   Review: Yes ☐ No ☐

5. Answer: b
   Why: Overall guidelines developed in an institution for all processes used and all personnel involved in patient care can be thought of as the program called Quality Improvement. These guidelines relate to customer satisfaction and accountability,

Box 2-1 Good Laboratory Practices

For more information see http://www.cms.hhs.gov/clia/downloads/wgoodlab.pdf

1. Keep and make available to the testing personnel the manufacturer's current product insert for the lab test being performed.
2. Follow the manufacturer's instructions for specimen collection and handling.
3. Properly identify the patient.
4. Label the patient's specimen for testing with an identifier unique to each patient.
5. Inform the patient of any test preparation such as fasting, clean-catch urines, etc.
6. Read the product insert prior to performing the test and achieving the optimal result.
7. Follow the storage requirements for the test kit.
8. Do not mix components of different kits.
9. Record the patient's test results in the proper place, such as the lab test log or the patient's chart.
10. Perform any instrument maintenance as directed by the manufacturer.

minimizing circumstances that jeopardize patient care and identifying situations that pose risk to employees as well. The Occupational Safety and Health Administration (OSHA) is concerned with safety and minimizing risk to employees but does not require or administer institutional QI programs.

Review: Yes ☐ No ☐

6. Answer: a

Why: Quality System Essentials (QSEs) are a core set of operations that can be applied to workflow steps necessary to deliver a product or service. See Table 2-1, Published Laboratory Quality Indicators for Arterial Blood Gases (ABG) Collection, for an example of QSEs and indicators that can be used to monitor the workflow process being evaluated.

Review: Yes ☐ No ☐

7. Answer: d

Why: The Center for Medicare and Medicaid Services (CMS) is an agency of the U.S. government that administers or manages federal healthcare programs for Medicare and Medicaid. The supervision of federal regulations passed by Congress called the Clinical Laboratory Improvement Amendments of 1988 (CLIA '88) also falls under its scope of authority. Although the CMS manages federal healthcare programs, it is not in the business of insuring medical personnel.

Review: Yes ☐ No ☐

Table 2-1 Published Laboratory Quality Indicators for Arterial Blood Gases (ABG) Collection

Quality System Essentials (QSEs)	Quality Indicators
Patient assessment	• Practice guideline implementation • Duplicate test ordering
Test request	• Ordering accuracy • Accuracy of order transmission • Verbal order evaluation
Specimen collection/labeling	• Wristband evaluation
Specimen transport	• Transit time • Stat transit time
Specimen receiving/processing	• Blood gas sample acceptability • Chemistry sample acceptability
QSE personnel	• Competence evaluation • Employee retention
QSE process control	• Safety
QSE occurrence management	• Incidents
QSE internal assessment	• On-site assessments • Self-assessments

Adapted from CLSI/NCCLS document H11-A4, *Procedures for the Collection of Arterial Blood Specimens; Approved Standard – Fourth Edition* with permission.

8. Answer: b
   Why: Giving a deposition is a process in which one party questions another under oath with both defense and prosecuting attorneys present. A court reporter records every word. Discovery is the process during which the attorneys for the defendant and plaintiff interrogate all parties involved in the legal dispute to determine the facts, which will be used in the trial phase. Civil actions are procedures in which the alleged injured party sues for monetary damages, and the tort is the most common civil action in healthcare.
   Review: Yes ☐ No ☐

9. Answer: a
   Why: The Procedure Manual states the policies and procedures that apply to each test or practice performed in the laboratory. It is a QA document that must be made available to all employees of the laboratory for standardization purposes. It contains, among other things, equipment used, purpose of the procedure, and all revision dates (Fig. 2-3). Corrective actions deal with personnel performance and are part of the performance improvement plan.
   Review: Yes ☐ No ☐

10. Answer: a
    Why: Risk is managed in two ways: controlling risk to avoid incidents and paying for occurrences after they have happened. Risk management focuses on minimizing the situations that could lead to occurrences for patients and employees. Sentinel event policies signal the need for immediate investigation and response to an occurrence that had unexpected results. Performance improvement plans and delta checks in an institution deal with quality assurance rather than risk management.
    Review: Yes ☐ No ☐

11. Answer: a
    Why: Not all laboratories perform the same level of testing. All laboratories subject to CLIA '88 regulations are required to obtain a CLIA certificate according to the complexity of testing performed there. Complexity of testing is based on the level of difficulty involved in performing a test and the degree of risk of harm to the patient if the test is performed incorrectly. The higher the complexity of testing performed, the more stringent the CLIA requirements are. Personnel qualifications are spelled out in the regulations but do not determine the type of certificate the laboratory will be awarded. Additionally, quality control standards and the size of the laboratory do not play a part in determining CLIA certification.
    Review: Yes ☐ No ☐

12. Answer: b
    Why: CLIA requirements are stringent for laboratories that perform moderate- and high-complexity testing. These laboratories are subject to routine inspections and must have written protocols for all procedures used. The laboratories are not federally funded. Personnel standards do not dictate that PhDs be hired as supervisors. The certificates do not need to be renewed annually.
    Review: Yes ☐ No ☐

13. Answer: a
    Why: The Joint Commission is committed to improving the safety of patients. The Joint Commission's quality improvement (QI) sentinel event policy is intended to identify unfavorable occurrences, initiate an immediate response, and take steps to prevent it from happening again. It stresses early identification of an event that may lead to death or serious physical or psychological injury or any deviation from practice that increases the chance that an undesirable outcome might recur. Because the intent of this policy is to protect the patients and residents, it can never be considered flexible.
    Review: Yes ☐ No ☐

SECTION: LABORATORY SERVICES

TOPIC: VENIPUNCTURE

REVIEWED: 3/95, 7/06

LAST REVISION: 3/93, 8/90, 3/88, 4/87, 8/04

APPROVAL:

1.0 PURPOSE

1.1 To provide our laboratory with quality blood specimens for testing.

2.0 POLICY

2.1 Blood collection by laboratory and hospital personnel will be performed according to our laboratory procedure.

3.0 PROCEDURE

3.1 Obtain computer labels generated by orders for tests requested. For registered outpatients, use faxed order from the Outpatient Order Log or prescription.

3.2 Upon entering the patient's room, identify yourself. State that you will be drawing blood for laboratory testing and gain the patient's confidence by behaving in a professional manner.

3.3 Ensure positive patient identification.

Inpatients

3.3.1 Identify the patient to be drawn by matching each label with the patient's hospital identification armband.

3.3.2 Check for the correct match of the patient's full name and hospital medical record number and account number.

3.3.3 In the case that there is no armband present, contact the patient's nurse or charge nurse for a armband to be placed on the patient.

3.3.4 Inpatients will **NOT** be drawn without a hospital armband.

Outpatients

3.3.5 For recurring outpatients without armbands, ask the patient for the spelling of their last name and their birth date. If the patient is a

FIGURE 2-3 Procedure manual page. (Courtesy John C. Lincoln Hospital & Health Center.)

14. Answer: d

Why: The intent of this policy is help healthcare organizations identify sentinel events and take steps to prevent them from happening again. The steps involve conducting a thorough analysis of the cause, initiating improvements to reduce the risk, and monitoring improvements for effectiveness. Healthcare organizations are not required to report these incidents to the Joint Commission.

Review: Yes ☐ No ☐

15. Answer: a
Why: A laboratory "path of workflow" is defined as the steps necessary to deliver a product or service. It includes preanalytical, analytical, and postanalytical processes and includes quality indicators (see Table 2-1) to monitor these processes. A workflow path does not include sending a periodic report to the hospital administrator.
Review: Yes ☐ No ☐

16. Answer: a
Why: Quality Assurance (QA) indicators can measure quality, adequacy, accuracy, timeliness, and customer satisfaction. They are designed to look at all areas of care and are used in conjunction with QSEs to monitor workflow and outcomes. Quality Improvement (QI) core measurements for hospitals have been set by the Joint Commission to document the results of care for individual patients and specific patient groups in certain diagnostic categories. Threshold values must be established for all clinical indicators.
Review: Yes ☐ No ☐

17. Answer: c
Why: The National Accrediting Agency for Clinical Laboratory Sciences (NAACLS) is an agency that approves phlebotomy programs. The Clinical Laboratory Improvement Amendments of 1988 (CLIA '88) are federal regulations aimed at ensuring the accuracy, reliability, and timeliness of patient test results regardless of laboratory size. The Clinical and Laboratory Standards Institute (CLSI) develops standards for laboratory procedures, including phlebotomy. The National Credentialing Agency (NCA) for Laboratory Personnel is one of several organizations that certify laboratory personnel, including phlebotomists.
Review: Yes ☐ No ☐

18. Answer: d
Why: Failure to exercise the level of care that a person of ordinary intelligence and good sense would exercise under the given circumstances is called negligence. If a medical procedure results in injury, the injured person has the right to sue for damages. Because the phlebotomist did not threaten or intend to harm the patient, there are no assault and battery charges; nor did the phlebotomist commit fraud because there was not a willful plan to deceive the patient.
Review: Yes ☐ No ☐

19. Answer: b
Why: The Clinical Laboratory Improvement Amendments of 1988 (CLIA '88) are federal regulations aimed at ensuring the accuracy, reliability, and timeliness of patient test results regardless of the size, type, or location of the laboratory. CLIA regulations pertain to all laboratories in the United States that perform laboratory testing used for the assessment of human health or the diagnosis, treatment, or prevention of disease. The Occupational Safety and Health Act (OSHA) mandates safe working conditions for employees and is enforced by the Occupational Safety and Health Administration (also OSHA). The Bloodborne Pathogen (BBP) Standard was instituted by OSHA to protect employees from exposure to bloodborne pathogens. The Hazard Communication Standard (HazCom) was developed by OSHA to protect employees from exposure to hazardous chemicals.
Review: Yes ☐ No ☐

20. Answer: b
Why: The Clinical and Laboratory Standards Institute (CLSI), formerly known as the National Committee for Clinical Laboratory Standards (NCCLS), is a global, nonprofit, standards-developing organization with representatives from the profession, industry, and government who use a consensus

process to develop guidelines and standards for all areas of the laboratory. The American Society for Clinical Pathology (ASCP), NCA, and NAACLS are organizations that contribute to the standards of phlebotomy practices by offering continuing education, certification exams, and phlebotomy program approval respectively.

Review: Yes ☐ No ☐

21. Answer: b
 Why: Patient identification, phlebotomy technique, and specimen handling are all areas of phlebotomy that are subject to QC procedures. Adjusting a patient's IV is not in the scope of practice for a phlebotomist. Even though it is necessary at times to have blood specimens withdrawn from intravenous devices, such as heparin or saline locks, it is not in the phlebotomist's scope of practice to handle such procedures unless specifically trained by the facility to do so. It is never appropriate to adjust an IV in a patient's arm or to put a tourniquet near that area.
 Review: Yes ☐ No ☐

22. Answer: a
 Why: Delta checks compare current results of a test with previous results for the same test on the same patient. Although some variation is to be expected, a major difference in results could indicate error and requires investigation.
 Review: Yes ☐ No ☐

23. Answer: b
 Why: The College of American Pathologists (CAP) is a national organization of board-certified pathologists that offers laboratory inspection and proficiency testing. OSHA inspections involve safety violations. The American Society for Clinical Pathology is an organization that certifies laboratory personnel. The Clinical and Laboratory Standards Institute (CLSI) develops standards and guidelines for laboratory procedures, including phlebotomy. OSHA mandates and enforces safe working conditions for employees.
 Review: Yes ☐ No ☐

24. Answer: c
 Why: Outdated tubes should never be used. The tube vacuum and the integrity of any additive that might be in the tube are guaranteed by the manufacturer, but only if the tube is used before the expiration date. After that date, the additive may break down and no longer function as intended. In addition, outdated tubes may lose some of the vacuum and no longer fill completely. In either situation, the results may be incorrect or erroneous. It has not been shown that the tube stoppers actually shrink when held past the expiration date.
 Review: Yes ☐ No ☐

25. Answer: a
 Why: The Joint Commission is a nongovernmental agency that establishes standards and provides accreditation for healthcare organizations. Their standards focus on improving the quality and safety of care provided and stress performance improvement by requiring healthcare facilities to be directly accountable to their customers. The Clinical and Laboratory Standards Institute (CLSI) develops standards for laboratory procedures, including phlebotomy. NAACLS develops phlebotomy competencies and has an approval process for phlebotomy programs. Laboratory personnel are certified by organizations such as ASCP, AMT, and NCA.
 Review: Yes ☐ No ☐

26. Answer: c
 Why: Quality control procedures involve checking all operational procedures to make certain they are performed correctly and include checking expiration dates, documenting centrifuge maintenance, and recording refrigerator temperatures. Filling out your

time sheet is important but is not considered a quality control procedure.

Review: Yes ☐ No ☐

27. Answer: a

Why: If the threshold of an indicator is exceeded, data is collected and organized to see if there is a problem. If a problem is identified, a corrective action plan is established and implemented (see Fig. 2-1).

Review: Yes ☐ No ☐

28. Answer: c

Why: QA procedures include checking for needle defects before use, following strict specimen-labeling requirements, and recording results of refrigerator temperature checks. Keeping a record of employee sick leave is an important personnel issue but is not a part of QA.

Review: Yes ☐ No ☐

29. Answer: b

Why: Preparing a patient for testing is not generally under the control of the phlebotomist. However, it is up to the phlebotomist to determine that preparation procedures have been followed. For example, if a test is ordered fasting, the phlebotomist must check to see that the patient is indeed fasting. The phlebotomist is responsible for obtaining proper patient identification, collecting the specimen, and handling the specimen properly after collection until turning it over to the laboratory for testing.

Review: Yes ☐ No ☐

30. Answer: b

Why: The medical record is a chronological record of a patient's care and serves as a valuable tool in evaluating medical treatment and communicating with all of the patient's caregivers. A delta check compares current results of a lab test with previous results for the same test on the same patient. A major difference in results could indicate error and requires investigation. A specimen label contains patient information that often includes a medical record number. A user manual gives specimen requirements and collection information.

Review: Yes ☐ No ☐

31. Answer: c

Why: Negligence is failure to exercise due care or perform duties according to the standards of the profession. If a medical procedure such as phlebotomy results in injury, a claim of negligence can be made by the injured party. Redirecting the needle multiple times in an attempt to locate a vein is called probing and is not considered due care because it can result in damage to nerves, arteries, and other tissues. Pain in the area where the venipuncture attempt was unsuccessful is an indication that the patient may have been physically harmed by the probing.

Review: Yes ☐ No ☐

32. Answer: d

Why: A document called a Performance Improvement Plan (Fig. 2-4) is used when counseling a person or when suspension is necessary. The document states the deficiency, describes a specific action plan for improvement, or indicates consequences such as termination or suspension. New guidelines are sometimes implemented as a result of an incident but are not included on the incident report form.

Review: Yes ☐ No ☐

33. Answer: d

Why: Following standard precaution guidelines, not wearing lab coats outside of work areas, and not eating, drinking, or smoking in lab work areas are all safety rules. QA indicators are not considered rules but are statements that serve as monitors of patient care. By setting a limit or threshold value, they serve as initiators of action plans, as shown in Fig. 2-1.

Review: Yes ☐ No ☐

HOSPITAL & HEALTH CENTER

PERFORMANCE IMPROVEMENT PLAN

Employee Name:	**Facility**	**Department**	**Job Title**
Previous Action:	**Type**	**Reason**	**Date**

Current Action: (please check one)
☐ Verbal Counseling ☐ Written Warning ☐ Final Written Warning
☐ Suspension – Date ☐ Termination (check reason below)

Termination Reason: ☐ Unexcused Absence/Tardiness ☐ Job Performance ☐ Conduct ☐ Other

I. Describe the performance deficiency giving rise to the counseling (include specific dates, times and policies violated, etc.):

II. Describe specific job performance expectations and areas for improvement:

III. Describe the agreed upon action plan for improvement including date of follow-up to review progress, if applicable:

IV. State the next step if job performance does not improve (warning, discharge, etc.):

V. Department Director/Supervisor Comments:

Department Director/Supervisor Signature:	Date

VI. Employee Comments:

I understand that all corrective action notices other than a verbal counseling will be placed in my personnel file. My signature below does not indicate agreement regarding the contents of the document; only that I have received a copy for my records.

Employee	**Date**	**Witness**	**Date**
Human Resources	**Date**	**Reason**	

FIGURE 2-4 Performance Improvement Plan. (Courtesy John C. Lincoln Hospital & Health Center.)

34. Answer: c
Why: The laboratory procedure manual is a reference book that describes in detail the step-by-step processes for specimen collection and other procedures performed in the laboratory. An example of a page from a procedure manual is shown in Fig. 2-3. Other manuals may contain information on safety, details on administrative duties, or data for the quality control program.
Review: Yes ☐ No ☐

35. Answer: a
Why: Drawing a person's blood without permission can be perceived as assault, which is the act or threat of intentionally causing a person to be in fear of harm to his or her person. If the act or threat is actually carried out, then it can also be perceived as battery. Battery is defined as the intentional harmful or offensive touching of a person without consent or legal justification. Breach of confidentiality involves failure to keep medical information private or confidential. Negligence requires doing something that a reasonable person would not do, or not doing something a reasonable person would do. Malpractice is negligence by a professional.
Review: Yes ☐ No ☐

36. Answer: d
Why: A "tort" is a wrongful act resulting in injury for which a civil, rather than criminal, action can be brought. A tort is committed against one's property, reputation, or other legally protected right, for which an individual is entitled to damages awarded by the court. Damages are generally in the form of monetary awards.
Review: Yes ☐ No ☐

37. Answer: a
Why: Risk management is a process that focuses on identifying and minimizing situations that pose a risk to patients and employees by using education and following procedures that are already in place. Breach of confidentiality caused by the unauthorized release of information concerning a patient can lead to the implementation of risk management techniques, but it is not one of the designated steps in the process, as the other choices are.
Review: Yes ☐ No ☐

38. Answer: d
Why: As a professional, the phlebotomist should recognize that all patient information, including disease status and laboratory test results, is absolutely private or confidential. However, letting other phlebotomists know where the best site is to obtain a blood sample on a patient who is a "difficult draw" is part of proper patient care and not considered a violation of patient confidentiality.
Review: Yes ☐ No ☐

39. Answer: c
Why: Unauthorized release of confidential patient information is called invasion of privacy and can result in a civil lawsuit. It may also be considered breach of confidentiality if medical information is involved. It is not considered a type of negligence or failure to use due care, or called a violation of discovery.
Review: Yes ☐ No ☐

40. Answer: a
Why: Civil actions involve legal proceedings between private parties. The most common civil actions involve tort. For example, a claim of malpractice because of harm or injury to a patient by a phlebotomist is a civil wrong, or tort. Crimes against the state or that violate laws established by governments are criminal actions for which a guilty individual may be imprisoned.
Review: Yes ☐ No ☐

41. Answer: b
Why: Malpractice can be described as improper or negligent treatment resulting in injury, loss, or damage. Breach of confidentiality involves failure to keep medical information private or confidential, as opposed

to invasion of privacy, which involves physical intrusion or the unauthorized publishing or releasing of private information. Res ipsa loquitur is a Latin phrase that means "the thing speaks for itself" and applies to the rule of evidence in cases of negligence in which a breach of duty is obvious.

Review: Yes ☐ No ☐

42. Answer: d

Why: Forgetting to return a bedrail to its upright position, failing to discard needles properly (such as dropping them in the trash instead of the sharps container), and not reporting an obvious problem with a patient's condition (such as severe breathing difficulties or inability to awaken) could all lead to serious consequences and are examples of negligence or failure to exercise reasonable care. Inability to obtain a specimen from a patient is not negligence. In addition, collecting a specimen from a combative patient against his or her will could be considered assault and battery.

Review: Yes ☐ No ☐

43. Answer: a

Why: Assault involves the act or threat of causing an individual to be in fear of harm. Threatening to restrain the patient can be considered assault. Restraining the patient and collecting a blood specimen can be considered assault and battery.

Review: Yes ☐ No ☐

44. Answer: b

Why: Informed consent implies voluntary and competent permission for a medical procedure, test, or medication and requires that the patient be given adequate information as to the method, risks, and consequences involved before consent is given. In implied consent, the patient's actions or condition (as in an emergency situation in which the patient is unconscious) indicate consent rather than a verbal or written statement.

Review: Yes ☐ No ☐

45. Answer: c

Why: Statute of limitations is the particular number of years within which one party can sue another. Binding arbitration is a way that equitable settlements over a controversy are made outside the courts. It is one of the pathways used in the litigation process, which is defined as a course of action used to settle legal disputes. Tort interval is not a legal term.

Review: Yes ☐ No ☐

46. Answer: b

Why: The definition of a minor is anyone who has not reached the age of majority. The age of majority is determined by state law and normally ranges from 18 to 21 years of age regardless of whether the individual is self-supporting.

Review: Yes ☐ No ☐

47. Answer: b

Why: The standard of care is a level of care that protects clients from harm because it follows established standards of the profession and expectations of society. It requires that duties be performed the same way any other reasonable and prudent person with the same experience and training would perform those duties. Risk management is a process that focuses on identifying and minimizing risks so as to protect clients from harm.

Review: Yes ☐ No ☐

48. Answer: d

Why: Negligence involves doing something that a reasonable and prudent person would not do, or not doing something that a reasonable and prudent person would do. Battery is the intentional harmful or offensive touching of another person without consent or legal justification. Discovery is process of taking depositions or interrogating parties involved in a lawsuit. Fraud is deceitful practice or false portrayal of facts by word or conduct.

Review: Yes ☐ No ☐

49. Answer: b
Why: With implied consent, the patient's actions or condition (as in an emergency situation in which the patient is unconscious) indicate consent, rather than a verbal or written statement. A patient who extends his arm and rolls up his sleeve after being told that the phlebotomist is there to collect a blood specimen is implying consent with his actions. The patient is obviously not refusing consent, or he might have pulled his arm away and kept his sleeve down. To be expressed consent, the patient would have to give a written or verbal statement of consent. Implied consent can be informed consent; however, implied consent is the best choice because it is a more specific answer to the situation.
Review: Yes ☐ No ☐

50. Answer: a
Why: A 12-year-old is not old enough to give consent for a medical procedure such as phlebotomy. A phlebotomist who collects a blood specimen from a minor without permission from a parent risks being charged with assault and battery. As long as no harm to the patient was involved, this would not be considered negligence or malpractice. The patient refused blood collection, so this is not considered implied consent.
Review: Yes ☐ No ☐

51. Answer: b
Why: The Clinical and Laboratory Standards Institute (CLSI) is a global nonprofit organization that publishes standards for phlebotomy procedures. These standards are recognized as the legal standard of care for phlebotomy procedures. CAP sets standards for laboratories, but not specifically for phlebotomy procedures. OSHA sets and enforces standards regarding the safety of employees. NAACLS approves phlebotomy programs.
Review: Yes ☐ No ☐

52. Answer: a
Why: To claim negligence, the following elements must be present: a legal obligation or duty owed by one person to another, a breaking of that duty or obligation, and harm done as a result of that breach of duty. Informing the patient of test results is the physician's responsibility but is not considered negligence. Watching for implied consent from a patient is necessary in some cases. Documenting an unusual happening during venipuncture is a good habit to get into in case there are future complaints.
Review: Yes ☐ No ☐

53. Answer: c
Why: The process of gathering information by taking statements and interrogating parties involved in a lawsuit is called discovery. It involves taking depositions (questioning parties under oath). Some collaboration may be involved, but it is not the term used to describe this process. Litigation is the process used to settle disputes, and discovery is part of this process.
Review: Yes ☐ No ☐

54. Answer: d
Why: The Joint Commission is presently the largest healthcare standards-setting body in the world. All departments of a healthcare facility, including the laboratory, must comply with their standards to receive accreditation. The Environmental Protection Agency (EPA) and the Food and Drug Administration (FDA) are agencies of the federal government that are designed to protect the public in their respective areas. The Health Insurance Portability and Accountability Act (HIPAA) is a federal law designed to protect patient information.
Review: Yes ☐ No ☐

55. Answer: b
Why: The person against whom a complaint has been filed is the defendant. The person

who complains of injury is the plaintiff and will become the prosecuting attorney's client.

Review: Yes ☐ No ☐

56. Answer: b
Why: The number of contaminated blood culture draws was highest in May (see Fig. 2-1).
Review: Yes ☐ No ☐

57. Answer: a
Why: The report on the form in Fig. 2-1 clearly states that the emergency room (ER) is over threshold for each month of the quarter. The % contaminated draws for the ER went as high as 11.5% in May. The report shows the comparison between laboratory draws and those in the ER. This QA indicator tool is an objective measurement of phlebotomist technique.
Review: Yes ☐ No ☐

58. Answer: b
Why: The date this QA monitoring began was in 1990 (see Fig. 2-1). This long-term tracking serves to point out valuable patterns in collection and gives insight into corrective actions that can be taken.
Review: Yes ☐ No ☐

59. Answer: d
Why: As shown in the report (Fig. 2-1), during the 3 months being monitored, the laboratory staff did not exceed the allowable contamination rate of 3% during blood culture collection.
Review: Yes ☐ No ☐

60. Answer: a
Why: The anti-thrombin III activity is a test ordered to evaluate a specific coagulation factor that is not stable at room temperature. Consequently, the specimen should be centrifuged and separated and the plasma frozen immediately, as indicated on the page from the nursing services manual (Fig. 2-2).
Review: Yes ☐ No ☐

61. Answer: b
Why: The APTT test is drawn to monitor heparin therapy. As stated in the nursing services manual (Figure 2-2), if the patient is receiving heparin therapy at the time of the draw, the collection should be timed so that the blood is not drawn immediately after the dose is given.
Review: Yes ☐ No ☐

62. Answer: b
Directions in the Nursing Services Manual (Fig. 2-2) clearly state that a red top tube must be drawn before collecting the blue top tube for an APTT. The red top is collected first so that any tissue fluid that contains thromboplastin, a clot activator, is removed from the needle before collecting the APTT coagulation test.
Review: Yes ☐ No ☐

INFECTION CONTROL, SAFETY, FIRST AID, AND PERSONAL WELLNESS

CHAPTER 3

study tip

Questions in this chapter assesses the ability to describe the process of infection, and identify the components of the chain of infection, required safety equipment, and infection control procedures. They also test the ability to recognize biological, electrical, radiation, and chemical hazards and identify the safety precautions, rules, and procedures necessary to eliminate or minimize them. First aid issues tested include control of external hemorrhage and how to recognize and treat shock victims. Wellness issues addressed include back injury prevention, benefits of exercise, and dealing with stress.

overview

This chapter tests knowledge of infection control, safety, first aid, and personal wellness. A thorough knowledge in these areas is necessary for phlebotomists to protect themselves, patients, coworkers, and others from infection or injury, react quickly and skillfully in emergency situations, and stay healthy both physically and emotionally, all without compromising the quality of patient care.

REVIEW QUESTIONS

Choose the BEST answer.

1. These are the initials of the U.S. government agency that mandates and enforces safe working conditions for employees.
   a. CDC
   b. HICPAC
   c. NIOSH
   d. OSHA

2. The series of components that lead to infection are referred to as the:
   a. chain of infection.
   b. immune response.
   c. infection cycle.
   d. pathogenic series.

3. The pathogen responsible for causing an infection is called the infectious:
   a. agent.
   b. host.
   c. vector.
   d. vehicle.

4. The term "pathogenic" means:
   a. highly communicable.
   b. possessing virulence.
   c. productive of disease.
   d. systemic in nature.

5. A specimen processor removes the stopper from a tube without barrier protection and feels a mist of specimen touch the eyes. What type of exposure occurs through eye contact?
   a. airborne
   b. non-intact skin
   c. percutaneous
   d. permucosal

6. Isolation procedures are used to separate patients from contact with others if they:
   a. are a carrier of a bloodborne pathogen.
   b. have highly transmissible infections.
   c. require blood or body fluid precautions.
   d. were exposed to a contagious disease.

7. Microbes include all of the following EXCEPT:
   a. bacteria.
   b. fungi.
   c. ova.
   d. viruses.

8. All of the following can leave a patient more susceptible to infection EXCEPT:
   a. antibiotic treatment.
   b. chemotherapy drugs.
   c. previous vaccination.
   d. surgical procedures.

9. An individual who has little resistance to an infectious microbe is referred to as a susceptible:
   a. agent.
   b. host.
   c. pathway.
   d. reservoir.

10. MSDS information includes:
    a. general and emergency information.
    b. highly technical chemical formulas.
    c. information on competitor products.
    d. product manufacturing conditions.

11. Transmission-based precautions must be followed for patients with:
    a. compromised immune systems.
    b. highly transmissible diseases.
    c. severe gastrointestinal distress.
    d. symptoms of acute appendicitis.

12. Which of the following patients would require contact precautions pending a diagnosis?
    a. child with a maculopapular rash highly suggestive of rubeola (measles)
    b. diapered patient with symptoms of infection with an enteric pathogen
    c. HIV-positive patient who has a cough, fever, and pulmonary infiltrate
    d. man with a severe persistent cough indicative of *Bordetella pertussis*

13. An individual is infected with *Escherichia coli* (*E. coli*) after eating contaminated spinach. What type of infection transmission is involved?
    a. contact
    b. droplet
    c. vector
    d. vehicle

14. An avulsion is a:
    a. hematoma in an extremity.
    b. situation that is repulsive.
    c. tearing away of a body part.
    d. type of operation on a bone.

15. This type of precaution is required for a patient with *Mycoplasma pneumonia.*
    a. airborne
    b. contact
    c. droplet
    d. standard

16. Proper neonatal intensive care unit blood-drawing procedure includes:
    a. never awaken an infant to draw a blood specimen.
    b. place the phlebotomy tray right next to the isolette.
    c. use povidone-iodine to clean a skin puncture site.
    d. wash hands and put on a gown, mask, and gloves.

17. What does the NFPA codeword *RACE* mean?
    a. react, activate, cover, extinguish
    b. rescue, alarm, confine, extinguish
    c. respond, activate, confine, escape
    d. run, alarm, counter, extinguish

18. All of the following statements concerning an employee bloodborne pathogen exposure incident are true EXCEPT:
    a. employees are entitled to free confidential medical evaluation.
    b. exposures should be documented on an incident report form.
    c. incidents should be immediately reported to a supervisor.
    d. source patients, if known, must be tested for HIV and HBV.

19. When the chain of infection is broken, an:
    a. individual is immune to that microbe.
    b. individual is susceptible to infection.
    c. infection is prevented from happening.
    d. infection will most likely be the result.

20. The focus of infection control turned from preventing patient-to-patient transmission to preventing patient-to-personnel transmission with the introduction of this concept.
    a. body substance isolation (BSI)
    b. category-specific isolation
    c. disease-specific isolation
    d. universal precautions (UP)

21. The term used to describe an infection that infects the entire body is:
    a. communicable.
    b. local.
    c. nosocomial.
    d. systemic.

22. Which type of precautions would be used for a patient who has pulmonary tuberculosis?
    a. airborne
    b. droplet
    c. contact
    d. reverse

23. Exercise reduces stress by:
    a. decreasing buildup of lactic acid.
    b. increasing utilization of glucose.
    c. promoting glycogen production.
    d. triggering release of endorphins.

24. The abbreviation for the virus that causes acquired immune deficiency syndrome (AIDS) is:
    a. HAV.
    b. HBV.
    c. HCV.
    d. HIV.

25. A person who has recovered from a particular virus and has developed antibodies against that virus is said to be:
    a. a carrier.
    b. immune.
    c. infectious.
    d. susceptible.

26. According to standard first aid procedures, severe external hemorrhage is *best* controlled by:
    a. applying direct pressure and elevating the extremity.
    b. keeping the injured extremity well below heart level.
    c. placing a tourniquet directly above the affected area.
    d. raising the patient's head above the level of the injury.

27. The main purpose of an infection control program is to:
    a. identify the source of communicable infections.
    b. separate infectious patients from other patients.
    c. prevent the spread of infection in the hospital.
    d. protect patients from outside contamination.

28. All pathogens are:
    a. communicable microorganisms.
    b. microbes that can cause disease.
    c. microorganisms that live in soil.
    d. normal flora found on the skin.

29. All of the following diseases involve a bloodborne pathogen EXCEPT:
    a. hepatitis B.
    b. malaria.
    c. syphilis.
    d. tuberculosis.

30. Proper hand-washing procedure involves all of the following steps EXCEPT:
    a. stand back so clothing does not touch the sink.
    b. wet hands with water before applying the soap.
    c. wash hands thoroughly for at least 15 seconds.
    d. use one towel to dry hands and turn off faucets.

31. An example of a disease requiring droplet isolation is:
    a. pertussis.
    b. rubeola.
    c. scabies.
    d. varicella.

32. Class C fires involve:
    a. combustible metals.
    b. electrical equipment.
    c. flammable liquids.
    d. ordinary materials.

33. Standard precautions should be followed:
    a. for anyone with hepatitis B.
    b. if a patient is HIV positive.
    c. while a patient is in isolation.
    d. with all patients, at all times.

34. Hepatitis B vaccination normally involves:
    a. a first shot of vaccine, one a month later, and one 6 months after the first.
    b. a single shot of vaccine that confers immunity for the individual's lifetime.
    c. three shots of vaccine, each 3 months apart, then yearly booster shots.
    d. two shots of vaccine 6 months apart, then a booster shot every 5 years.

35. Objects that can harbor and transmit infectious material are called:
    a. fomites.
    b. hosts.
    c. pathogens.
    d. vectors.

36. The HazCom Standard is also commonly called the:
    a. Full Disclosure Law.
    b. Material Safety Law.
    c. "Right to Know" Law.
    d. Universal Safety Law.

37. The body organ targeted by HBV is the:
    a. brain.
    b. heart.
    c. liver.
    d. lungs.

38. These are the initials of the two organizations responsible for the latest *Guideline for Isolation Precautions in Hospitals*.
    a. CDC and HICPAC
    b. CLSI and OSHA
    c. HICPAC and NIOSH
    d. NIOSH and OSHA

39. The primary purpose of wearing gloves during phlebotomy procedures is to protect the:
    a. patient from contamination by the phlebotomist.
    b. phlebotomist from exposure to the patient's blood.
    c. specimen from contamination by the phlebotomist.
    d. venipuncture site from contamination by the hands.

40. The first three components of fire that were traditionally referred to as the fire triangle are:
    a. carbon, air, and static.
    b. fuel, oxygen, and heat.
    c. oxygen, energy, and fuel.
    d. vapor, heat, and static.

41. All of the following can help break the chain of infection EXCEPT:
    a. implementing isolation procedures.
    b. opening exit pathways for pathogens.
    c. practicing stress reduction techniques.
    d. washing hands and wearing gloves.

42. Which of the following statements complies with electrical safety guidelines?
    a. electrical equipment should be unplugged while being serviced
    b. extension cords should be used to conveniently place equipment
    c. it is safe to use an electrical cord if it is only slightly frayed
    d. use electrical equipment carefully if it is starting to malfunction

43. Standard precautions apply to all body fluids EXCEPT:
    a. joint fluid.
    b. saliva.
    c. sweat.
    d. urine.

44. The ability of a microorganism to survive on contaminated articles and equipment has to do with its:
    a. susceptibility.
    b. transmission.
    c. viability.
    d. virulence.

45. The fourth component that turns the fire triangle into a fire tetrahedron is a:
    a. chain of ignition.
    b. chemical reaction.
    c. combustible item.
    d. temperature boost.

46. This equipment is required when collecting a specimen from a patient in airborne isolation.
    a. eye protection
    b. full face shield
    c. mask and goggles
    d. N95 respirator

47. Most exposures to HIV in healthcare settings are the result of:
    a. accidental needlesticks.
    b. splashes during surgery.
    c. tainted blood transfusions.
    d. touching AIDS patients.

48. The most common type of nosocomial infection in the United States is:
    a. bedsore infection.
    b. hepatitis B infection.
    c. respiratory infection.
    d. urinary tract infection.

49. These are the initials of the organization that instituted and enforces the Bloodborne Pathogen Standard (BBP).
    a. CAP
    b. CDC
    c. NIOSH
    d. OSHA

50. All of the following are proper laboratory safety procedures EXCEPT:
    a. keep your lab coat on at all times.
    b. never eat or apply makeup in the lab.
    c. secure long hair away from the face.
    d. wear closed-toe shoes when in the lab.

51. You accidentally splash a bleach solution in your eyes while preparing it for cleaning purposes. What is the first thing to do?
    a. dry your eyes quickly with a clean paper towel or tissue
    b. flush your eyes with water for a minimum of 15 minutes
    c. proceed to the emergency room as quickly as possible
    d. put 10 to 20 drops of saline in your eyes immediately

52. What is the best way to clean up blood that has dripped on the arm of a phlebotomy chair?
    a. absorb it with a gauze pad and clean the area with disinfectant
    b. rub it with a damp cloth and wash the area with soap and water
    c. wait for it to dry and then scrape it into a biohazard container
    d. wipe it with an alcohol pad using an outward circular motion

53. An example of employee screening for infection control is requiring employees to have:
    a. hepatitis B vaccinations.
    b. measles vaccinations.
    c. PPD (or TB) testing.
    d. tetanus booster shots.

54. Which mode of infection transmission occurs from touching contaminated bed linens?
    a. direct contact
    b. droplet contact
    c. indirect contact
    d. vehicle contact

55. All of the following can be transmitted through blood transfusion EXCEPT:
    a. cytomegalovirus.
    b. diabetes mellitus.
    c. hepatitis C virus.
    d. *Treponema pallidum.*

56. Which of the following is required by the Bloodborne Pathogen (BBP) Standard?
    a. providing isolation of patients known to be HIV positive
    b. gowning before entering rooms of AIDS patients
    c. having warning labels on specimens from AIDS patients
    d. wearing gloves when performing phlebotomy

57. What is the meaning of the symbol ₩ in Figure 3-1?
    a. water based
    b. water neutral
    c. water reactive
    d. water soluble

58. Neutropenic isolation is a type of reverse isolation used for patients with:
    a. a low WBC count.
    b. tuberculosis (TB).
    c. very severe burns.
    d. viral meningitis.

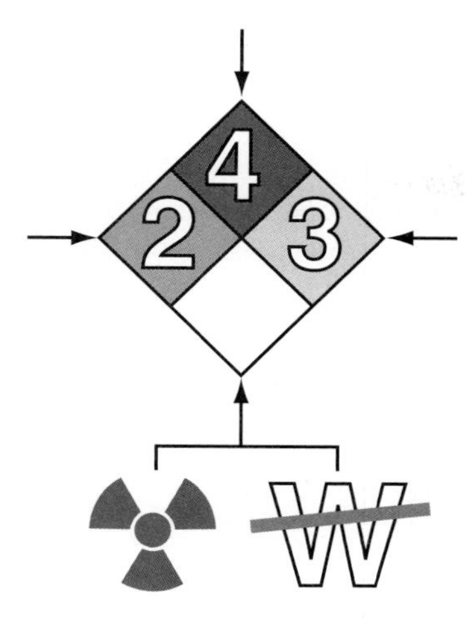

FIGURE 3-1 National Fire Protection Association 704 marking system.

59. What should the phlebotomist do if the outside of a patient specimen tube has blood on it?
    a. discard it and draw a new tube
    b. label it with a biohazard sticker
    c. put the specimen in a new tube
    d. wipe the tube with disinfectant

60. A laboratory or patient care activity that requires goggles to prevent exposure from sprays or splashes also requires this protective attire.
    a. earplugs
    b. gown
    c. mask
    d. respirator

61. Which of the following conditions would *not* necessarily lead to work restrictions for a hospital employee?
    a. a positive PPD test
    b. acute conjunctivitis
    c. German measles
    d. mononucleosis

62. How many classes of fire are identified by the National Fire Protection Association (NFPA)?
    a. two
    b. three
    c. four
    d. five

63. Which of the following would be the *best* means of preventing nosocomial infection?
    a. current immunization
    b. glove use if indicated
    c. isolation procedures
    d. proper hand hygiene

64. The purpose of "reverse" isolation is to:
    a. prevent airborne transmission of infectious microbes.
    b. protect susceptible patients from outside contamination.
    c. separate contagious patients from contact with others.
    d. provide the safest environment for psychiatric patients.

65. Which of the following could result in exposure to a bloodborne pathogen by a "percutaneous" exposure route?
    a. drawing blood without using a needle safety device
    b. handling specimens with ungloved, chapped hands
    c. licking your fingers while turning lab manual pages
    d. rubbing your eyes while processing blood specimens

66. In which instance could an electrical shock to a patient most likely occur?
    a. collecting a blood specimen during a bad electrical storm
    b. performing phlebotomy while the patient is on the phone
    c. standing on a wet floor while drawing a blood specimen
    d. touching some electrical equipment during a blood draw

67. The "Right to Know" Law primarily deals with:
   a. electrical safety issues.
   b. exposure to pathogens.
   c. hazard communication.
   d. labeling of specimens.

68. The *best* course of action when entering an isolation room is:
   a. ask the patient's nurse what to do.
   b. do whatever you did the last time.
   c. follow the posted precautions.
   d. put on gloves and a respirator.

69. Which one of the following diseases involves a bloodborne pathogen?
   a. diphtheria
   b. influenza
   c. malaria
   d. rubella

70. The degree to which a microorganism is capable of causing disease is the definition of:
   a. resistance.
   b. susceptibility.
   c. viability.
   d. virulence.

71. A material or substance harmful to health is the definition of a:
   a. biohazard.
   b. contaminant.
   c. pathogen.
   d. toxic agent.

72. What is the proper order for putting on protective clothing?
   a. gloves first, then gown, mask last
   b. gown first, then gloves, mask last
   c. gown first, then mask, gloves last
   d. mask first, then gown, gloves last

73. The blue quadrant of the NFPA diamond-shaped symbol for hazardous materials (Fig. 3-1) indicates a:
   a. fire hazard.
   b. health hazard.
   c. reactivity hazard.
   d. specific hazard.

74. These are the initials of the agency that developed a hazard labeling system that is a diamond-shaped sign containing the United Nations hazard class number and a symbol representing the hazard.
   a. CDC
   b. DOT
   c. NFPA
   d. OSHA

75. All of the following are acceptable chemical safety procedures EXCEPT:
   a. adding the acid to the water when diluting an acid.
   b. familiarizing oneself with the MSDS of a new reagent.
   c. mixing bleach solutions with other types of cleaners.
   d. reporting a faulty safety shower to a proper authority.

76. Federal law requires that hepatitis B vaccination be made available to employees assigned to duties with occupational exposure risk:
   a. after any probationary period is over.
   b. immediately or as soon as possible.
   c. within 1 month of their employment.
   d. within 10 working days of assignment.

77. What is the *first* thing a phlebotomist should do if he or she is accidentally stuck by a needle used to draw blood from a patient?
   a. check the patient's medical records for HIV test results
   b. clean the site with soap and water for at least 30 seconds
   c. go to the employee health service and get a tetanus booster
   d. leave the area so the patient does not notice the injury

78. All of the following are symptoms of shock EXCEPT:
   a. an expressionless face.
   b. increased shallow breathing.
   c. pale, cold, clammy skin.
   d. slow, strong, pulse rate.

79. The main principles involved in radiation exposure are:
   a. exposure rate, dose, and shelter.
   b. distance, time, and shielding.
   c. source, amount, and duration.
   d. strength, location, and protection.

80. Which of the following is a role of the Joint Commission?
   a. accreditation of healthcare facilities
   b. development of BBP exposure plans
   c. enforcement of safety requirements
   d. prevention of work-related injuries

81. Which of the following would be considered a nosocomial infection?
   a. a catheter site of a patient in the intensive care unit (ICU) becomes infected
   b. a child breaks out with measles on admission day
   c. a healthcare worker comes down with hepatitis B
   d. a patient is admitted with Hantavirus infection

82. Of every 100 hospitalized patients in the United States, approximately how many acquire a nosocomial infection?
   a. 2
   b. 5
   c. 15
   d. 25

83. The free availability of personal protective equipment (PPE) for employee use in the medical laboratory is mandated by the:
   a. Clinical Laboratory Improvement Amendments.
   b. *Guideline for Isolation Precautions in Hospitals.*
   c. OSHA Bloodborne Pathogens (BBP) Standard.
   d. OSHA Hazard Communication (HazCom) Standard.

84. The latest American Heart Association (AHA) recommendations for cardiopulmonary resuscitation (CPR) on adults by laypersons include all the following EXCEPT:
   a. advocating a blind finger-sweep of the mouth before initiating CPR.
   b. deleting the pulse check from layperson CPR training.
   c. public training in the use of automatic external defibrillators (AEDs).
   d. standardizing the chest compressions-to-rescue breaths ratio to 15:1.

85. The most frequently occurring laboratory-acquired infection is caused by:
   a. HAV.
   b. HBV.
   c. HCV.
   d. HIV.

86. All of the following are required parts of an exposure control plan EXCEPT:
   a. an exposure determination.
   b. communication of hazards.
   c. isolation procedure policies.
   d. methods of implementation.

87. Which class of fire occurs with combustible metals?
   a. Class A
   b. Class B
   c. Class C
   d. Class D

88. What precautions are to be used for a patient who has an enteric pathogen?
   a. airborne
   b. contact
   c. droplet
   d. standard

89. All of the following are examples of possible "parenteral" means of transmission EXCEPT:
    a. drinking water from a glass that is contaminated.
    b. getting stuck by a needle used on an AIDS patient.
    c. rubbing the eyes without first washing the hands.
    d. touching infectious material with chapped hands.

90. All of the following affect a person's general susceptibility to infection EXCEPT:
    a. age.
    b. gender.
    c. health.
    d. immune status.

91. An example of vector infection transmission is contracting:
    a. HIV from a tainted blood transfusion.
    b. hepatitis B from a contaminated countertop.
    c. the plague from the bite of a rodent flea.
    d. tuberculosis after inhaling droplet nuclei.

92. A patient might be placed in protective isolation if he or she has:
    a. chickenpox.
    b. hepatitis C.
    c. severe burns.
    d. tuberculosis.

93. What is the correct order for removing protective clothing?
    a. gloves, mask, gown
    b. gown, gloves, mask
    c. gown, mask, gloves
    d. mask, gown, gloves

94. The substance abbreviated as HBsAg when detected in a patient's serum confirms:
    a. hepatitis B immunity.
    b. hepatitis B infection.
    c. hepatitis B susceptibility.
    d. hepatitis B vaccination.

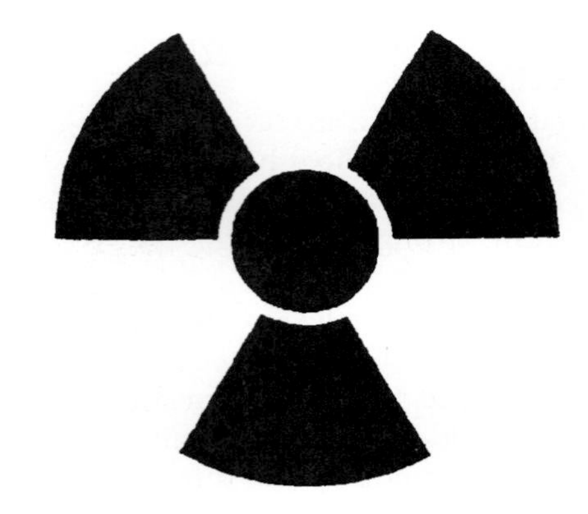

FIGURE 3-2 Radiation hazard symbol.

95. A radiation hazard symbol (Fig. 3-2) on a patient's door signifies a patient who:
    a. has been sent to the radiology department.
    b. has had x-rays taken in the past few days.
    c. is being treated with radioactive isotopes.
    d. is scheduled for a radiology procedure.

96. Which of the following is an example of a work practice control that reduces risk of exposure to bloodborne pathogens?
    a. ordering self-sheathing needles
    b. reading the exposure control plan
    c. receiving an HBV vaccination
    d. Wearing gloves to draw blood

97. These are the initials of the organization that introduced universal precautions, the precursor to standard precautions.
    a. CAP
    b. CDC
    c. NIOSH
    d. OSHA

98. Healthcare workers are considered immune to a disease if they:
    a. eat right and get enough rest and exercise.
    b. have a normal number of white blood cells.
    c. have had the disease and recovered.
    d. received gamma globulin in the past year.

99. What is the best way to extinguish a flammable liquid fire?
a. douse it with large amounts of water
b. smother it with a special fire blanket
c. spray it with a Class A extinguisher
d. spray it with a Class B extinguisher

100. These are the initials of the federal agency that instituted and enforces regulations requiring the labeling of hazardous materials.
a. CDC
b. EPA
c. NFPA
d. OSHA

101. Which mode of infection transmission involves transfer of an infective microbe to the mucous membranes of a susceptible individual by means of a cough or sneeze?
a. contact
b. droplet
c. fomite
d. vehicle

102. All of the following are links (components) in the chain of infection EXCEPT:
a. exit pathway.
b. reservoir.
c. surveillance.
d. susceptible host.

103. This is the abbreviation for the organization that is specifically charged with the investigation and control of disease.
a. CDC
b. HICPAC
c. NIOSH
d. OSHA

104. What is the first action to take to help a patient in shock?
a. call for assistance
b. control any bleeding
c. keep the patient lying down
d. maintain an open airway

105. All of the following are healthy ways to deal with stress EXCEPT:
a. exercise regularly.
b. learn how to relax.
c. make a major life change.
d. take time to plan your day.

106. A nosocomial infection is one that is:
a. caught by a healthcare worker.
b. communicable in nature.
c. healthcare facility acquired.
d. present without symptoms.

107. This mode of transmission involves contaminated food, water, drugs, or blood transfusions.
a. airborne
b. contact
c. vector
d. vehicle

108. A phlebotomist who has just been diagnosed with strep throat should be:
a. allowed to work if no symptoms are currently being exhibited.
b. evaluated by an employee health nurse before resuming duties.
c. off work until on an antibiotic for 24 hours and symptom-free.
d. required to wear a mask when having any contact with patients.

109. The manufacturer must supply a material safety data sheet (MSDS) for:
a. distilled water.
b. laboratory coats.
c. isopropyl alcohol.
d. isotonic saline.

110. Devices required by the OSHA that remove BBP hazards from the workplace are called:
a. biohazard controls.
b. engineering controls.
c. pathogen controls.
d. work practice controls.

111. Chemical manufacturers are required to supply material safety data sheets (MSDS) for their products, if applicable, by the:
   a. Chemical Manufacturers Association Guideline.
   b. National Fire Protection Association Act.
   c. OSHA Hazard Communication Standard.
   d. United Nations Placard Recognition System.

112. What term is used to describe a type of infection that can be spread from person to person?
   a. communicable
   b. nonpathogenic
   c. nosocomial
   d. systemic

113. Which class of fire occurs with flammable liquids?
   a. Class B
   b. Class C
   c. Class D
   d. Class K

114. The first thing to do in the event of electrical shock to a coworker or patient is:
   a. call for medical assistance.
   b. keep the patient warm.
   c. shut off the electricity source.
   d. start CPR if indicated.

115. The main purpose of PPE is to:
   a. help project a professional appearance.
   b. prevent infection transmission to patients.
   c. protect street clothes from getting soiled.
   d. provide the user a barrier against infection.

116. The acronym used to remember the actions to take when using a fire extinguisher is:
   a. ACT.
   b. HELP.
   c. PASS.
   d. RACE.

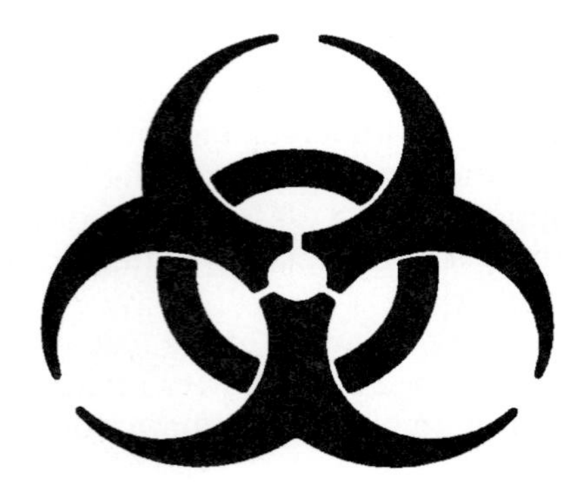

FIGURE 3-3

117. Which of the following is the *best* action to take if a coworker's clothing is on fire?
   a. have the individual roll on the floor
   b. smother the fire with a fire blanket
   c. spray it with a Class A extinguisher
   d. tear off everything that is burning

118. What type of hazard is identified by the symbol in Fig. 3-3?
   a. biohazard
   b. electrical
   c. explosive
   d. radiation

119. Which of the following bleach dilutions is recommended for cleaning contaminated specimen collection area surfaces?
   a. 1:1
   b. 1:2
   c. 1:10
   d. 1:25

120. Alcohol-based antiseptic hand cleaners can be used in place of hand washing if:
   a. gloves were worn during the prior activity.
   b. hands are first cleaned with detergent wipes.
   c. hands were washed after the prior activity.
   d. no dirt or organic matter is seen on the hands.

121. All of the following actions violate laboratory safety rules EXCEPT:
   a. chewing on a pencil while processing specimens.
   b. stashing your lunch in a lab specimen refrigerator.
   c. unplugging a centrifuge while it is still rotating.
   d. wearing open-toed shoes while working in the lab.

122. Approximately how many workplace injuries and illness are related to back injuries?
   a. 10%
   b. 20%
   c. 30%
   d. 40%

123. HBV in dried blood on work surfaces, equipment, telephones, and other objects can survive up to:
   a. 24 hours.
   b. 3 days.
   c. 7 days.
   d. 2 months.

124. The most common chronic bloodborne illness in the United States is:
   a. HAV
   b. HBV
   c. HCV
   d. HDV

125. Respirators used to enter rooms of patients with airborne diseases must be approved by this agency.
   a. CDC
   b. HICPAC
   c. NIOSH
   d. OSHA

ANSWERS AND EXPLANATIONS

1. Answer: d

   Why: OSHA stands for the Occupational Safety and Health Administration. This agency enforces the Occupational Safety and Health Act (also OSHA), a federal law that requires employers to ensure safe working conditions. The Centers for Disease Control and Prevention (CDC) is charged with the investigation and control of certain communicable diseases with epidemic potential. The Healthcare Infection Control Practices Advisory Committee (HICPAC) is a federal committee of experts who provide advice and guidance to the CDC and the Department of Health and Human Services (HHS) regarding infection control. The National Institute for Occupational Safety and Health (NIOSH), a federal agency that is part of the CDC, is responsible for conducting research and making recommendations for the prevention of work-related injury and illness.

   Review: Yes ☐ No ☐

2. Answer: a

   Why: Infection transmission requires the presence of six key components, which form the links in what is commonly referred to as the chain of infection (Fig. 3-4). The components are an infectious agent, reservoir, exit pathway, means of transmission, entry pathway, and susceptible host.

   Review: Yes ☐ No ☐

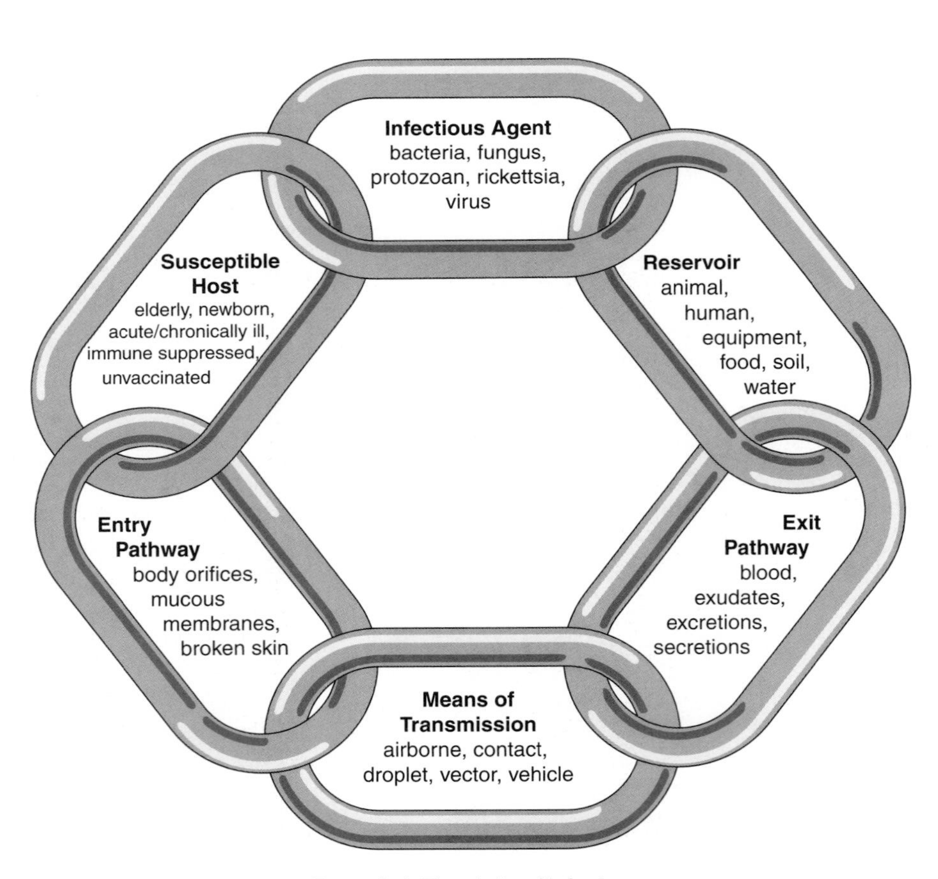

FIGURE 3-4 The chain of infection.

3. Answer: a
Why: A pathogen is a microbe that is capable of causing disease. The microbe that is responsible for an infection is referred to as the infectious or causative agent. In human infection transmission, a host is a susceptible individual or one that harbors an infectious agent. A vector is an insect, arthropod, or animal that harbors an infectious agent. A vehicle is food, water, or drugs that are contaminated with the infectious agent.
Review: Yes ☐ No ☐

4. Answer: c
Why: The term pathogenic means "causing or productive of disease." A microorganism that is capable of causing disease is said to be pathogenic. Communicable is an adjective used to describe infections that can spread from person to person. Virulence is the degree to which an organism is capable of causing disease. Systemic means pertaining to the entire body.
Review: Yes ☐ No ☐

5. Answer: d
Why: Permucosal means through or across mucous membranes, moist tissue layers that line areas of the body open to the environment such as eyes, nose, and mouth. Mucous membranes can be an entry pathway for infectious agents if aerosols or splashes land on them. Airborne exposure occurs if an infectious agent is inhaled. Non-intact skin exposure occurs through visible or invisible pre-existing breaks in the skin. Percutaneous exposure occurs when a sharp object penetrates previously intact skin.
Review: Yes ☐ No ☐

6. Answer: b
Why: Isolation procedures minimize the spread of infection by separating patients with highly transmissible infections from contact with other patients and limiting their contact with hospital personnel and visitors. Simply being a carrier of a bloodborne pathogen or having been exposed to a contagious disease does not warrant isolation procedures. Standard precautions, which encompass blood and body fluid precautions, are used in the care of all patients.
Review: Yes ☐ No ☐

7. Answer: c
Why: Microbes (a short term for microorganisms) are tiny life forms that cannot be seen with the naked eye. They include bacteria, fungi, protozoa, and viruses. Ova (gametes or eggs) are reproductive cells, and although they may be microscopic they are not microorganisms.
Review: Yes ☐ No ☐

8. Answer: c
Why: Antibiotic treatment, chemotherapy drugs, and surgical procedures can all increase a patient's susceptibility to infection. Vaccination against a particular microbe decreases the likelihood of infection with that microbe. Previous vaccination does not increase an individual's present susceptibility to other types of infection.
Review: Yes ☐ No ☐

9. Answer: b
Why: In healthcare, a susceptible host is someone with decreased ability to resist infection. A microbe responsible for an infection is called the causative or infectious agent. An exit or entry pathway is the way an infectious microbe is able, respectively, to leave or to enter a host. A reservoir is a place where an infectious microbe can survive and multiply and includes humans, animals, food, water, soil, contaminated articles, and equipment.
Review: Yes ☐ No ☐

10. Answer: a
Why: MSDS stands for material safety data sheet, a document that contains general, precautionary, and emergency information for a product with a hazardous warning on the label. The OSHA Hazard Communication (HazCom) Standard requires manufacturers to supply MSDS for their products. Employers are required to obtain the MSDS for every hazardous chemical present in the workplace and have all MSDS readily accessible to employees.
Review: Yes ☐ No ☐

11. Answer: b
Why: Transmission-based precautions are used in addition to standard precautions only for patients who are known or suspected to be infected or colonized with highly transmissible or epidemiologically significant pathogens.
Review: Yes ☐ No ☐

12. Answer: b
Why: According to transmission-based precautions, symptoms of infection with an enteric pathogen in an incontinent or diapered patient warrant contact precautions pending diagnosis. A child with a rash suggestive of rubeola requires airborne precautions. A cough, fever, and pulmonary infiltrate in a patient with HIV are suggestive of TB infection and require airborne precautions. A cough indicative of *Bordetella pertussis* requires droplet precautions.
Review: Yes ☐ No ☐

13. Answer: d
Why: Transmission of an infective agent through contaminated food, water, or drugs is called vehicle transmission. Contact transmission involves direct transmission of an infectious microbe to a susceptible host through close or intimate contact such as kissing, or indirect transmission of the microbe by personal contact with a contaminated inanimate object. Droplet transmission involves the transfer of the microbe to the mucous membranes of a susceptible host by activities such as sneezing, coughing, or talking by an infected person. Vector transmission typically involves the transfer of the microbe by an insect, arthropod, or animal.
Review: Yes ☐ No ☐

14. Answer: c
Why: An avulsion is the forceful tearing away or amputation of a body part.
Review: Yes ☐ No ☐

15. Answer: c
Why: A patient with *Mycoplasma pneumoniae* requires droplet precautions, one of three types of transmission-based precautions used for patients known or suspected to be colonized or infected with certain highly transmissible pathogens. Droplet precautions protect against microbes transmitted in droplets generated when a person talks, coughs, or sneezes, and during certain procedures such as suctioning. The other two transmission-based precautions are airborne and contact. Airborne precautions protect against microbes transmitted in droplet nuclei, the residue of evaporated droplets. Contact precautions protect against microbes transmitted by contact with a patient, or contaminated items and surfaces. Transmission-based precautions are used in addition to the standard precautions, which are used in the care of all patients.
Review: Yes ☐ No ☐

16. Answer: d
Why: Because newborns are more susceptible to infection than older children or adults, strict infection control techniques are required for those working with them. Typical nursery and neonatal ICU infection control techniques include washing the hands with an antiseptic hand cleaner and putting on a mask, gown, and gloves. Infants

sometimes have to be awakened to collect specimens. Only the equipment needed is brought into the room, not the phlebotomy tray. Povidone-iodine (example, Betadine) should not be used to clean a skin puncture site because it interferes with some tests.

Review: Yes ☐ No ☐

17. Answer: b

Why: The code word or acronym *RACE* was established by the National Fire Protection Association (NFPA) as a way to remember the order of action steps in the event of a fire. The "R" stands for *rescue* individuals in danger (Step 1). The "A" stands for sound the *alarm* (Step 2). The "C" stands for *confine* the fire by closing doors and windows (Step 3). The "E" stands for *extinguish* the fire with the nearest fire extinguisher (Step 4).

Review: Yes ☐ No ☐

18. Answer: d

Why: It is not mandatory for the source patient to submit to HIV or HBV testing. The source patient will be asked to submit to testing, and it is hoped that he or she will do so.

Review: Yes ☐ No ☐

19. Answer: c

Why: The process of infection requires the chain of infection (Fig. 3-4) to be complete. Stopping or interrupting the process by such things as wearing gloves, immunizing susceptible individuals, or instituting isolation procedures breaks the chain and prevents infection.

Review: Yes ☐ No ☐

20. Answer: d

Why: The concept that the blood and certain body fluids of all patients potentially contain bloodborne pathogens originated with the introduction of universal precautions (UP) by the CDC. This concept changed the focus of infection control from prevention of patient-to-patient transmission to prevention of patient-to-personnel transmission. Category-specific and disease-specific precautions focused on patient-to-patient transmission. BSI focused on patient-to-personnel transmission but came after UP.

Review: Yes ☐ No ☐

21. Answer: d

Why: Systemic means "pertaining to a whole body rather than one of its parts." A systemic infection infects the entire body. A communicable infection is one that is spread from person to person. A local infection is restricted to a small area of the body. A nosocomial infection is a healthcare facility–acquired infection.

Review: Yes ☐ No ☐

22. Answer: a

Why: Under transmission-based precautions, airborne isolation is required in addition to standard precautions for a patient who has pulmonary tuberculosis (TB). With airborne precautions, anyone entering the patient's room is required to wear an N95 respirator (Fig. 3-5).

Review: Yes ☐ No ☐

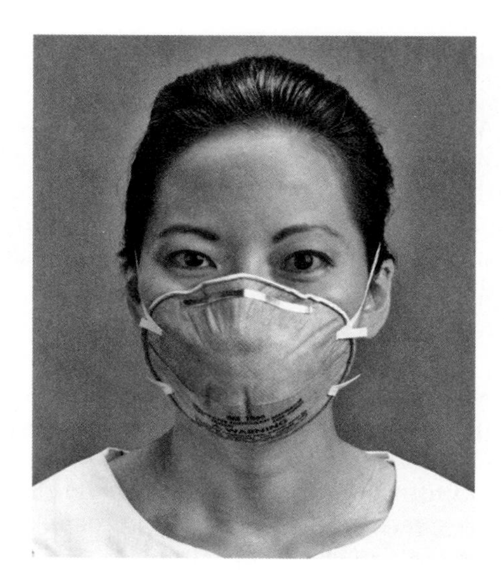

FIGURE 3-5 N95 respirator. (Courtesy 3M Occupational Health and Environmental Safety Division. St. Paul, MN.)

23. Answer: d
    Why: Exercise reduces stress by triggering the release of substances called endorphins, which create an exhilarating yet peaceful state.
    Review: Yes ☐ No ☐

24. Answer: d
    Why: Human immunodeficiency virus (HIV) is the leading cause of AIDS. Hepatitis A virus (HAV), hepatitis B virus (HBV), and hepatitis C virus (HCV) cause hepatitis A, hepatitis B, and hepatitis C, respectively.
    Review: Yes ☐ No ☐

25. Answer: b
    Why: Immunity to a particular virus normally exists when a person's blood has antibodies directed against that virus. A person who has recovered from infection with a virus has antibodies directed against it and is considered immune. A person who does not display symptoms of a virus such as hepatitis B, but whose blood contains the virus, is capable of transmitting it to others and is called a carrier. A person who is susceptible to a virus has no antibodies against it.
    Review: Yes ☐ No ☐

26. Answer: a
    Why: Control of external profuse bleeding (hemorrhage) is most effectively accomplished by applying direct pressure to the wound and elevating the affected part above the level of the heart.
    Review: Yes ☐ No ☐

27. Answer: c
    Why: An infection control program is responsible for implementing procedures designed to break the chain of infection and prevent the spread of infection in the hospital.
    Review: Yes ☐ No ☐

28. Answer: b
    Why: Microorganisms (microbes) that are capable of causing disease are called pathogens. Communicable microorganisms are pathogens that can be spread from person to person. Only some pathogenic microbes live in the soil. Normal flora (microorganisms that live on the skin) do not cause disease under normal conditions.
    Review: Yes ☐ No ☐

29. Answer: d
    Why: The microbes that cause hepatitis B, malaria, and syphilis are all bloodborne pathogens. Tuberculosis is an infectious disease caused by *Mycobacterium tuberculosis*. This organism is not normally present in the blood of infected individuals. It can be present in their respiratory secretions, however, in which case it is spread by droplets and airborne droplet nuclei.
    Review: Yes ☐ No ☐

30. Answer: d
    Why: A clean paper towel should be used to turn off the faucet after hand washing. Using the same paper towel to dry the hands and turn off the faucets can contaminate the faucet handles and the hands.
    Review: Yes ☐ No ☐

31. Answer: a
    Why: Pertussis (whooping cough) is a respiratory disease transmitted by droplets. Varicella (chickenpox) and rubeola are highly contagious and require airborne precautions. Varicella requires contact precautions in addition to airborne precautions. Scabies requires contact precautions.
    Review: Yes ☐ No ☐

32. Answer: b
    Why: Fires are classified by fuel source. Class C fires occur with electrical equipment. Class A fires involve ordinary combustible

materials, Class B fires involve flammable liquids, and Class D fires involve combustible metals. Class K fires involve cooking oils, fat, or grease.

Review: Yes ☐ No ☐

33. Answer: d
Why: Standard precautions should be followed for all patients at all times with no exceptions. When standard precautions are followed, it is not necessary to know if the patient has hepatitis B or is HIV positive. Patients in normal isolation require transmission-based precautions in addition to standard precautions. Reverse isolation requires precautions to protect the patient in addition to standard precautions.
Review: Yes ☐ No ☐

34. Answer: a
Why: Hepatitis B vaccination involves three separate injections: an initial dose, another dose 1 month later, and a final dose 6 months from the original dose.
Review: Yes ☐ No ☐

35. Answer: a
Why: Fomites are objects capable of adhering to infectious material and transmitting disease. Fomites can include telephones, computer terminals, and countertops. Hosts, as related to healthcare infection control, are individuals who harbor infectious agents. A pathogen is a microbe that is capable of causing disease. A vector is an insect, arthropod, or animal involved in the transmission of an infective microbe.
Review: Yes ☐ No ☐

36. Answer: c
Why: The OSHA HazCom Standard is known as the "Right to Know" Law because it requires all chemicals to be evaluated for health hazards, all chemicals found to be hazardous to be labeled as such, and the information communicated to employees.
Review: Yes ☐ No ☐

37. Answer: c
Why: Hepatitis means inflammation of the liver. (The word root "hepat" means *liver,* and the suffix "itis" means *inflammation.*) Hepatitis B virus (HBV) and the other hepatitis viruses target the liver, causing liver inflammation.
Review: Yes ☐ No ☐

38. Answer: a
Why: The CDC and HICPAC together developed the latest *Guideline for Isolation Precautions in Hospitals.* The guideline identifies two tiers of precautions; standard precautions to be used in the care of all patients and transmission-based precautions to be used in addition to standard precautions for patients with certain highly transmissible diseases.
Review: Yes ☐ No ☐

39. Answer: b
Why: The OSHA Bloodborne Pathogen (BBP) standard requires glove use during phlebotomy procedures to protect the phlebotomist from bloodborne pathogen contamination. Gloves do not necessarily protect the patient; in fact, they can be a source of contamination to the patient if the phlebotomist touches contaminated articles before touching the patient's arm. Gloves can also be a source of contamination to capillary puncture specimens. Rather than protecting the venipuncture site, gloves can contaminate it if the phlebotomist touches the site after it is cleaned.
Review: Yes ☐ No ☐

40. Answer: b
Why: Four components must be present for fire to occur. Three of them are the traditional

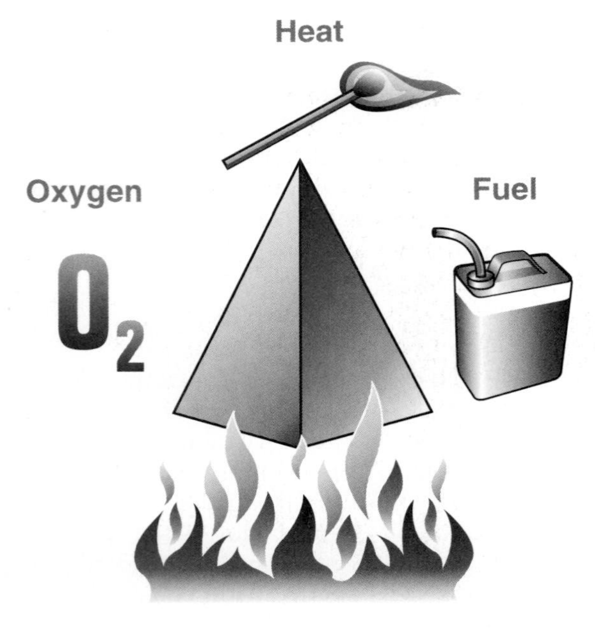

FIGURE 3-6 Fire tetrahedron.

fire triangle components of fuel (material that will burn), heat (to raise the temperature of the material to a point where it will ignite), and oxygen (to maintain combustion). The fourth component is the chemical reaction that produces the fire. Addition of the fourth component to the original fire triangle created the fire tetrahedron (Fig. 3-6).

Review: Yes ☐ No ☐

41. Answer: b

Why: An exit pathway is the way an infectious agent is able to leave a reservoir host and be transmitted to a new susceptible individual, and should be blocked, not opened. Infectious agents can exit a reservoir host in secretions from the eyes, nose or mouth; exudates from wounds; tissue specimens; blood from venipuncture and skin puncture sites; and excretions of feces, and urine. Blocking a pathogen exit pathway by protecting yourself from secretions, excretions, exudates, and other potentially infectious body substances can break the chain of infection.

Review: Yes ☐ No ☐

42. Answer: a

Why: Electrical equipment should be unplugged before servicing to avoid electrical shock. The use of extension cords should be avoided because they lead to circuit overload, incomplete connections, and potential clutter in the path of workers. Frayed electrical cords are dangerous and should be replaced rather than used. Malfunctioning equipment should be unplugged and not used until fixed.

Review: Yes ☐ No ☐

43. Answer: c

Why: Standard precautions apply to all body fluids, excretions, and secretions except sweat.

Review: Yes ☐ No ☐

44. Answer: c

Why: The ability of a microorganism to survive on contaminated articles and equipment has to do with its viability, which is the ability to survive, or live, grow, and develop.

Review: Yes ☐ No ☐

45. Answer: b

Why: Fuel, oxygen, and heat make up the fire triangle. The fourth component, the chemical reaction that produces fire, creates a fire tetrahedron (Fig. 3-6), the latest way of looking at the chemistry of fire.

Review: Yes ☐ No ☐

46. Answer: d

Why: Anyone entering the room of a patient with airborne precautions must wear an N95 respirator (Fig. 3-5), unless the precautions are for rubeola or varicella and the individual entering the room is immune.

Review: Yes ☐ No ☐

47. Answer: a
Why: Statistics compiled by the CDC have shown that accidental needlesticks are the leading cause of HIV exposures that have occurred so far among healthcare workers.
Review: Yes ☐ No ☐

48. Answer: d
Why: Approximately 5% of all hospitalized patients in the United States develop some type of nosocomial infection. The most common type of nosocomial infection developed is urinary tract infection (UTI).
Review: Yes ☐ No ☐

49. Answer: d
Why: The BBP Standard was instituted by OSHA when it was determined that healthcare employees face a serious health risk as a result of occupational exposure to bloodborne pathogens. The standard is part of Federal law, and OSHA is responsible for its enforcement.
Review: Yes ☐ No ☐

50. Answer: a
Why: Laboratory safety procedures include securing long hair away from the face; never eating, drinking, or applying makeup in the laboratory; and wearing closed-toe shoes. A laboratory coat is considered personal protective equipment and as such may become contaminated. It should be worn during procedures that require it, but it should not be worn on break, to lunch, or when leaving the lab to go home.
Review: Yes ☐ No ☐

51. Answer: b
Why: The immediate thing to do in the event of a chemical splash to the eyes is to flush them with water for 15 minutes at the nearest eyewash station (Fig. 3-7).
Review: Yes ☐ No ☐

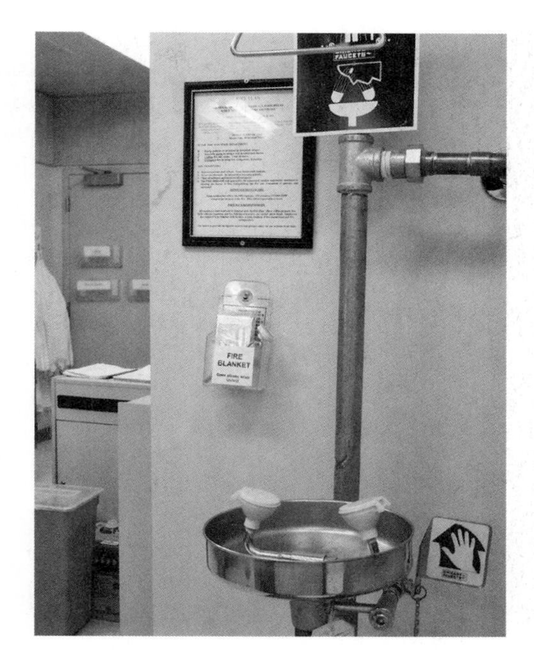

FIGURE 3-7 Eyewash station.

52. Answer: a
Why: The best way to clean up small amounts of blood is to absorb them with a paper towel or gauze pad and then clean the area with a disinfectant, being careful not to spread the blood over a wider area than the original spill. Dried spills should be moistened with disinfectant to avoid scraping, which could disperse infectious organisms into the air. Do not wipe in an outward circular motion because it can spread the contamination. Alcohol is not a disinfectant, nor is soap and water.
Review: Yes ☐ No ☐

53. Answer: c
Why: Purified protein derivative (PPD) is the antigen used in a tuberculosis (TB) test. Both PPD and TB are abbreviations used for the test, which screens for exposure to tuberculosis. Hepatitis B vaccination, measles vaccinations, and tetanus booster shots are examples of employee immunizations that prevent the spread of infection.
Review: Yes ☐ No ☐

54. Answer: c
Why: The indirect contact mode of infection transmission occurs when a susceptible individual touches contaminated inanimate objects such as bed linens. Direct contact transmission involves direct, physical transfer of an infective microbe through close or intimate contact such as touching or kissing. Droplet transmission involves the transfer of an infective microbe to the mucous membranes of a susceptible individual through sneezing, coughing, or talking. Vehicle transmission involves contaminated food, water, drugs, or blood for transfusion.
Review: Yes ☐ No ☐

55. Answer: c
Why: Diabetes mellitus is an endocrine disorder involving improper carbohydrate metabolism. It is not caused by a bloodborne pathogen and is not transmitted through blood transfusion. Cytomegalovirus, hepatitis C virus, and *Treponema pallidum,* the organism that causes syphilis, are bloodborne pathogens that can be transmitted through blood transfusion if present in the transfused blood.
Review: Yes ☐ No ☐

56. Answer: d
Why: According to the OSHA Bloodborne Pathogens Standard, gloves are to be worn when performing vascular access procedures. This means that gloves are required for phlebotomy procedures. HIV-positive patients are not normally isolated unless they have AIDS and their immune systems are severely weakened, in which case they may be placed in protective isolation. A gown may be required in certain situations but is not normally required when working with AIDS patients. It is against the law to label specimens from patients with bloodborne pathogens any differently than other specimens.
Review: Yes ☐ No ☐

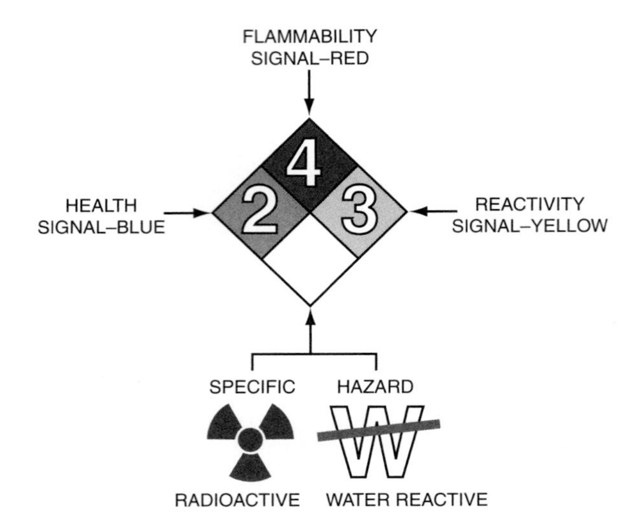

FIGURE 3-8 National Fire Protection Association 704 marking system.

57. Answer: c
Why: Figure 3-1 represents the National Fire Protection Association (NFPA) 704 marking system used to identify areas where hazardous chemicals are present. The symbol W̶ means "water reactive" and identifies material that should not come in contact with water. (See Fig. 3-8.)
Review: Yes ☐ No ☐

58. Answer: a
Why: Reverse isolation is designed to protect patients who have compromised immune systems. Neutropenic is a term used to describe a condition in which there is an abnormally low number of white blood cells (neutrophils). A patient with a low white blood cell count has increased susceptibility to infection and may be placed in a type of protective or reverse isolation called neutropenic isolation. Persons with severe burns may be put in reverse isolation because the burns make them susceptible to infection, but it is not called neutropenic isolation.
Review: Yes ☐ No ☐

59. Answer: d
Why: To prevent contamination of other articles in the phlebotomist's tray or other workers who may handle it, a tube that has blood on it should be wiped with disinfectant and placed in a biohazard bag before being placed in the tray.
Review: Yes ☐ No ☐

60. Answer: c
Why: If a laboratory or patient care activity requires a healthcare worker to wear goggles to prevent exposure from sprays or splashes, a mask must also be worn to prevent mucous membrane exposure of the nose and mouth.
Review: Yes ☐ No ☐

61. Answer: a
Why: A positive PPD test means that an individual has been exposed to tuberculosis (TB) and developed antibodies against it. It does not necessarily mean that the individual has TB. An employee with a positive PPD test result would not have restrictions on working if the results of chest x-rays to detect signs of TB were negative. An employee with pinkeye (acute conjunctivitis), German measles, or mononucleosis could spread the infection to others and would have work restrictions.
Review: Yes ☐ No ☐

62. Answer: d
Why: Five classes of fire are recognized by the NFPA. Fires are classified by fuel source. Class C fires occur with electrical equipment. Class A fires involve ordinary combustible materials. Class B fires involve flammable liquids. Class D fires involve combustible metals. Class K fires (the newest class) occur with cooking oils, grease, or fat.
Review: Yes ☐ No ☐

63. Answer: d
Why: Nosocomial infections can result from contact with infected personnel, other patients, visitors, or equipment. Studies have shown that the best way to prevent transmission of pathogenic microorganisms is proper hand hygiene, which includes the frequent use of antiseptic hand cleaners or hand washing, depending on the degree of contamination. Following isolation procedures and being up to date on immunizations are important in preventing specific infections. Wearing gloves when required plays a role in infection control, but proper hand hygiene measures are still required after glove removal.
Review: Yes ☐ No ☐

64. Answer: b
Why: Also called "protective" isolation, reverse isolation is a special kind of isolation that is used for patients who are highly susceptible to infections. Examples of patients requiring protective isolation are patients with compromised immune systems such as neutropenic patients (those with abnormally low white blood cell counts), severely burned patients, and patients with compromised immune systems, such as patients with AIDS.
Review: Yes ☐ No ☐

65. Answer: a
Why: Percutaneous means "through the skin." Percutaneous exposure routes involve direct inoculation of infectious material through previously intact skin, such as occurs with accidental needlesticks and injuries from other sharp objects. Drawing blood without using a needle safety device increases the risk of an accidental needlestick. The exposure route involved when handling blood specimens with ungloved, badly chapped hands is non-intact skin contact. Licking your fingers before turning pages of a lab manual could lead to ingestion of infectious material. Rubbing your eyes during specimen processing activities could lead to mucous membrane contact with infectious material, or permucosal route of exposure.
Review: Yes ☐ No ☐

66. Answer: d
Why: Touching electrical equipment while drawing a patient's blood could conceivably cause a short to travel through the needle and shock the patient. Drawing a patient's blood when he or she is talking on the phone, during an electrical storm, or while you are standing on a wet floor will not cause electrical shock to the patient.
Review: Yes ☐ No ☐

67. Answer: c
Why: The OSHA HazCom Standard, which is called the "Right to Know Law," requires manufacturers of hazardous materials to provide MSDS for their products. An MSDS contains general, precautionary, and emergency information about the product.
Review: Yes ☐ No ☐

68. Answer: c
Why: Because different types of isolation require the use of different types of personal protective equipment, the *best* thing to do before entering an isolation room is to follow the directions on the precaution sign on the door. Precautions needed are usually indicated on the sign, or you may be directed to check with the patient's nurse before entering the room. You must check the sign even if you have entered that room before, because precautions may have changed.
Review: Yes ☐ No ☐

69. Answer: c
Why: Bloodborne pathogen is a term applied to any infectious microorganism present in blood and other body fluids and tissues. It most commonly refers to HBV and HIV but also includes the organisms that cause syphilis, malaria, relapsing fever, and Creutzfeldt-Jakob disease. The microorganisms that cause diphtheria, influenza, and rubella are not found in the blood.
Review: Yes ☐ No ☐

70. Answer: d
Why: The virulence of a microorganism is the degree to which it is capable of causing disease. Resistance and susceptibility have to do with the immune system of the host and are affected by such things as age and health. Viability is the ability of the microorganism to survive on a source.
Review: Yes ☐ No ☐

71. Answer: a
Why: Biohazard is defined as any material or substance that is harmful to health. Federal regulations require any material that is a biohazard to be marked with a special biohazard symbol (Fig. 3-9).
Review: Yes ☐ No ☐

72. Answer: c
Why: When putting on protective clothing, the phlebotomist puts on the gown first, being careful to touch only the inside surface. The mask is put on next. Gloves are applied last and pulled over the cuffs of the gown.
Review: Yes ☐ No ☐

73. Answer: b
Why: In the NFPA hazardous materials rating system (Fig. 3-8), health hazards are indicated in the blue quadrant on the left. The upper red quadrant indicates fire hazards.

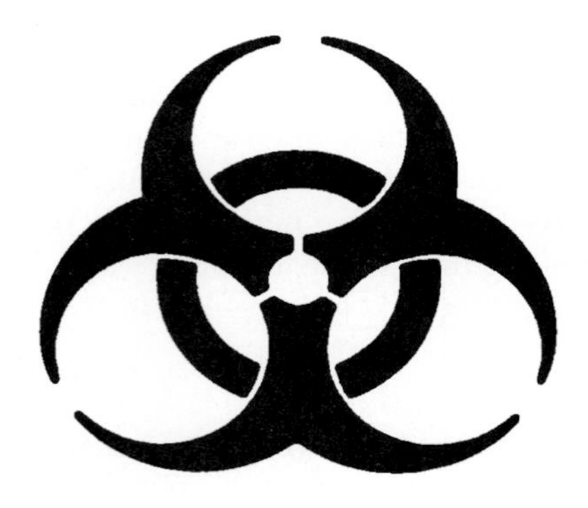

FIGURE 3-9 Biohazard symbol.

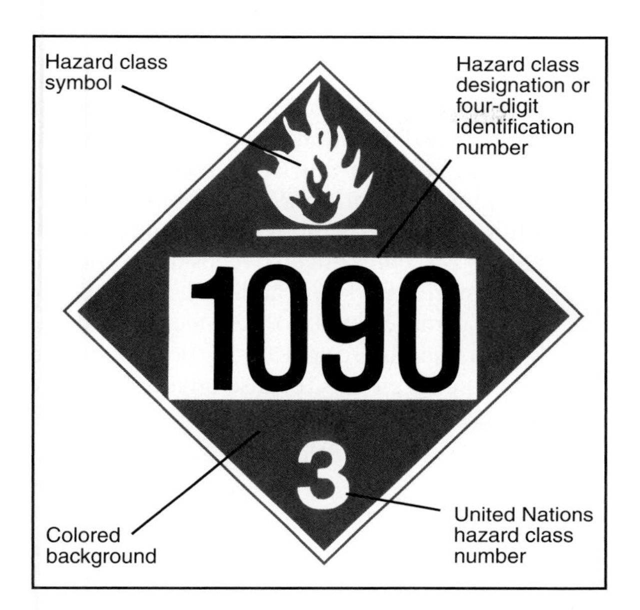

FIGURE 3-10 Example of DOT hazardous material labels (flammable, poison, corrosive, etc.). (From *Jones SA, Weigel A, White RD, McSwain NE, Breiter M, eds. Advanced Emergency Care for Paramedics Practice (1992). Philadelphia: JB Lippincott.*

Stability or reactivity hazards are indicated in the yellow quadrant on the right, and other specific hazards are indicated in the white quadrant on the bottom.

Review: Yes ☐ No ☐

74. Answer: b
Why: The Department of Transportation (DOT) labeling system (Fig 3-10) uses a diamond-shaped warning sign incorporating the United Nations hazard class number and symbol as well as a four-digit identification number. This symbol should not be confused with the NFPA diamond-shaped sign divided into four quadrants used to signify specific hazards.
Review: Yes ☐ No ☐

75. Answer: c
Why: Bleach or bleach solutions should never be mixed with other cleaners because doing so can release dangerous gases.
Review: Yes ☐ No ☐

76. Answer: d
Why: OSHA regulations require employers to offer HBV vaccination free of charge to employees within 10 days of their assignment to duties with risk of exposure.
Review: Yes ☐ No ☐

77. Answer: b
Why: If an accidental needlestick occurs, it is very important to decontaminate the site immediately. The exposure should then be reported to the supervisor and an incident report filled out. The phlebotomist should also report to the employee health department for medical evaluation and possible treatment. Checking the patient's medical record cannot be done because it would violate the Health Insurance Portability and Accountability Act (HIPAA) confidentiality regulations.
Review: Yes ☐ No ☐

78. Answer: d
Why: The symptoms of shock are an expressionless face and staring eyes; increased shallow breathing; pale, cold, clammy skin; and a rapid, weak pulse, not a slow, strong pulse.
Review: Yes ☐ No ☐

79. Answer: b
Why: Distance, shielding, and time are the principles involved in radiation exposure. This means that the amount of radiation you are exposed to depends on how far you are from the source of radioactivity, what protection you have from it, and how long you are exposed to it.
Review: Yes ☐ No ☐

80. Answer: a
Why: The Joint Commission (formerly JCAHO, the Joint Commission on Accreditation of Healthcare Organizations) accredits healthcare facilities. Development of BBP exposure plans is a healthcare facility obligation. OSHA enforces safety

requirements. The National Institute for Occupational Safety and Health (NIOSH) conducts research and makes recommendations for the prevention of work-related disease and injury.

Review: Yes ☐ No ☐

81. Answer: a
Why: A nosocomial infection is an infection that is acquired by a patient after admission to a healthcare facility. Consequently, a catheter site that becomes infected while a patient is in the ICU is a nosocomial infection. Because the incubation period for measles is longer than 1 day, the patient with measles acquired the infection before being admitted to the hospital. Infection of a healthcare worker is not considered a nosocomial infection. The patient admitted with Hantavirus obviously acquired the virus before admission.
Review: Yes ☐ No ☐

82. Answer: b
Why: Statistics show that approximately 5% (5 of 100) of hospitalized patients in the United States are exposed to and contract some type of infection while they are in the hospital. A healthcare facility-acquired infection is called a nosocomial infection.
Review: Yes ☐ No ☐

83. Answer: c
Why: Availability of PPE for use in the laboratory is mandated by the BBP Standard to minimize occupational exposure to HBV, HIV, and other bloodborne pathogens. CLIA '88 is concerned with laboratory testing. The CDC and Hospital Infection Control Practices Advisory Committee (HICPAC) *Guideline for Isolation Precautions in Hospitals* describes what PPE to use for the different categories of precautions but has no authority to regulate availability of PPE. The OSHA HazCom Standard deals with communicating hazards to employees.
Review: Yes ☐ No ☐

84. Answer: a
Why: The latest American Heart Association (AHA) recommendations for CPR no longer recommend a blind finger-sweep of the mouth before starting CPR. In fact, they now recommend that CPR on an unconscious adult be started without conducting abdominal thrusts, blind finger-sweeps of the mouth, or a pulse check. In addition, the ratio of chest compressions to rescue breaths has been standardized to 15:1 for both one- and two-rescuer CPR. AHA also advocates public access to and training in the use of AEDs.
Review: Yes ☐ No ☐

85. Answer: b
Why: According to OSHA, thousands of healthcare workers contract hepatitis B (HBV) every year, and approximately 200 die as a result. This makes HBV the most frequently occurring laboratory-associated infection and a major infectious health hazard. Hepatitis A virus (HAV), hepatitis C Virus (HCV), and human immunodeficiency virus (HIV) are also hazards to healthcare workers, but they do not occur as frequently as HBV.
Review: Yes ☐ No ☐

86. Answer: c
Why: To comply with OSHA standards, an exposure control plan must contain an exposure determination, communication of hazards, and methods of implementation. Isolation guidelines are not a required part of an exposure control plan.
Review: Yes ☐ No ☐

87. Answer: d
Why: Class D fires occur with combustible or reactive metals such as sodium, potassium, magnesium, and lithium. Class A fires occur with ordinary combustible materials. Class B fires occur with flammable liquids, and Class C fires occur with electrical equipment.
Review: Yes ☐ No ☐

88. Answer: b
Why: The word "enteric" is defined as pertaining to the small intestine. The route of exposure for enteric pathogens is ingestion. According to guidelines for transmission-based precautions, contact precautions should be followed in addition to standard precautions for patients with enteric pathogens.
Review: Yes ☐ No ☐

89. Answer: a
Why: The word "parenteral" means *other than the digestive tract.* Therefore, something that is *not* parenteral involves the digestive tract. Drinking water involves the digestive tract and is therefore *not* parenteral. The other choices *are* examples of parenteral transmission.
Review: Yes ☐ No ☐

90. Answer: b
Why: Gender does not play a role in a person's general susceptibility to infection. Age, health, and immune status do. Gender may, however, play a role in the site of infection because of differences in male and female anatomy.
Review: Yes ☐ No ☐

91. Answer: c
Why: Vector transmission involves transfer of the microbe by an insect, arthropod, or animal; for example, the bite of a rodent flea. HIV acquired from a blood transfusion is vehicle transmission. Contracting hepatitis B infection from a contaminated countertop is indirect contact transmission involving a fomite. Contracting tuberculosis from droplet nuclei is airborne transmission.
Review: Yes ☐ No ☐

92. Answer: c
Why: Protective, or reverse, isolation is used for patients who are highly susceptible to infections, as in the case with a severely burned patient. Hepatitis C requires standard precautions. Chickenpox and tuberculosis require airborne precautions in addition to standard precautions.
Review: Yes ☐ No ☐

93. Answer: a
Why: Protective clothing is removed in the opposite order that it is put on. For phlebotomy procedures, the gloves are considered the most contaminated article and are removed first. They are removed by grasping one glove at the wrist and pulling it inside-out off the hand and holding it in the gloved hand. The second glove is removed by slipping several fingers under it at the wrist and pulling it inside-out over the first glove, which ends up inside of it. The mask is removed next, by touching only the strings. The gown is removed last by sliding one's arms out of the sleeves, holding the gown away from the body, and folding it with the outside (contaminated side) in.
Review: Yes ☐ No ☐

94. Answer: b
Why: HBV infection is indicated by the presence of hepatitis B surface antigen (HBsAg) in the patient's serum. HBV immunity and proof of successful vaccination are both indicated by a certain titer (level) of hepatitis B antibody (HBsAb) in the patient's serum. HBV susceptibility is indicated by the absence of hepatitis antibody or an insufficient level of antibody to confer immunity.
Review: Yes ☐ No ☐

95. Answer: c
Why: A radiation hazard sign on a patient's door means the patient has been injected with radioactive dyes or has radioactive implants. Although they are inside the patient, these radioactive isotopes can be hazardous to the fetus of a pregnant healthcare worker. In addition, a blood specimen collected at this time may be radioactive.
Review: Yes ☐ No ☐

96. Answer: d
Why: Work practice controls are routines that alter the manner in which a task is performed to reduce likelihood of exposure to bloodborne pathogens (BBPs). Wearing gloves to draw blood reduces the chance of exposure to BBPs. Ordering self-sheathing needles, reading the exposure control plan, and receiving an HBV vaccination all are important in reducing the risk of exposure to BBPs but do not in themselves alter the actual performance of a task and are not considered work practice controls.
Review: Yes ☐ No ☐

97. Answer: b
Why: The CDC introduced the concept of universal precautions because it is not always possible to know if a patient is infected with a bloodborne pathogen.
Review: Yes ☐ No ☐

98. Answer: c
Why: Immunity to a particular disease is conferred by having had the disease and therefore developing antibodies against the disease-causing organism, or by vaccination against the particular organism. Eating right, getting enough rest, and exercising all are important to staying healthy and reducing susceptibility to disease but will not make an individual immune to a disease. A normal white blood cell count is necessary to fight infection, but it is not an indication of immunity. A shot of gamma globulin or immune globulin confers temporary immunity.
Review: Yes ☐ No ☐

99. Answer: d
Why: The Class B fire extinguisher was designed to put out flammable liquid fires. A flammable liquid or vapor fire requires blocking the source of oxygen or smothering the fuel to extinguish the fire. A Class B extinguisher uses dry chemicals to smother the fire and is intended for use on flammable liquid fires.
Review: Yes ☐ No ☐

100. Answer: d
Why: OSHA instituted and enforces the HazCom Standard. This federal law requires the labeling of hazardous materials. In addition, labeling must comply with requirements set by the Manufacturers Chemical Association (MCA).
Review: Yes ☐ No ☐

101. Answer: b
Why: Droplet contact transmission involves the transfer of infective microbes to the mucous membranes of the mouth, nose, or eyes of a susceptible individual by the sneezing, coughing, or talking by an infected person. The common cold is an example of infection that can be transmitted by droplets through coughing or sneezing.
Review: Yes ☐ No ☐

102. Answer: c
Why: An exit pathway, a reservoir where the organism can survive, and a susceptible host are all "links" in the chain of infection (Fig. 3-4). Surveillance is a means of monitoring and preventing infection or breaking the chain of infection.
Review: Yes ☐ No ☐

103. Answer: a
Why: The Centers for Disease Control and Prevention (CDC) is a division of the U.S. Public Health Service that is charged with the investigation and control of various diseases, especially those that are communicable and have epidemic potential.
Review: Yes ☐ No ☐

104. Answer: d
Why: An immediate and proper first aid response to shock is important and includes the following, in order: maintain an open

airway, call for assistance, keep the patient lying down with the head lower than the rest of the body, attempt to control bleeding or other cause of shock if known, and keep the patient warm until help arrives.

Review: Yes ☐ No ☐

105. Answer: c

Why: Healthy ways to deal with stress include exercising regularly, learning how to relax, and planning your day. Making a major life change can be a source of stress.

Review: Yes ☐ No ☐

106. Answer: c

Why: Approximately 5% of patients in the United States contract (acquire) some sort of infection after admission to a healthcare facility. Such infections are called nosocomial infections. An infection caught by a healthcare worker would not be considered a nosocomial infection, but it could become a source of nosocomial infection in patients. A nosocomial infection can be, but is not normally, a communicable infection. Nosocomial infections are not normally without symptoms.

Review: Yes ☐ No ☐

107. Answer: d

Why: Vehicle transmission involves the transmission of an infective microbe through contaminated food, water, drugs, or blood products. *Shigella* infection from contaminated water and hepatitis infection from blood products are examples of vehicle transmission. Airborne infection involves droplet nuclei. Contact transmission involves close or intimate contact with an infectious patient or articles contaminated by the patient. Vector transmission involves the transfer of an infectious microbe by an insect, arthropod, or animal.

Review: Yes ☐ No ☐

108. Answer: c

Why: A phlebotomist diagnosed with strep throat is not allowed to work until he or she has taken antibiotics for a minimum of 24 hours and is not exhibiting symptoms. Once the phlebotomist is allowed to return to work, a mask is not necessary and neither is an evaluation by infection control personnel.

Review: Yes ☐ No ☐

109. Answer: c

Why: Any product that has a hazardous warning on the label must have an MSDS supplied by the manufacturer. Isopropyl alcohol has a hazardous warning on the label and requires an MSDS. Laboratory coats, saline, and most medications do not have hazard warnings and do not require an MSDS.

Review: Yes ☐ No ☐

110. Answer: b

Why: The Bloodborne Pathogen Standard requires the use of engineering controls to reduce the risk of bloodborne pathogen (BBP) exposure. OSHA defines engineering controls as items or devices that isolate or remove a BBP hazard from the workplace. Examples of engineering controls include sharps containers and shelf-sheathing needles.

Review: Yes ☐ No ☐

111. Answer: c

Why: The OSHA HazCom Standard requires chemical manufacturers to supply an MSDS for any product with a hazardous warning on the label. An MSDS contains general information as well as precautionary and emergency information for the product.

Review: Yes ☐ No ☐

112. Answer: a

Why: An infection or disease that can spread from person to person is called a communicable infection. A nonpathogenic microorganism is not capable of causing disease or

infection. A nosocomial infection is a healthcare facility-acquired infection. Systemic is a term used to describe an infection that infects the entire body.
Review: Yes ☐ No ☐

113. Answer: a
Why: Class B fires occur with flammable liquids and vapors such as paint, oil, grease, or gasoline. Class C fires occur with electrical equipment, Class D fires occur with combustible or reactive metals, and Class K fires occur with cooking oils, grease, or fat.
Review: Yes ☐ No ☐

114. Answer: c
Why: The first thing to do when someone is the victim of electrical shock is shut off the source of electricity. (A typical first reaction is to try to remove the person from the source of the electricity, but that can result in shock to the rescuer if the source of electricity is still there). Other actions to take after the source of electricity is shut off are to call for medical assistance, start CPR if indicated, and keep the patient warm.
Review: Yes ☐ No ☐

115. Answer: d
Why: Personal protective equipment (PPE) includes all items worn to provide a barrier against infection and other hazards in situations when exposure to hazardous agents is likely. PPE includes gloves, gowns, lab coats, aprons, face shields, masks, and resuscitation mouthpieces that minimize the risk of BBP infection. OSHA requires PPE in situations where there is potential exposure to bloodborne pathogens.
Review: Yes ☐ No ☐

116. Answer: c
Why: The acronym PASS provides an easy way to remember the actions to take when using a fire extinguisher. The "P" stands for "Pull the Pin"; the "A" stands for "Aim Nozzle"; the first "S" stands for "Squeeze the Trigger"; and the second "S" stands for "Sweep Nozzle."
Review: Yes ☐ No ☐

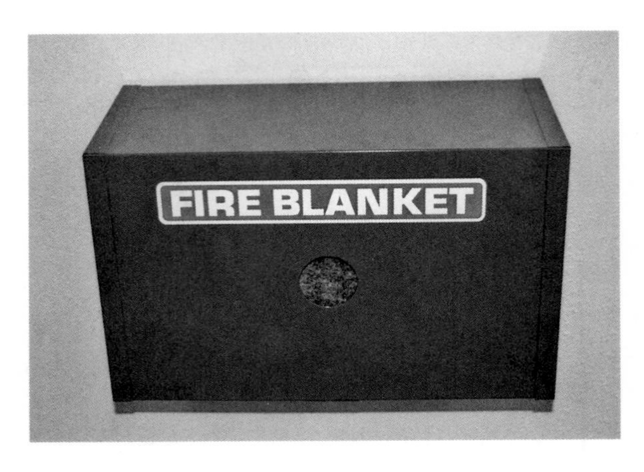

FIGURE 3-11 Fire blanket storage box.

117. Answer: b
Why: The best way to extinguish a fire in a coworker's clothing is to smother the fire by wrapping the person in a fire blanket (Fig. 3-11). Although it could be an option if no fire blanket were available, rolling on the floor is not the best option because it could spread the fire. Spraying the person with a fire extinguisher could injure him or her. Trying to take off a coworker's burning clothes could spread the fire to you or surrounding areas and could even result in your actions being misinterpreted as assault or harassment.
Review: Yes ☐ No ☐

118. Answer: a
Why: The symbol in Fig. 3-3 is a biohazard symbol, which identifies something that is hazardous to health.
Review: Yes ☐ No ☐

119. Answer: c
Why: OSHA requires surfaces in specimen collection and processing areas to be decontaminated at the end of each shift

and whenever surfaces are visibly contaminated by cleaning them with a 1:10 bleach solution or other disinfectant approved by the Environmental Protection Agency (EPA). Bleach solutions should be prepared daily.

Review: Yes ☐ No ☐

120. Answer: d

Why: CDC and Hospital Infection Control Practices Advisory Committee (HICPAC) infection control recommendations allow the use of alcohol-based antiseptic hand cleaners such as foams, gels, and lotions in place of hand washing if there is no visible dirt or organic material such as blood or other body substances on the hands. Hands must be cleaned even if gloves are worn because gloves can have defects that allow contaminants to leak through them. Cleaning with detergent-containing wipes followed by the use of an alcohol-based cleaner is recommended if hands are heavily contaminated and hand washing facilities are not available. Hand-washing after a prior activity has no bearing on how hands should be decontaminated for a current activity.

Review: Yes ☐ No ☐

121. Answer: c

Why: Unplugging a centrifuge while it is still rotating is not normal procedure but may be necessary in the event of an electrical fire, fluid spill, or malfunction connected with it. Chewing on pencils or pens and putting your lunch in a reagent or specimen refrigerator risks exposure to toxic or infectious substances. Open-toed shoes leave the wearer vulnerable to spills of hazardous or infectious substances or sharps injury from broken glass and other sharp objects.

Review: Yes ☐ No ☐

122. Answer: b

Why: It has been estimated that approximately 20% of all workplace illnesses involve back injuries. Healthcare workers are at risk of back injuries from work they are required to do (such as lift and move patients) and the stressful environment often associated with healthcare.

Review: Yes ☐ No ☐

123. Answer: c

Why: Studies have shown that hepatitis B virus (HBV) can survive up to a week in dried blood on work surfaces, equipment, telephones, and other objects.

Review: Yes ☐ No ☐

124. Answer: c

Why: According to the CDC, hepatitis C (HCV infection) has become the most widespread chronic bloodborne illness in the United States. Infection primarily occurs after large or multiple exposures. HCV symptoms are similar to those of HBV infection, although only 25% to 30% of infections even display symptoms. No vaccine is currently available.

Review: Yes ☐ No ☐

125. Answer: c

Why: NIOSH conducts research and makes recommendations for the prevention of work-related injury and illness. CDC and HICPAC transmission-based precautions recommend the wearing of properly fitting, NIOSH-approved N95 respirators when entering rooms of patients with airborne infections. Manufacturers apply to NIOSH for certificates of approval for their respirators. NIOSH-approved respirators are marked with the manufacturer's name, the part number (PN), the protection provided by the filter (e.g., N95), and "NIOSH."

Review: Yes ☐ No ☐

MEDICAL TERMINOLOGY

CHAPTER 4

study tip

Questions in this chapter test the ability to identify word elements and determine the general meaning of medical terms. Questions also test knowledge of pronunciation guidelines, unique plural endings, and abbreviations.

overview

Medical terminology is a special vocabulary of scientific and technical terms used in the healthcare professions. Knowledge of medical terminology is necessary for healthcare workers to speak and write effectively and precisely. Medical terms typically contain two or more basic word elements that are primarily derived from Greek and Latin words. These word elements are word roots, prefixes, suffixes, and combining forms.

REVIEW QUESTIONS

Choose the BEST answer.

1. A suffix is an element of a word that:
   a. establishes its basic meaning.
   b. follows the root of the word.
   c. makes pronunciation easier.
   d. precedes the root of the word.

2. The meaning of a medical term is usually determined by identifying the:
   a. combining form first, suffix next, and prefix last.
   b. prefix first, word root next, and suffix last.
   c. suffix first, prefix next, and word root last.
   d. word root first, suffix next, and prefix last.

3. What word is used to describe the breakdown of red blood cells?
   a. erythema
   b. erythrocytosis
   c. hemostasis
   d. hemolysis

4. The balanced or "steady state" of the body is called:
   a. hematology.
   b. homeostasis.
   c. hemopoiesis.
   d. hemostasis.

5. The combining form *erythro* means:
   a. cell.
   b. earthlike.
   c. oxygen.
   d. red.

6. The singular form of atria is:
   a. atris.
   b. atrium.
   c. atrion.
   d. atrius.

7. The plural form of lumen is:
   a. lumena.
   b. lumeni.
   c. lumina.
   d. lumini.

8. What word means "large cell"?
   a. acromegaly
   b. cystocele
   c. macrocyte
   d. myelocyte

9. What word means "controlling blood flow"?
   a. hemolysis
   b. hemostasis
   c. homeostasis
   d. venostasis

10. In which of the following pairs of letters is each letter pronounced separately?
    a. "ae" as in vena cavae
    b. "ch" as in chloride
    c. "pn" as in dyspnea
    d. "ps" in psychology

11. The "e" at the end is pronounced separately in:
    a. centriole.
    b. clavicle.
    c. supine.
    d. syncope.

12. Which of the following is a suffix?
    a. an
    b. neo
    c. osis
    d. ren

13. In the term "bicuspid," bi- is a:
    a. combining form.
    b. prefix.
    c. suffix.
    d. word root.

14. The "c" has the sound of "s" in the term:
    a. brachial.
    b. cirrhosis.
    c. glycolysis.
    d. pancreas.

15. Which of the following is the abbreviation for a type of cell?
    a. CMV
    b. ESR
    c. RBC
    d. TSH

16. "Myalgia" means:
    a. bone condition.
    b. muscle pain.
    c. nerve sheath.
    d. small algae.

17. Which of the following word roots means "vessel"?
    a. arteri
    b. bronch
    c. vas
    d. ven

18. This prefix means "outside."
    a. anti
    b. exo
    c. dys
    d. mal

19. Which of the following word parts means "recording" or "writing"?
    a. gram
    b. meter
    c. rrhage
    d. tomy

20. A hematologist is a specialist in the branch of medicine that deals with:
    a. blood disorders.
    b. eye problems.
    c. lung diseases.
    d. benign tumors.

21. According to the meanings of its word parts, "phlebotomy" means:
    a. cutting a vein.
    b. drawing blood.
    c. piercing a vessel.
    d. suctioning of fluid.

22. What is the meaning of the word root in the term "hyperglycemia"?
    a. condition
    b. sugar
    c. low
    d. under

23. Which of the following terms means "pertaining to the skin"?
    a. dermal
    b. dermatitis
    c. epidermis
    d. scleroderma

24. Which of the following abbreviations is on the Joint Commission "Do Not Use" list?
    a. diff
    b. IU
    c. mL
    d. QNS

25. The abbreviation for microgram (μ) may be added to the Joint Commission "Do Not Use" list in the future because it can be mistaken for:
    a. cc.
    b. mg.
    c. U.
    d. #7.

26. The Greek word root *nephr* means kidney. What is the Latin word root for kidney?
    a. cyst
    b. kid
    c. nep
    d. ren

27. The prefix "inter" means:
    a. between.
    b. entrance.
    c. inside.
    d. within.

28. Which of the following word parts are prefixes?
    a. al, lysis, pnea
    b. gastr, lip, onc
    c. ices, ina, nges
    d. iso, neo, tachy

29. Identify the combining form among the following word parts.
    a. iso
    b. hypo
    c. lipo
    d. neo

30. Which of the following abbreviations identifies a type of blood cell?
    a. diff
    b. Hct
    c. seg
    d. trig

31. The meanings of the suffix, prefix, and word root (in that order) of the medical term "anisocytosis" are:
    a. condition, unequal, cell.
    b. deficiency, blue, skin.
    c. disorder, without, cold.
    d. pertaining to, many, bladder.

32. Which of the following word parts means "blood condition"?
    a. emia
    b. ism
    c. oma
    d. osis

33. Which of the following is the word part of "cardiomyopathy" that means "disease"?
    a. cardio
    b. diom
    c. myo
    d. pathy

34. Which of the following are abbreviations for lab tests?
    a. ABGs, ASO, LDL, TIBC
    b. CAD, CML, COPD, SLE
    c. CCU, OR, PEDs, RR
    d. PP, PRN, Sx, TPR

35. Which body organ is primarily affected in a person with pulmonary disease?
    a. brain
    b. kidney
    c. lungs
    d. stomach

36. "Hepatitis" means:
    a. blood cell disorder.
    b. kidney infection.
    c. liver inflammation.
    d. muscle weakness.

37. The lab abbreviation PT stands for:
    a. partial thromboplastin.
    b. patient temperature.
    c. prothrombin time.
    d. prenatal therapy.

38. The word root of the term "oncologist" means:
    a. cancer.
    b. tumor.
    c. study of.
    d. without.

39. The word root of the medical term "thoracic" is:
    a. acic.
    b. oraci.
    c. racic.
    d. thorac.

40. Which of the following word parts means "cold"?
    a. cry
    b. cyan
    c. hypo
    d. sub

ANSWERS AND EXPLANATIONS

1. Answer: b
   Why: A suffix is a word ending. It follows a word root and either changes or adds to the meaning of the word root.
   Review: Yes ☐ No ☐

2. Answer: c
   Why: Generally the best way to determine the meaning of a medical term is to start with the meaning of the suffix, then the prefix and identify the meaning of the word root or roots last.
   Review: Yes ☐ No ☐

3. Answer: d
   Why: Hemolysis is the breakdown of red blood cells. The combining form *hemo* means blood. The suffix *-lysis* means "breakdown."
   Review: Yes ☐ No ☐

4. Answer: b
   Why: Homeostasis is the term used to describe the state of equilibrium or "steady state" that the body strives to maintain. The word part *homeo* means "the same," and *stasis* means controlling, standing, or stopping.
   Review: Yes ☐ No ☐

5. Answer: d
   Why: The combining form *erythro* means "red," as in the word "erythrocyte," which means "red blood cell."
   Review: Yes ☐ No ☐

6. Answer: b
   Why: Atrium is the singular form for atria, the name for the upper chambers of the heart.
   Review: Yes ☐ No ☐

7. Answer: c
   Why: Lumina is the plural form of lumen, the internal space of a tubular structure such as a vein or a blood collection needle.
   Review: Yes ☐ No ☐

8. Answer: c
   Why: The term "macrocyte" means "large cell," from *macro,* meaning large, and *cyte,* which means "cell."
   Review: Yes ☐ No ☐

9. Answer: b
   Why: Hemostasis is the stoppage or control of bleeding and another name for the coagulation process. The combining form *hemo* means "blood." The suffix *-stasis* means controlling, standing, or stopping.
   Review: Yes ☐ No ☐

10. Answer: c
    Why: When "pn" is in the middle of a word, it is pronounced as a "p" and an "n," as in dyspnea and apnea. Only the "e" of the "ae" at the end of vena cavae is pronounced. The "ch" in chloride is pronounced as a "k." The "p" in psychology is silent; only the "s" is pronounced.
    Review: Yes ☐ No ☐

11. Answer: d
    Why: The "e" at the end of some words such as syncope and systole is pronounced separately. The "e" at the end of centriole, clavicle, and supine is silent.
    Review: Yes ☐ No ☐

12. Answer: c
    Why: The word part *-osis* is a suffix, as in the word "necrosis," which means "the death of cells, tissues, or organs." The word part *an* is a prefix meaning "without" that is used before a word beginning with a vowel, as in anaerobic. The word part *neo* is also a prefix meaning new, as in neonatal. The word part *ren* is a word root meaning kidney, as in renal.
    Review: Yes ☐ No ☐

13. Answer: b
    Why: In the term "bicuspid," *bi-* is a prefix that means two. "Bicuspid" means having two cusps.
    Review: Yes ☐ No ☐

14. Answer: b
    Why: The letter "c" before an "e," "i,", or "y" is pronounced like an "s," as in the term "cirrhosis." The letter "c" before other vowels has the sound of a "k," as in brachial, glycolysis, and pancreas.
    Review: Yes ☐ No ☐

15. Answer: c
    Why: RBC is the abbreviation for red blood cell. CMV is the abbreviation for cytomegalovirus. ESR is the abbreviation for erythrocyte sedimentation rate. TSH is the abbreviation for thyroid stimulating hormone.
    Review: Yes ☐ No ☐

16. Answer: b
    Why: "Myalgia" means muscle pain. The word root *my* means "muscle." The suffix*algia* means pain.
    Review: Yes ☐ No ☐

17. Answer: c
    Why: The word root *vas* means vessel, as in "vascular," which means "pertaining to or composed of blood vessels." The word root *arteri* means "artery," *bronch* means "bronchus," and *ven* means "vein."
    Review: Yes ☐ No ☐

18. Answer: b
    Why: The prefix *exo-* means "outside," as in exocrine, a term used to describe a gland that secretes to the outside of the body through ducts. The prefix *anti-* means "against," *dys-* means "difficult," and *mal* means "poor."
    Review: Yes ☐ No ☐

19. Answer: a
    Why: The word part *gram* means recording or writing, as in the term "electrocardiogram," which is a recording of the electrical activity of the heart. The word part *meter* means "an instrument that measures," *rrhage* means "bursting forth," and *tomy* means "cutting or incision."
    Review: Yes ☐ No ☐

20. Answer: a
    Why: The word "hematologist" means a specialist in the study of blood disorders. The word root *hemat* means "blood." The suffix*logist* means "specialist in the study of."
    Review: Yes ☐ No ☐

21. Answer: a
    Why: The word "phleb" means vein. The term "tomy" means cutting or incision.
    Review: Yes ☐ No ☐

22. Answer: b
    Why: The word root of the term "hyperglycemia" is *glyc,* which means "sugar or glucose." "Hyperglycemia" means a condition of too much glucose (sugar) in the blood.
    Review: Yes ☐ No ☐

23. Answer: a
    Why: Dermal means "pertaining to the skin." The word root *derm* means "skin." The suffix *-al* means "pertaining to." Dermatitis is inflammation of the skin. Epidermis is the outer layer of the skin. Scleroderma is a skin disorder that causes abnormal thickening of the skin.
    Review: Yes ☐ No ☐

24. Answer: b
    Why: The abbreviation for international units (IU) is on the Joint Commission "Do Not Use" list because it can be mistaken for IV, the abbreviation for "intravenous," or it can be mistaken for the number 10. The Joint Commission wants it to be written out as "international units" instead.
    Review: Yes ☐ No ☐

25. Answer: b
Why: The abbreviation for microgram (μ) can be mistaken for the abbreviation for milligrams (mg), resulting in an overdose of a thousand times the requested dose. The Joint Commission wants it to be written "mcg" or "micrograms" instead.
Review: Yes ☐ No ☐

26. Answer: d
Why: The Latin word root for kidney is *ren,* as in "renal," which means "pertaining to the kidney."
Review: Yes ☐ No ☐

27. Answer: a
Why: The prefix *inter-* means between; as in "interstitial fluid," which is fluid between the cells.
Review: Yes ☐ No ☐

28. Answer: d
Why: The word parts *iso-*, *neo-*, and *tachy-* are prefixes. The word parts *-al, -lysis,* and *-pnea* are suffixes; *gastr, lip,* and *onc* are word roots; and *ices, ina,* and *nges* are plural endings.
Review: Yes ☐ No ☐

29. Answer: c
Why: A combining form is a word root combined with a vowel. The word part *lipo* is the word root *lip,* which means "fat," combined with the vowel "o." The word parts *iso-, hypo-,* and *neo-* are prefixes that end in "o."
Review: Yes ☐ No ☐

30. Answer: c
Why: The abbreviation "seg" stands for segmented neutrophil, a type of white blood cell. The abbreviation "diff" stands for differential, a test that determines the number and type of blood cells in a specimen. Hct is the abbreviation for hematocrit, a test that determines the percentage by volume of red blood cells in whole blood. Trig is the abbreviation for triglycerides, a type of fat, or lipid, in the blood.
Review: Yes ☐ No ☐

31. Answer: a
Why: Anisocytosis is a condition in which the red blood cells are unequal in size. The suffix is *-osis,* which means "condition." The prefix is *aniso-,* which means "unequal." The word root is *cyte,* which means "cell."
Review: Yes ☐ No ☐

32. Answer: a
Why: The suffix *-emia* means "blood condition." It is more specific than the suffix *-ism,* which simply means "condition." The suffix *-osis* means "state of." The suffix *-oma* means tumor.
Review: Yes ☐ No ☐

33. Answer: d
Why: Cardiomyopathy means "disease of the myocardium (heart muscle)." *Cardio* is a combining form that means "heart," *myo* is a combining form that means "muscle," and *-pathy* is a suffix that means "disease." *Diom* is not a recognized word part.
Review: Yes ☐ No ☐

34. Answer: a
Why: Arterial blood gases (ABGs), antistreptolysin O (ASO), low density lipoprotein (LDL), and total iron binding capacity (TIBC) are laboratory tests. CAD, CML, COPD, and SLE are abbreviations for diseases. CCU, OR, PEDs, and RT are abbreviations for hospital departments. PP, PRN, Sx, and TPR are abbreviations seen in physician's orders and notes.
Review: Yes ☐ No ☐

35. Answer: c
Why: Pulmonary disease affects the lungs. The word root *pulmon* means "lungs." The suffix *-ary* means "pertaining to."
Review: Yes ☐ No ☐

36. Answer: c
Why: Hepatitis means "liver inflammation." The word root *hepat* means "liver." The suffix *-itis* means "inflammation."
Review: Yes ☐ No ☐

37. Answer: c
Why: PT is a laboratory abbreviation for prothrombin time (or protime for short).
Review: Yes ☐ No ☐

38. Answer: b
Why: The word root of the medical term "oncologist" is *onc,* which means "tumor." An oncologist is a physician who is a specialist in the study of tumors, both malignant and benign.
Review: Yes ☐ No ☐

39. Answer: d
Why: Thoracic means "pertaining to the chest." The word root is *thorac,* which means "chest." The suffix *-ic* means "pertaining to."
Review: Yes ☐ No ☐

40. Answer: a
Why: The word part *cry* means cold. An example is cryoglobulin, an abnormal protein (globulin) that precipitates when cooled. The word part *cyan* means "blue." The word part *hypo* means "low" or "under." The word part *sub* means "below" or "under."
Review: Yes ☐ No ☐

HUMAN ANATOMY AND PHYSIOLOGY REVIEW

CHAPTER 5

study tip

Basic anatomy and physiology (A & P) questions in this chapter test the ability to describe body positions, identify areas of the body with respect to body planes, refer to areas of the body using directional terms, and locate the various body cavities and the organs and structures within them. Questions also test ability to identify and describe the cells, tissues, organs, and systems into which the body is organized, and the specific functions, structures, disorders, and diagnostic tests associated with all body systems except the circulatory system.

overview

This chapter deals with the anatomy and physiology (A & P) of the human body, including general body organization and function, anatomic terminology, and 9 of 10 body systems. Because of its special importance to phlebotomy, the 10th system (the circulatory system) is covered separately in Chapter 6. A fundamental knowledge of anatomy (structural composition) and physiology (function) of the human body is an asset to anyone working in a healthcare setting, and especially helps the phlebotomist understand the importance of the role laboratory tests play in monitoring body system functions and diagnosing disorders.

REVIEW QUESTIONS

Choose the BEST answer.

1. Human anatomy deals with:
   a. chemical reactions within the body.
   b. functioning of all the body systems.
   c. homeostatic equilibrium processes.
   d. structural composition of the body.

2. A person who is standing erect with arms at the side and eyes and palms facing forward is said to be in the:
   a. anatomic position.
   b. prone position.
   c. supine position.
   d. syncope position.

3. Pronation of the hand is the act of:
   a. extending the hand out to the side.
   b. flexing the hand at the wrist.
   c. rotating the hand so that it is vertical.
   d. turning the hand palm down.

4. Which body plane divides the body into equal portions?
   a. frontal
   b. midsagittal
   c. sagittal
   d. transverse

5. When you are facing someone in normal anatomic position, at which body plane are you looking?
   a. frontal
   b. midsagittal
   c. sagittal
   d. transverse

6. Which body plane divides the body into upper and lower portions?
   a. frontal
   b. midsagittal
   c. sagittal
   d. transverse

7. Which of the following is a true statement?
   a. a man who is supine is lying on his stomach
   b. the big toe is on the medial side of the foot
   c. the hand is at the proximal end of the arm
   d. the posterior curvature is a heelstick site

8. Which of these statements is true?
   a. the abdominal cavity is inferior to the diaphragm
   b. the elbow is on the ventral surface of the forearm
   c. the head is described as being inferior to the neck
   d. the little finger is on the medial surface of the hand

9. The term "distal" means:
   a. farthest from the point of attachment.
   b. higher or above, or toward the head.
   c. nearest the central portion of the body.
   d. to the back of the body or body part.

10. The plantar surface of the foot is the:
    a. area of the arch.
    b. heel portion.
    c. sole or bottom.
    d. top of the foot.

11. An example of a dorsal body cavity is the:
    a. abdominal cavity.
    b. pelvic cavity.
    c. spinal cavity.
    d. thoracic cavity.

12. The heart and lungs are located in this body cavity.
    a. abdominal
    b. cranial
    c. spinal
    d. thoracic

13. Which body cavities are separated by the diaphragm?
    a. abdominal and thoracic
    b. cranial and spinal
    c. pelvic and abdominal
    d. thoracic and cranial

14. Simple compounds are transformed by the body into complex substances in the process called:
    a. anabolism.
    b. catabolism.
    c. digestion.
    d. homeostasis.

15. This term describes the balanced or "steady state" condition normally maintained by the body.
    a. anabolism
    b. catabolism
    c. hemostasis
    d. homeostasis

16. The result of all chemical and physical reactions in the body that are necessary to sustain life is called:
    a. anabolism.
    b. cannibalism.
    c. catabolism.
    d. metabolism.

17. Human chromosomes are:
    a. networks of tubules in the cytosol.
    b. rod-shaped bodies near the nucleus.
    c. strands of deoxyribonucleic acid.
    d. structures within the cytoplasm.

18. Which one of the following cellular structures plays a role in assembling proteins from amino acids?
    a. lysosome
    b. mitochondria
    c. nucleus
    d. ribosome

19. This cellular structure contains the chromosomes and is called the command center of the cell.
    a. centriole
    b. cytoplasm
    c. nucleus
    d. nucleolus

20. These are oval or rod-shaped organelles that play a role in energy production.
    a. Golgi apparatus
    b. lysosomes
    c. mitochondria
    d. ribosomes

21. Which of the following is adipose tissue?
    a. bone
    b. cells
    c. fat
    d. skin

22. The skeletal system produces:
    a. blood cells.
    b. calcium.
    c. lactic acid.
    d. vitamin D.

23. Which of the following is a disorder associated with the skeletal system?
    a. atrophy
    b. cholecystitis
    c. multiple sclerosis
    d. osteochondritis

24. Which of the following laboratory tests is associated with the skeletal system?
    a. alkaline phosphatase
    b. creatine kinase (CK)
    c. cholinesterase
    d. lactic dehydrogenase

25. Skeletal system structures include:
    a. dendrites.
    b. papillae.
    c. phalanges.
    d. ureters.

26. Which of the following bones are categorized as short bones?
    a. carpals
    b. femurs
    c. ribs
    d. vertebrae

27. Which of the following is one way muscle type is determined?
    a. enzymes released
    b. heat production
    c. layer thickness
    d. nervous control

28. Which of the following is an abbreviation for a test that is associated with the muscular system?
    a. BUN
    b. CK
    c. CSF
    d. TSH

29. Wasting or decrease in size of a muscle because of inactivity is called:
    a. atrophy.
    b. myalgia.
    c. rickets.
    d. uremia.

30. Which type of muscle is under voluntary nervous control?
    a. cardiac
    b. skeletal
    c. smooth
    d. visceral

31. Which of the following is a function of the muscular system?
    a. absorb nutrients
    b. create blood cells
    c. maintain posture
    d. produce vitamin D

32. In numerical order, the skin layers or structures identified by numbers 1, 2, and 3 in Fig. 5-1 are:
    a. corium, stratum basale, and epidermis.
    b. dermis, epidermis, and adipose tissue.
    c. epidermis, dermis, and subcutaneous.
    d. papillary dermis, dermis, and corneum.

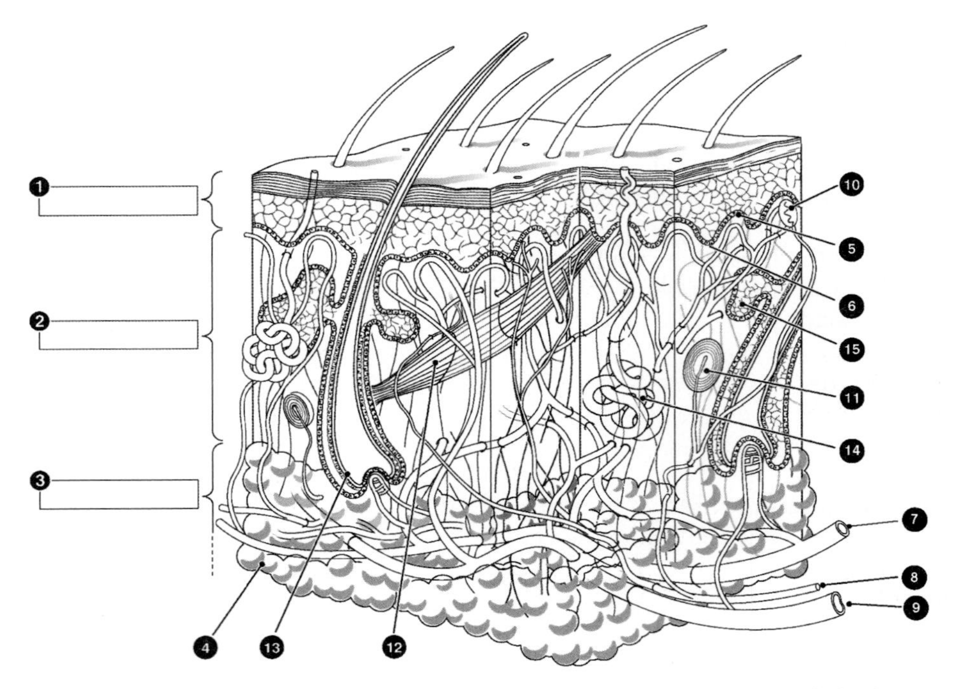

FIGURE 5-1 Cross section of the skin. (Used with permission from Cohen BJ, Hull KL, *Study Guide for Memmler's The Human Body in Health and Disease* 10th ed. 2005. Philadelphia: Lippincott Williams & Wilkins, p. 85.)

33. In numerical order, the skin structures identified by numbers 12, 13, 14, and 15 in Fig. 5-1 are:
 a. arrector pili muscle, hair follicle, sweat gland, and oil gland.
 b. nerve ending, sweat gland, hair follicle, and pressure receptor.
 c. papilla, sebaceous gland, sudoriferous gland, and pore opening.
 d. touch receptor, nerve ending, sweat gland, and dermal papilla.

34. Which of the following is a function of the skin?
 a. hormone production
 b. posture maintenance
 c. temperature regulation
 d. vitamin C manufacture

35. Which skin structures give rise to fingerprints?
 a. arrector pili
 b. hair follicles
 c. oil glands
 d. papillae

36. Blood vessels of the skin are found only in the:
 a. corium and subcutaneous.
 b. dermis and germinativum.
 c. epidermis and adipose layer.
 d. germinativum and corneum.

37. Which of the following tests is often associated with the integumentary system?
 a. aldosterone
 b. occult blood
 c. fungal culture
 d. serum gastrin

38. Mitosis takes place in this skin structure.
 a. adipose tissue layer
 b. papillary dermis
 c. stratum germinativum
 d. subcutaneous tissue

39. Which of the following is an integumentary system disorder?
 a. diabetes
 b. impetigo
 c. meningitis
 d. rhinitis

40. This skin layer is avascular.
 a. corneum
 b. dermis
 c. epidermis
 d. subcutaneous

41. The integumentary system produces:
 a. melanin.
 b. melatonin.
 c. surfactant.
 d. trypsin.

42. Cells in this skin structure can be described as stratified, keratinized, epithelial cells.
 a. adipose tissue
 b. dermis
 c. epidermis
 d. subcutaneous

43. The brain and spinal cord comprise the:
 a. autonomic nervous system.
 b. central nervous system.
 c. peripheral nervous system.
 d. somatic nervous system.

44. Which of the following is a nervous system test?
 a. AFB culture
 b. CK isoenzymes
 c. C-reactive protein
 d. CSF analysis

45. In numerical order, the structures identified by numbers 1, 2, 3, and 4 in Fig. 5-2 are:
 a. axons, dendrites, cell body, and myelin sheath.
 b. dendrites, cell body, cell nucleus, and axon.
 c. myelin sheath, cell body, axon branch, and node.
 d. neurilemma, nodes, nucleus, and axon branches.

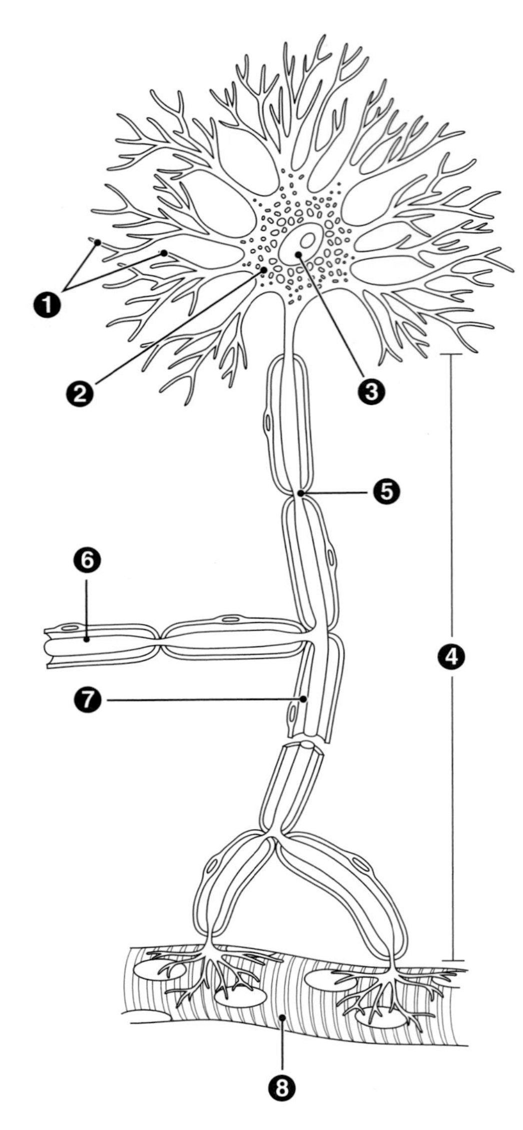

FIGURE 5-2 Diagram of a motor neuron. (Used with permission from Cohen BJ, Hull KL, *Study Guide for Memmler's The Human Body in Health and Disease* 10th ed. 2005. Philadelphia: Lippincott Williams & Wilkins, p. 143.)

46. Which of the following is a nervous system disorder?
   a. encephalitis
   b. gigantism
   c. myxedema
   d. pediculosis

47. The spinal cavity is enclosed and protected by three layers of connective tissue called:
   a. bursae.
   b. calcaneus.
   c. glomeruli.
   d. meninges.

48. Which of the following structures belong in the peripheral nervous system?
   a. afferent nerves
   b. brain
   c. meninges
   d. spinal cord

49. The fundamental units of the nervous system are the:
   a. axons.
   b. meninges.
   c. nephrons.
   d. neurons.

50. This disorder involves destruction of the myelin sheath of nerves.
   a. Cushing's syndrome
   b. hydrocephalus
   c. multiple sclerosis
   d. Parkinson's disease

51. Which of the following glands is an integumentary system structure?
   a. adrenal
   b. pituitary
   c. sebaceous
   d. thyroid

52. Erythropoietin is a hormone secreted by the:
   a. adrenals.
   b. kidneys.
   c. ovaries.
   d. thyroid.

53. Excessive growth hormone in adulthood can cause:
   a. acromegaly.
   b. emphysema.
   c. encephalitis.
   d. myxedema.

54. A disorder in which the pancreas is unable to produce insulin is:
    a. diabetes insipidus.
    b. diabetes mellitus type I.
    c. diabetes mellitus type II.
    d. gestational diabetes.

55. All of the following organs have endocrine function EXCEPT the:
    a. bronchi.
    b. kidneys.
    c. placenta.
    d. stomach.

56. In numerical order, the glands identified by numbers 2, 3, 5, and 6 in Fig. 5-3 are the:
    a. adrenals, pineal, thymus, and parathyroids.
    b. hypophysis, thyroid, thymus, and adrenals.
    c. pineal, adrenals, parathyroids, and thymus.
    d. pituitary, parathyroid, thymus, and pineal.

57. T_4 and TSH are abbreviations for tests that measure the function of the:
    a. adrenals.
    b. ovaries.
    c. pancreas.
    d. thyroid.

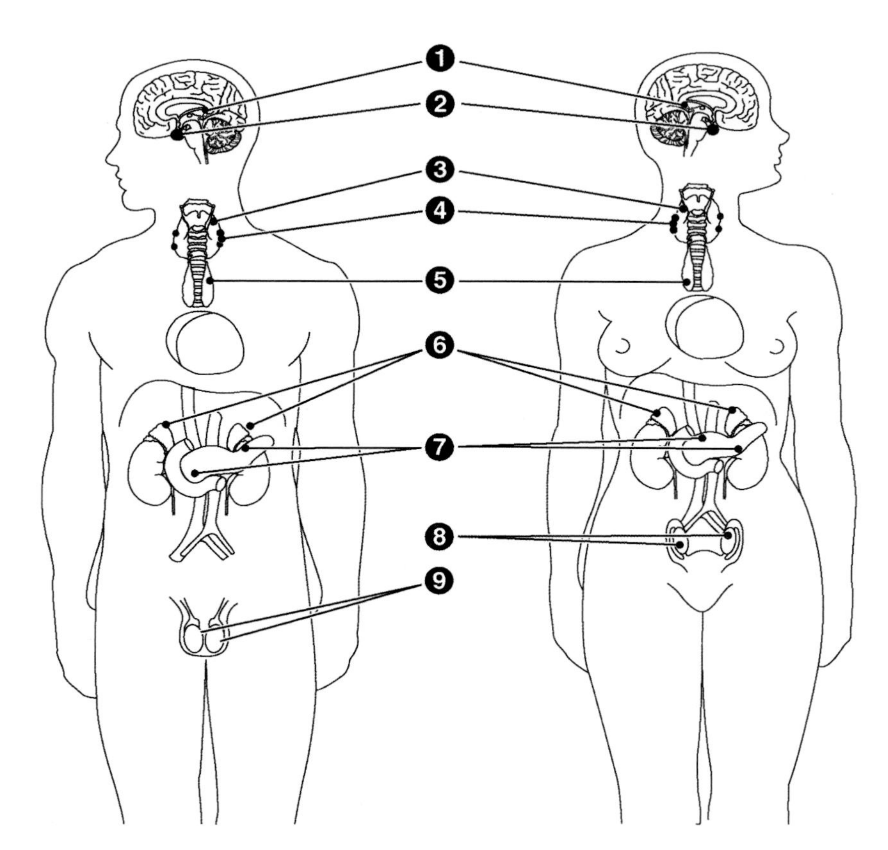

FIGURE 5-3 Endocrine system. (Used with permission from Cohen BJ, Hull KL, *Study Guide for Memmler's The Human Body in Health and Disease* 10th ed. 2005. Philadelphia: Lippincott Williams & Wilkins, p. 194.)

58. This gland is called the "master gland" of the endocrine system.
a. pineal
b. pituitary
c. thymus
d. thyroid

59. Growth hormone (GH) levels test the function of the:
a. adrenals.
b. ovaries.
c. pancreas.
d. pituitary.

60. Which of the following substances is secreted by the islets of Langerhans?
a. adrenaline
b. cortisol
c. estrogen
d. glucagon

61. Antidiuretic hormone (ADH) is also called:
a. aldosterone.
b. epinephrine.
c. noradrenaline.
d. vasopressin.

62. This gland produces "fight or flight" hormones.
a. adrenal
b. pancreas
c. pituitary
d. thyroid

63. Calcitonin levels test the function of the:
a. adrenals.
b. pituitary.
c. thymus.
d. thyroid.

64. Which gland is most active before birth and during childhood?
a. pineal
b. pituitary
c. thymus
d. thyroid

65. This gland is affected by light and helps create the diurnal rhythm of the sleep-wake cycle.
a. adrenal
b. pineal
c. thymus
d. thyroid

66. This hormone increases metabolism.
a. cortisol
b. glucagon
c. melatonin
d. thyroxine

67. Which of the following structures is part of the digestive system?
a. arrector pili
b. bronchiole
c. gallbladder
d. glomerulus

68. Which of the following is a test of a digestive system organ?
a. bilirubin
b. cortisol
c. myoglobin
d. uric acid

69. Hepatitis is a disorder that primarily affects the:
a. colon.
b. kidneys.
c. liver.
d. spleen.

70. Bile is stored in the:
a. duodenum.
b. epididymis.
c. gallbladder.
d. glomerulus.

71. Diagnostic tests of the digestive system include:
a. amylase and lipase.
b. calcium and uric acid.
c. cortisol and glucagon.
d. Dilantin and serotonin.

72. Digestive system structures include the:
    a. esophagus and salivary glands.
    b. neurilemma and axon branches.
    c. seminal ducts and vas deferens.
    d. stratum corneum and papillae.

73. Reproductive system functions include production of:
    a. gametes.
    b. gastrin.
    c. melanin.
    d. sputum.

74. Which of the following is a structure of the male reproductive system?
    a. alveolar sac
    b. epididymis
    c. fallopian tube
    d. renal artery

75. Which of the following is an abbreviation for a test of the male, but not the female, reproductive system?
    a. ALP
    b. BMP
    c. PSA
    d. RPR

76. Which of the following are male gametes?
    a. gonads
    b. ovum
    c. sperm
    d. testes

77. Female gametes are produced in the:
    a. cervix.
    b. fallopian tubes.
    c. ovaries.
    d. uterus.

78. Which of the following is an abbreviation for a female reproductive system test?
    a. CEA
    b. FSH
    c. GTT
    d. PSA

79. Which of the following is a structure of the female reproductive system?
    a. oviduct
    b. pharynx
    c. sacrum
    d. ureter

80. This disease is associated with the reproductive system.
    a. cholecystitis
    b. gonorrhea
    c. myxedema
    d. shingles

81. Which of the following is a urinary system test?
    a. alkaline phosphatase
    b. creatinine clearance
    c. lactic dehydrogenase
    d. rapid plasma reagin

82. Which of the following are all urinary system structures?
    a. axons, myelin sheath, prostate
    b. centriole, nuclei, Golgi apparatus
    c. glomeruli, nephrons, ureters
    d. neurons, renal arteries, urethra

83. Which of the following is a function of the urinary system?
    a. electrolyte balance
    b. heat production
    c. stimuli reception
    d. removal of gases

84. Which of the following is normally a urinary system disorder?
    a. cystitis
    b. gastritis
    c. neuritis
    d. pruritus

85. This substance secreted by the kidneys plays a role in increasing blood pressure.
    a. melanin
    b. renin
    c. sebum
    d. uric acid

86. These structures are tufts of capillaries that are the filtering components of the urinary system.
    a. fallopian tubes
    b. glomeruli
    c. nephrons
    d. ureters

87. Which of the following is an abbreviation for a respiratory system test?
    a. ABG
    b. KOH
    c. TSH
    d. UA

88. During internal respiration:
    a. carbon dioxide enters the tissue cells.
    b. carbon dioxide exits the bloodstream.
    c. oxygen enters the blood in the lungs.
    d. oxygen enters the cells in the tissues.

89. During normal respiratory function, bicarbonate ion acts as a buffer to keep blood pH within a steady range of:
    a. 7.25 to 7.75.
    b. 7.35 to 7.45.
    c. 7.50 to 8.00.
    d. 8.00 to 8.10.

90. Acidosis can result from:
    a. high carbon dioxide levels.
    b. increased blood pH levels.
    c. increased rate of respiration.
    d. prolonged hyperventilation.

91. The ability of oxygen to combine with this substance in the red blood cells increases the amount of oxygen that can be carried in the blood by up to 70 times.
    a. carbon dioxide
    b. glucose
    c. hemoglobin
    d. potassium

92. A major cause of respiratory distress in infants and young children is:
    a. airway blockage associated with emphysema.
    b. dyspnea as a consequence of cystic fibrosis.
    c. infection with *Mycobacterium tuberculosis.*
    d. respiratory syncytial virus (RSV) infection.

93. Which of the following are respiratory system structures?
    a. bronchioles, epiglottis, pleura
    b. calcaneus, mandible, phalanges
    c. corium, corneum, adipose cells
    d. neurons, meninges, myelin sheath

94. The exchange of O_2 and CO_2 in the lungs takes place in the:
    a. alveoli.
    b. bronchi.
    c. larynx.
    d. trachea.

95. Decreased partial pressure of oxygen (PO_2) in the capillaries of the tissues causes:
    a. carbon dioxide to diffuse into the tissues.
    b. carbon dioxide to release from hemoglobin.
    c. oxygen to associate with hemoglobin.
    d. oxygen to disassociate from hemoglobin.

96. Infant respiratory distress syndrome (IRDS) in premature infants is most often caused by a lack of:
    a. alveolar sacs.
    b. carbon dioxide.
    c. hemoglobin.
    d. surfactant.

97. This is the abbreviation for a respiratory system disorder caused by an acid-fast bacillus.
    a. COPD
    b. IRDS
    c. RSV
    d. TB

98. A person is having difficulty breathing. The term used to describe this condition is:
    a. asthma.
    b. dyspnea.
    c. emphysema.
    d. pneumonia.

99. Which body system controls and coordinates the activities of all the other body systems?
    a. muscular
    b. nervous
    c. respiratory
    d. skeletal

100. Elimination of waste products is a function of this body system.
    a. digestive
    b. endocrine
    c. nervous
    d. skeletal

101. The medical term for elevated blood sugar is:
    a. diabetes mellitus.
    b. diabetes insipidus.
    c. hyperglycemia.
    d. hyperinsulinism.

102. This body system is responsible for releasing hormones directly into the bloodstream.
    a. circulatory
    b. endocrine
    c. integumentary
    d. respiratory

103. Pancreatitis is a disorder of this system.
    a. digestive
    b. reproductive
    c. respiratory
    d. skeletal

104. Powerful chemical substances secreted directly into the bloodstream by certain glands are called:
    a. electrolytes.
    b. hormones.
    c. lysosomes.
    d. surfactants.

105. Hematopoiesis is a function of this body system.
    a. endocrine
    b. muscular
    c. skeletal
    d. urinary

ANSWERS AND EXPLANATIONS

1. Answer: d
   Why: Human anatomy is defined as the branch of science that deals with the structural composition of the body. Human physiology deals with body function, including chemical reactions and homeostatic processes.
   Review: Yes ☐ No ☐

2. Answer: a
   Why: Anatomic position is defined as standing erect, arms at the side, with eyes and palms facing forward. When describing the direction or the location of a given point on the body, medical personnel normally refer to the body as if the patient is in the anatomic position, regardless of actual body position. Prone is lying face down. Supine is lying face up. Syncope is a medical term for fainting.
   Review: Yes ☐ No ☐

3. Answer: d
   Why: Pronation is defined as the condition of being prone or the act of assuming a prone position. A hand that is prone is palm down. Consequently, pronation of the hand can be defined as the act of turning the hand palm down. Extending the hand out to the side of the body is called abduction. The act of flexing the hand at the wrist is called flexion of the wrist. The act of rotating the hand called rotation.
   Review: Yes ☐ No ☐

4. Answer: b
   Why: A sagittal plane (Fig. 5-4) divides the body into right and left portions, but they are not necessarily equal. A midsagittal plane is a type of sagittal plane that divides

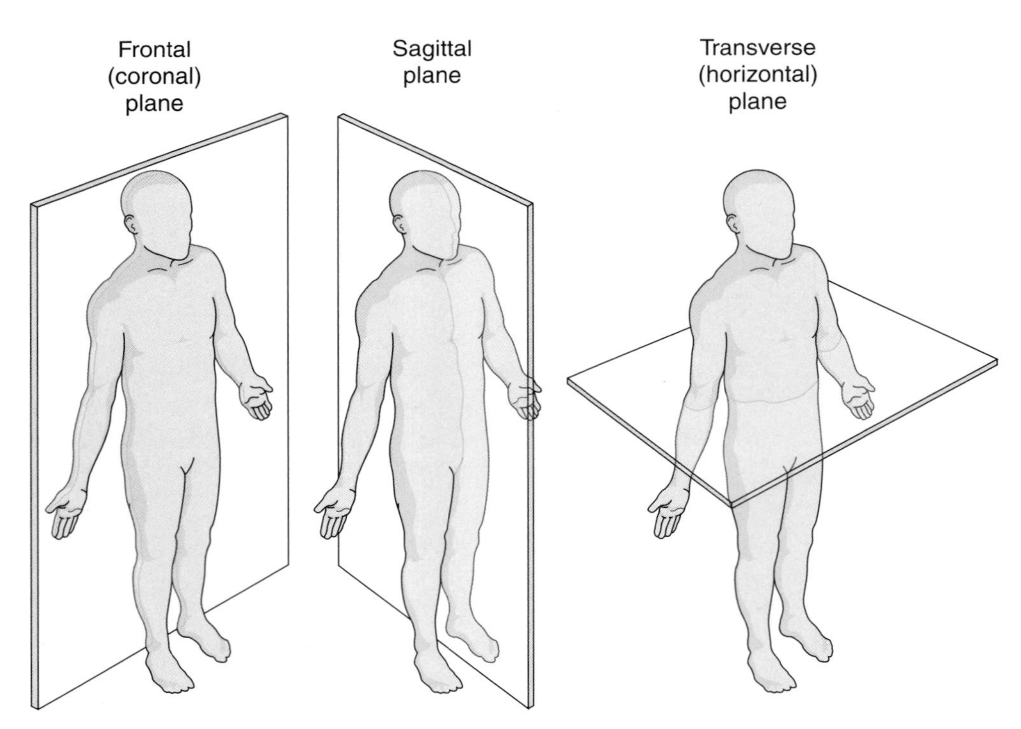

FIGURE 5-4 Body planes. (Used with permission from Cohen BJ, Taylor J. *Memmler's Structure and Function of the Human Body.* 8th ed. 2005. Philadelphia: Lippincott Williams & Wilkins, p. 9.)

the body into equal right and left portions. A frontal plane divides the body vertically into front and back portions. A transverse plane divides the body into upper and lower portions.

Review: Yes ☐ No ☐

5. Answer: a

Why: The frontal plane (Fig. 5-4) divides the body vertically into front and back portions. When you are facing someone in normal anatomic position, he or she is also facing you, which means you are seeing a frontal plane. A midsagittal plane divides a body into equal right and left portions. A sagittal plane divides the body into right and left portions that are not necessarily equal. A transverse plane divides the body into upper and lower portions.

Review: Yes ☐ No ☐

6. Answer: d

Why: A transverse plane (Fig. 5-4) is defined as a plane that divides the body into upper and lower portions. A frontal plane divides the body vertically into front and back portions. A sagittal plane divides the body into right and left portions. A midsagittal plane divides the body into equal right and left portions.

Review: Yes ☐ No ☐

7. Answer: b

Why: Medial means "toward the midline of the body" (Fig. 5-5). The big toe is on the inner side of the foot, which is the side closest to the midline of the body. A man who is in a supine position is lying on his back. The hand is at the distal end of the arm. The posterior curvature of the heel is *not* a recommended site for heel puncture.

Review: Yes ☐ No ☐

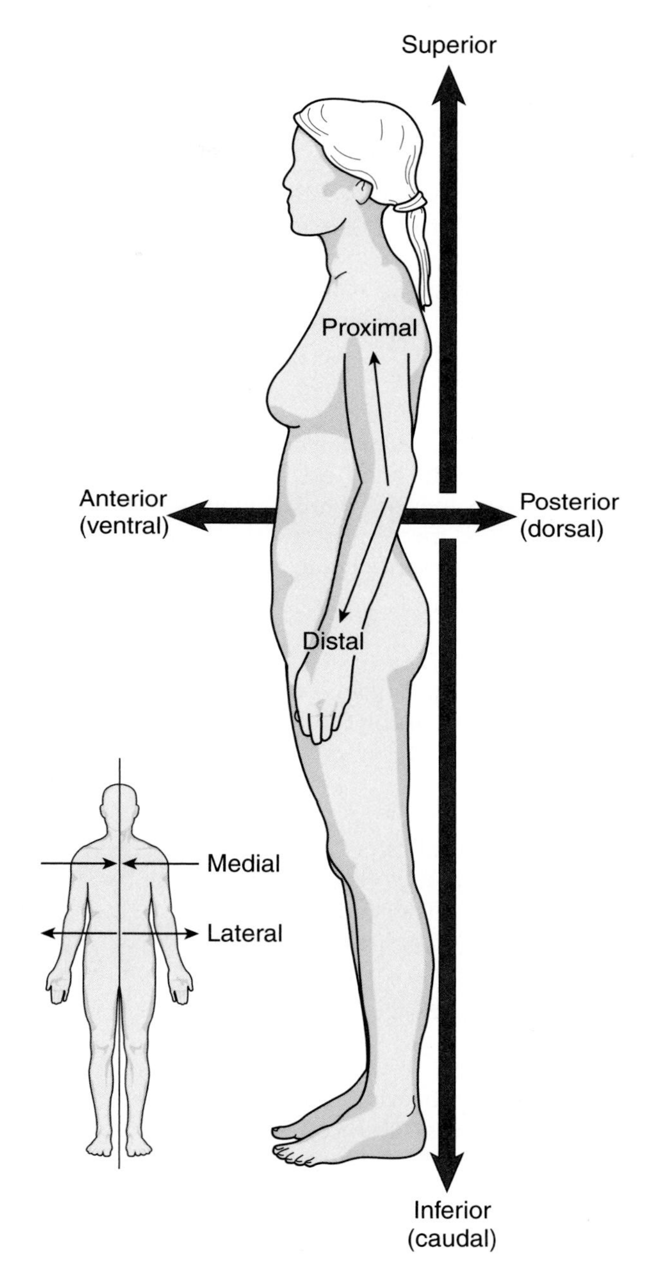

FIGURE 5-5 Directional terms. (Used with permission from Cohen BJ, Taylor J. *Memmler's Structure and Function of the Human Body*. 8th ed. 2005. Philadelphia: Lippincott Williams & Wilkins, p. 8.)

8. Answer: a
   Why: The diaphragm separates the thoracic cavity from the abdominal cavity. The meaning of inferior is "beneath or lower." The abdominal cavity is beneath the thoracic cavity and therefore beneath the diaphragm also. The elbow is on the back, or dorsal, surface of the arm. The head is above or superior to the neck. The little finger is on the lateral side of the hand.
   Review: Yes ☐ No ☐

9. Answer: a
   Why: Distal is defined as farthest from the center of the body, origin, or point of attachment. Superior means "higher or above." Proximal means "nearest to the center of the body." Dorsal refers to the back (Fig. 5-5).
   Review: Yes ☐ No ☐

10. Answer: c
    Why: Plantar means "concerning the sole or bottom of the foot."
    Review: Yes ☐ No ☐

11. Answer: c
    Why: Dorsal refers to the back (Fig. 5-5). Dorsal cavities (Fig. 5-6) are to the back of the body. The spinal and cranial cavities are dorsal cavities. The abdominal, pelvic, and thoracic cavities are ventral cavities.
    Review: Yes ☐ No ☐

12. Answer: d
    Why: The heart and lungs are located in a cavity in the chest called the thoracic cavity (Fig. 5-6).The word thoracic comes from *thorac,* which means "chest," and *-ic,* which means "pertaining to."
    Review: Yes ☐ No ☐

13. Answer: a
    Why: The diaphragm (Fig. 5-6) is the name of the muscular partition between the thoracic cavity and the abdominal cavity.
    Review: Yes ☐ No ☐

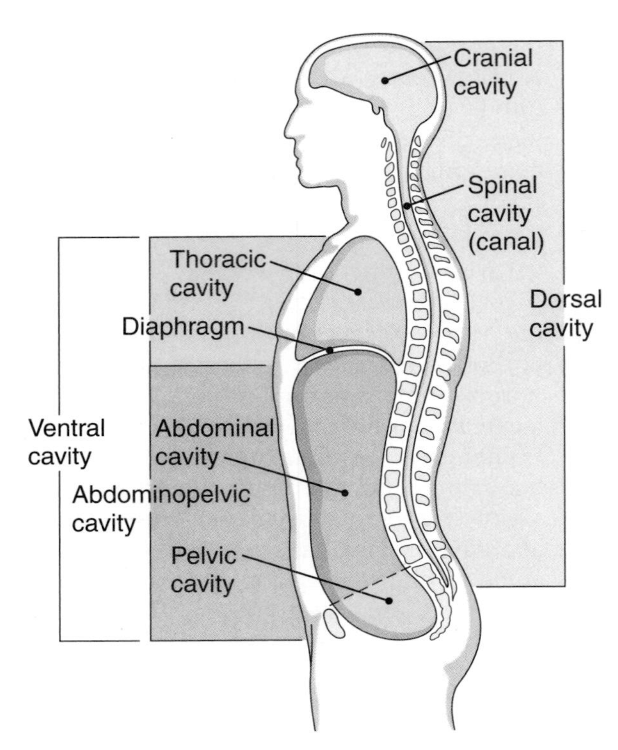

FIGURE 5-6 Body cavities, lateral view. (Used with permission from Cohen BJ, Taylor J. *Memmler's Structure and Function of the Human Body.* 8th ed. 2005. Philadelphia: Lippincott Williams & Wilkins, p. 11.)

14. Answer: a
    Why: Anabolism is the name for the constructive process in which simple compounds are transformed into complex substances. Catabolism is a destructive process by which complex substances are broken into simple ones. Digestion is the process by which food is broken into simple usable components. Homeostasis means "staying the same," and is the term is used to describe the state of equilibrium or balance the body strives to maintain
    Review: Yes ☐ No ☐

15. Answer: d
    Why: Homeostasis means "staying the same." The term is used to describe the state of equilibrium or balance, referred to as "steady state," that the body strives to

maintain. Anabolism is the part of the metabolism process in which the body converts simple compounds into complex substances. Catabolism is the process by which the body breaks complex substances into simple ones. Hemostasis refers to the stagnation or stopping of the flow of blood within the circulatory system.

Review: Yes ☐ No ☐

16. Answer: d

Why: Metabolism is defined as the sum of all the chemical and physical reactions necessary to sustain life. Anabolism is the part of the metabolism process in which the body converts simple compounds into complex substances. Cannibalism is the eating of human flesh. Catabolism is the process by which the body breaks complex substances into simple ones.

Review: Yes ☐ No ☐

17. Answer: c

Why: Chromosomes (Fig. 5-7) are the genetic material of the cell found in the nucleus. They are long strands of deoxyribonucleic acid (DNA) that are organized into units called genes. Humans normally have 26 identical pairs of chromosomes (46 individual ones). The endoplasmic reticulum is a network of tubules in the cytosol (fluid of the cytoplasm). The rod-shaped bodies near the nucleus are the centrioles. Structures within the cytoplasm are called organelles.

Review: Yes ☐ No ☐

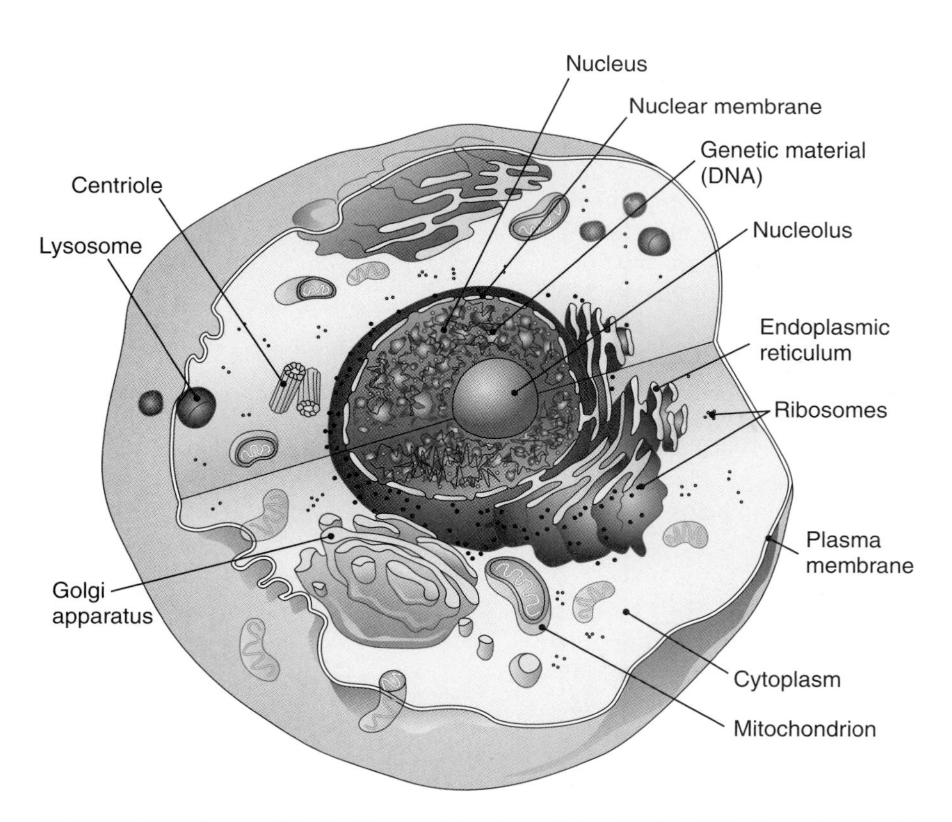

FIGURE 5-7 Cell diagram. (Used with permission from Cohen BJ, Wood DL. *Memmler's The Human Body in Health and Disease.* 9th ed. 2000. Philadelphia: Lippincott Williams & Wilkins, p. 29.)

18. Answer: d
Why: Ribosomes (Fig. 5-7) are tiny organelles in the fluid portion of cells where amino acid assembly takes place. Lysosomes digest substances within the cell. The mitochondria play a role in energy production. The nucleus is the command center of the cell and contains the chromosomes.
Review: Yes ☐ No ☐

19. Answer: c
Why: The chromosomes are found in the large, dark-staining organelle called the nucleus that is found near the center of the cell (Figure 5-7). Because the nucleus contains the chromosomes, which govern all cellular activities, it is referred to as the command center of the cell.
Review: Yes ☐ No ☐

20. Answer: c
Why: Organelles are specialized structures in the fluid portion of the cell (Fig. 5-7). Although mitochondria, Golgi apparatus, lysosomes, and ribosomes are all organelles, the mitochondria are oval or rod-shaped and are the site of energy production. The Golgi apparatus are layers of membranes that make, sort, and prepare protein compounds for transport. Lysosomes are small sacs of enzymes that digest substances within the cell. Ribosomes are tiny bodies that that play a role in assembling proteins from amino acids.
Review: Yes ☐ No ☐

21. Answer: c
Why: Adipose means "fat or pertaining to fat." Adipose tissue consists mainly of fat cells. Adipose tissue, bone, and blood are types of connective tissue. Cells are the basic structural unit of all life. Skin is epithelial tissue.
Review: Yes ☐ No ☐

22. Answer: a
Why: Blood cells are produced in the bone marrow, which is part of the skeletal system (Fig. 5-8). The skeletal system does not produce calcium; it stores calcium. Lactic acid is produced in muscle and other

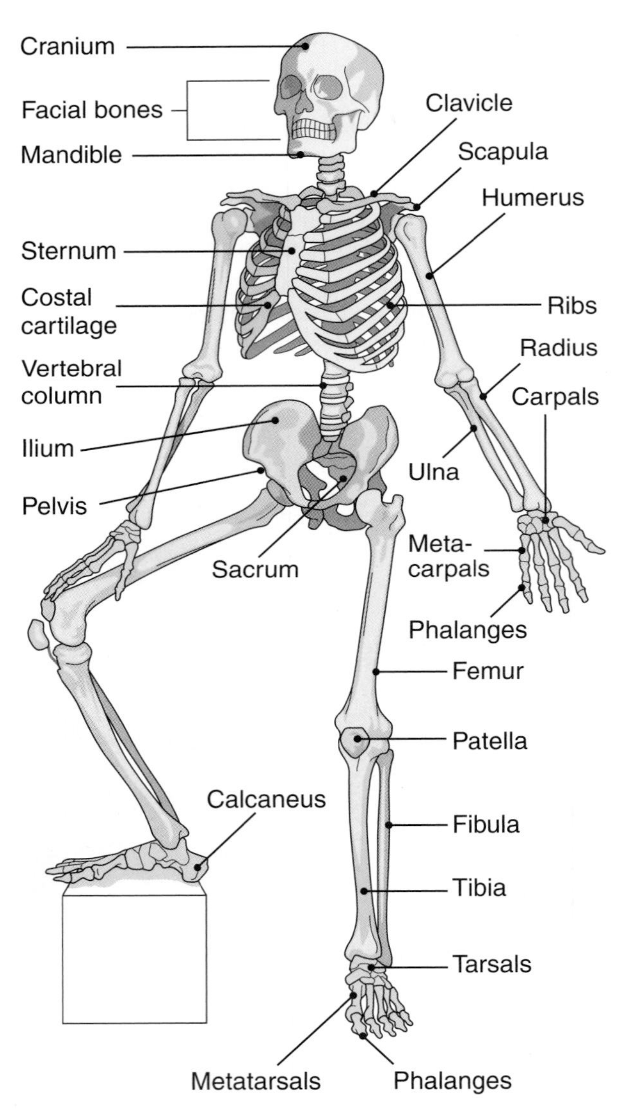

FIGURE 5-8 Human skeleton. (Used with permission from Cohen BJ, Taylor J. *Memmler's Structure and Function of the Human Body.* 8th ed. 2005. Philadelphia: Lippincott Williams & Wilkins, p. 66.)

tissues in the process of carbohydrate metabolism. Vitamin D is produced in the skin.
Review: Yes ☐ No ☐

23. Answer: d
Why: Osteochondritis means "inflammation of the bone and cartilage," which are skeletal system (Fig. 5-8) structures. Atrophy, a disorder of the muscular system, is muscle wasting. Cholecystitis is gallbladder inflammation. The gallbladder is an accessory organ of the digestive system. Multiple sclerosis is an inflammatory disease of the nervous system that causes degeneration of the myelin sheath of the nerves.
Review: Yes ☐ No ☐

24. Answer: a
Why: Alkaline phosphatase is an enzyme that functions in the mineralization of bone. Creatine kinase and lactic dehydrogenase are muscular system tests. Cholinesterase is a nervous system test.
Review: Yes ☐ No ☐

25. Answer: c
Why: Phalanges are finger bones, and part of the skeletal system (Fig. 5-8). Dendrites are nervous system structures. Papillae are integumentary system structures. Ureters are urinary system structures.
Review: Yes ☐ No ☐

26. Answer: a
Why: Bones are categorized by shape. Carpals (wrist bones) are categorized as short bones. Femurs are categorized as long bones. Ribs are categorized as flat bones. Vertebrae are categorized as irregular bones. (See skeletal system Fig. 5-8.)
Review: Yes ☐ No ☐

27. Answer: d
Why: Muscle type (Table 5-1) is determined according to where the muscle is located, its histologic (microscopic) cellular characteristics, and whether nervous control of the muscle is voluntary or involuntary.
Review: Yes ☐ No ☐

28. Answer: b
Why: Creatine kinase (CK) is an enzyme present in skeletal and heart muscle. Blood urea nitrogen (BUN) is a urinary system test. CSF stands for cerebrospinal fluid. CSF analysis is a nervous system test. Thyroid-stimulating hormone (TSH) is an endocrine system test.
Review: Yes ☐ No ☐

29. Answer: a
Why: Atrophy means "muscle wasting." Myalgia means "muscle pain." Rickets is abnormal bone formation from lack of vitamin D. Uremia is impaired kidney function with a buildup of waste products in the blood.
Review: Yes ☐ No ☐

30. Answer: b
Why: Skeletal muscles are made to contract by conscious thought, which means their nervous control is voluntary. Cardiac and visceral (smooth) muscles function automatically, which means their nervous control is involuntary. (See Table 5-1.)
Review: Yes ☐ No ☐

31. Answer: c
Why: Muscular system functions include maintaining posture, producing heat, and enabling movement. Nutrient absorption is a function of the digestive system. Blood cells are produced in the skeletal system. Vitamin D is manufactured in the skin of the integumentary system.
Review: Yes ☐ No ☐

32. Answer: c
Why: There are two main layers of the skin (Fig. 5-9) and a subcutaneous (under the skin) layer. The epidermis is the outer

Table 5-1 Comparison of the Different Types of Muscle

	Smooth	Cardiac	Skeletal
Location	Wall of hollow organs, vessels, respiratory passageways	Wall of heart	Attached to bones
Cell characteristics	Tapered at each end, branching networks, nonstriated 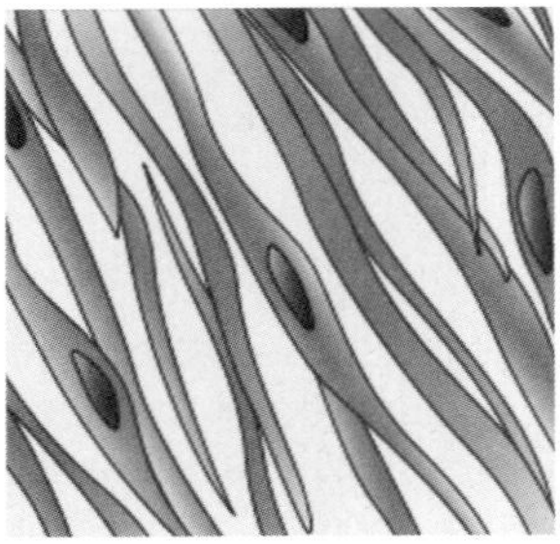	Branching networks; special membranes (intercalated disks) between cells; single nucleus; lightly striated 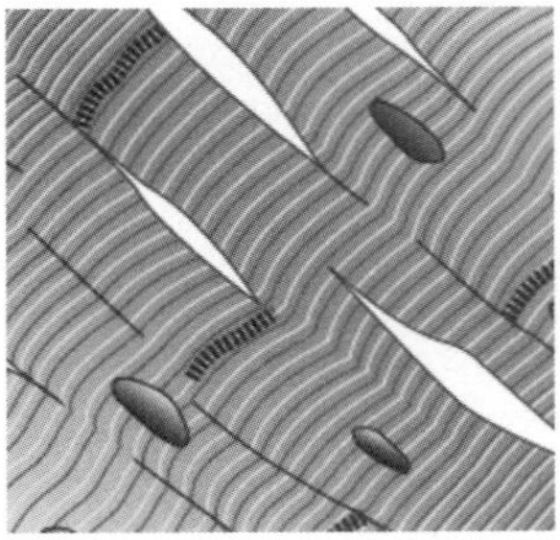	Long and cylindrical; multinucleated; heavily striated 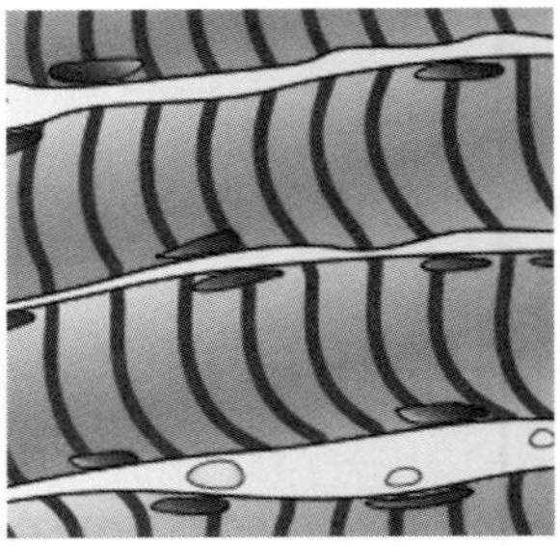
Control	Involuntary	Involuntary	Voluntary
Action	Produces peristalsis; contracts and relaxes slowly; may sustain contraction	Pumps blood out of heart; self-excitatory but influenced by nervous system and hormones	Produces movement at joints; stimulated by nervous system; contracts and relaxes rapidly

layer of the skin. The dermis is the inner layer of the skin. The subcutaneous layer connects the skin to the surface of muscles.

Review: Yes ☐ No ☐

33. Answer: a
Why: The skin structures identified in Figure 5-1 are an arrector pili muscle (#12), a hair follicle (#13), a sudoriferous (sweat) gland (#14), and a sebaceous (oil) gland (#15). (See Fig. 5-9.)
Review: Yes ☐ No ☐

34. Answer: c
Why: The skin plays a role in temperature regulation by helping give off excess heat and protecting the body against the cold. Hormones are produced by endocrine system glands and tissues with endocrine function. The muscular system gives the body the ability to maintain posture. The skin manufactures vitamin D, not vitamin C.
Review: Yes ☐ No ☐

35. Answer: d
Why: Elevations called papillae (Fig. 5-9), and resulting depressions in the dermis

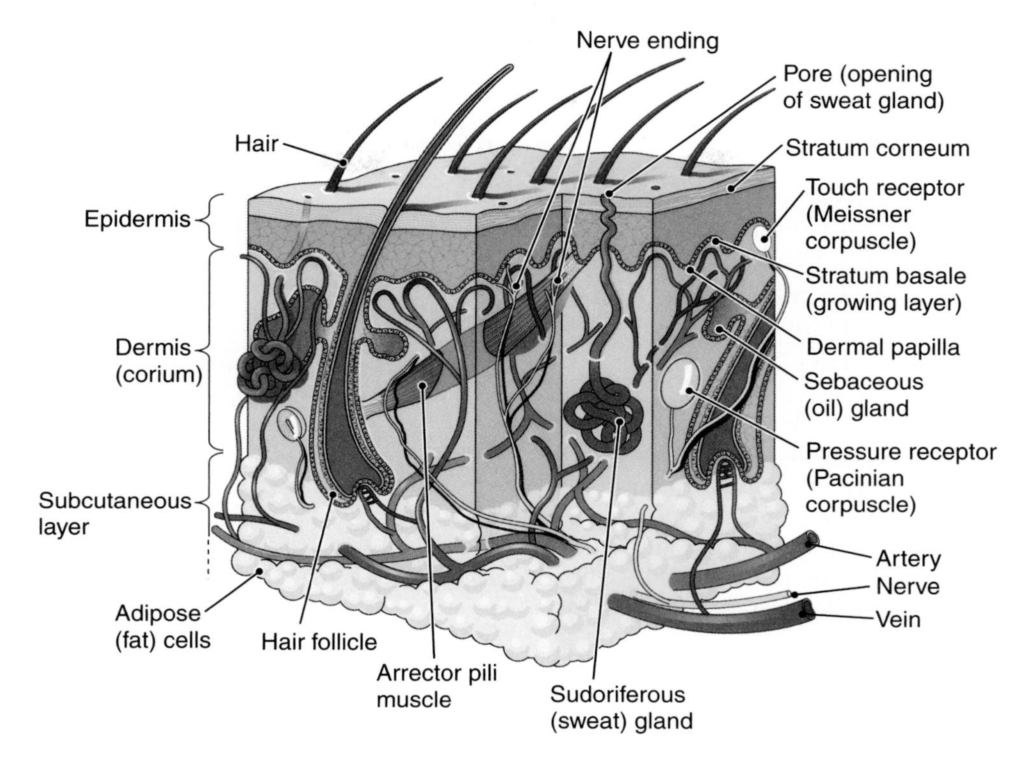

FIGURE 5-9 Cross section of the skin. (Used with permission from Cohen BJ, Taylor J. *Memmler's Structure and Function of the Human Body.* 8th ed. 2005. Philadelphia: Lippincott Williams & Wilkins, p. 74.)

where it meets the epidermis, form the ridges and grooves of fingerprints.

Review: Yes ☐ No ☐

36. Answer: a

Why: Blood vessels are found in the corium (dermis) and subcutaneous layers of the skin (Fig. 5-9). The epidermis is avascular, which means it does not contain blood vessels. The stratum germinativum (SYN stratum basale) and stratum corneum are layers of the epidermis. Adipose (fat) cells are found in the subcutaneous.

Review: Yes ☐ No ☐

37. Answer: c

Why: Fungal cultures are often performed on skin scrapings. The skin is part of the integumentary system. Aldosterone is an endocrine system test. Occult blood (a test for hidden blood in feces) and serum gastrin are digestive system tests.

Review: Yes ☐ No ☐

38. Answer: c

Why: Mitosis occurs in the stratum germinativum (SYN. stratum basale), the deepest and only layer of living cells in the epidermis.

Review: Yes ☐ No ☐

39. Answer: b

Why: Impetigo is an inflammatory condition of the skin most often caused by staphylococcus or streptococcus infection. It is characterized by isolated blisters that rupture and crust over. The skin is part of the integumentary system. Diabetes is an endocrine system disorder. Meningitis is a

nervous system disorder. Rhinitis is a respiratory system disorder.
Review: Yes ☐ No ☐

40. Answer: c
Why: Avascular means "without blood vessels." The epidermis of the skin (Fig. 5-9) does not contain blood vessels. The blood vessels are in the dermis (corium) and subcutaneous layers of the skin.
Review: Yes ☐ No ☐

41. Answer: a
Why: Melanin is a skin pigment that is produced in the stratum germinativum (SYN. stratum basale) of the epidermis (Fig. 5-9.) Melatonin plays a role in promoting sleep and is secreted by the pineal gland of the endocrine system. Surfactant is a substance that coats the walls of the alveoli of the respiratory system. Trypsin is a digestive system enzyme.
Review: Yes ☐ No ☐

42. Answer: c
Why: The epidermis consists mainly of stratified (layered) epithelial cells. New cells form in the stratum germinativum (SYN. Stratum basale), its deepest layer. As the cells push to the surface of the skin they become keratinized (hardened), which helps to thicken and protect the skin.
Review: Yes ☐ No ☐

43. Answer: b
Why: The central nervous system (Fig. 5-10) is composed of the brain and spinal cord. The autonomic and somatic nervous systems are part of the peripheral nervous system.
Review: Yes ☐ No ☐

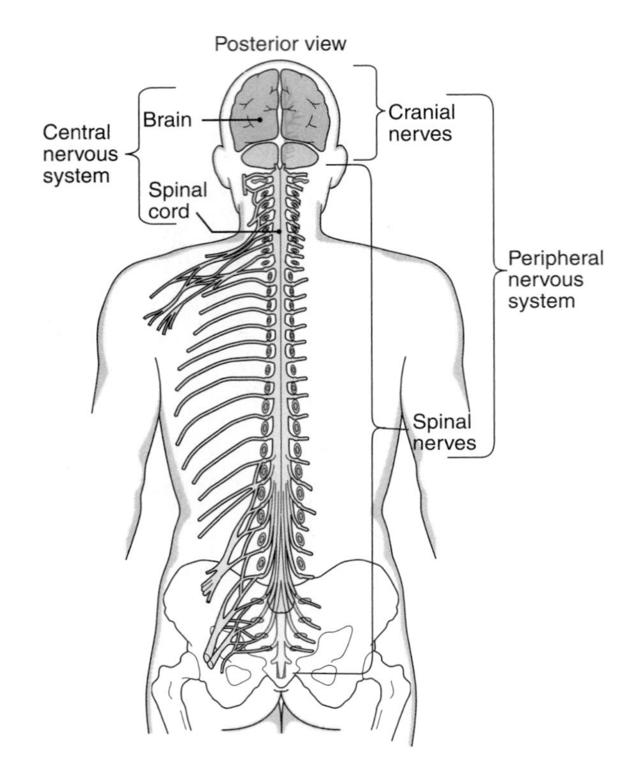

FIGURE 5-10 Structural divisions of the nervous system. (Used with permission from Cohen BJ, Taylor J. *Memmler's Structure and Function of the Human Body.* 8th ed. 2005. Philadelphia: Lippincott Williams & Wilkins, p. 138.)

44. Answer: d
Why: Cerebrospinal fluid (CSF) is the fluid that surrounds and cushions the brain and spinal cord. Acid-fast bacillus (AFB) culture is a respiratory system test. The CK isoenzymes test is a muscular system test. C-reactive protein (CRP) is a substance that is often elevated in the serum of individuals with certain inflammatory and infectious diseases.
Review: Yes ☐ No ☐

45. Answer: b
Why: Figure 5-2 is a motor neuron. Dendrites (#1) carry messages to the nerve cell body (#2). The cell nucleus (#3) is the nerve cell command center. The axon (#4), which has a myelin sheath, carries messages away from the nerve cell body. (See Figure 5-11)
Review: Yes ☐ No ☐

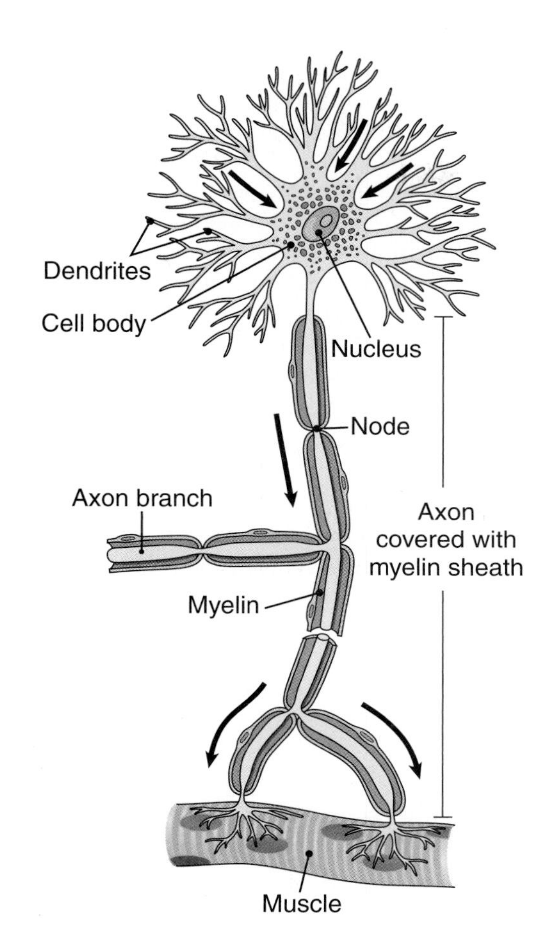

FIGURE 5-11 Diagram of a motor neuron. (Used with permission from Cohen BJ, Taylor J. *Memmler's Structure and Function of the Human Body.* 8th ed. 2005. Philadelphia: Lippincott Williams & Wilkins, p. 139.)

46. Answer: a
Why: Encephalitis means "inflammation of the brain," which is a nervous system structure. Gigantism is a pituitary disorder. Myxedema is a thyroid disorder. The pituitary and thyroid are endocrine system glands. Pediculosis (lice infestation) is an integumentary system disorder.
Review: Yes ☐ No ☐

47. Answer: d
Why: The meninges are layers of connective tissue that completely surround and protect the brain and spinal cavities. Bursae are synovial fluid-filled sacs near joints. Calcaneus is the medical term for the heel bone. Glomeruli are filtering structures in the nephrons of the kidneys.
Review: Yes ☐ No ☐

48. Answer: a
Why: The peripheral nervous system (PNS) consists of all the nerves outside of the central nervous system (CNS). Afferent (sensory) nerves, which conduct impulses toward the brain, are part of the peripheral nervous system. The brain, spinal cord, and meninges are structures of the central nervous system.
Review: Yes ☐ No ☐

49. Answer: d
Why: Neurons (Fig. 5-11) are highly complex cells that are the primary functioning components of the nervous system. Axons are structural parts of neurons. The meninges are the covering of the brain and spinal cord. Nephrons are the functional units of the kidneys.
Review: Yes ☐ No ☐

50. Answer: d
Why: Multiple sclerosis is a disorder of the nervous system in which there is destruction of portions of the myelin sheath and disruption of the conduction of nerve impulses within several regions of the brain and spinal cord. Cushing's syndrome is an endocrine system disorder involving excess production of cortisone. Hydrocephalus is the accumulation of cerebrospinal fluid in the brain. Parkinson's disease is a chronic nervous system disease characterized by muscle weakness and tremors.
Review: Yes ☐ No ☐

51. Answer: c
Why: Sebaceous glands are located in the skin (Fig. 5-9), which is a major part of the

integumentary system. They secrete an oily substance called sebum that helps lubricate the skin. The adrenal, pituitary, and thyroid glands secrete hormones and are part of the endocrine system.
Review: Yes ☐ No ☐

52. Answer: b
Why: The kidneys secrete erythropoietin, a hormone that stimulates red blood cell production.
Review: Yes ☐ No ☐

53. Answer: a
Why: Acromegaly is a condition characterized by the overgrowth of bones in the hands, feet, and face caused by excessive growth hormone in adulthood. Emphysema is chronic obstructive pulmonary disease. Encephalitis means "inflammation of the brain." Myxedema is hypothyroid syndrome, a disorder caused by decreased functioning of the thyroid gland.
Review: Yes ☐ No ☐

54. Answer: b
Why: Diabetes mellitus type I, also called insulin-dependent diabetes, is a disorder in which the body is unable to produce insulin. In diabetes mellitus type II, or non–insulin-dependent diabetes, the body is able to produce insulin, but either the amount produced is not sufficient or the insulin is not properly used by the body. Diabetes insipidus, a condition characterized by increased thirst and increased urine production, is caused by inadequate secretion of antidiuretic hormone. Gestational diabetes is impaired glucose tolerance that develops during pregnancy.
Review: Yes ☐ No ☐

55. Answer: a
Why: The bronchi, which are respiratory system structures, do not have endocrine function. Although they are not endocrine system glands, the kidneys, placenta, and stomach all have endocrine function because they produce substances that affect other tissues. The kidneys secrete erythropoietin, which stimulates red blood cell production. The placenta secretes several hormones that function during pregnancy, including the human chorionic gonadotropin (HCG), which is detected in pregnancy tests. The lining of the stomach secretes gastrin, which stimulates digestion.
Review: Yes ☐ No ☐

56. Answer: b
Why: The hypophysis (#2) is another name for the pituitary gland, which is located in the brain. The thyroid (#3) is located in the neck. The thymus (#5) is located in the chest behind the sternum (breastbone). There are two adrenals (#6), one on top of each kidney. All of the choices in this question are adrenal system glands (Fig. 5-12).
Review: Yes ☐ No ☐

57. Answer: d
Why: Thyroxine (T_4) is a hormone released by the thyroid gland (Fig. 5-12) that increases metabolic rate. TSH is released by the pituitary to stimulate the thyroid. Both T_4 and TSH are common tests of thyroid function.
Review: Yes ☐ No ☐

58. Answer: b
Why: The pituitary gland (Fig. 5-12) is referred to as the "master gland" of the endocrine system because it releases hormones that stimulate other glands.
Review: Yes ☐ No ☐

59. Answer: d
Why: Growth hormone (GH) is secreted by the pituitary gland. The adrenals secrete several hormones including epinephrine, norepinephrine, cortisol, and aldosterone.

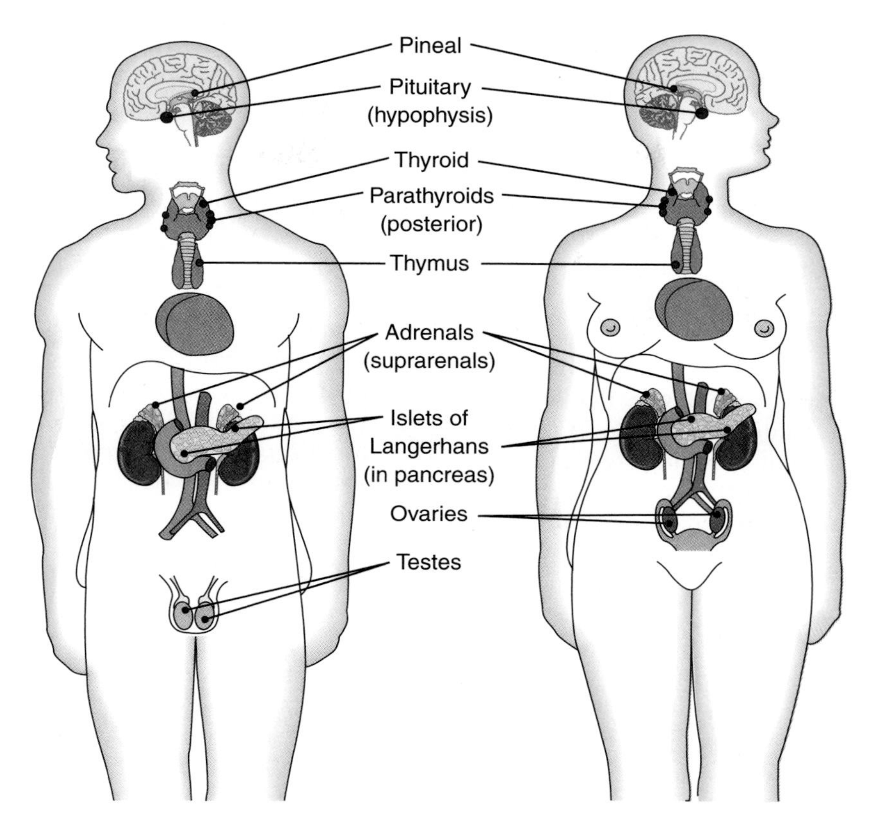

FIGURE 5-12 Endocrine system. (Used with permission from Cohen BJ, Taylor J. *Memmler's Structure and Function of the Human Body.* 8th ed. 2005. Philadelphia: Lippincott Williams & Wilkins, p. 199.)

The ovaries secrete several hormones, including estrogen and progesterone. The islets of Langerhans in the pancreas secrete insulin and glucagon. (See Fig. 5-12.)

Review: Yes ☐ No ☐

60. Answer: d

Why: The islets of Langerhans are located in the pancreas and are part of the endocrine system (Fig. 5-12). They secrete insulin and glucagon. Insulin reduces blood glucose levels by helping move glucose into the cells. Glucagon increases blood glucose levels by stimulating the liver to release glucose into the bloodstream. Adrenaline and cortisol are secreted by the adrenal glands. Estrogen is secreted by the reproductive system.

Review: Yes ☐ No ☐

61. Answer: d

Why: Vasopressin is another name for ADH, which is secreted by the pituitary (Fig. 5-12) and decreases urine production.

Review: Yes ☐ No ☐

62. Answer: a

Why: The adrenals secrete the hormones epinephrine (adrenaline) and norepinephrine (noradrenaline), also referred to as the "fight or flight" hormones because of their effects on the body when it is under stress.

There are two adrenal glands, one atop each kidney (Fig. 5-12).
Review: Yes ☐ No ☐

63. Answer: d
Why: Calcitonin is a hormone secreted by the thyroid (Fig. 5-12) that regulates the amount of calcium in the blood.
Review: Yes ☐ No ☐

64. Answer: c
Why: The thymus gland (Fig. 5-12), located in the chest behind the sternum, functions in the development of immunity and is most active before birth and during childhood until puberty, when it begins to shrink.
Review: Yes ☐ No ☐

65. Answer: b
Why: The pineal gland (Fig. 5-12) secretes the hormone melatonin. Melatonin secretion is inhibited by light and enhanced by darkness. Blood levels of melatonin create the diurnal (daily) rhythm of the sleep-wake cycle, with levels lowest around noon and highest at night.
Review: Yes ☐ No ☐

66. Answer: d
Why: Thyroxine is a hormone released by the thyroid (Fig. 5-12) that increases the metabolic rate. Cortisol is an adrenal hormone that suppresses inflammation. Glucagon is produced by the islets of Langerhans of the pancreas and stimulates the liver to release glucose (from glycogen stores) into the bloodstream. Melatonin, a hormone released by the pineal gland, plays a role in diurnal (daily) rhythms.
Review: Yes ☐ No ☐

67. Answer: c
Why: The gallbladder stores and concentrates bile, which is needed for the digestion of fat. Consequently, it is considered an accessory organ of the digestive system (Fig. 5-13). Arrector pili are structures in the skin. A bronchiole is a structure of the respiratory system. The glomerulus (plural, glomeruli) is a structure of the urinary system.
Review: Yes ☐ No ☐

68. Answer: a
Why: Bilirubin is a liver function test. The liver is an accessory organ of the digestive system (Fig. 5-13). Cortisol is an adrenal function test. The adrenals are endocrine system glands. Myoglobin is a muscular system test. Uric acid is a skeletal system test.
Review: Yes ☐ No ☐

69. Answer: c
Why: Hepatitis means "liver inflammation." The term comes from the Greek word *hepatos,* meaning liver. The suffix *-itis* means "inflammation." The term for inflammation of the colon is colitis. Kidney inflammation is called nephritis. Splenitis is inflammation of the spleen.
Review: Yes ☐ No ☐

70. Answer: c
Why: Bile is secreted by the liver and stored in the gallbladder, an accessory organ of the digestive system (Fig. 5-13). Bile emulsifies fats and facilitates their digestion.
Review: Yes ☐ No ☐

71. Answer: a
Why: Amylase and lipase are digestive enzymes produced by the pancreas. Calcium and uric acid are skeletal system tests. Cortisol and glucagon are endocrine system tests. Dilantin and serotonin are nervous system tests.
Review: Yes ☐ No ☐

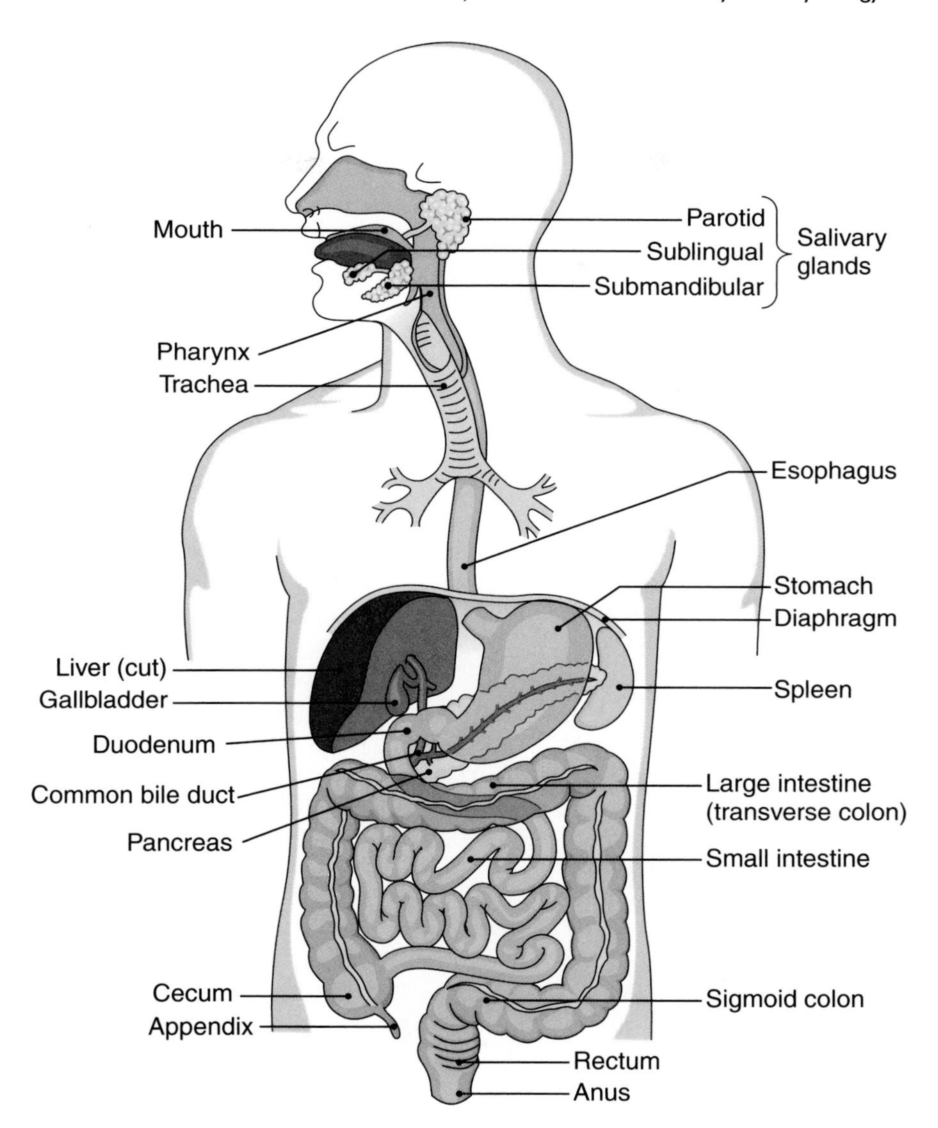

FIGURE 5-13 The digestive system. (Used with permission from Cohen BJ, Taylor J. *Memmler's Structure and Function of the Human Body.* 8th ed. 2005. Philadelphia: Lippincott Williams & Wilkins, p. 309.)

72. Answer: a
Why: The esophagus is part of the gastrointestinal (GI) tract of the digestive system (Fig. 5-13). Salivary glands are accessory structures of the digestive system. Neurilemma and axon branches are nervous system structures. Seminal ducts and the vas deferens are male reproductive system structures. The stratum corneum and papillae are integumentary system structures.
Review: Yes ☐ No ☐

73. Answer: a
Why: Gametes are the sex cells needed to create a new human being. They are produced by the reproductive system (Fig. 5-14). The male reproductive system produces gametes called sperm. The female reproductive system produces gametes called ova (eggs). Gastrin is produced by endocrine tissue in the stomach. Melanin is produced in the skin. Sputum is produced by the respiratory system.
Review: Yes ☐ No ☐

74. Answer: b
Why: The epididymis is a tightly coiled duct in the male reproductive system (Fig. 5-14A) that carries sperm from the testes to the vas deferens. An alveolar sac is a cluster of alveoli in the lungs of the respiratory system. A fallopian tube is a structure of the female reproductive system (Fig. 5-14B). The renal artery carries blood to the kidneys and is part of the urinary system.
Review: Yes ☐ No ☐

75. Answer: c
Why: The prostate-specific antigen (PSA) test identifies the level of a protein produced by the prostate, a male reproductive system structure. ALP is an abbreviation for alkaline phosphatase, a test associated with the skeletal system. A basic metabolic panel or profile (BMP) is a group of tests that cover several body systems. The rapid plasma reagin (RPR) is a syphilis test and is a test of both the male and female reproductive systems.
Review: Yes ☐ No ☐

76. Answer: c
Why: Male gametes (sex cells) are called spermatozoa (sperm). An ovum is a female gamete. Gonads are the glands that produce gametes. The male gonads are the testes.
Review: Yes ☐ No ☐

77. Answer: c
Why: Female gametes (ova) are produced in the ovaries. The cervix is the neck of the uterus. The fallopian tubes are the pathway through which the ova reach the uterus. The uterus is another name for the womb. (See Fig. 5-14B.)
Review: Yes ☐ No ☐

78. Answer: b
Why: Follicle-stimulating hormone (FSH) is a female reproductive system test. Carcinoembryonic antigen (CEA) is a digestive system test associated with the diagnosis of colon cancer. A glucose tolerance test (GTT) is a digestive and an endocrine system test. Prostate-specific antigen (PSA) is a male reproductive system test.
Review: Yes ☐ No ☐

79. Answer: a
Why: Oviduct is another name for fallopian tube, a structure of the female reproductive system (Fig. 5-14B). Each ovary has an oviduct that extends from the ovary to the uterus. The pharynx is a digestive system structure. The sacrum is a skeletal system structure. A ureter is a urinary system structure.
Review: Yes ☐ No ☐

80. Answer: b
Why: Gonorrhea is a sexually transmitted disease (STD). Cholecystitis is inflammation of the gallbladder, which is an accessory organ of the digestive system. Myxedema is an endocrine system disorder that results from decreased thyroid function. Shingles, a nervous system disorder, is an acute eruption of herpes blisters along the length of a peripheral nerve.
Review: Yes ☐ No ☐

81. Answer: b
Why: Creatinine, a byproduct of muscle metabolism, is produced at a constant rate

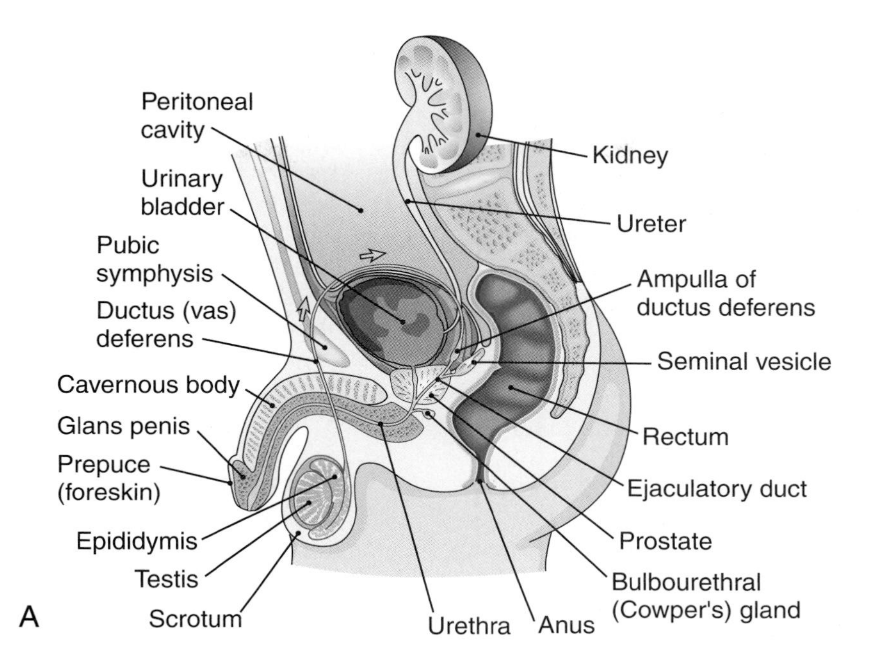

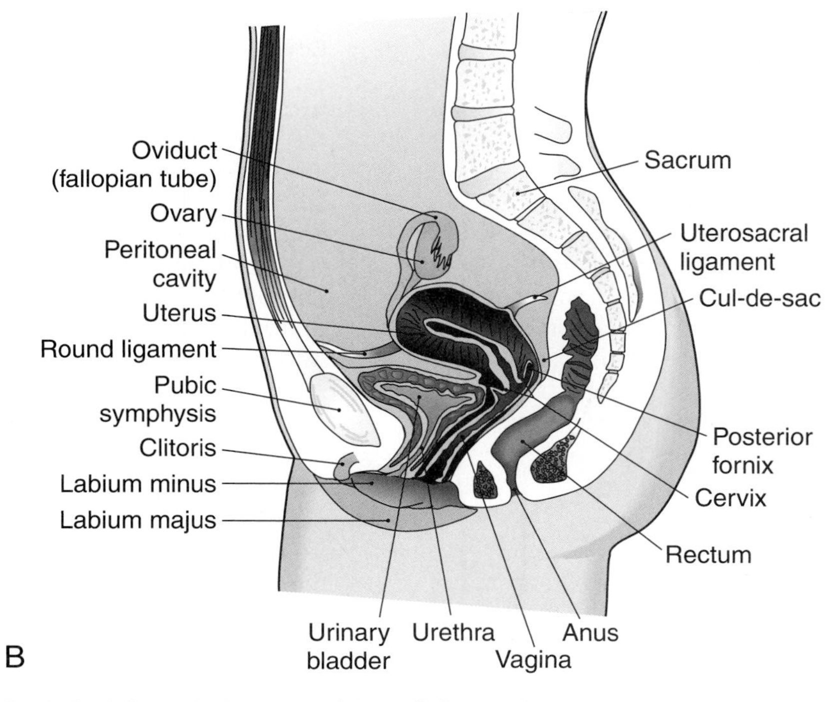

FIGURE 5-14 Reproductive system. **A.** Male. **B.** Female. (Used with permission from Cohen BJ, Wood DL. *Memmler's Structure and Function of the Human Body.* (2000). 7th ed. Philadelphia: Lippincott Williams & Wilkins, pp. 314, 321.)

and is cleared from the blood by the kidneys. The creatinine clearance test measures the rate that creatinine is cleared from the blood by the kidneys as a test of kidney function. Alkaline phosphatase is a skeletal system test. Lactic dehydrogenase is a muscular system test. Rapid plasma reagin is a reproductive system test.
Review: Yes ☐ No ☐

82. Answer: c
Why: Glomeruli are the filtering structures in the nephrons. Ureters are the tubes that carry urine from the kidneys to the bladder (see the Urinary System, Fig. 5-15). The prostate is a male reproductive system structure, but the axons and myelin sheath are nervous system structures. Centrioles, nuclei, and Golgi apparatus are all structures within cells. Renal arteries and the urethra are structures of the urinary system, but neurons are nervous system structures.
Review: Yes ☐ No ☐

83. Answer: a
Why: The primary function of the kidneys, which are a part of the urinary system (Fig. 5-15), is to maintain water and electrolyte balance. (Electrolytes include sodium, potassium, chloride, and bicarbonate.) Heat production is a function of the muscular system. The nervous system and structures in the skin receive environmental stimuli. The circulatory system removes carbon dioxide gas.
Review: Yes ☐ No ☐

84. Answer: a
Why: Cystitis is inflammation of the urinary bladder. Gastritis is inflammation of the stomach lining, a digestive system disorder. Neuritis is nerve inflammation, a nervous system disorder. Pruritus (itching) is typically an integumentary system disorder.
Review: Yes ☐ No ☐

85. Answer: b
Why: Renin is an enzyme secreted by the kidneys that plays a role in the formation of angiotensin, a family of substances that cause vasoconstriction and an increase in blood pressure. Melanin is a pigment produced in the skin. Sebum is an oily substance produced by the sebaceous glands in the skin. Uric acid is an end product of purine metabolism that increases in certain disorders such as gout, a skeletal system disorder.
Review: Yes ☐ No ☐

86. Answer: b
Why: Glomeruli are tufts of capillaries within the nephrons of the kidneys that filter water and dissolved substances, including wastes, from the blood. Fallopian tubes are female reproductive system structures. Ureters are the two tubes (one per kidney) that carry urine from the kidneys to the bladder.
Review: Yes ☐ No ☐

87. Answer: a
Why: An arterial blood gas (ABG) test assesses a patient's oxygenation and ventilation, which are respiratory system functions. A potassium hydroxide (KOH) prep is typically an integumentary system test. Thyroid-stimulating hormone (TSH) is a thyroid function test. Urinalysis (UA) is a urinary system test.
Review: Yes ☐ No ☐

88. Answer: d
Why: Internal respiration takes place in the tissues. During internal respiration, oxygen from the bloodstream enters the cells in the tissues, and carbon dioxide from the tissues enters the bloodstream to be carried back to the lungs. During external respiration, oxygen enters the blood in the lungs and carbon dioxide exits the bloodstream in the lungs.
Review: Yes ☐ No ☐

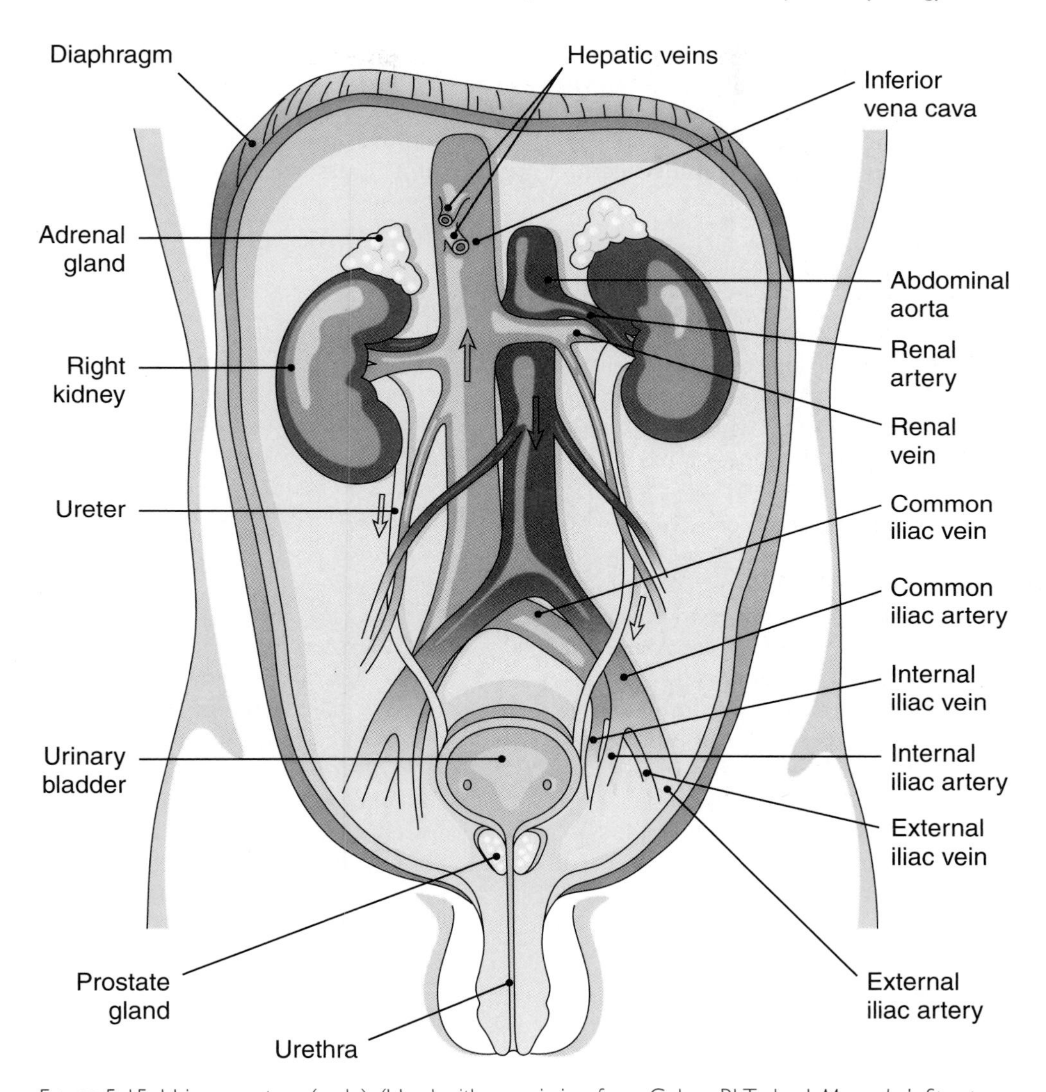

FIGURE 5-15 Urinary system (male). (Used with permission from Cohen BJ, Taylor J. *Memmler's Structure and Function of the Human Body.* 8th ed. 2005. Philadelphia: Lippincott Williams & Wilkins, p. 338.)

89. Answer: b
Why: Normal blood pH is maintained within a narrow range of 7.35 to 7.45. A decrease below normal levels results in acidosis. An increase above normal levels is alkalosis. Both are dangerous conditions.
Review: Yes ☐ No ☐

90. Answer: a
Why: Carbon dioxide (CO_2) levels play a major role in acid-base balance. As CO_2 levels increase, blood pH decreases (becomes more acidic), which can lead to a condition called acidosis.
Review: Yes ☐ No ☐

91. Answer: c
Why: The ability of oxygen to combine with a protein in red blood cells called hemoglobin increases the oxygen-carrying capacity of the blood. Hemoglobin combined with oxygen is called oxyhemoglobin.
Review: Yes ☐ No ☐

92. Answer: d
Why: Infection with respiratory syncytial virus causes acute respiratory problems in children. Cystic fibrosis, emphysema, and *Mycobacterium tuberculosis* can cause respiratory distress in children but are not nearly as common.
Review: Yes ☐ No ☐

93. Answer: a
Why: Bronchioles are small branches of the bronchi. The epiglottis is the structure that covers the entrance of the larynx during swallowing. The pleura are thin layers of membrane that encase the lungs. All of these structures are part of the respiratory system (Fig. 5-16). The calcaneus, mandible, and phalanges are skeletal system bones. The corium, corneum, and adipose cells are structures of the skin. The neurons, meninges, and myelin sheath are nervous system structures.
Review: Yes ☐ No ☐

94. Answer: a
Why: The alveoli, bronchi, larynx, and trachea are all respiratory system (Fig. 5-16) structures, but the exchange of oxygen and carbon dioxide occurs through the walls of the alveoli in the lungs.
Review: Yes ☐ No ☐

95. Answer: d
Why: Partial pressure (P) is the pressure exerted by one gas in a mixture of gases. Whether oxygen or carbon dioxide associates (combines) with or disassociates (releases) from hemoglobin depends on the partial pressure of each gas. In the tissues, the PO_2 of oxygen is decreased, so oxygen releases from hemoglobin and defuses into the tissues. PCO_2 is increased in the tissues, so carbon dioxide from the tissues associates with hemoglobin.
Review: Yes ☐ No ☐

96. Answer: d
Why: Surfactant is a fluid substance that coats the thin walls of the alveoli to help keep them from collapsing. Premature infants often lack or do not have sufficient surfactant to keep their lungs from collapsing. The resulting condition is called infant respiratory distress syndrome (IRDS).
Review: Yes ☐ No ☐

97. Answer: d
Why: Tuberculosis (TB) is caused by *Mycobacterium tuberculosis,* a microorganism that is called an acid-fast bacillus (AFB) because it is not decolorized by acid-alcohol after being stained with a dark dye. Chronic obstructive pulmonary disease (COPD) is a condition associated with breathing difficulties resulting from lung damage. Infant respiratory distress syndrome (IRDS) is a condition caused by a lack of surfactant. RSV stands for respiratory syncytial virus, a virus that affects the lungs.
Review: Yes ☐ No ☐

98. Answer: b
Why: Dyspnea is the medical term for difficult breathing. (The prefix *dys-* means "difficult." *Pnea* means "breathing.") Asthma is a condition characterized by dyspnea accompanied by wheezing. Emphysema is a chronic obstructive pulmonary disease. Pneumonia is inflammation of the lungs most commonly caused by bacteria, viruses, or chemical irritation.
Review: Yes ☐ No ☐

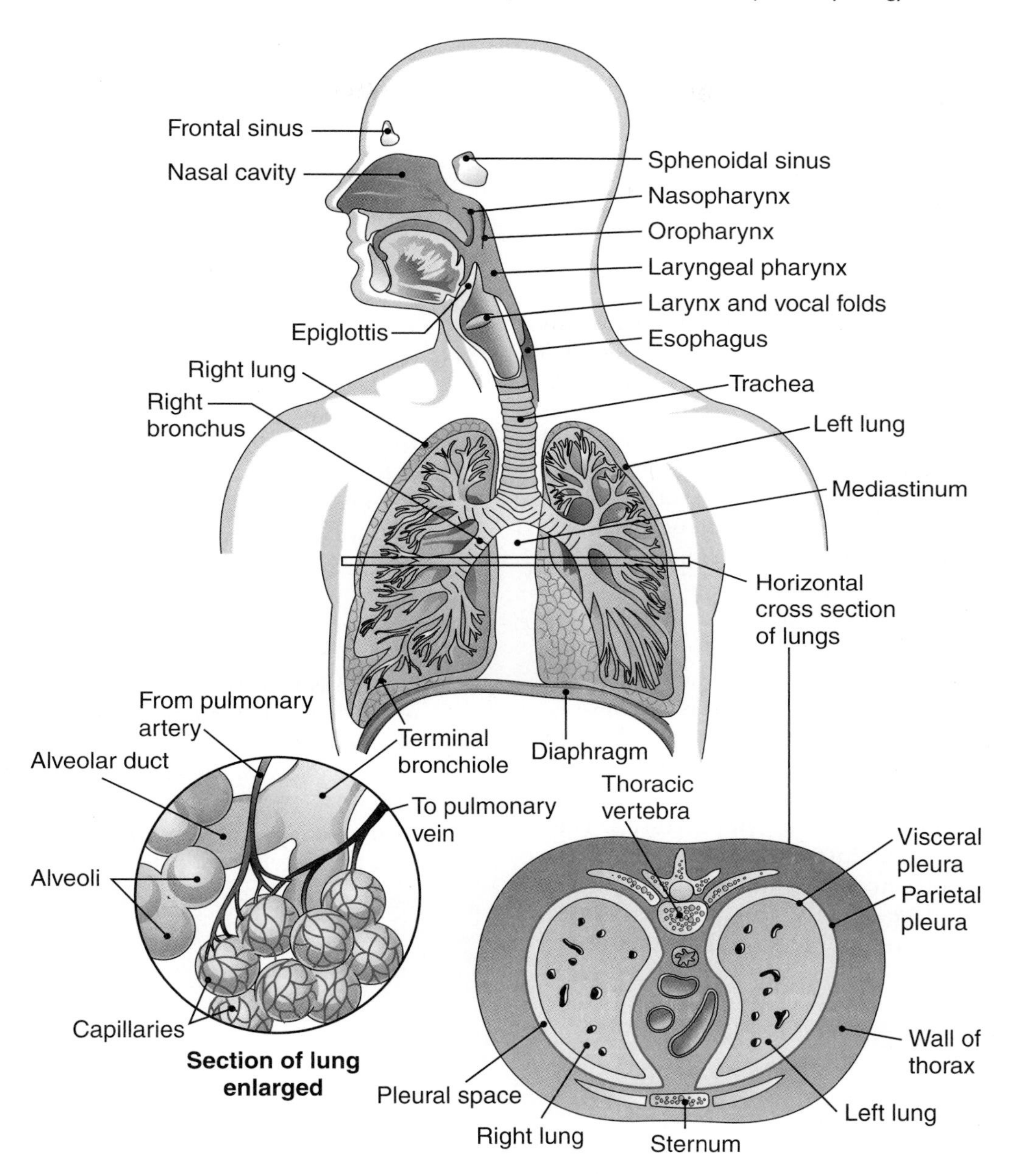

FIGURE 5-16 Respiratory system. (Used with permission from Cohen BJ, Taylor J. *Memmler's Structure and Function of the Human Body*. 8th ed. 2005. Philadelphia: Lippincott Williams & Wilkins, p. 291.)

99. Answer: b
Why: The nervous system controls and coordinates the activities of all body systems by means of electrical impulses and chemical substances sent to and received from all parts of the body.
Review: Yes ☐ No ☐

100. Answer: a
Why: Functions of the digestive system (Fig. 5-13) include taking in food, breaking it down into usable components, and eliminating waste products from this process.
Review: Yes ☐ No ☐

101. Answer: c
Why: Hyperglycemia is the medical term for abnormally increased blood sugar. The prefix *hyper-* means too much or high. *Glyc* is the word root for glucose (sugar). The suffix-*emia* means "blood condition." Diabetes mellitus is a disorder characterized by abnormal glucose metabolism. Diabetes insipidus is a disorder characterized by abnormally increased urination. Hyperinsulinism is an excess of insulin in the blood.
Review: Yes ☐ No ☐

102. Answer: b
Why: The endocrine system is a series of glands that produce hormones and release them directly into the bloodstream. The circulatory system is primarily composed of the heart, blood, and lymph vessels. The glands of the integumentary system release their substances through ducts leading to the surface of the skin. The respiratory system is responsible for delivering oxygen to the cells and removing carbon dioxide from the cells.
Review: Yes ☐ No ☐

103. Answer: a
Why: Pancreatitis means inflammation of the pancreas, which is an accessory organ of the digestive system (Fig. 5-13).
Review: Yes ☐ No ☐

104. Answer: b
Why: Hormones are powerful chemical substances secreted directly into the bloodstream by endocrine system glands. Individual endocrine glands secrete unique hormones that control specific body functions.
Review: Yes ☐ No ☐

105. Answer: c
Why: Hematopoiesis (also called hemopoiesis) is the production and development of the formed elements (blood cells and platelets). Hematopoiesis occurs in the bone marrow of the skeletal system. The urinary system produces the hormone erythropoietin, which stimulates erythrocyte (red blood cell) production.
Review: Yes ☐ No ☐

THE CIRCULATORY SYSTEM

CHAPTER

study tip

Questions in this chapter test the ability to identify and describe cardiovascular system components and the functions, structures, disorders, and diagnostic tests associated with them. Questions also cover knowledge of blood types, the different kinds of blood specimens, and the coagulation process that helps protect the system from blood loss.

overview

This chapter assesses knowledge of the circulatory system, which consists of the cardiovascular system (heart, blood, and blood vessels) and the lymphatic system (lymph, lymph vessels, and nodes). A thorough knowledge of this system is especially important to the phlebotomist who must access it when collect blood specimens for analysis. It also helps the phlebotomist understand the importance of the many tests associated with it.

REVIEW QUESTIONS

Choose the BEST answer.

1. In numerical order, the structures indicated by numbers 1 and 8 in Fig. 6-1 are the:
   a. aortic arch and the left pulmonary arteries.
   b. aortic arch and the right pulmonary arteries.
   c. left pulmonary artery and left pulmonary veins.
   d. superior vena cava and right pulmonary arteries.

2. In numerical order, the structures indicated by numbers 11 and 17 in Fig. 6-1 are the:
   a. left pulmonary arteries and right pulmonary veins.
   b. left pulmonary veins and the arch of the aorta.

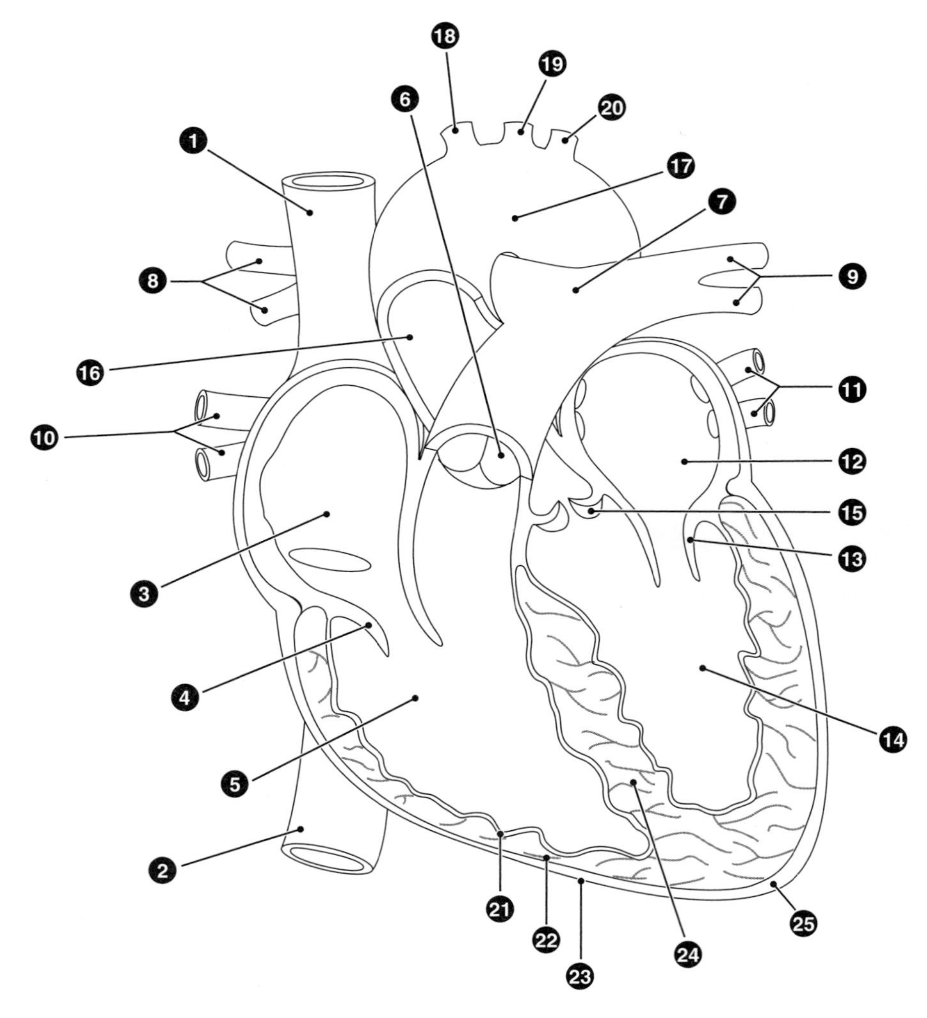

FIGURE 6-1 Heart and great vessels. (Used with permission from Cohen BJ, Hull KL *Study Guide for Memmler's The Human Body in Health and Disease.* (2005). 10th ed. Philadelphia: Lippincott Williams & Wilkins, p. 225.)

c. right pulmonary arteries and superior vena cava.
d. right pulmonary veins and inferior vena cava.

3. In numerical order, the structures indicated by numbers 4 and 15 in Fig. 6-1 are the:
a. aortic valve and the bicuspid valve.
b. mitral valve and the pulmonic valve.
c. right and left atrioventricular valves.
d. tricuspid valve and the aortic valve.

4. In numerical order, the structures indicated by numbers 5 and 12 in Fig. 6-1 are the:
a. left atrium and right ventricle.
b. left ventricle and right atrium.
c. right atrium and left ventricle.
d. right ventricle and left atrium.

5. Which of the following is a function of the circulatory system?
a. carry oxygen to the tissue cells
b. convey afferent nerve impulses
c. excrete wastes from the body
d. produce the formed elements

6. The heart is surrounded by a thin, fluid-filled sac called the:
a. endocardium.
b. epicardium.
c. myocardium.
d. pericardium.

7. The middle layer of the heart is called the:
a. endocardium.
b. epicardium.
c. myocardium.
d. pericardium.

8. How many chambers are in the human heart?
a. 1
b. 2
c. 4
d. 6

9. This heart chamber delivers oxygen-rich blood to the ascending aorta.
a. left atrium
b. left ventricle
c. right atrium
d. right ventricle

10. This heart chamber receives blood from the systemic system.
a. left atrium
b. left ventricle
c. right atrium
d. right ventricle

11. The semilunar valves are located:
a. at the exits of both of the ventricles.
b. between the atria and the ventricles.
c. where the aortic arch becomes the aorta.
d. within the veins of the systemic system.

12. The right atrioventricular valve is also called the:
a. bicuspid valve.
b. pulmonic valve.
c. semilunar valve.
d. tricuspid valve.

13. This valve gets its name from a resemblance to a bishop's hat.
a. aortic valve.
b. mitral valve.
c. pulmonic valve.
d. tricuspid valve.

14. The structure that separates the right and left ventricles of the heart is called the:
a. atrioventricular septum.
b. interatrial septum.
c. interventricular septum.
d. myocardial septum.

15. The heart muscle gets its blood supply from the:
    a. carotid arteries.
    b. coronary arteries.
    c. pulmonary arteries.
    d. pulmonary veins.

16. These structures keep the atrioventricular valves from flipping back into the atria.
    a. chordae tendineae
    b. myocardial septa
    c. Purkinje fibers
    d. semilunar cusps

17. Myocardial ischemia is a condition that results from:
    a. complete blockage of a coronary artery.
    b. death of a portion of myocardial tissue.
    c. malfunction of an atrioventricular valve.
    d. partial obstruction of a coronary artery.

18. The medical term for a heart attack is myocardial:
    a. arrhythmia.
    b. infarction.
    c. ischemia.
    d. tachycardia.

19. The heart's "pacemaker" is the:
    a. bundle of His.
    b. chorda tendinea.
    c. papillary muscle.
    d. sinoatrial node.

20. This is an abbreviation for a test that traces the electrical impulses of the heart.
    a. ALT
    b. ECG
    c. EEG
    d. TnT

21. One complete contraction and subsequent relaxation of the heart is called one cardiac:
    a. cycle.
    b. diastole.
    c. output.
    d. systole.

22. Systole is the:
    a. closing of the semilunar valves.
    b. completion of one cardiac cycle.
    c. contracting phase of the heart.
    d. relaxation stage of the heart.

23. A cardiac cycle lasts approximately:
    a. 0.5 seconds.
    b. 0.8 seconds.
    c. 1.5 seconds.
    d. 8.0 seconds.

24. On an electrocardiogram, atrial activity is represented by the:
    a. P wave.
    b. QRS complex.
    c. T wave.
    d. T and P waves.

25. On an electrocardiogram, which wave represents the activity of the ventricles?
    a. P
    b. P and T
    c. QRS and P
    d. QRS and T

26. The first sound of the heartbeat is created by the:
    a. closing of the atrioventricular valves.
    b. opening of the semilunar valves.
    c. resonation of the chordae tendineae.
    d. ventricular muscle contraction echo.

27. Abnormal heart sounds are called:
    a. arrhythmias.
    b. extrasystoles.
    c. fibrillations.
    d. murmurs.

28. Average normal heart rate is:
    a. 63 beats per minute.
    b. 72 beats per minute.
    c. 81 beats per minute.
    d. 96 beats per minute.

29. An abnormally fast heart rate is called:
    a. bradycardia.
    b. extrasystole.
    c. fibrillation.
    d. tachycardia.

30. A person's pulse is created by a wave of pressure caused by:
    a. atrial contraction.
    b. atrial relaxation.
    c. ventricular contraction.
    d. ventricular relaxation.

31. The force exerted by the blood on the walls of the blood vessels is called:
    a. blood pressure.
    b. cardiac output.
    c. heart rhythm.
    d. pulse rate.

32. The technical term for this device is sphygmomanometer.
    a. artificial pacemaker
    b. brain wave detector
    c. blood pressure cuff
    d. heart wave monitor

33. Which of the following is a normal blood pressure reading?
    a. 60/40 mm Hg
    b. 80/120 mm Hg
    c. 100/120 mm Hg
    d. 120/80 mm Hg

34. Systolic pressure measures pressure in the arteries during:
    a. atrial contraction.
    b. atrial relaxation.
    c. ventricular contraction.
    d. ventricular relaxation.

35. An infection of the lining of the heart is called:
    a. angina pectoris.
    b. aortic stenosis.
    c. endocarditis.
    d. pericarditis.

36. Which of the following are abbreviations for cardiac enzyme tests?
    a. ALP, ALT
    b. BUN, PT
    c. CK, LDH
    d. GTT, ESR

37. The pulmonary circulation takes blood to the:
    a. arteries in the heart muscle.
    b. heart from the body tissues.
    c. internal organs to the body.
    d. lungs and back to the heart.

38. All of the following blood vessels are part of the systemic circulation EXCEPT:
    a. brachial artery.
    b. cephalic vein.
    c. pulmonary artery.
    d. inferior vena cava.

39. Blood vessels that carry blood away from the heart are called:
    a. arteries.
    b. capillaries.
    c. veins.
    d. venules.

40. Which of the following veins carry oxygen-rich blood?
    a. pulmonary
    b. saphenous
    c. subclavian
    d. vena cava

41. Normal systemic arterial blood is:
    a. dark blue.
    b. bright red.
    c. bluish red.
    d. dark red.

42. The largest artery in the body is the:
    a. aorta.
    b. carotid.
    c. femoral.
    d. vena cava.

43. The longest vein in the body is the:
    a. great saphenous.
    b. median cubital.
    c. inferior vena cava.
    d. right pulmonary.

44. What keeps the blood moving through the venous system?
    a. expansion and contraction of the systemic arteries.
    b. movement of fluid throughout the lymphatic system.
    c. pressure caused by contraction of the ventricles.
    d. skeletal muscle movement and valves in the veins.

45. The smallest branches of veins are called:
    a. arterioles.
    b. capillaries.
    c. lumina.
    d. venules.

46. These are tiny blood vessels that are only one cell thick.
    a. arteries
    b. arterioles
    c. capillaries
    d. venules

47. The tunica adventitia is the:
    a. external layer of a blood vessel.
    b. inside lining of a blood vessel.
    c. internal layer of a blood vessel.
    d. middle layer of a blood vessel.

48. The internal space of a blood vessel is called the:
    a. interna.
    b. intima.
    c. lumen.
    d. media.

49. The layers of arteries differ from the layers of veins in that the:
    a. inner lining is much thicker in veins.
    b. middle layer of veins is more elastic.
    c. muscle layer is thicker in arteries.
    d. outer layer of arteries is thinner.

50. Oxygen and nutrients diffuse through the walls of the:
    a. alveoli.
    b. arterioles.
    c. capillaries.
    d. venules.

51. Identify the structure on the right in Fig. 6-2 from the following choices.
    a. artery
    b. capillary
    c. lymph vessel
    d. vein

52. The right ventricle delivers blood to the:
    a. aorta
    b. left atrium
    c. pulmonary artery
    d. pulmonary vein

53. Which of the following blood vessels carries oxygenated blood?
    a. brachial vein
    b. pulmonary vein
    c. pulmonary artery
    d. inferior vena cava

54. Which of the following blood vessels are listed in the proper direction of blood flow?
    a. arteries, arterioles, capillaries
    b. arterioles, venules, capillaries
    c. capillaries, arterioles, arteries
    d. veins, venules, capillaries

55. The antecubital fossa is located:
    a. anterior and distal to the elbow.
    b. anterior and distal to the wrist.
    c. posterior and proximal to the elbow.
    d. posterior and proximal to the wrist.

56. All of the following are antecubital veins EXCEPT:
    a. accessory cephalic.
    b. median.

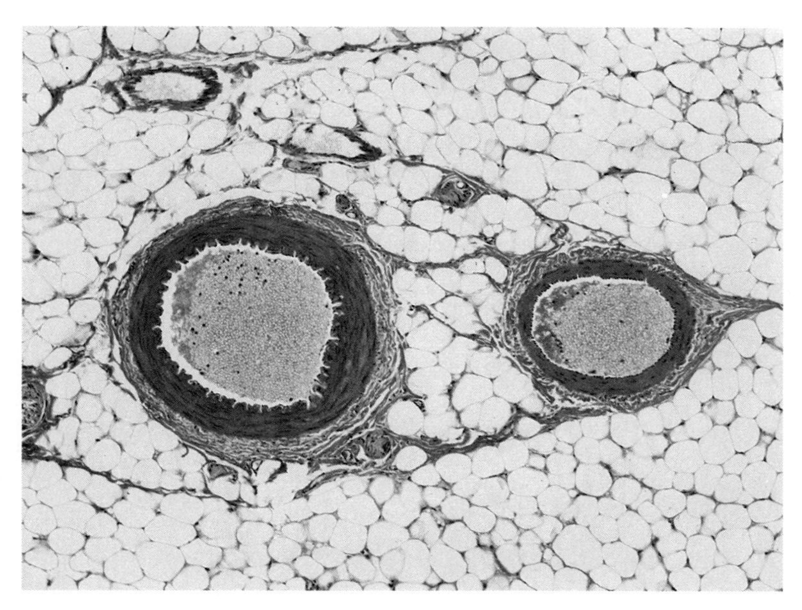

FIGURE 6-2 (Used with permission from Cormack DH. *Essential Histology.* (1993). Philadelphia: JB Lippincott, Plate 11-1.)

c. median basilic.
d. subclavian.

57. In numerical order, the veins identified by numbers 1, 6, and 7 in Fig. 6-3A are the:
a. basilic, median cubital, and cephalic.
b. cephalic, basilic, and median cubital.
c. median cubital, cephalic, and basilic.
d. subclavian, median cubital, and basilic.

58. In numerical order, the veins identified by numbers 16, 18, and 19 in Fig. 6-3B are:
a. accessory cephalic, median, and median basilic.
b. cephalic, median basilic, and accessory basilic.
c. median basilic, accessory cephalic, and median.
d. median cephalic, median, and median basilic.

59. In numerical order, the veins identified by numbers 26, 27, and 28 in Fig. 6-3C are the:
a. basilic, dorsal metacarpal, and cephalic.
b. brachial, dorsal metacarpal, and basilic.
c. cephalic, dorsal metacarpal, and basilic.
d. median, dorsal metacarpal, and cephalic.

60. The basilic vein is the last choice for venipuncture for all of the following reasons EXCEPT that it is:
a. fixed in the surrounding tissues.
b. located close to a major nerve.
c. more painful when punctured.
d. very near the brachial artery.

61. This major vein merges with the brachiocephalic vein in the chest.
a. cephalic
b. popliteal
c. saphenous
d. subclavian

62. Two median cutaneous nerves lie close to this vein.
a. basilic
b. cephalic
c. median
d. radial

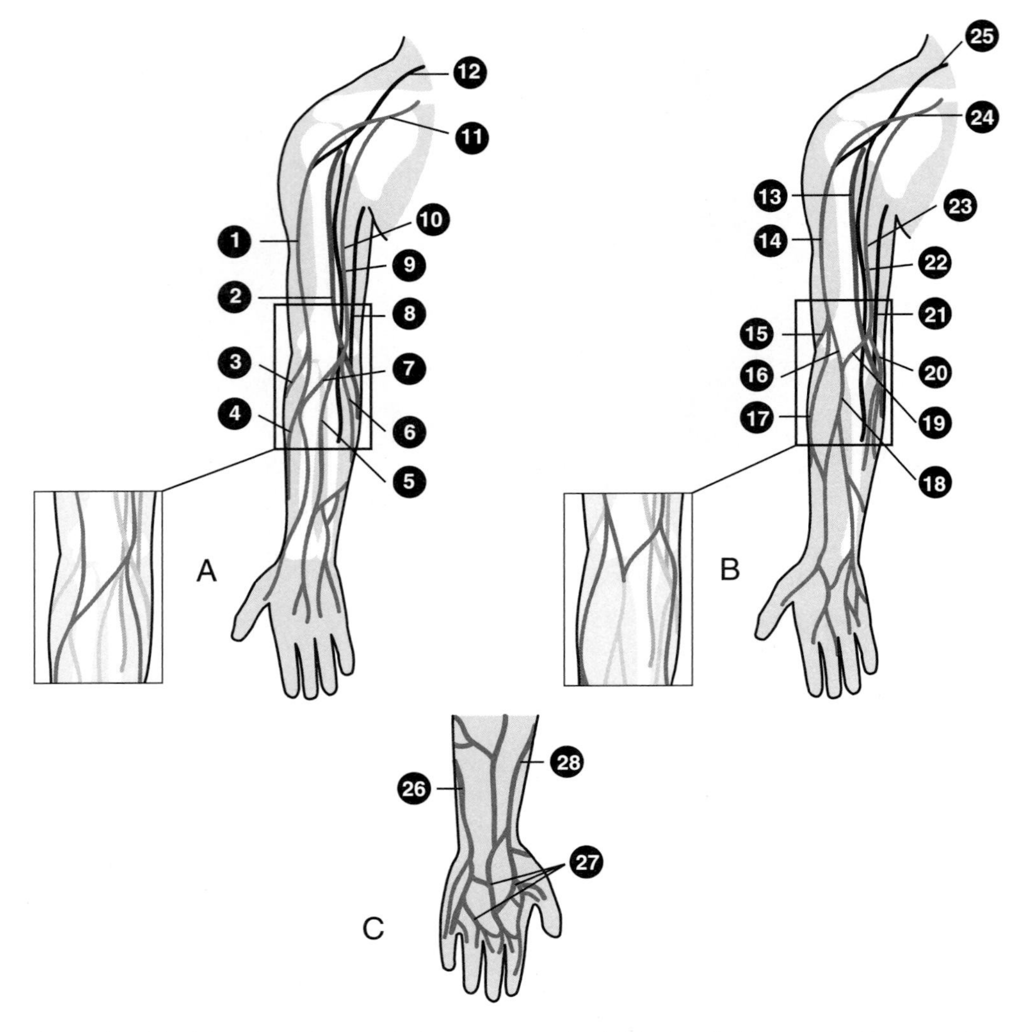

FIGURE 6-3 Principle veins of the arm including major antecubital veins. **A.** H-shaped pattern of antecubital veins of the right arm in anatomic position. **B.** M-shaped pattern of antecubital veins of the right arm in anatomic position. **C.** Right forearm, wrist, and hand veins in prone position.

63. Which of the following veins are listed in the proper order of selection for venipuncture?
    a. basilic, cephalic, median cubital
    b. cephalic, median cubital, basilic
    c. median, median basilic, cephalic
    d. median cubital, cephalic, basilic

64. When the hand is prone, the antecubital portion of the cephalic vein is normally located in line with the:
    a. index finger.
    b. little finger.
    c. radial artery.
    d. thumb.

65. According to the Clinical and Laboratory Standards Institute (CLSI), venipuncture should not be performed on leg, ankle or foot veins unless:
    a. both arms have intravenous lines or other vascular devices.
    b. permission of the patient's physician is obtained.
    c. there are no acceptable antecubital or hand veins.
    d. the patient does not have any coagulation problems.

66. The popliteal vein is found in the:
    a. arm.
    b. hand.
    c. heart.
    d. leg.

67. This is the medical term for a blood clot circulating in the bloodstream.
    a. aneurysm
    b. embolism
    c. embolus
    d. thrombus

68. The medical term for vein inflammation is:
    a. embolism
    b. hemostasis
    c. phlebitis
    d. thrombosis

69. Which of the following is an abbreviation used for a vascular system test?
    a. ADH
    b. CSF
    c. DIC
    d. RPR

70. Lipid accumulation on the intima of an artery is called:
    a. atherosclerosis.
    b. cholesterol.
    c. endocarditis.
    d. lipemia.

71. Which of the following is a localized dilation or bulging of an artery?
    a. aneurysm
    b. embolism
    c. phlebitis
    d. thrombus

72. Inflammation of a vein in conjunction with formation of a blood clot is called:
    a. atherosclerosis.
    b. phlebosclerosis.
    c. thrombophlebitis.
    d. vasculitis.

73. Normal adult blood volume is approximately:
    a. 2 L.
    b. 4 L.
    c. 5 L.
    d. 8 L.

74. The normal composition of blood is approximately:
    a. 10% plasma, 90% formed elements.
    b. 30% plasma, 70% formed elements.
    c. 55% plasma, 45% formed elements.
    d. 90% plasma, 10% formed elements.

75. Normal plasma is a:
    a. clear, colorless, watery fluid containing about 10% solutes.
    b. clear or slightly hazy, pale yellow fluid that is 90% water.
    c. cloudy, completely colorless fluid containing 45% solutes.
    d. slightly hazy, pale yellow fluid that is close to 55% water.

76. Which of the following are *not* normally found in the blood?
    a. antibodies
    b. bacteria
    c. blood cells
    d. platelets

77. Which blood cell contains a nucleus?
    a. erythrocyte
    b. leukocyte
    c. thrombocyte
    d. reticulocyte

78. A reticulocyte count identifies immature:
    a. lymphocytes.
    b. neutrophils.
    c. red blood cells.
    d. white blood cells.

79. Which blood cell increases in allergic reactions and pinworm infestations?
    a. basophil
    b. eosinophil
    c. lymphocyte
    d. neutrophil

80. How large is a normal erythrocyte?
    a. 4–5 microns
    b. 7–8 microns
    c. 8–10 microns
    d. 10–12 microns

81. Which of the following would be considered a normal erythrocyte count?
    a. 4.5 million/mm^3
    b. 6.0 million/mm^3
    c. 10.5 million/mm^3
    d. 20.0 million/mm^3

82. Red blood cells are produced in the:
    a. bloodstream.
    b. bone marrow.
    c. lymph nodes.
    d. thymus gland.

83. The primary function of red blood cells is to:
    a. deliver nutrients to the body tissues.
    b. produce antibodies to combat infection.
    c. transport carbon dioxide to the lungs.
    d. transport oxygen to cells in the body.

84. A leukocyte is a:
    a. lymphatic cell.
    b. platelet stem cell.
    c. red blood cell.
    d. white blood cell.

85. Which blood cell has the ability to pass through blood vessel walls?
    a. erythrocyte
    b. leukocyte
    c. reticulocyte
    d. thrombocyte

86. Which type of cell destroys pathogens by phagocytosis?
    a. erythrocyte
    b. neutrophil
    c. red blood cell
    d. thrombocyte

87. Which of the following is a short term for neutrophils?
    a. eos
    b. basos
    c. monos
    d. polys

88. Which formed element is the first to play a role in sealing an injury to a blood vessel?
    a. erythrocyte
    b. leukocyte
    c. platelet
    d. reticulocyte

89. Which of the following is an anuclear, biconcave disc?
    a. erythrocyte
    b. granulocyte
    c. leukocyte
    d. thrombocyte

90. Which type of cell is sometimes called a macrophage?
    a. eosinophil
    b. basophil
    c. lymphocyte
    d. monocyte

91. Some of these cells give rise to plasma cells.
 a. eosinophils
 b. lymphocytes
 c. monocytes
 d. neutrophils

92. Which of the following would be considered a normal platelet count?
 a. $20{,}000/mm^3$
 b. $70{,}000/mm^3$
 c. $300{,}000/mm^3$
 d. $600{,}000/mm^3$

93. Platelets are also called:
 a. erythrocytes.
 b. leukocytes.
 c. neutrophils.
 d. thrombocytes.

94. A platelet is actually a part of a bone marrow cell called a:
 a. granulocyte.
 b. macrophage.
 c. megakaryocyte.
 d. T lymphocyte.

95. Which of the following are normally the most numerous of the formed elements?
 a. platelets
 b. red blood cells
 c. reticulocytes
 d. white blood cells

96. A person's blood type is determined by the presence or absence of certain types of:
 a. antibodies on the surface of the red blood cells.
 b. antibodies on the surface of the white blood cells.
 c. antigens on the surface of the red blood cells.
 d. antigens on the surface of the white blood cells.

97. To prevent sensitization, Rh immunoglobulin is given to:
 a. pregnant women who bleed throughout the pregnancy.
 b. Rh-negative mothers who deliver Rh-positive babies.
 c. Rh-positive babies immediately after they are born.
 d. Rh-positive mothers who deliver Rh-negative babies.

98. A woman who becomes "sensitized" to the Rh factor:
 a. can produce antibodies against the Rh antigen.
 b. has Rh antigen circulating in her bloodstream.
 c. should not try to have more than one child.
 d. will test Rh-positive for months afterward.

99. A person who has A-negative blood has red blood cells that:
 a. have the A antigen and lack the Rh antigen.
 b. have both the A antigen and the Rh antigen.
 c. lack the A antigen and have the Rh antigen.
 d. lack both the A antigen and the Rh antigen.

100. Hemolytic disease of the newborn is most often caused by:
 a. ABO incompatibility between mother and infant.
 b. incompatible blood given to the infant in utero.
 c. previous sensitization of an Rh-negative mother.
 d. Rh incompatibility between the infant and father.

101. A whole blood specimen consists of:
 a. aggregated blood cells and water.
 b. blood cells suspended in serum.
 c. plasma and the formed elements.
 d. serum and clotted red blood cells.

102. The liquid portion of a clotted specimen is called:
 a. fibrinogen.
 b. plasma.
 c. saline.
 d. serum.

103. A whole blood specimen has an abnormally large buffy coat. This is an indication that the patient has:
 a. an elevated leukocyte or platelet count.
 b. an increased amount of red blood cells.
 c. large numbers of bacteria in the blood.
 d. recently eaten a meal with a lot of fat.

104. Fig. 6-4 shows a centrifuged whole blood specimen. Identify the portion of the specimen indicated by arrow 1.
 a. buffy coat
 b. plasma
 c. serum
 d. red blood cells

105. Identify the portion of the specimen indicated by arrow 2 in Fig. 6-4.
 a. buffy coat
 b. plasma
 c. serum
 d. red blood cells

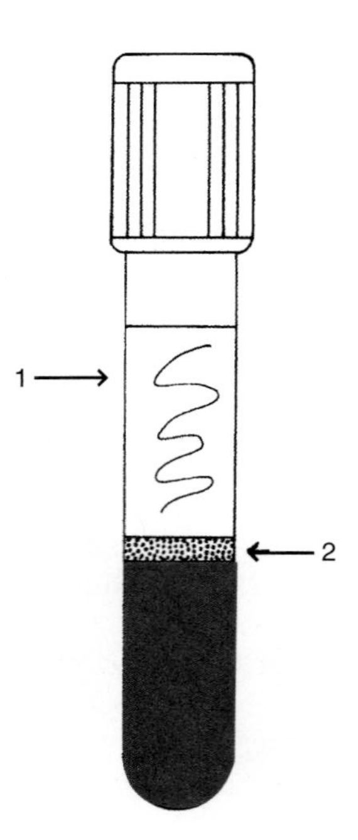

FIGURE 6-4 Centrifuged plasma specimen.

106. How can you visually tell serum from plasma?
 a. plasma is yellow, serum is colorless
 b. serum is clear, plasma is cloudy
 c. serum is fluid, plasma is gel-like
 d. you cannot visually tell them apart

107. A blood smear made using an ethylenediaminetetraacetate (EDTA) specimen should be prepared within:
 a. 5 minutes.
 b. 30 minutes.
 c. 60 minutes.
 d. 12 hours.

108. Most tests in this department are performed on plasma specimens.
 a. coagulation
 b. cytology
 c. hematology
 d. immunology

109. It is preferable to perform most STAT chemistry tests on plasma rather than serum because plasma:
 a. can be tested a lot sooner.
 b. gives more accurate results.
 c. is more stable than serum.
 d. tests require less specimen.

110. This is the abbreviation for a test that is always performed on whole blood.
 a. BUN
 b. CBC
 c. LDL
 d. PTT

111. This is the abbreviation for a test that can be done on plasma.
 a. CBC
 b. ESR
 c. Hgb
 d. PTT

112. All of the following statements are true of serum EXCEPT that it:
 a. can be used for most chemistry tests.
 b. contains the clotting factor fibrinogen.

c. is collected in a nonanticoagulant tube
d. normally is a clear, pale yellow fluid

113. A person with thrombocytosis has abnormally:
a. decreased platelets.
b. functioning platelets.
c. increased platelets.
d. large-sized platelets.

114. A disease that is often characterized by an abnormally low red blood cell count is:
a. anemia.
b. leukemia.
c. neutropenia.
d. polycythemia.

115. Which of the following is the abbreviation for a test of the formed elements?
a. ASO
b. CBC
c. lytes
d. SPEP

116. An abnormal increase in white blood cells is called:
a. leukemia.
b. leukocytosis.
c. leukopenia.
d. leukopoiesis.

117. All of the following tests are used to diagnose blood cell disorders EXCEPT:
a. creatinine.
b. ferritin.
c. hematocrit.
d. hemoglobin.

118. The process of coagulation is also called:
a. hemolysis.
b. hemopoiesis.
c. hemostasis.
d. homeostasis.

119. The ability of platelets to stick to each other is called platelet:
a. aggregation.
b. adhesion.
c. cohesion.
d. inhibition.

120. This ion is essential to the coagulation process.
a. calcium
b. chloride
c. potassium
d. sodium

121. The extrinsic pathway of coagulation is initiated by:
a. activation of plasma coagulation factors.
b. commencement of platelet aggregation.
c. events occurring within the bloodstream.
d. injury with tissue thromboplastin release.

122. The first stage in the hemostatic process is:
a. fibrin formation.
b. fibrin degradation.
c. platelet adhesion.
d. vasoconstriction.

123. Which stages of the coagulation process are called primary hemostasis?
a. coagulation factor activation and fibrinolysis
b. fibrin clot formation and the coagulation cascade
c. platelet plug formation and fibrin clot formation
d. vasoconstriction and platelet plug formation

124. This is the abbreviation for a test that assesses platelet plug formation.
a. BT
b. FDP
c. PT
d. PTT

125. A disorder caused most often by lack of factor VIII is:
a. hemophilia.
b. intravascular coagulation.
c. thrombocytopenia.
d. varicose veins.

126. Coagulation problems may result from liver disease because the liver:
 a. filters impurities from the blood.
 b. manufactures coagulation factors.
 c. removes damaged red blood cells.
 d. stores and releases calcium ions.

127. Which stage of the coagulation process involves the action of the enzyme plasmin?
 a. fibrin clot formation
 b. fibrinolysis
 c. platelet plug formation
 d. vasoconstriction

128. The coagulation process is kept in check by:
 a. fibrin degradation.
 b. natural inhibitors.
 c. plasminogen enzymes.
 d. prothrombin activators.

129. Tests of primary hemostasis include:
 a. bleeding time and platelet count.
 b. D-dimer and partial thromboplastin time.
 c. factor assays and prothrombin time.
 d. fibrin split products and protime.

130. A venipuncture site is normally healed by:
 a. factor VIII activation.
 b. fibrin clot formation.
 c. platelet plug formation.
 d. vasoconstriction.

131. Obstruction of a blood vessel by an embolus:
 a. causes vessel necrosis.
 b. leads to an aneurysm.
 c. results in an embolism.
 d. produces atherosclerosis.

132. Which of the following is a coagulation test?
 a. digoxin
 b. hemogram
 c. myoglobin
 d. protime

133. Lymph fluid is most like:
 a. serum.
 b. plasma.
 c. urine.
 d. whole blood.

134. Lymph fluid originates from excess:
 a. blood plasma.
 b. digestive liquid.
 c. tissue fluid.
 d. urinary filtrate.

135. Lymph fluid keeps moving in the right direction because of:
 a. functioning of the lymphatic ducts.
 b. lymphatic capillary structure.
 c. pressure from the arterial system.
 d. valves within the lymph vessels.

136. Lymphatic system functions include all of the following EXCEPT:
 a. deliver fats to the blood.
 b. make clotting factors.
 c. process lymphocytes.
 d. trap and destroy bacteria.

137. Lymph node tissue has the ability to:
 a. create red blood cells.
 b. produce tissue fluid.
 c. remove impurities.
 d. secrete antibodies.

138. Lymphoid tissue is also found in the:
 a. heart.
 b. kidneys.
 c. lungs.
 d. thymus.

139. A malignant lymphoid tumor is called:
 a. lymphadenopathy.
 b. lymphangitis.
 c. lymphoma.
 d. lymphosarcoma.

140. This test is associated with the lymph system.
 a. carotene
 b. cholinesterase
 c. lipoprotein
 d. mononucleosis

ANSWERS AND EXPLANATIONS

1. Answer: d
   Why: Number 1 points to the superior vena cava, the major vein that returns blood to the heart from the upper part of the body. Number 8 points to the right pulmonary arteries that take blood from the heart to the lungs (Fig. 6-5).
   Review: Yes ☐ No ☐

2. Answer: b
   Why: Number 11 points to the left pulmonary veins that carry oxygen-rich blood from the lungs back to the left atrium of the heart. Number 17 points to the aortic arch, through which oxygenated blood travels from the heart to the systemic system (Fig. 6-5).
   Review: Yes ☐ No ☐

3. Answer: d
   Why: Number 4 points to the tricuspid valve, also called the right atrioventricular valve, because it is between the right atrium and the right ventricle. Number 15 points to the aortic valve located at the exit of the left ventricle, where blood is delivered to the aorta (Fig. 6-5).
   Review: Yes ☐ No ☐

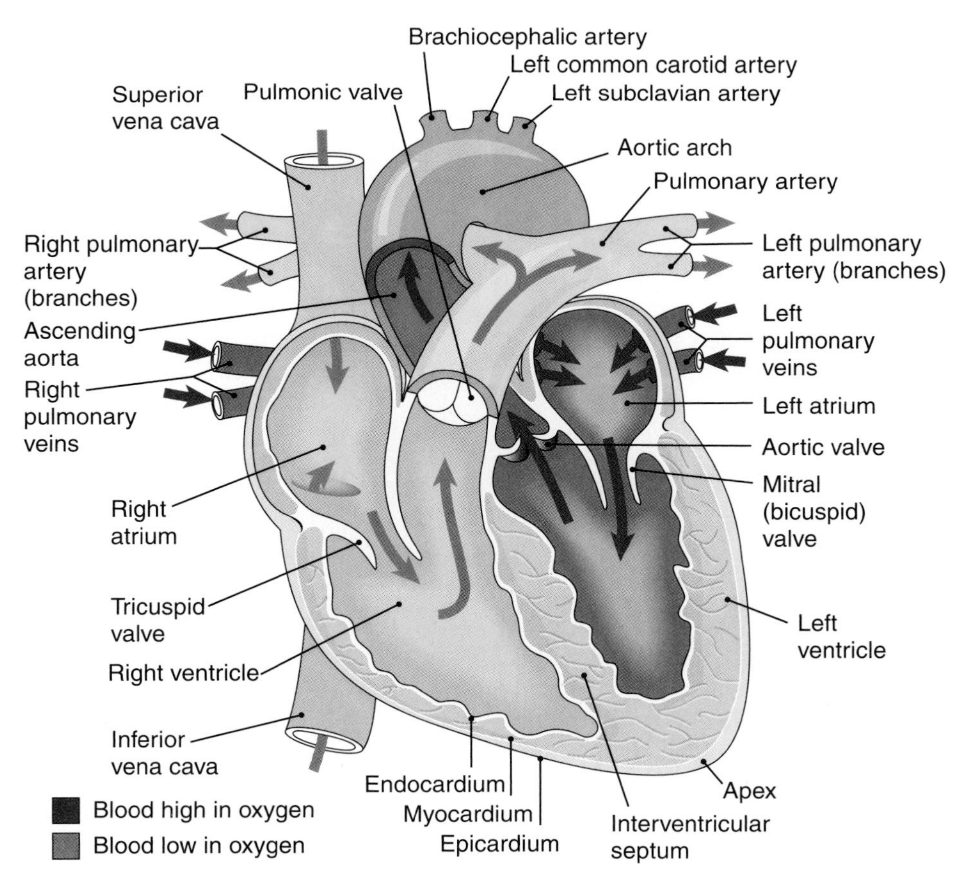

FIGURE 6-5 Heart and great vessels. (Used with permission from Cohen BJ, Taylor JJ. *Memmler's The Human Body in Health and Disease.* (2005). 10th ed. Philadelphia: Lippincott Williams & Wilkins, p. 287.)

4. Answer: d
Why: Number 5 points to the right ventricle, which receives blood from the right atrium and delivers it to the pulmonary system. Number 12 points to the left atrium, which receives oxygen-rich blood from the pulmonary system and delivers it to the left ventricle (Fig. 6-5).
Review: Yes ☐ No ☐

5. Answer: a
Why: A major role of the circulatory system is to carry oxygen to the cells and take carbon dioxide away from the cells to the lungs for expiration. The nervous system conveys nerve impulses. Wastes are primarily excreted by the digestive system. Some waste is excreted by sweat glands of the skin. The formed elements (blood cells) are produced in the bone marrow of the skeletal system.
Review: Yes ☐ No ☐

6. Answer: d
Why: The pericardium is a double-layered sac that encloses the heart. The space between the layers is filled with fluid that reduces friction as the heart beats. The endocardium is a thin membrane lining the inside of the heart. The epicardium is the thin outer layer of the heart. The myocardium is the thick muscular middle layer of the heart.
Review: Yes ☐ No ☐

7. Answer: c
Why: The heart (Fig. 6-5) has three layers. The myocardium is the thick muscular middle layer of the heart. The endocardium, the inner layer, is the thin membrane that lines the inside of the heart. The epicardium is the thin outer layer of the heart. The pericardium is the fluid-filled sac that surrounds the heart.
Review: Yes ☐ No ☐

8. Answer: c
Why: The human heart (Fig. 6-5) has two sides, a right and a left. Each side has two chambers, an upper and a lower. The right and left upper chambers are called atria (singular, atrium) and the right and left lower chambers are called ventricles.
Review: Yes ☐ No ☐

9. Answer: b
Why: The ventricles, the lower chambers of the heart, are called delivering chambers because they deliver blood to the pulmonary and systemic systems. The left ventricle (Fig. 6-5) delivers oxygen-rich blood through the aortic semilunar valve to the ascending aorta, which is the beginning of the systemic system. The right ventricle delivers deoxygenated blood through the pulmonary semilunar valve to the pulmonary artery. The right and left atria receive blood from the systemic and pulmonary systems, respectively.
Review: Yes ☐ No ☐

10. Answer: c
Why: The atria (singular, atrium), the upper chambers of the heart (Fig. 6-5), are called receiving chambers because they receive blood from the systemic and pulmonary systems. The right atrium receives blood from the systemic system via the superior (upper) and inferior (lower) vena cavae. The left atrium receives blood from the pulmonary system. The right and left ventricles deliver blood to the pulmonary and systemic systems, respectively.
Review: Yes ☐ No ☐

11. Answer: a
Why: The valves at the exits of the ventricles (Fig. 6-5) are called semilunar valves because each flap resembles a half-moon. The pulmonary semilunar valve is located at the exit of the right ventricle and the aortic

semilunar valve is located at the exit of the left ventricle. There is no valve between the aortic arch and the aorta. The valves in the veins of the systemic system are similar to semilunar valves but are not called semilunar valves.

Review: Yes ☐ No ☐

12. Answer: d

Why: The right atrioventricular (AV) valve, located between the right atrium and the right ventricle (Fig. 6-5), is also called the tricuspid valve because it has three flaps, or cusps. The bicuspid (two cusps) valve, also called the mitral valve, is located between the left atrium and the left ventricle. The pulmonic valve is located at the exit of the right ventricle. The pulmonic valve and the aortic valve, which are located at the exit of the left atrium, are called semilunar valves because they are crescent-shaped, like a half-moon.

Review: Yes ☐ No ☐

13. Answer: b

Why: The left atrioventricular (AV) valve (Fig. 6-5) is called the bicuspid valve because it has two cusps (flaps). It is also called the mitral valve, because the two cusps resemble a miter, the two-sided pointed hat worn by bishops.

Review: Yes ☐ No ☐

14. Answer: c

Why: A wall that divides two cavities is called a septum. The wall that separates the right and left ventricles of the heart is called the interventricular septum (Fig. 6-5). The interatrial septum separates the right and left atria. The walls of the heart, including the septa, have a thick middle layer of muscle called myocardium. The atrioventricular septum is a small section of septum that separates the right atrium from the left ventricle.

Review: Yes ☐ No ☐

15. Answer: b

Why: The heart does not receive oxygen or nourishment from the blood passing through it. The heart receives its blood supply from the right and left coronary arteries, which are the first branches off of the aorta, just beyond the aortic semilunar valve. The carotid arteries carry blood to the brain. The pulmonary arteries carry blood from the right ventricle to the lungs. The pulmonary veins carry blood from the lungs back to the left atrium.

Review: Yes ☐ No ☐

16. Answer: a

Why: The atrioventricular valves are attached to the walls of the ventricles by thin threads of tissue called chordae tendineae (Fig. 6-6). The chordae tendineae keep the valves from flipping back into the atria, which helps them close properly so that blood does not flow backward into the atria.

Review: Yes ☐ No ☐

17. Answer: d

Why: Partial obstruction of a coronary artery or one of its branches can reduce blood flow to a point where it can no longer meet the oxygen needs of the heart muscle, a condition called myocardial ischemia.

Review: Yes ☐ No ☐

18. Answer: b

Why: A heart attack is the death of heart muscle from lack of oxygen. The medical term for this is myocardial infarction (MI). (Myocardial means "pertaining to the heart muscle." Infarction means "death of tissue resulting from oxygen deprivation.") MI can be caused by complete obstruction of a coronary artery or prolonged ischemia (See answer to question 17). Arrhythmia is an irregularity in the heart rate, rhythm, or beat. Tachycardia is the term for a fast heart rate of more than 100 beats per minute.

Review: Yes ☐ No ☐

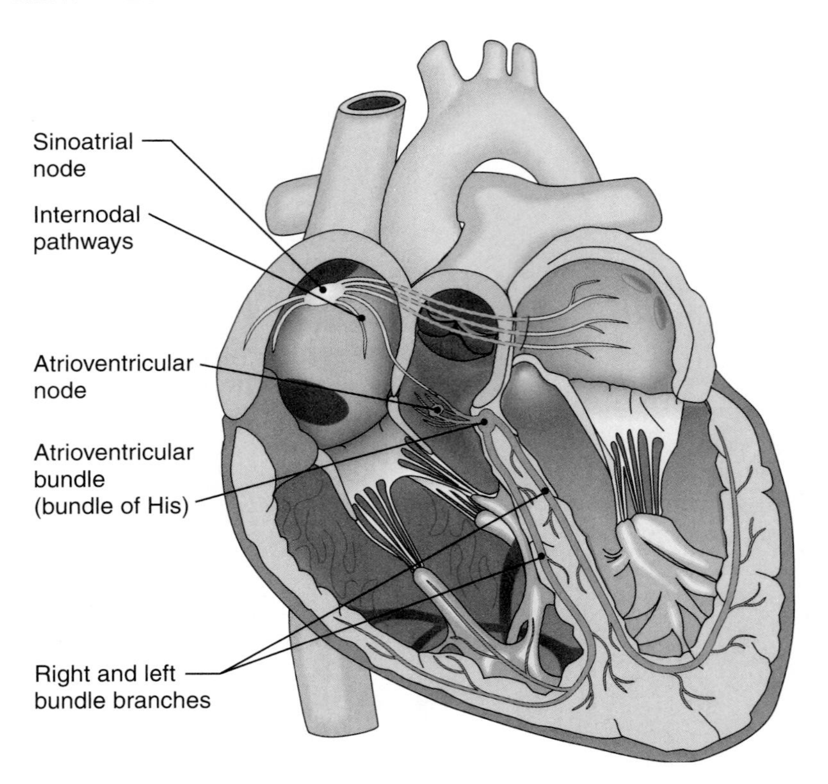

FIGURE 6-6 Electrical conduction system of the heart. (Used with permission from Cohen BJ, Wood DL. *Memmler's Structure and Function of the Human Body.* (2000). 7th ed. Philadelphia: Lippincott Williams & Wilkins, p. 201.)

19. Answer: d

    Why: Heart contraction is initiated by an electrical impulse generated by the sinoatrial (SA) node located in the upper wall of the right atrium (Fig. 6-6). It is called the pacemaker because it influences the rhythm and rate of the heartbeat. The bundle of His is part of the relay system that spreads the electrical impulse throughout the heart muscle. Chorda tendinea (plural, chordae tendineae) is the name for the thin thread of tissue that keeps an atrioventricular valve from flipping back into the atrium. A papillary muscle is attached to a chorda tendinea and helps open and close it.

    Review: Yes ☐ No ☐

20. Answer: b

    Why: An electrocardiogram (ECG or EKG) is the actual record of electrical currents that correspond to each event in heart muscle contraction. Alanine aminotransferase (ALT) is an enzyme associated with liver function. An electroencephalogram (EEG) measures electrical currents from the brain. Troponin T (TnT) is a protein released during muscle damage. Cardiac TnT (cTNT) is specific to heart muscle.

Review: Yes ☐ No ☐

21. Answer: a
Why: A cardiac cycle is defined as one complete contraction and relaxation of the heart. Diastole is the relaxing phase of the heart. Cardiac output is the volume of blood pumped by the heart in 1 minute. Systole is the contracting phase of the heart.
Review: Yes ☐ No ☐

22. Answer: c
Why: The medical term for the contracting phase of the cardiac cycle is systole. The closing of the semilunar valves is what creates the second sound of the heartbeat. A cardiac cycle is one complete contraction and subsequent relaxation of the heart. The relaxation phase of the heart is called diastole.
Review: Yes ☐ No ☐

23. Answer: b
Why: The complete cardiac cycle involving the simultaneous contraction of both atria pushing the blood into the ventricles followed by the simultaneous contraction of the ventricles pushing the blood into the exit arteries and then the relaxation of both takes approximately 0.8 seconds.
Review: Yes ☐ No ☐

24. Answer: a
Why: The P wave on an electrocardiogram tracing (Fig. 6-7) represents the activity of the atria and is usually the first wave seen. The QRS complex (a collection of three waves) along with the T wave represents the activity of ventricles. The atria are called receiving chambers.
Review: Yes ☐ No ☐

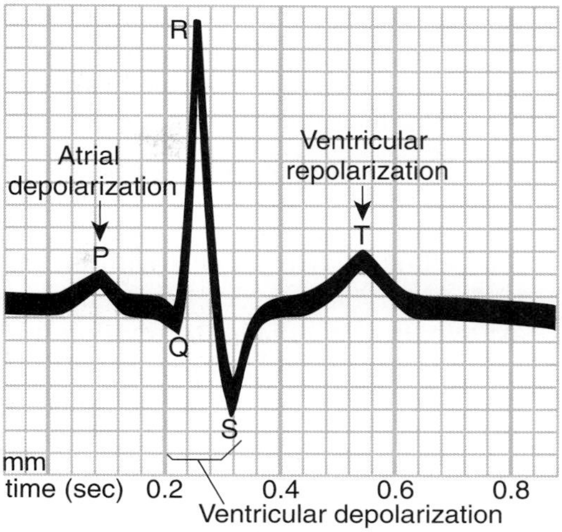

FIGURE 6-7 Normal ECG tracing showing one cardiac cycle. (Used with permission from Cohen BJ, Taylor J. *Memmler's The Human Body in Health and Disease.* 7th ed. 2005. Philadelphia: Lippincott Williams & Wilkins, p. 299)

25. Answer: d
Why: On an electrocardiogram tracing (Fig. 6-7), the QRS complex along with the T wave represents the electrical activity of the ventricles, whereas the P wave by itself represents the activity of the atria.
Review: Yes ☐ No ☐

26. Answer: a
Why: The closing of the atrioventricular valves as the ventricles contract results in the first sound of the heartbeat, which is a long, low-pitched sound described as a "lubb." The second sound of the heartbeat comes from the closing of the semilunar valves and is a shorter, sharper sound described as a "dupp."
Review: Yes ☐ No ☐

27. Answer: d
Why: Murmurs are abnormal heart sounds, usually caused by faulty valve action. Arrhythmias, extrasystoles, and fibrillations are abnormal contractions, not sounds.
Review: Yes ☐ No ☐

28. Answer: b
Why: The heart rate is the number of beats per minute. Average normal heart rate is around 72 beats per minute.
Review: Yes ☐ No ☐

29. Answer: d
Why: All of the choices deal with heart rate or rhythm. Tachycardia is an abnormally fast rate. Bradycardia is an abnormally slow rate. An extrasystole is an extra beat before the normal beat. Fibrillation is the term for rapid, uncoordinated contractions.
Review: Yes ☐ No ☐

30. Answer: c
Why: The wave of pressure created as the ventricles contract and blood is forced out of the heart and through the arteries creates the throbbing beat known as the pulse.
Review: Yes ☐ No ☐

31. Answer: a
Why: Blood pressure is defined as the force (pressure) exerted by the blood on the walls of the blood vessels. Cardiac output is the volume of blood pumped by the heart in 1 minute. Heart rhythm is the regularity of heart action or function. Pulse rate is the number of pulses per minute and normally reflects the heart rate, or number of heartbeats per minute.
Review: Yes ☐ No ☐

32. Answer: c
Why: Sphygmomanometer is the technical term for a blood pressure cuff. An artificial pacemaker is an implanted electrical device that automatically generates electrical impulses to initiate the heartbeat. A machine that records brain waves is used in electroencephalography (EEG). An electrocardiogram (ECG) is a record (tracing) of the electrical currents or waves that correspond to muscle contractions of the heart.
Review: Yes ☐ No ☐

33. Answer: d
Why: Blood pressure is a measure of the pressure exerted on the walls of a blood vessel. It is commonly measured in a large artery, such as the brachial. Blood pressure is expressed in millimeters of mercury and has two components: the systolic pressure, which is the highest pressure reached during ventricular contraction, and the diastolic pressure, which occurs during relaxation of the ventricles. Systolic pressure for the normal, relaxed, sitting adult averages 120 mm Hg, whereas diastolic averages 80 mm Hg.
Review: Yes ☐ No ☐

34. Answer: c
Why: Systolic pressure is the pressure in the arteries during contraction of the ventricles. Diastolic pressure is the arterial pressure when the ventricles are relaxed. Because atrial contraction is so very close to ventricle contraction, blood pressure during atrial contraction and relaxation cannot easily be detected and is not normaly measured.
Review: Yes ☐ No ☐

35. Answer: c
Why: Endocarditis means "inflammation of the endocardium." The endocardium is the thin membrane lining the inner surface of the heart. Angina pectoris refers to pain in the area of the heart caused by decreased blood flow to the muscle layer of the heart. Aortic stenosis is the term used to describe a narrowing of the aorta or its opening. Pericarditis is inflammation of the pericardium, the thin, fluid-filled sac that surrounds the heart.
Review: Yes ☐ No ☐

36. Answer: c
Why: Creatine kinase (CK) and lactate dehydrogenase (LDH) are enzymes present in cardiac muscle. They are released during myocardial infarction. Alkaline phosphatase

(ALP) and alanine aminotransferase (ALT) are enzymes measured most commonly to determine liver function. Blood urea nitrogen (BUN) is a kidney function test, and prothrombin time (PT) is a coagulation test used to monitor anticoagulant therapy. A glucose tolerance test (GTT) measures glucose metabolism, and erythrocyte sedimentation rate (ESR) is a nonspecific indicator of disease, especially inflammatory conditions such as arthritis.

Review: Yes ☐ No ☐

37. Answer: d

Why: Pulmonary circulation carries deoxygenated blood from the right ventricle of the heart to the lungs via the pulmonary artery. It also returns oxygenated blood from the lungs to the left atrium of the heart via the pulmonary vein. The left ventricle pumps the oxygenated blood into the arterial systemic circulation via the aorta. The arterial systemic circulation delivers the blood to the tissues. The venous systemic circulation returns deoxygenated blood to the heart (Fig. 6-8).

Review: Yes ☐ No ☐

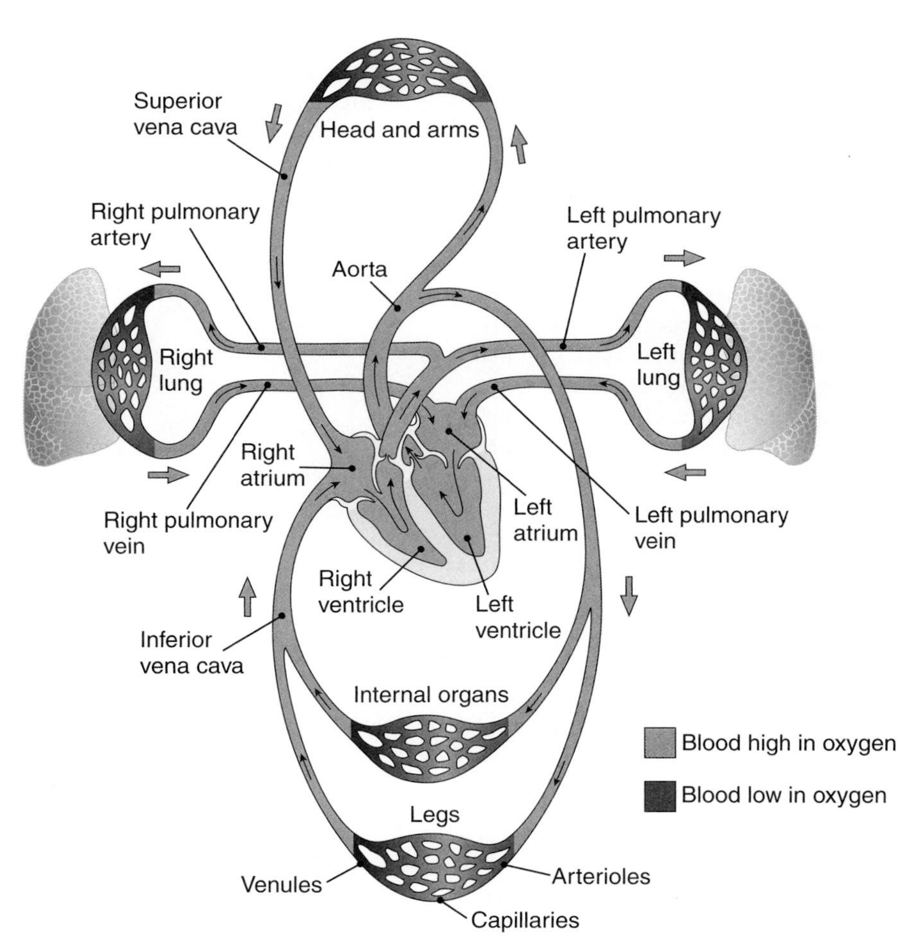

FIGURE 6-8 Representation of the vascular flow. (Used with permission from Cohen BJ, Taylor J. *Memmler's Structure and Function of the Human Body*. 8th ed. 2005. Philadelphia: Lippincott Williams & Wilkins, p. 235.)

38. Answer: c
Why: The pulmonary artery, as its name implies, is part of the pulmonary circulation. The brachial artery, cephalic vein, and vena cava are all part of the systemic circulation.
Review: Yes ☐ No ☐

39. Answer: a
Why: Arteries are vessels that carry blood away from the heart. (A way to remember this is, think AA for arteries away) Veins, such as the vena cava, carry blood to the heart. Capillaries are vessels that connect the ends of the smallest arteries (arterioles) to the smallest veins (venules).
Review: Yes ☐ No ☐

40. Answer: a
Why: The pulmonary vein carries oxygenated (oxygen-rich) blood from the lungs back to the heart. All vessels that return blood to the heart are called veins. All vessels that carry blood away from the heart are called arteries. The general rule of thumb that arteries carry oxygenated blood is only true for the systemic circulation. In the pulmonary circulation, the vessel that carries oxygenated (oxygen-rich) blood from the lungs is called a vein because it is returning the blood to the heart.
Review: Yes ☐ No ☐

41. Answer: b
Why: Because it is full of oxygen, normal systemic arterial blood is bright red. Normal systemic venous blood is dark red with a bluish tinge. Regardless of what some people think, no one has blue blood.
Review: Yes ☐ No ☐

42. Answer: a
Why: The aorta, at the start of the systemic arterial circulation, is almost 1 inch wide and is the largest artery in the body. The carotid artery in the neck and the femoral artery in the leg are large arteries but not as large as the aorta. The vena cavae (singular, vena cava) are the largest veins in the body.
Review: Yes ☐ No ☐

43. Answer: a
Why: The great saphenous vein runs the entire length of the leg (Fig. 6-9) and is considered the longest vein in the body. The median cubital is a relatively short vein located in the antecubital fossa of the arm. The inferior vena cava, which returns systemic blood to the lower right atrium, is one of the largest veins in the body, but not the longest. The right pulmonary vein returns oxygen-rich blood to the heart from the lungs and is nowhere near as long as the great saphenous.
Review: Yes ☐ No ☐

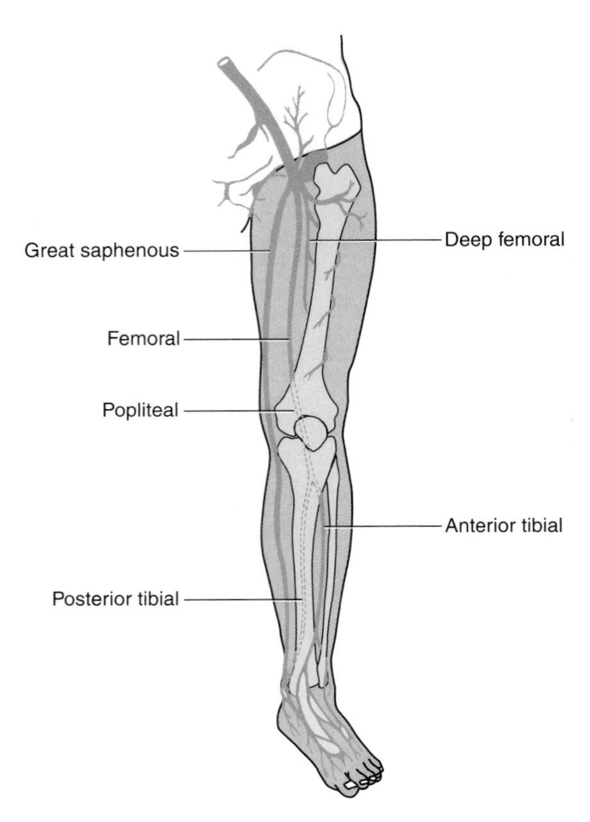

FIGURE 6-9 Major leg and foot veins.

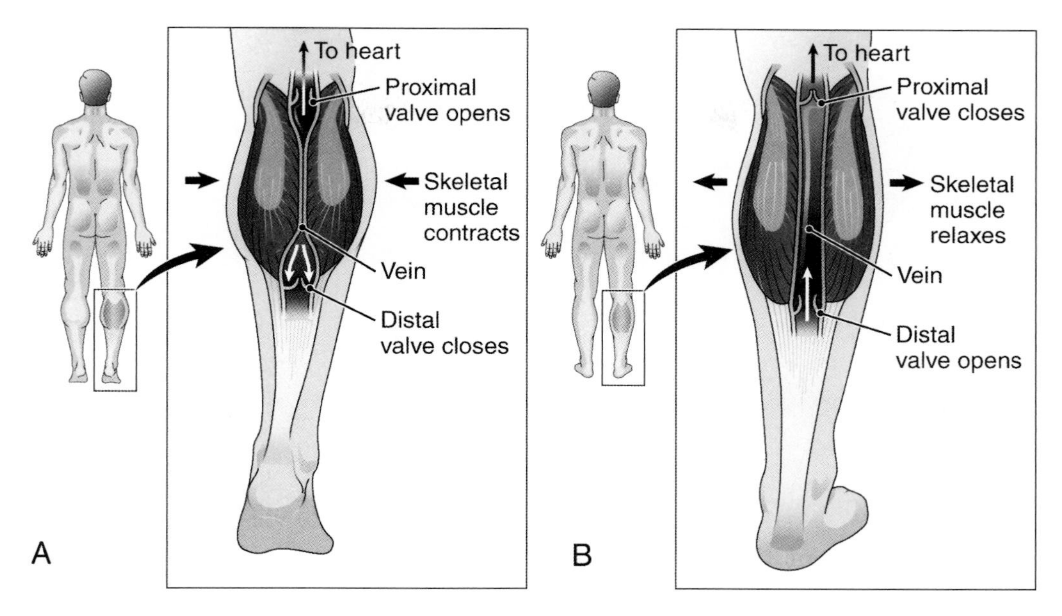

FIGURE 6-10 Role of skeletal muscles and valves in blood return. **A.** Contracting skeletal muscle compresses the vein and drives blood forward, opening the proximal valve, while the distal valve closes to prevent backflow of blood. **B.** When the muscle relaxes again, the distal valve opens, and the proximal valve closes until blood moving in the vein forces it open again. (Used with permission from Cohen BJ, Taylor J. *Memmler's Structure and Function of the Human Body.* 8th ed. 2005. Philadelphia: Lippincott Williams & Wilkins, p. 261.)

44. Answer: d
Why: Unlike the arterial system, veins do not have sufficient pressure from the heart's contractions to keep the blood moving through them. Veins rely on movement of nearby skeletal muscles and the opening and closing of the valves within them to keep the blood moving toward the heart (Fig. 6-10). The presence of valves in veins but not arteries is a major structural difference between arteries and veins.
Review: Yes ☐ No ☐

45. Answer: d
Why: Venules is the medical term for the smallest veins. The medical term for the smallest arteries is arterioles. Capillaries connect the arterioles (which are the end of the arterial system) to the venules (which are the beginning of venous system). Lumen (plural, lumina) is the term for the internal space of any tubular vessel.
Review: Yes ☐ No ☐

46. Answer: c
Why: Capillaries are tiny blood vessels that form the fine network that delivers oxygen and nutrients to the tissues and carries carbon dioxide and other waste products away. They are only one cell thick, which allows gases and nutrients to diffuse through their walls. Arteries, arterioles, and venules have multiple layers and are many cells thick.
Review: Yes ☐ No ☐

47. Answer: a
Why: Blood vessels have three main layers (Fig. 6-11). The tunica adventitia (also called tunica externa) is the term applied to the outer layer of an artery or a vein. It is made

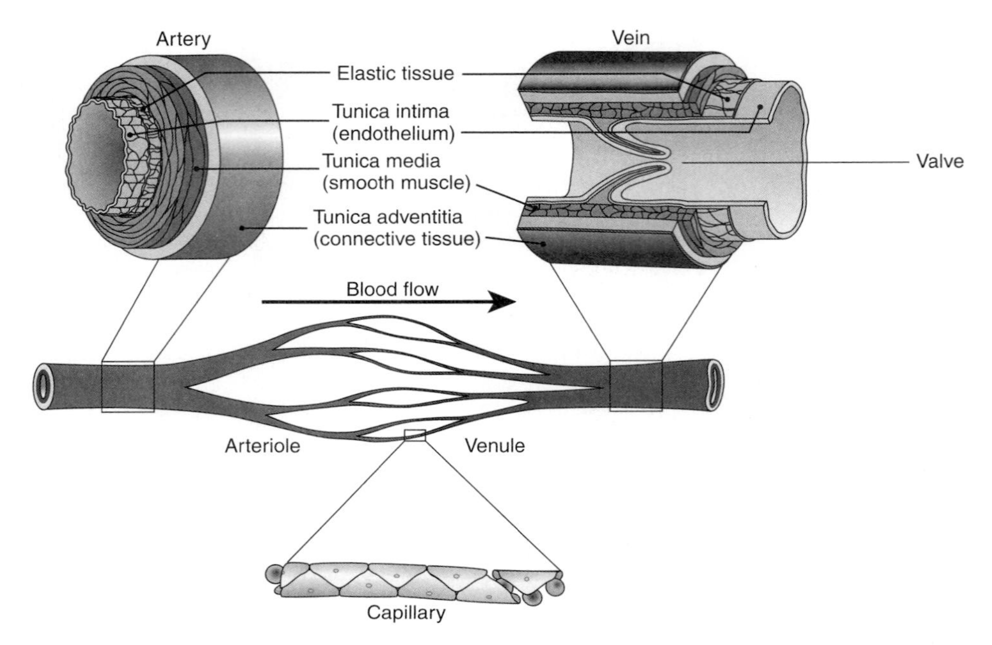

FIGURE 6-11 Artery, vein, and capillary structure. (Used with permission from Cohen BJ, Taylor J, Memmler's *The Human Body in Health and Disease.* 2005. 10th ed. Philadelphia: Lippincott Williams & Wilkins, p. 309.)

up of connective tissue and is thicker in arteries than veins. The tunica intima (also called tunica interna) is the inner layer or lining of a blood vessel and is composed of a single layer of endothelial cells with an underlying basement membrane, connective tissue layer, and elastic membrane. The tunica media is the middle layer, composed of smooth muscle and some elastic fibers. The tunica media is much thicker in arteries than in veins.

Review: Yes ☐ No ☐

48. Answer: c

Why: Lumen is the term for the space within a hollow tubular structure such as a blood vessel, intestine, or blood collection needle. The intima, interna, and media are terms used in identifying blood vessel layers. The tunica intima (also called tunica interna) is the inner layer of a blood vessel. The tunica media is the middle layer of a blood vessel.

Review: Yes ☐ No ☐

49. Answer: c

Why: The smooth muscle of the tunica media (middle layer) is much thicker in arteries than in veins (Fig. 6-11). The tunica adventitia, or outer layer, is also thicker in arteries. Both veins and arteries are lined with a single layer of endothelial cells. Arteries typically have more elastic tissue than veins.

Review: Yes ☐ No ☐

50. Answer: c

Why: Capillaries (Fig. 6-11) are the smallest blood vessels. They are one cell thick, which allows the exchange of oxygen, carbon dioxide, nutrients, and wastes between the tissue cells and the blood to take place through their walls. Alveoli are thin-walled, saclike chambers within the lungs where oxygen and carbon dioxide are exchanged between the air and blood. Arterioles are tiny arteries that connect with and deliver blood to the capillaries. Venules are tiny veins at the junction where the capillaries merge with the venous circulation.

Review: Yes ☐ No ☐

51. Answer: d

Why: Figure 6-2 is a cross section of an artery and a vein (see Fig. 6-12). The structure on the right is a vein. If you look closely you can see the valve against the wall on the left. Arteries do not have valves. Also, the structure on the left has a very thick middle layer, which is characteristic of arteries. See Fig. 6-11 for a comparison diagram of artery, vein, and capillary structure.

Review: Yes ☐ No ☐

52. Answer: c

Why: The right ventricle delivers blood to the pulmonary artery, which takes it to the lungs to pick up oxygen. The left ventricle delivers blood to the aorta by way of the aortic arch. The pulmonary veins carry oxygenated blood from the lungs to the left atrium of the heart (Fig. 6-8).

Review: Yes ☐ No ☐

53. Answer: b

Why: The pulmonary vein, part of the pulmonary circulation, carries oxygenated blood from the lungs to the heart so that it can be delivered to the systemic circulation. The inferior vena cava delivers deoxygenated blood from the systemic venous circulation to the lower right atrium of the heart. The brachial vein is part of the systemic venous

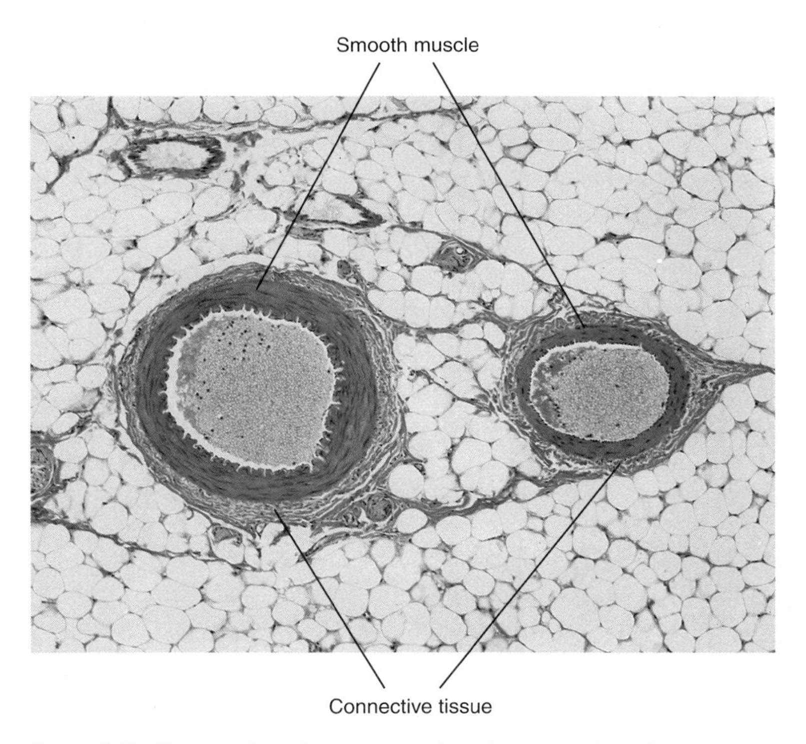

FIGURE 6-12 Cross section of an artery and a vein as seen through a microscope. (Used with permission from Cormack DH. *Essential Histology*. (1993). Philadelphia: JB Lippincott, Plate 11-1.)

circulation carrying deoxygenated blood. The pulmonary artery carries deoxygenated blood from the heart to the lungs.

Review: Yes ☐ No ☐

54. Answer: a
Why: Blood flows from the heart into arteries, which branch into smaller and smaller arteries, the smallest of which are called arterioles. Arterioles connect to the capillaries. Capillaries form the bridge between the arterial and venous circulation and are where the exchange of gases, nutrients, and waste products takes place. The opposite ends of the capillaries connect to the smallest veins, which are called venules. Venules merge with larger and larger veins until the blood returns to the heart. Choice "b" is obviously incorrect. In choices "c" and "d" the blood would be traveling in the wrong direction (Fig. 6-8).
Review: Yes ☐ No ☐

55. Answer: a
Why: The antecubital fossa is the area of the arm that is located in front of (anterior to) the elbow.
Review: Yes ☐ No ☐

56. Answer: d
Why: The subclavian vein begins in the shoulder area and leads into the chest. The accessory cephalic, basilic, and median veins all have portions that are in the antecubital fossa.
Review: Yes ☐ No ☐

57. Answer: b
Why: The vein identified by number 1 is the cephalic vein. The vein identified by number 6 is the basilic vein. The vein identified by number 7 is the median cubital vein. (See the H pattern veins in Fig. 6-13A.)
Review: Yes ☐ No ☐

58. Answer: d
Why: The vein identified by number 16 is the median cephalic vein. The vein identified by number 18 is the median vein. The vein identified by number 19 is the median basilic vein. (See the M pattern veins in Fig. 6-13B.)
Review: Yes ☐ No ☐

59. Answer: a
Why: The vein identified by number 26 is the basilic vein. The veins identified by number 27 are the dorsal metacarpal veins. The vein identified by number 28 is the cephalic vein. (See Figure 6-13C.)
Review: Yes ☐ No ☐

60. Answer: a
Why: Being fixed in the surrounding tissues is a good thing for a vein because it keeps it from rolling. One of the reasons the basilic vein is the last choice for venipuncture is because it is *not* well-fixed and rolls easily. Other reasons include that it is located close to a major nerve and the brachial artery and that it tends to be more painful to puncture.
Review: Yes ☐ No ☐

61. Answer: d
Why: The subclavian vein is in the shoulder area of the arm (Fig. 6-13) and merges with the brachiocephalic vein in the chest (Fig. 6-14). The cephalic vein merges with the subclavian vein. The popliteal and saphenous veins are in the leg (Fig. 6-9).
Review: Yes ☐ No ☐

62. Answer: a
Why: The anterior and posterior median cutaneous nerves are both very close to the basilic vein and are a major reason this vein is the very last choice for venipuncture (Fig. 6-13).
Review: Yes ☐ No ☐

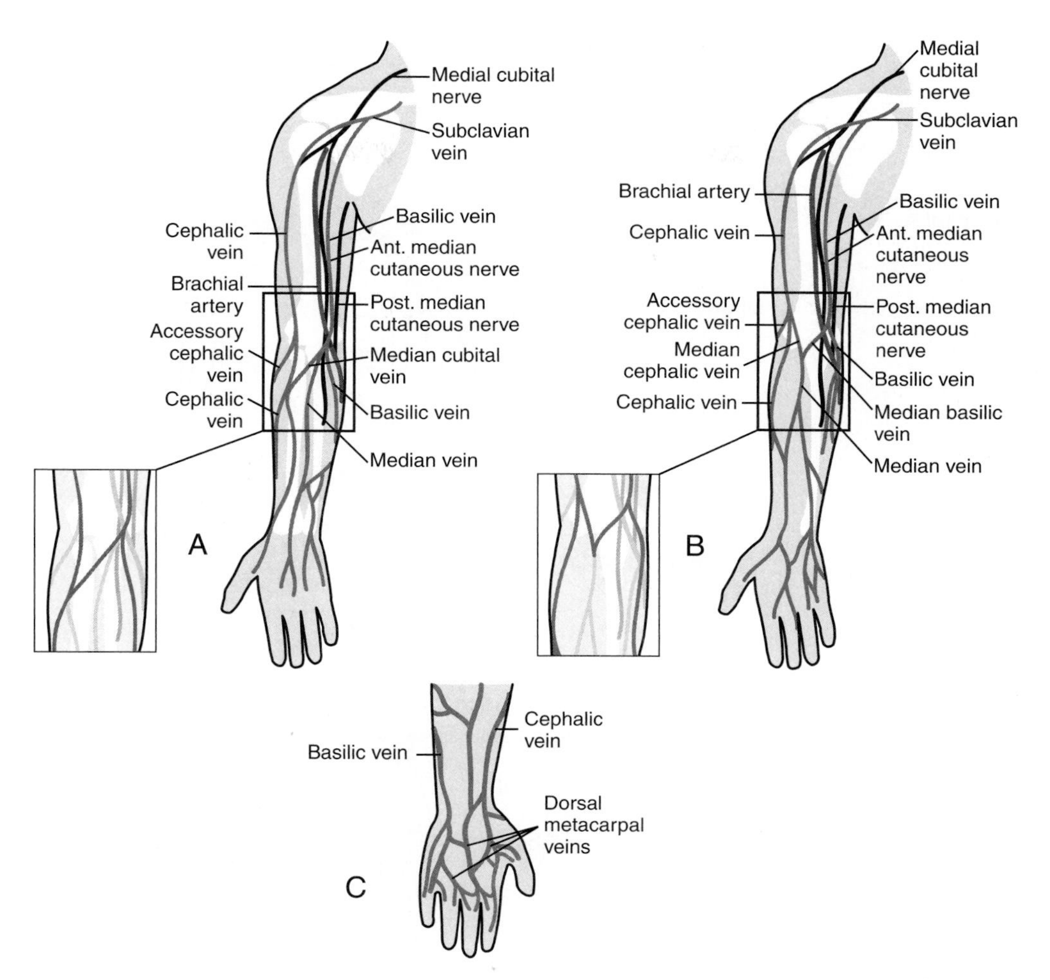

FIGURE 6-13 Principle veins of the arm including major antecubital veins. **A.** H-shaped pattern of antecubital veins of the right arm in anatomic position. **B.** M-shaped pattern of antecubital veins of the right arm in anatomic position. **C.** Right forearm, wrist, and hand veins in prone position.

63. Answer: d

Why: The median cubital, cephalic, and basilic are in the correct order of selection for veins in the H pattern. In choosing the best vein in the H pattern, the first selection is the median cubital because it is large and well anchored and therefore doesn't bruise easily and is least painful to puncture. The cephalic vein is the next choice because it is fairly well anchored and less painful to puncture than the basilic. The basilic vein is the last choice because it rolls and bruises easily, is more painful to puncture, and there is the possibility of accidentally hitting the brachial artery and a major nerve when accessing it (Fig. 6-13). According to CLSI, the basilic vein should not be selected unless the other veins on both arms have been eliminated. The median basilic is an M pattern vein.

Review: Yes ☐ No ☐

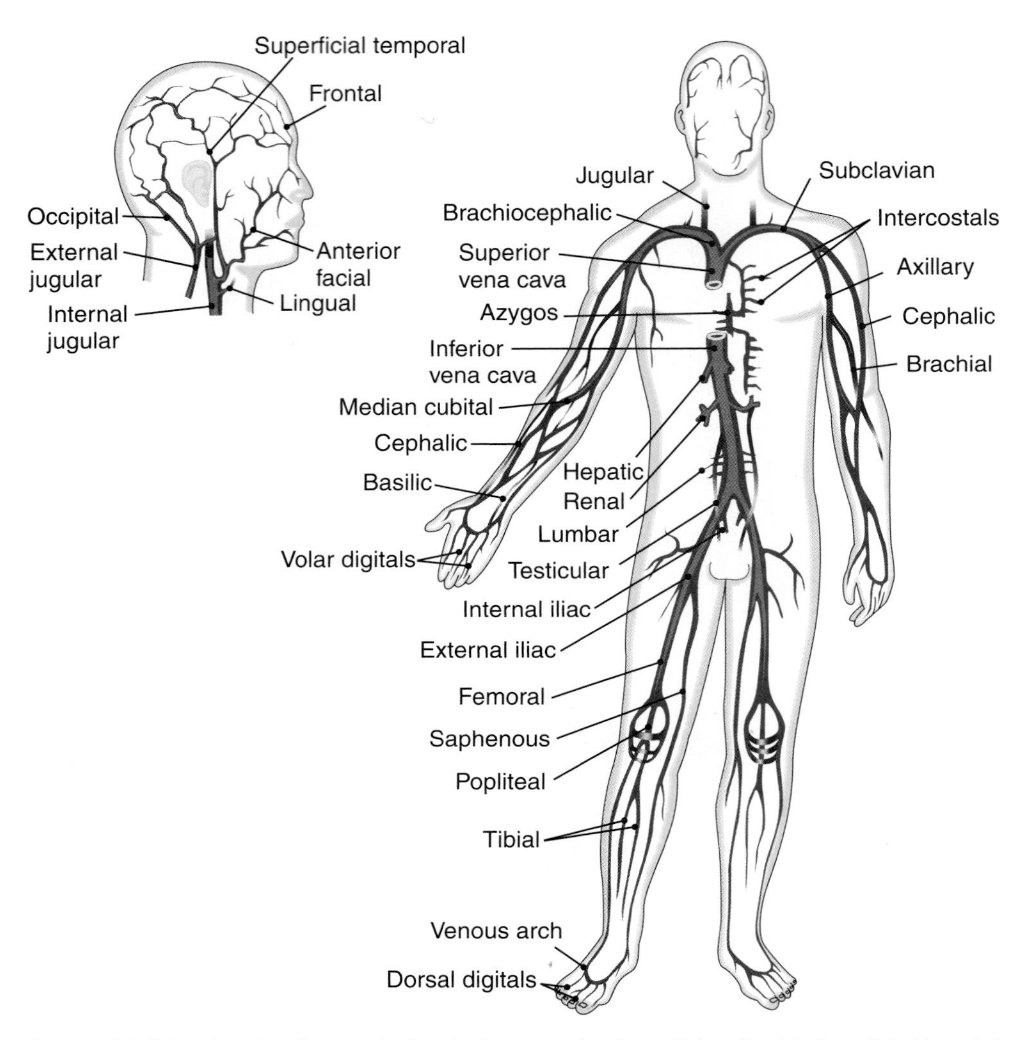

FIGURE 6-14 Principle veins of the body. (Used with permission from Cohen, B. J. & Wood, D. L. *Memmler's Structure and Function of the Human Body* (2000) 7th ed. Philadelphia: Lippincott Williams & Wilkins, p. 218)

64. Answer: b
Why: When the hand is prone the palm faces downward, causing the antecubital portion of the cephalic vein to be in line with the little finger. When the arm is in the normal anatomic position, the palm is up and the cephalic vein is on the same side as the thumb.
Review: Yes ☐ No ☐

65. Answer: b
Why: Leg ankle and foot veins should *never* be punctured routinely. Serious problems can result if ankle or foot veins of patients with coagulation problems or poor circulation are used for venipuncture. Test results can also be affected. If no other sites are available, the patient's physician *must* be consulted and permission obtained before performing venipuncture on the ankle or foot vein of *any* patient.
Review: Yes ☐ No ☐

66. Answer: d
Why: The popliteal vein is located deep in the leg (Fig. 6-9) in the area behind the knee. It is a continuation of the femoral vein.
Review: Yes ☐ No ☐

67. Answer: c
Why: Embolus is the medical term for a blood clot or other undissolved matter circulating in the bloodstream. An aneurysm is a bulging or dilation of a blood vessel. An embolism is the obstruction of a blood vessel by an embolus. A thrombus is a stationary blood clot that obstructs or partially obstructs a blood vessel.
Review: Yes ☐ No ☐

68. Answer: c
Why: Phlebitis is the medical term for vein inflammation. The term comes from the word root *phleb*, which means vein, and the suffix *-itis*, which means inflammation. An embolism is the obstruction of a blood vessel by a blood clot or other undissolved foreign matter. Hemostasis is the process by which bleeding is stopped. Thrombosis means the formation or existence of a blood clot in the vascular system.
Review: Yes ☐ No ☐

69. Answer: c
Why: DIC is the abbreviation for disseminated intravascular coagulation. A DIC test or screen is actually a series of tests used to detect diffuse uncontrolled coagulation throughout the vascular system. In DIC situations, continuous generation of thrombin causes depletion of several clotting factors to such an extent that generalized bleeding may occur. Antidiuretic hormone (ADH) is an endocrine system test. A cerebrospinal fluid (CSF) analysis test is a nervous system test. Rapid plasma reagin (RPR), a syphilis test, is a reproductive system test.
Review: Yes ☐ No ☐

70. Answer: a
Why: Atherosclerosis is a form of arteriosclerosis involving changes in the intima of the artery caused by the accumulation of lipid, cholesterol, and calcium material. Cholesterol is a substance produced by the liver and also found in animal products such as meat and eggs. It is an essential part of lipid metabolism, but high blood levels increase the risk of developing atherosclerosis. Endocarditis means inflammation of the membrane that lines the inside of the heart. Lipemia is a condition in which there is an abnormal amount of fat in the blood.
Review: Yes ☐ No ☐

71. Answer: a
Why: Aneurysm is a medical term for a localized dilation or bulging of a blood vessel, usually an artery. An embolism is the obstruction of a blood vessel by a blood clot or other undissolved foreign matter. Arteriosclerosis is a hardening or thickening and loss of elasticity of the wall of the artery. Thrombophlebitis is defined as inflammation of the vein in conjunction with the formation of a blood clot.
Review: Yes ☐ No ☐

72. Answer: c
Why: The word root *thromb* means "clot." Phlebitis is vein inflammation. The meaning of thrombophlebitis is "inflammation of a vein in conjunction with the formation of a blood clot." Atherosclerosis is a form of arteriosclerosis involving changes in the intima of the artery. Phlebosclerosis is the fibrous hardening of vein walls. Vasculitis is a general term meaning "inflammation of blood vessels."
Review: Yes ☐ No ☐

73. Answer: c
Why: The average 154-lb adult has approximately 5 liters (L), or 5.2 quarts, of blood.

A more exact blood volume can be calculated based on the fact that the average adult has 70 mL of blood per each kilogram of weight.
Review: Yes ☐ No ☐

74. Answer: c
Why: The normal ratio of plasma to formed elements is approximately 55% plasma and 45% cells. That means approximately half of a normal blood specimen is serum (in a clot tube) or plasma (in an anticoagulant tube). This is important when determining how much blood to collect for testing purposes.
Review: Yes ☐ No ☐

75. Answer: b
Why: A plasma specimen is obtained by centrifuging blood collected in an anticoagulant tube. Centrifugation separates the cells from the liquid (plasma) portion of the specimen, which is a clear to slightly hazy (due to fibrinogen), pale yellow fluid that is 90% water and 10% solutes (dissolved substances).
Review: Yes ☐ No ☐

76. Answer: b
Why: Blood is a mixture of fluid and cells. The fluid portion, *plasma,* is approximately 90% water and 10% dissolved substances such as antibodies, nutrients, minerals, and gases. Red blood cells, white blood cells, and platelets make up the cellular portion of blood referred to as the *formed elements*. Bacteria are not found in the blood under normal circumstances because the immune system recognizes them as foreign and destroys them.
Review: Yes ☐ No ☐

77. Answer: b
Why: All leukocytes (white blood cells) contain nuclei. Thrombocytes (platelets) and mature erythrocytes (red blood cells) do not have nuclei. A reticulocyte is an immature red blood cell that contains remnants of nuclear material but not a complete nucleus.
Review: Yes ☐ No ☐

78. Answer: c
Why: Reticulocytes are immature red blood cells that contain remnants of RNA and other material from their nuclear phase in the bone marrow. The remnants can be seen when blood is stained with a special stain used to perform a manual reticulocyte count.
Review: Yes ☐ No ☐

79. Answer: b
Why: An eosinophil (Fig. 6-15B) is a type of granulocytic white blood cell that can ingest and detoxify foreign protein and help turn off immune reactions. Consequently, eosinophils (Eos) increase in numbers during allergic reactions and infestations of parasites such as pinworms.
Review: Yes ☐ No ☐

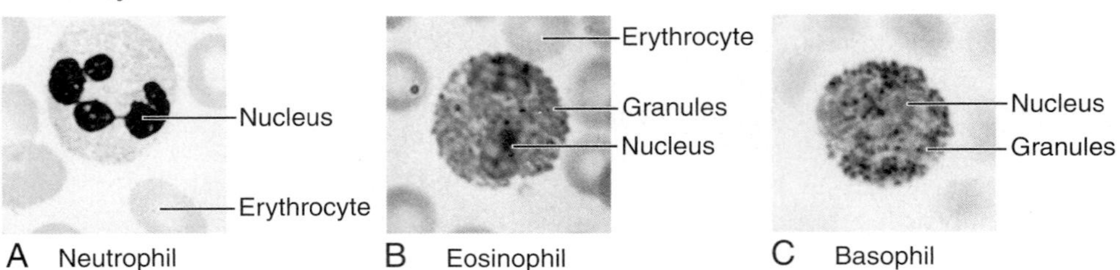

FIGURE 6-15 Granulocytes. **A.** Neutrophil. **B.** Eosinophil. **C.** Basophil. (Used with permission from Cohen BJ, *Memmler's The Human Body in Health and Disease.* 10th ed. 2005. Philadelphia: Lippincott Williams & Wilkins p. 268.)

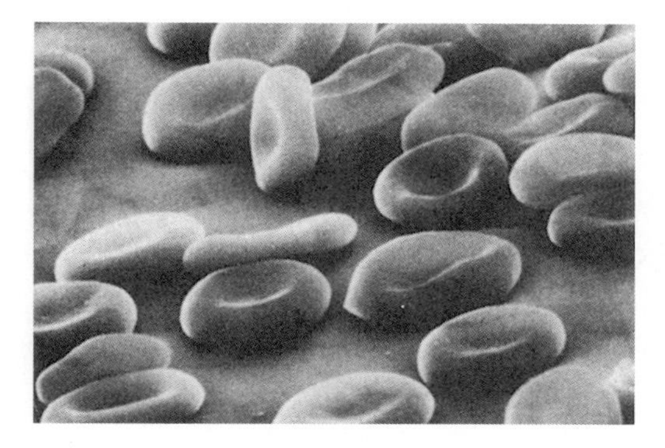

FIGURE 6-16 Red blood cells as seen under a scanning electron microscope. (Used with permission from Cohen BJ, Memmler's The Human Body in Health and Disease. 10th ed. 2005. Philadelphia: Lippincott Williams & Wilkins p. 266.)

80. Answer: b
Why: Normal erythrocytes (Fig. 6-16) are described as anuclear, biconcave disks that are approximately 7–8 microns in diameter.
Review: Yes ☐ No ☐

81. Answer: a
Why: Red blood cells (erythrocytes) are normally the most numerous formed element in the blood (Fig. 6-17), averaging 4.5 to 5.0 million per cubic millimeter of blood. Therefore, an erythrocyte count of 4.5 million/mm^3 would be considered normal.
Review: Yes ☐ No ☐

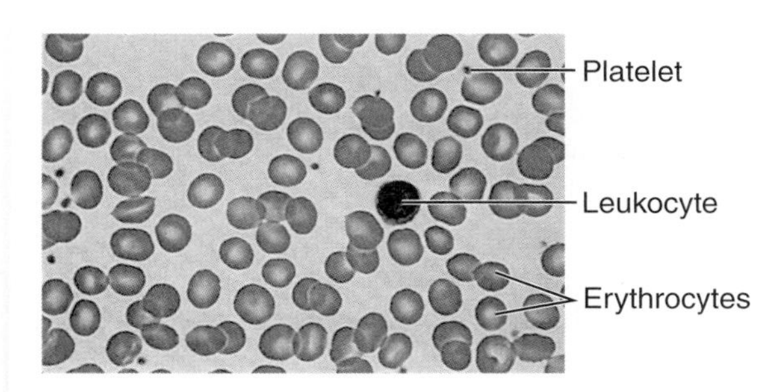

FIGURE 6-17 Blood cells in a stained blood smear as seen under a microscope. (Used with permission from Cohen BJ, *Memmler's The Human Body in Health and Disease.* 10th ed. 2005. Philadelphia: Lippincott Williams & Wilkins p. 266.)

82. Answer: b
Why: The production and development of red blood cells (erythrocytes) occurs in the bone marrow by a process called erythropoiesis.
Review: Yes ☐ No ☐

83. Answer: d
Why: The primary function of red blood cells is to transport oxygen from the lungs to the tissues. A secondary function of red blood cells is to transport carbon dioxide from the tissues to the lungs. Nutrients are dissolved in the plasma, not transported by red blood cells. Certain white blood cells produce antibodies, not red blood cells.
Review: Yes ☐ No ☐

84. Answer: d
Why: The medical term for a white blood cell is leukocyte. The word root *leuk* means white, and the suffix *-cyte* means cell.
Review: Yes ☐ No ☐

85. Answer: b
Why: Leukocytes have extravascular function, which means they do their job outside of the bloodstream. They are able to leave the bloodstream and pass through the spaces between the cells in the walls of blood vessels by a process called diapedesis. Erythrocytes, reticulocytes, and thrombocytes have intravascular function and cannot pass through intact blood vessel walls.
Review: Yes ☐ No ☐

86. Answer: b
Why: The main function of white blood cells (WBCs) is to neutralize or destroy pathogens. Neutrophils (Fig. 6-15A) are a type of WBC that destroys pathogens by phagocytosis, a process in which a pathogen or other foreign matter is surrounded and engulfed and destroyed by the WBC.

This process is also used to remove disintegrated tissue.
Review: Yes ☐ No ☐

87. Answer: d
Why: Neutrophils (Fig 6-15A) are polymorphonuclear (PMN), which means they have a nucleus that has several lobes connected by thin strands. Another term for this type of nucleus is segmented. Consequently, neutrophils are often called polys, PMNs, or segs for short.
Review: Yes ☐ No ☐

88. Answer: c
Why: Injury to a blood vessel exposes protein material in the vessel wall. Contact with this material causes platelets (Fig. 6-18) to degranulate and stick to one another (platelet aggregation) and to the injured area (platelet adhesion). This results in the formation of a platelet plug that temporarily seals off the injury. If the injury is large, a fibrin clot that includes all of the formed elements (RBCs, WBCs, and platelets) is eventually generated.
Review: Yes ☐ No ☐

89. Answer: a
Why: Erythrocytes (red blood cells) (Fig. 6-16 and 6-18) are described as being anuclear (non-nucleated), biconcave (curved inward on both sides) discs approximately 7–8 microns in diameter.
Review: Yes ☐ No ☐

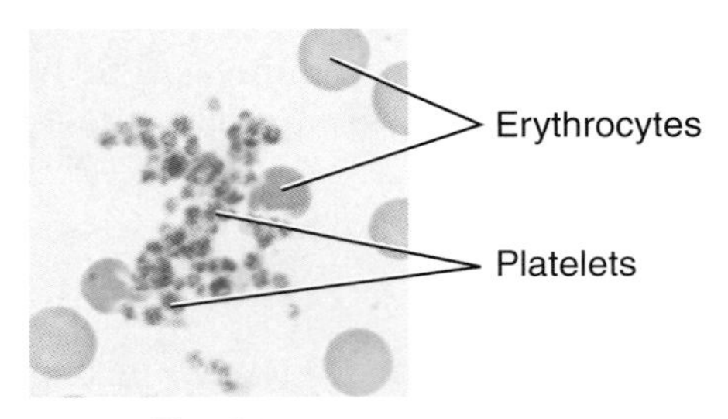

FIGURE 6-18 Platelets (thrombocytes) in a stained blood smear. (Used with permission from Cohen BJ, *Memmler's The Human Body in Health and Disease.* 10th ed. 2005. Philadelphia: Lippincott Williams & Wilkins p. 269.)

Agranulocytes

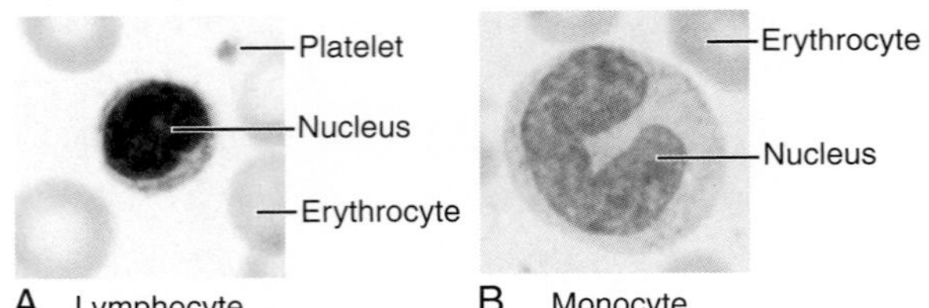

FIGURE 6-19 Agranulocytes. **A.** Lymphocyte. **B.** Monocyte. (Used with permission from Cohen BJ, *Memmler's The Human Body in Health and Disease.* 10th ed. 2005. Philadelphia: Lippincott Williams & Wilkins p. 268.)

90. Answer: d
Why: Monocytes (Fig. 6-19) that have left the bloodstream are sometimes referred to as macrophages because they are found in loose connective tissue where they phagocytize (engulf and destroy) particles much like cells of the reticuloendothlial (RE) system.
Review: Yes ☐ No ☐

91. Answer: b
Why: Lymphocytes (Fig. 6-19) play a role in immunity and are the second most numerous WBC. There are two main types of lymphocytes: T lymphocytes, which directly attack infected cells, and B lymphocytes, which differentiate into plasma cells. Plasma cells produce antibodies that are released into the bloodstream, where they circulate and attack foreign antigens.
Review: Yes ☐ No ☐

92. Answer: c
Why: The number of platelets in the blood of the average adult is between 150,000 and 400,000 per cubic millimeter (mm^3). Therefore, a platelet count of 300,000/mm^3 is considered normal.
Review: Yes ☐ No ☐

93. Answer: d
Why: Thromb means clotting, and *cyte* means cell. Thrombocyte is the medical term for platelets, which are cells that function in the clotting process.
Review: Yes ☐ No ☐

94. Answer: c
Why: A platelet is not a true cell but a fragment of a large bone marrow cell called a megakaryocyte. When separated into parts (mega-karyo-cyte), this term means "large-nucleated cell."
Review: Yes ☐ No ☐

95. Answer: b
Why: The formed elements are red blood cells, white blood cells, and platelets. The erythrocyte (red blood cell) is normally the most numerous formed element in the blood, averaging 4.5–5.0 million per cubic millimeter of blood.
Review: Yes ☐ No ☐

96. Answer: c
Why: Human blood type, which is inherited, is determined by the presence or absence of certain types of antigens on the surface of the red blood cells. The ABO blood group system recognizes four blood types based on two antigens called A and B. Type A individuals have the A antigen; type B have the B antigen; type AB have both antigens; and type O have neither A nor B. The Rh system is based on the presence or absence of the Rh antigen. Rh-positive individuals have the Rh antigen, and Rh-negative individuals lack the Rh antigen.
Review: Yes ☐ No ☐

97. Answer: b
Why: Rh sensitization means an Rh-negative individual has been exposed to Rh-positive blood and is thus able to produce antibodies directed against the Rh factor. To prevent sensitization from an Rh-positive fetus, an Rh-negative woman may be given Rh immunoglobulin at certain times during her pregnancy as well as immediately after the baby's birth. Rh immunoglobulin destroys any Rh-positive fetal cells that may have entered her bloodstream, thus preventing sensitization. Only an Rh-negative person can become sensitized to the Rh factor. Carrying an Rh-negative fetus will not cause sensitization.
Review: Yes ☐ No ☐

98. Answer: a
Why: Becoming sensitized means that the individual may produce antibodies against the Rh factor. Rh antibodies produced by the mother and circulating in her bloodstream can cross the placenta into the fetal circulation and cause the destruction of red blood cells of an Rh-positive fetus.
Review: Yes ☐ No ☐

99. Answer: a
Why: The red blood cells of an individual whose blood type is A-negative have the A antigen but lack the Rh antigen. (See the answer to question 96.)
Review: Yes ☐ No ☐

100. Answer: c
Why: Hemolytic disease of the newborn (HDN) is most often the result of an Rh-negative mother being sensitized by a previous Rh-positive fetus, causing her to form Rh antibodies. During a subsequent pregnancy, these antibodies can cross the placenta into the fetal circulation, attack the red blood cells of the fetus, and cause hemolysis.
Review: Yes ☐ No ☐

101. Answer: c
Why: Whole blood, like blood circulating in the bloodstream, consists of liquid called plasma with the formed elements (red blood cells, white blood cells, and platelets) suspended in it. The liquid is called plasma

because it still contains fibrinogen and other coagulation factors.
Review: Yes ☐ No ☐

102. Answer: d
Why: A clotted blood specimen is actually made up of two parts, a clotted portion containing cells enmeshed in fibrin, and a liquid portion called serum. The liquid portion is called serum because it does not contain fibrinogen. The fibrinogen was used up in the process of clot formation.
Review: Yes ☐ No ☐

103. Answer: a
Why: The buffy coat of a whole blood specimen is made up of white blood cells and platelets. Therefore, a specimen with an abnormally large buffy coat has either a high white blood cell count or a high platelet count.
Review: Yes ☐ No ☐

104. Answer: b
Why: A whole blood specimen is collected in an anticoagulant such as EDTA to keep it from clotting. If the specimen is centrifuged or allowed to settle, the clear liquid portion at the top of the specimen is called plasma. Arrow number 1 in Figure 6-4 points to the top portion of the specimen, which is the plasma.
Review: Yes ☐ No ☐

105. Answer: a
Why: Arrow number 2 in Figure 6-4 points to the thin layer of white blood cells and platelets on top of the red blood cells that is commonly called the buffy coat.
Review: Yes ☐ No ☐

106. Answer: d
Why: You cannot visually tell serum from plasma because both serum and plasma are mostly clear, pale yellow fluids. Plasma is sometimes slightly hazy because of the fibrinogen in it, but serum may also be slightly hazy when fats are present, a condition called lipemia.
Review: Yes ☐ No ☐

107. Answer: c
Why: Although EDTA is the anticoagulant of choice for hematology studies, a blood smear made from an EDTA specimen should be made within 1 hour of collection because prolonged contact with EDTA can change the staining characteristics of the formed elements.
Review: Yes ☐ No ☐

108. Answer: a
Why: Coagulation tests are concerned with the blood-clotting process, which involves the activation and interaction of a series of components called coagulation factors. Most coagulation tests (except some point-of-care tests that are performed on whole blood) are performed on plasma because it contains coagulation factors. Serum is obtained from clotted blood and cannot be used for most coagulation tests because the coagulation factors are consumed (i.e., fibrinogen), or partially consumed when blood clots.
Review: Yes ☐ No ☐

109. Answer: a
Why: A fast turnaround time (TAT) is vitally important for STAT requests. Although serum is ideal for most chemistry tests because nothing has been added to the blood during collection, to obtain serum a normal blood specimen must be allowed to clot completely before it can be centrifuged. This can take from 30 to 60 minutes. Blood from patients receiving blood thinners may take even longer. The 30 minutes or more can mean the difference between life and death in a STAT situation. With the exception of fibrinogen and other coagulation factors, plasma contains the same analytes as serum. However, because a plasma specimen does not clot, it can be spun immediately upon

reaching the laboratory and therefore tested much sooner.

Review: Yes ☐ No ☐

110. Answer: b

Why: A complete blood count (CBC) is a multipart test that includes erythrocyte, leukocyte, and platelet counts. It is always performed on whole blood because the cells cannot be identified or counted in blood that is clotted. A blood urea nitrogen (BUN) and lactate dehydrogenase (LDL) are chemistry tests that are typically performed on serum. A PTT test is a coagulation test that is performed on plasma because it contains clotting factors. A PTT can also be performed on whole blood from a finger stick using a special machine.

Review: Yes ☐ No ☐

111. Answer: d

Why: A partial thromboplastin test (PTT) is a coagulation test that is performed on plasma because plasma contains clotting factors. A PTT can also be performed on whole blood from a finger stick using a special machine. A CBC, erythrocyte sedimentation rate (ESR), and hemoglobin (Hgb) are hematology tests that require a whole blood EDTA specimen.

Review: Yes ☐ No ☐

112. Answer: b

Why: To obtain serum, blood must be allowed to clot. During the clotting process, fibrinogen is split into fibrin, which enmeshes the cells to form the clot. Once the clotting is complete, the specimen is centrifuged and the clear liquid obtained is called serum. Serum does not contain fibrinogen because it was used up in the clotting process.

Review: Yes ☐ No ☐

113. Answer: c

Why: Thromb, cyt, and *osis* mean "clotting," "cell," and "condition," respectively. Thrombocytosis is a condition in which the clotting cells (platelets) are abnormally increased.

Review: Yes ☐ No ☐

114. Answer: a

Why: Anemia is a blood disorder usually characterized by an abnormal reduction in the number of red blood cells in the circulating blood. Leukemia is a disorder characterized by an abnormal increase in white blood cell (WBC) numbers along with an increase in abnormal forms of WBCs. Polycythemia is overproduction of red blood cells. Thrombocytopenia is abnormally decreased platelets.

Review: Yes ☐ No ☐

115. Answer: b

Why: The formed elements are red blood cells, white blood cells, and platelets. Assessing the formed elements is part of a hematology test called a complete blood count (CBC). The antistreptolysin (ASO) is a test for the antibody against streptolysin O, a red blood cell-destroying substance produced by a certain type of streptococci. Electrolytes (lytes) are a panel of chemistry tests that measure ions in the blood, most commonly sodium, potassium, chloride, and bicarbonate. Serum protein electrophoresis (SPEP) is a chemistry test that identifies various protein components in a serum specimen.

Review: Yes ☐ No ☐

116. Answer: b

Why: When broken into parts, "leuko-cyt-osis" means *white-cell-condition.* The term is used to describe an abnormal increase of white blood cells. Leukemia is a disorder characterized by an abnormal increase in WBC numbers along with an increase in abnormal WBC forms. Leukopenia is an abnormal decrease in WBC numbers. Leukopoiesis is leukocyte production.

Review: Yes ☐ No ☐

117. Answer: a
Why: Creatinine is a kidney function test performed in the chemistry department. Hematocrit and hemoglobin are hematology tests used to assess blood disorders. Ferritin, the form in which iron is stored in the tissues, is a whole blood chemistry test that is also used in the diagnosis of blood disorders.
Review: Yes ☐ No ☐

118. Answer: c
Why: Hemostasis means "stopping or controlling the flow of blood" and is a medical term for the coagulation process. Hemolysis is destruction of red blood cells. Hemopoiesis is the production and maturation of red blood cells. Homeostasis is the state of equilibrium or balance the body strives to maintain.
Review: Yes ☐ No ☐

119. Answer: a
Why: Platelet aggregation is the terminology used to describe the ability of platelets to stick to each other. Platelet adhesion is the ability of platelets to stick to surfaces. The property of adhering is called cohesion. Inhibition is the stopping or suppression of a function.
Review: Yes ☐ No ☐

120. Answer: a
Why: Ions are particles that carry an electrical charge. The coagulation process requires the presence of calcium ions, which have a positive charge, for proper function. Chloride sodium and potassium are also ions. They function in other body processes, however.
Review: Yes ☐ No ☐

121. Answer: d
Why: The word *extrinsic* means "from or coming from outside." The extrinsic coagulation pathway is initiated outside the bloodstream by tissue injury, which causes the release of thromboplastin (factor III) and the activation of factor VII. The intrinsic pathway of coagulation is initiated by events within the bloodstream and the activation of coagulation factors circulating in the plasma. Platelet aggregation is part of platelet plug formation, the second stage in the coagulation process that occurs before the initiation of either pathway.
Review: Yes ☐ No ☐

122. Answer: d
Why: There are four stages to hemostasis (Fig. 6-20). The initial stage is the constriction of blood vessels (vasoconstriction) to slow down blood loss. The second stage is platelet plug formation, which involves platelet aggregation and adhesion. These first two stages are called primary hemostasis. Stage 3 is fibrin clot formation, which involves activation of the intrinsic and extrinsic pathways of the coagulation cascade. Stage 4 is fibrinolysis, the process by which the fibrin clot is dissolved.
Review: Yes ☐ No ☐

123. Answer: d
Why: The word *primary* means "first." The first two stages of the hemostasis/coagulation process (Fig. 6-20) are vasoconstriction and platelet plug formation. These first two stages combined are called primary hemostasis and are sometimes all that is needed to stop blood loss, so the process goes no further.
Review: Yes ☐ No ☐

124. Answer: a
Why: A bleeding time (BT) test assesses the ability of the platelet to aggregate (degranulate and stick to one another) and form a platelet plug. FDP, PT, and PTT test other parts of the coagulation process.
Review: Yes ☐ No ☐

125. Answer: a
Why: Hemophilia is a hereditary blood disorder characterized by very long bleeding times. The most common type of hemophilia is caused by the lack of clotting factor VIII. Disseminated intravascular coagulation (DIC) is a pathologic form of diffuse rather than local coagulation in which coagulation

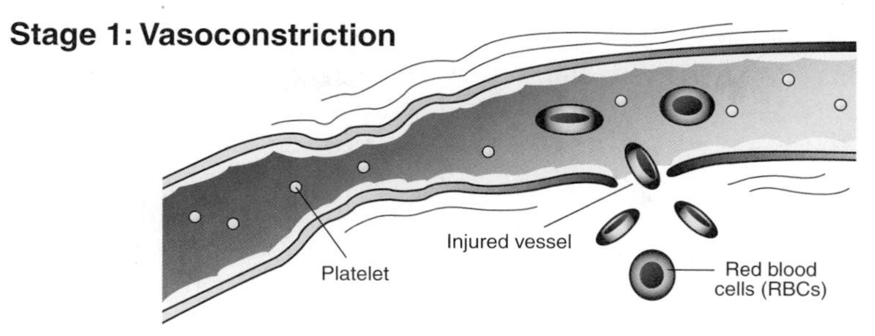

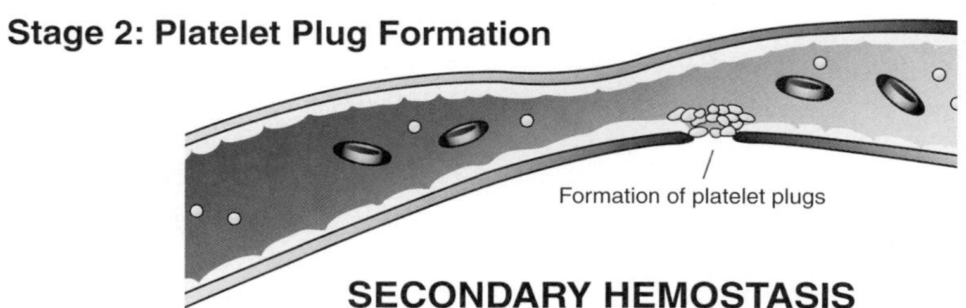

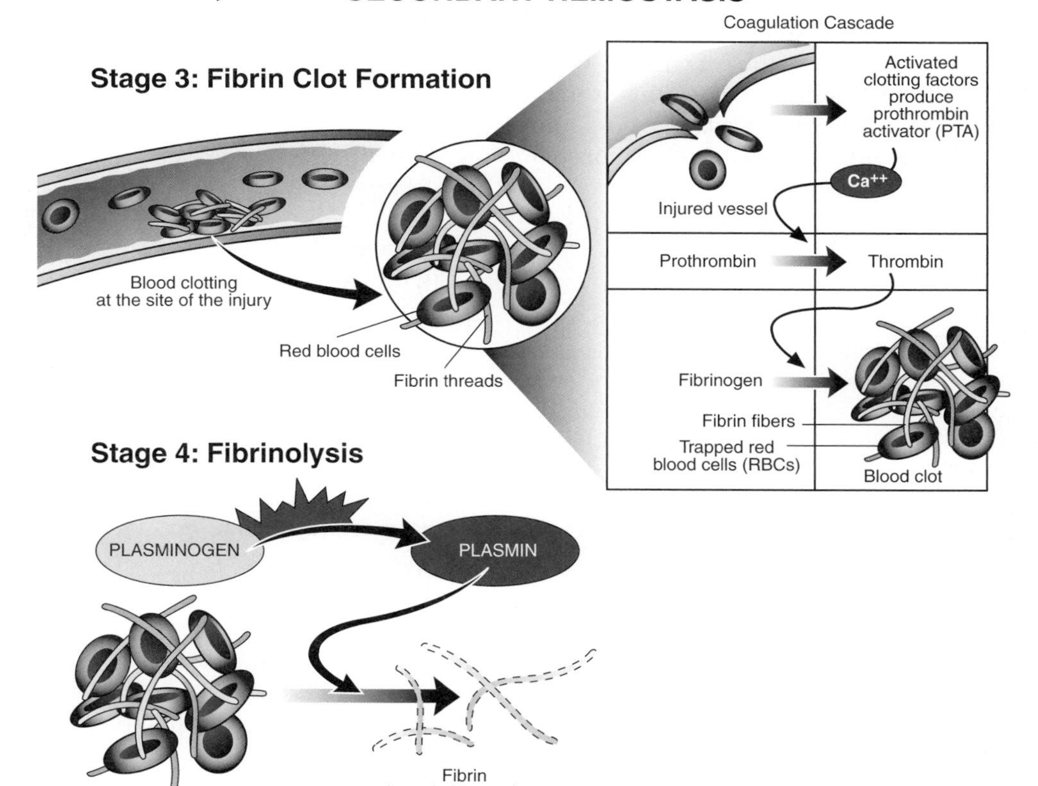

FIGURE 6-20 The process of hemostasis.

factors are consumed to such an extent that bleeding occurs. Thrombocytopenia is an abnormally decreased number of platelets. Varicose veins, swollen, knotted veins, are not a coagulation disorder.

Review: Yes ☐ No ☐

126. Answer: b

Why: The liver plays a major role in coagulation. It synthesizes the clotting factors fibrinogen and prothrombin and is the source of heparin, a naturally formed anticoagulant found in the bloodstream.

Review: Yes ☐ No ☐

127. Answer: b

Why: The last stage of the coagulation process (Fig. 6-20) is called fibrinolysis and involves the removal of the fibrin clot after healing has occurred. In this stage the protein plasminogen is converted to the enzyme plasmin. Plasmin splits the fibrin in the clot into small fragments called fibrin degradation products (FDP), which are removed by phagocytic cells of the reticuloendothelial system.

Review: Yes ☐ No ☐

128. Answer: b

Why: Substances called natural inhibitors circulate in the plasma along with the coagulation factors. They normally keep the coagulation process in check and limited to local sites by binding with activated coagulation factors that escape the clotting site and any that remain after clotting is complete.

Review: Yes ☐ No ☐

129. Answer: a

Why: Primary hemostasis ends with platelet plug formation (Fig. 6-20). Tests that evaluate platelet plug formation include bleeding time and platelet count. D-dimer, partial thromboplastin time, prothrombin time (protime), factor assays and fibrin split products (FSP), measure the functioning of secondary hemostasis.

Review: Yes ☐ No ☐

130. Answer: c

Why: For some injuries such as a needle puncture to a vein, platelet plug formation (stage 2 of the coagulation process and the end of primary hemostasis) is enough to seal the site until healing occurs, in which case the coagulation process goes no further. For larger injuries the process continues to secondary hemostasis, which involves activation of a series of coagulation factors (including factor VIII) and the formation of a fibrin clot. Vasoconstriction (stage 1) plays a role in reducing blood flow in the immediate area of injury to prevent blood from escaping from the site of injury, but by itself is not enough to seal an injury.

Review: Yes ☐ No ☐

131. Answer: c

Why: A circulating blood clot, part of a clot, or other mass of undissolved matter is called an embolus. The sudden obstruction of a blood vessel by an embolus is called an embolism.

Review: Yes ☐ No ☐

132. Answer: d

Why: A protime (PT), also called a prothrombin time, is a coagulation test. Digoxin is a chemistry test for a drug of the same name that is used in patients with certain heart problems. A hemogram is a type of hematology report that lists the results of a complete blood count. Myoglobin is an oxygen-binding protein found in cardiac and skeletal muscle.

Review: Yes ☐ No ☐

133. Answer: b

Why: Lymph fluid is similar to plasma but is 95% water instead of 90%. Plasma is unlike serum because it contains fibrinogen, and serum does not. The composition of lymph fluid is very different from the composition of whole blood and urine.

Review: Yes ☐ No ☐

134. Answer: c
Why: Body cells are bathed in tissue fluid acquired from the bloodstream. Much of the fluid diffuses back into the capillaries along with waste products of metabolism. Excess tissue fluid filters into lymphatic capillaries, where it is called lymph.
Review: Yes ☐ No ☐

135. Answer: d
Why: Lymph fluid moves through lymph vessels primarily by skeletal muscle contraction, much like blood moves through the veins. Like veins, the lymph vessels have valves to keep the lymph flowing in the right direction.
Review: Yes ☐ No ☐

136. Answer: b
Why: Functions of the lymphatic system (Fig. 6-21) include delivering fats to the bloodstream, processing lymphocytes, and trapping and destroying bacteria and other impurities. The lymphatic system *does not* make coagulation factors.
Review: Yes ☐ No ☐

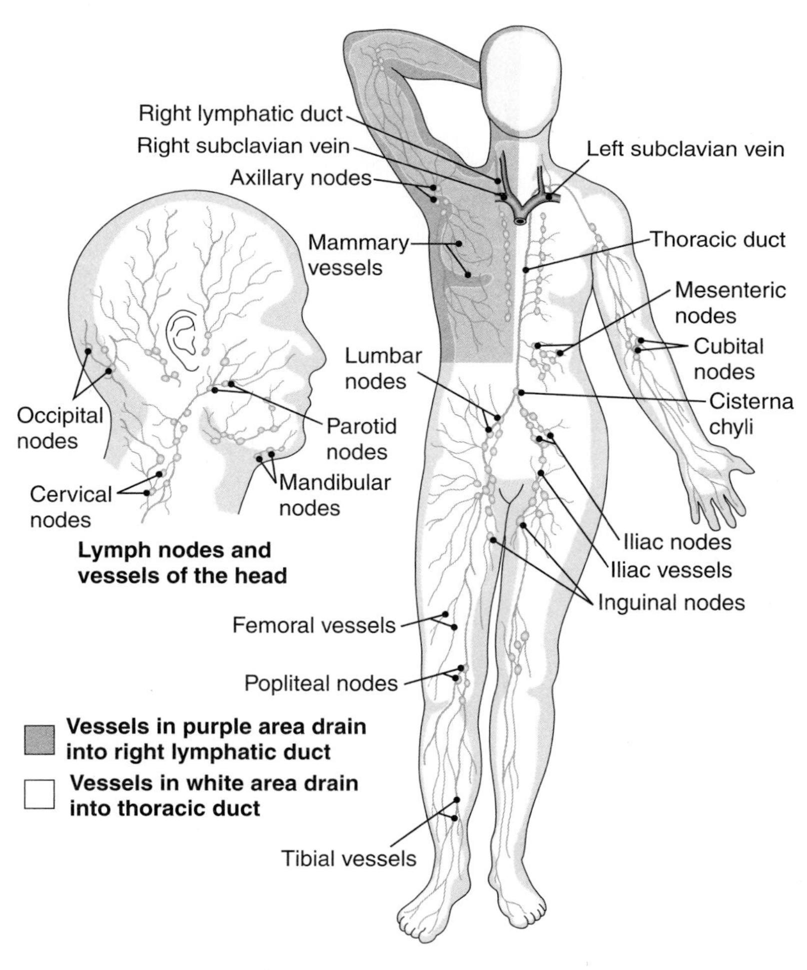

FIGURE 6-21 Lymphatic system. (Used with permission from Cohen BJ, Wood, DL, *The Human Body in Health and Disease* (2000), 9th ed. Philadelphia: Lippincott Williams & Wilkins, p.296.)

137. Answer: c
Why: Lymph node tissue (lymphoid tissue) is a special kind of tissue that is able to trap microorganisms, remove impurities, and process lymphocytes. It does *not* have the ability to create red blood cells, produce tissue fluid, or secrete antibodies.
Review: Yes ☐ No ☐

138. Answer: d
Why: Lymphoid tissue is also found in other areas of the body, including the thymus, tonsils, gastrointestinal tract, and spleen. It is not found in the heart, lungs, or kidneys.
Review: Yes ☐ No ☐

139. Answer: d
Why: Lymphosarcoma is the medical term for a malignant lymphoid tumor. The word parts, "lympho-sarc-oma" combine to mean *lymphoid-fleshy-malignant tumor.*
Review: Yes ☐ No ☐

140. Answer: d
Why: Mononucleosis is an acute infectious disease that primarily affects lymphoid tissue. The mononucleosis (mono) test is the most common test associated with the lymph system.
Review: Yes ☐ No ☐

BLOOD COLLECTION EQUIPMENT, ADDITIVES, AND ORDER OF DRAW

CHAPTER 7

study tip

Questions in this chapter test the ability to identify general blood collection equipment and supplies as well as evacuated tube system (ETS) and syringe system equipment used in venipuncture. Questions also test the ability to identify the various types of ETS tube additives, describe how they work, name the stopper colors of the tubes that contain them, and collect tubes during venipuncture or fill tubes from a syringe in the appropriate order of draw.

overview

The primary duty of the phlebotomist is to collect blood specimens for laboratory testing. Blood is collected by several methods, including arterial puncture, capillary puncture, and venipuncture. This chapter assesses knowledge of general blood collection equipment and supplies, specific equipment and supplies used for venipuncture, additives used in blood collection, and the order of draw for collecting or filling blood specimen tubes. A phlebotomist needs to be familiar with all the types of equipment to select appropriate collection devices for the type and condition of the patient's vein and the type and amount of specimen required for the test. Safe collection of quality blood specimens is assured when the appropriate tools are chosen and they are used correctly.

REVIEW QUESTIONS

Choose the BEST answer.

1. What additive in a blood sample can inhibit the metabolism of glucose by the cells?
   a. EDTA
   b. heparin
   c. NaF
   d. oxalate

2. All of the following items are used when performing a routine venipuncture EXCEPT:
   a. disinfectant.
   b. evacuated tubes.
   c. safety needle.
   d. tourniquet.

3. A serum specimen is requested. Which of the following evacuated tubes can be used to collect it?
   a. EDTA
   b. PPT
   c. PST
   d. SST

4. Which of the following are all anticoagulants that remove calcium from the specimen by forming insoluble calcium salts, and therefore prevent coagulation?
   a. EDTA, lithium heparin, citrate
   b. NaF, sodium heparin, EDTA
   c. oxalate, SPS, sodium heparin
   d. sodium citrate, EDTA, oxalate

5. In a successful venipuncture, evacuated tubes fill automatically as soon as the tube is pierced because of:
   a. equal pressure in the vein and tube.
   b. premeasured vacuum in each tube.
   c. pressure from the arterial system.
   d. tourniquet pressure on the vein.

6. Lavender stopper or closure tubes are most commonly used to collect:
   a. chemistry tests.
   b. coagulation tests.
   c. hematology tests.
   d. immunology tests.

7. The evacuated tube system (ETS) is the preferred blood collection system for all of the reasons stated EXCEPT:
   a. exposure of the blood to contaminants is avoided.
   b. it is easier to see the flash when entering a vein.
   c. the collector's exposure to blood is minimized.
   d. there are safety concerns when a syringe is used.

8. Lithium heparin is a suitable anticoagulant for which of the following tests?
   a. complete blood count
   b. basic metabolic panel
   c. partial thromboplastin time
   d. plasma lithium value

9. Which one of the following additives can be found in a royal blue top collection tube?
   a. citrate
   b. EDTA
   c. fluoride
   d. oxalate

10. Measurement of copper, a trace element, requires blood collection in a tube with a:
    a. green top.
    b. lavender top.
    c. light blue top.
    d. royal blue top.

11. All of the following are true of glove powder EXCEPT that it can:
    a. cause an allergic reaction.
    b. contaminate specimens.
    c. make gloves last longer.
    d. suspend latex bits in air.

12. If phlebotomists have dermatitis, they should:
    a. change their gloves more frequently.
    b. use sanitizer instead of soap and water.

c. wash their hands thoroughly and often.
d. wear a barrier hand cream or lotion.

13. Decontamination of hands after glove removal is essential for all of the following reasons EXCEPT:
    a. decontamination is needed to quickly restore normal flora.
    b. glove powder must be removed as a contamination source.
    c. gloves may contain defects and not be an adequate barrier.
    d. hand contamination may not be visible to the naked eye.

14. All of the following are antiseptics used in blood collection EXCEPT:
    a. benzylkonium chloride.
    b. chlorhexidine gluconate.
    c. household bleach.
    d. hydrogen peroxide.

15. Which disinfectant is preferred by the HICPAC for use on surfaces and instruments?
    a. CDC-approved solution of 2% phenol
    b. commercial brand of Lysol disinfectant
    c. manufactured povidone-iodine dilution
    d. EPA-registered sodium hypochlorite product

16. After a blood spill, a disinfectant is applied and must have at least _________minutes of contact time for cleanup to be effective.
    a. 2 minutes
    b. 5 minutes
    c. 10 minutes
    d. 30 minutes

17. If hands are heavily contaminated with organic material, and a sink is not available, the phlebotomist should clean them with:
    a. alcohol-based hand cleaner and sterile gauze pads.
    b. detergent-containing wipes followed by a sanitizer.
    c. hydrogen peroxide followed by a hand sanitizer.
    d. three separate 70% isopropyl swabs used in a row.

18. What is a venoscope?
    a. machine used to input patient information
    b. puncture device with its own light source
    c. tool attached to a catheter to aid insertion
    d. transillumination device for locating veins

19. Properly applied tourniquets should do all of the following EXCEPT:
    a. distend or inflate the veins of choice.
    b. make veins larger and easier to find.
    c. restrict venous and arterial blood flow.
    d. stretch vein walls so they are thinner.

20. This gauge of needle is used primarily as a transfer needle rather than for blood collection.
    a. 16
    b. 18
    c. 21
    d. 23

21. Safety features on needles work by all of the following methods EXCEPT:
    a. covering or shielding the needle.
    b. plugging the needle with silicon.
    c. retracting the needle after use.
    d. using a device to blunt the needle.

22. Occupational Safety and Health Administration (OSHA) regulations require that after use the:
    a. needle be automatically ejected into the sharps container.
    b. needle be removed from the holder and put in the sharps container.
    c. tube holder be sanitized soon after the needle is removed.
    d. tube holder with needle attached be disposed of as a unit.

23. The headspace in an evacuated tube is:
    a. a consistent amount of air space left when a tube is filled properly.
    b. due to premature depletion of tube vacuum when a vein is missed.
    c. room left in a tube if the tube is not completely filled with blood.
    d. space inside a colored tube stopper that should not touch the blood.

24. Tubes designed by the manufacturer to be "short draw" are:
    a. bad for coagulation testing.
    b. made to fill only partially.
    c. smaller than regular tubes.
    d. tubes without anticoagulants.

25. ETS tube additives are all of the following EXCEPT:
    a. clot activators.
    b. anticoagulants.
    c. silicon gels.
    d. tube coatings.

26. Plastic red top tubes used to collect blood specimens contain:
    a. anticoagulants.
    b. clot activators.
    c. no additives.
    d. preservatives.

27. Improper handling or storage of evacuated tubes can affect all of the following EXCEPT:
    a. additive integrity.
    b. inert gel quality.
    c. shape of the tube.
    d. vacuum of a tube.

28. Which test can be affected by cross-contamination from a light blue tube?
    a. acid phosphatase
    b. calcium
    c. lithium
    d. potassium

29. Which of the following tests might be affected by carryover from an EDTA tube?
    a. activated clotting time
    b. amylase
    c. creatine kinase
    d. lithium

30. All of the following additives can potentially affect an alkaline phosphatase test EXCEPT:
    a. citrate.
    b. EDTA.
    c. heparin.
    d. oxalate.

31. The partial thromboplastin time is potentially affected by all of the following additives EXCEPT:
    a. EDTA.
    b. heparin.
    c. NaF.
    d. silica.

32. This antiseptic has been traditionally used to obtain the high degree of skin antisepsis required when collecting blood cultures.
    a. 70% ethyl alcohol
    b. 70% isopropanol
    c. hydrogen peroxide
    d. povidone-iodine

33. Which of the following is the *preferred* solution to use to clean up blood spills?
    a. 5.25% sodium hypochlorite
    b. an EPA-approved bleach product
    c. fresh solution of soap and water
    d. undiluted 70% isopropyl alcohol

34. Disinfectants are all of the following EXCEPT:
    a. corrosive chemical compounds.
    b. safe for use on human skin.
    c. used on surfaces and instruments.
    d. used to kill pathogenic microbes.

35. A solution used to clean the site before routine venipuncture is:
a. 5.25% sodium hypochlorite.
b. 70% isopropyl alcohol.
c. 70% methanol.
d. povidone-iodine.

36. Why are gauze pads a better choice than cotton balls for covering the site and holding pressure following venipuncture?
a. cotton balls are not very absorbent
b. cotton ball fibers can stick to the site
c. gauze pads are a more sterile choice
d. gauze pads deliver more pressure

37. All of the following can be used on infants and children younger than 2 years of age EXCEPT:
a. adhesive bandages.
b. evacuated tubes.
c. isopropyl alcohol.
d. vinyl tourniquets.

38. Which one of the following is *not* a required characteristic of a sharps container?
a. leak-proof
b. lid that locks
c. puncture-resistant
d. red in color

39. When a disposable latex or vinyl tourniquet becomes soiled with blood, it is best to:
a. autoclave it before reuse.
b. toss it in biohazard trash.
c. wash it in a bleach solution.
d. wipe it down with alcohol.

40. Wearing gloves during phlebotomy procedures is mandated by the following agency:
a. CDC
b. FDA
c. HICPAC
d. OSHA

41. What criterion is used to decide which needle gauge to use for venipuncture?
a. depth of the selected vein
b. size and condition of the vein
c. type of test being collected
d. your personal preference

42. To what does the "gauge" of a needle relate?
a. diameter
b. length
c. strength
d. volume

43. Which needle gauge has the largest bore or lumen?
a. 18
b. 20
c. 21
d. 22

44. Multisample needles are typically available in these gauges.
a. 16–18
b. 18–20
c. 20–22
d. 22–24

45. The slanted tip of a needle is called the:
a. bevel.
b. hub.
c. lumen.
d. shaft.

46. The purpose of the rubber sleeve that covers the tube end of a multiple-sample needle is to:
a. enable smooth tube placement and removal.
b. maintain the sterile condition of the sample.
c. prevent leakage of blood during tube changes.
d. protect the needle and help keep it sharp.

47. A phlebotomy needle that does *not* have a safety feature:
    a. cannot be used for any venipuncture procedure.
    b. must be used with a holder that has a safety feature.
    c. requires immediate recapping after venipuncture.
    d. should be removed from the holder before disposal.

48. All of the following are considerations for what size tubes to use for ETS blood collection EXCEPT the:
    a. age and weight of the patient.
    b. patient's allergy to antiseptics.
    c. sample size needed for testing.
    d. size and condition of the veins.

49. Glass evacuated tubes are coated with silicon to:
    a. allow a number of tubes to fill more quickly.
    b. inhibit glycolysis during the clotting phase.
    c. keep blood from clinging to the tube interior.
    d. prevent reflux of tube contents into the vein.

50. Which of the following stopper colors identifies a tube used for coagulation testing?
    a. green
    b. lavender
    c. light blue
    d. red

51. Which of the following tubes will yield a serum sample?
    a. green top
    b. lavender top
    c. light blue top
    d. red top

52. The cleaning agent in hand sanitizers used in healthcare is:
    a. alcohol-based.
    b. phenol-based.
    c. sodium hypochlorite.
    d. Zephiran Chloride.

53. All of the following tube stopper colors indicate the presence (or absence) and type of additive in the tube EXCEPT:
    a. green.
    b. lavender.
    c. light blue.
    d. royal blue.

54. Heparin prevents blood from clotting by:
    a. activating calcium.
    b. binding calcium.
    c. chelating thrombin.
    d. inhibiting thrombin.

55. Which department would most likely perform the test on a specimen collected in an SPS tube?
    a. chemistry
    b. coagulation
    c. hematology
    d. microbiology

56. A royal blue top tube with green color-coding on the label contains:
    a. EDTA.
    b. heparin.
    c. no additive.
    d. sodium citrate.

57. Which one of the following substances is an anticoagulant?
    a. oxalate
    b. phosphate
    c. silica
    d. thrombin

58. It is important to fill oxalate tubes to the stated fill capacity because excess oxalate:
    a. causes hemolysis of blood specimens.
    b. changes WBC staining characteristics.
    c. erroneously increases potassium levels.
    d. leads to the formation of microclots.

59. Which of the following substances is contained in a serum separator tube?
    a. K_3EDTA
    b. lithium heparin
    c. sodium citrate
    d. thixotropic gel

60. What is the purpose of an antiglycolytic agent?
    a. enhance the clotting process
    b. inhibit electrolyte breakdown
    c. preserve glucose
    d. prevent clotting

61. Glass particles present in serum separator tubes:
    a. activate clotting.
    b. deter clotting.
    c. inhibit glycolysis.
    d. prevent hemolysis.

62. Which is the *best* tube for collecting an ETOH (ethanol) specimen?
    a. gray top
    b. green top
    c. lavender top
    d. light blue top

63. Identify the tubes needed to collect a CBC, PTT, and STAT potassium by color and in the proper order of collection for a multitube draw.
    a. gold top, yellow top, light blue top
    b. lavender top, SST royal blue top
    c. light blue top, green top, lavender top
    d. red top, gray top, light blue top

64. During venipuncture the tourni quet should not be left on longer than:
    a. 30 seconds.
    b. 1 minute.
    c. 2 minutes.
    d. 5 minutes.

65. Which one of the following tubes is filled first when multiple tubes are filled from a syringe?
    a. blood culture tube
    b. complete blood count tube
    c. nonadditive tube
    d. STAT potassium tube

66. This test is collected in a light blue top tube.
    a. glucose
    b. platelet count
    c. prothrombin time
    d. red blood count

67. Which of the following STAT tests is typically collected in a lithium heparin tube?
    a. blood type and screen
    b. complete blood count
    c. electrolytepanel
    d. prothrombin time (PTT)

68. This tube stopper color indicates that the tube contains EDTA.
    a. green
    b. lavender
    c. light blue
    d. royal blue

69. What anticoagulant is contained in a plasma separator (gel-barrier) tube?
    a. ACD
    b. citrate
    c. heparin
    d. oxalate

70. The purpose of sodium citrate in specimen collection is to:
    a. accelerate coagulation.
    b. inhibit glucose breakdown.
    c. preserve glucose values.
    d. protect coagulation factors.

71. The part of a syringe that shows measurements in cc or mL is called the:
    a. adapter.
    b. barrel.
    c. hub.
    d. plunger.

72. This part of the evacuated tube holder is meant to aid in smooth tube removal.
    a. barrel
    b. flange
    c. hub
    d. sleeve

73. The *best* choice of equipment for drawing difficult veins is a:
    a. butterfly and ETS holder.
    b. lancet and microtainer.
    c. needle and ETS holder.
    d. needle and 10-cc syringe.

74. Mixing equipment from different manufacturers can result in all of the following EXCEPT:
    a. improper fit of the needle.
    b. needles coming unscrewed.
    c. tubes popping off of needles.
    d. wrong choices of additives.

75. You are *most* likely to increase the chance of hemolyzing a specimen if you use a:
    a. 21-gauge needle and ETS tube to collect a specimen from a median vein.
    b. 22-gauge needle and syringe to collect a specimen from a difficult vein.
    c. 23-gauge butterfly needle to collect a specimen from a hand vein.
    d. 25-gauge butterfly needle to collect a specimen from a small child.

76. The purpose of a tourniquet in the venipuncture procedure is to:
    a. block the flow of arterial blood into the area.
    b. enlarge veins so they are easier to find and enter.
    c. obstruct blood flow to concentrate the analyte.
    d. redirect more blood flow to the venipuncture site.

77. If a blood pressure cuff is used for venipuncture in place of a tourniquet, the pressure used must be:
    a. below the patient's diastolic pressure.
    b. between the diastolic and systolic pressure.
    c. equal to the patient's systolic pressure.
    d. equal to the patient's venous pressure.

78. An anticoagulant works in all of the following ways EXCEPT:
    a. binds calcium or inhibits thrombin.
    b. inhibits the metabolism of glucose.
    c. keeps the blood in its natural state.
    d. prevents the specimen from clotting.

79. Needle safety devices are required to have all of the following qualities EXCEPT:
    a. allow the phlebotomist to use one hand to activate the device.
    b. create a barrier between the user's hand and the needle after use.
    c. permit the user's hand to remain behind the needle at all times.
    d. provide temporary containment of the used venipuncture needle.

80. This gel separator tube contains EDTA.
    a. EST
    b. PPT
    c. PST
    d. SST

81. Which additive contains a substance that inhibits phagocytosis of bacteria by white blood cells?
    a. silica (glass) clot activator
    b. sodium or lithium heparin
    c. sodium polyanethol sulfonate
    d. thixotropic silicon barrier gel

82. Which type of test is most affected by tissue thromboplastin contamination?
    a. chemistry
    b. coagulation
    c. microbiology
    d. serology

83. Which of the following tests would be most affected by carryover of K_2EDTA?
    a. BUN
    b. glucose

c. potassium
d. sodium

84. Which of the following microcollection containers should be filled first if collected by skin puncture?
a. gray stopper
b. green stopper
c. lavender stopper
d. red stopper

85. The intent of the alternate syringe order of draw is to:
a. decrease the clotting time in serum separator tubes.
b. minimize microclot formation in anticoagulant tubes.
c. prevent additive carryover when filling other tubes.
d. reduce the likelihood of microbial contamination.

86. A pink top tube containing EDTA is primarily used for:
a. blood bank tests.
b. chemistry tests.
c. coagulation tests.
d. microbiology tests.

87. Which of the following is *not* true of the blood collection equipment shown in Fig. 7-1? It can be used:
a. as a syringe.
b. as a VAD.
c. as an ETS.
d. with a butterfly.

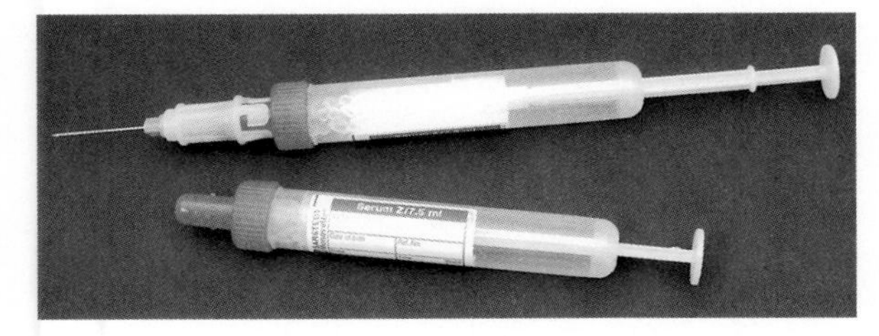

FIGURE 7-1 S-Monovette Blood Collection System. (Sarstedt, Inc., Newton, NC.)

88. Identify the tubes needed to collect a PT, STAT lytes, and BC in the proper order of collection.
a. gold, yellow, light blue
b light blue, lavender, yellow
c. SST, yellow, light blue
d. yellow, light blue, PST

89. Which one of the following tubes contains an additive?
a. red glass
b. red/light gray plastic
c. red plastic
d. royal blue glass/red label

90. Which chemistry tube could contain either of two different forms of an anticoagulant salt because both have the same stopper color?
a. blue
b. gray
c. green
d. tan

91. Which additive can be found in four separate tubes with different stopper colors?
a. EDTA
b. heparin
c. potassium oxalate
d. sodium citrate

92. Which stopper color is the same for two completely different types of additives used by two different departments?
a. blue
b. green
c. tan
d. yellow

93. How many tubes with different colored stoppers can sometimes go to the chemistry department?
a. 5
b. 9
c. 12
d. 14

94. Which of the following additives is used for chemistry tests?
   a. ACD
   b. citrate
   c. heparin
   d. SPS

95. An ETS holder and a syringe transfer device look very similar. What is the difference between the two?
   a. the hub on the transfer device attaches to a multisample needle or syringe barrel
   b. the transfer device is smaller in size than the regular holder and has no flanges
   c. there is a permanently attached needle with a sleeve inside the transfer device
   d. there is no difference between the ETS holder and the syringe transfer device

96. A prothrombin time (PT) and platelet count are ordered on an 80-year-old female patient. Deciding to use a butterfly and "short draw" evacuated tubes on the tiny cephalic vein on the dorsal side of the right arm, the phlebotomist collects the light blue tube first and the lavender last. Why would you suspect that the PT test results might be incorrect and the platelet count unaffected?
   a. no tube was drawn to remove air in the butterfly tubing
   b. PTs should never be collected using "short draw" tubes
   c. the tubes were drawn in the wrong collection sequence
   d. venipuncture of the tiny vein led to specimen hemolysis

97. A home care phlebotomist had a requisition to collect a complete blood count (CBC), plasma K, partial thromboplastin time (PTT), and prothrombin time (PT). He collected the tubes from the client, who was lying on the sofa with her arm elevated above her shoulder on a table next to the sofa. As he collected the tests in the following order: CBC, K, and finally the PT and PTT, he was careful to invert the tubes as specified. Later that day, the lab called the phlebotomist to say that three of the tests would have to be redrawn. Which three tests had questionable results?
   a. CBC, PT, and potassium
   b. potassium, PTT, and PT
   c. PTT, potassium, and CBC
   d. PTT, PT, and CBC

98. While collecting a STAT blood culture and electrolytes on a child in the emergency room, the physician asked the phlebotomist to get an extra tube of blood to check for metal poisoning. Which one of the following tubes would the phlebotomist add to the ones already being collected?
   a. gold
   b. gray
   c. pink
   d. royal blue

99. Which one of the following tubes/additives would be used to collect a DNA test?
   a. gold/clot activator
   b. light green/heparin
   c. yellow/ACD
   d. yellow/SPS

100. Electrolytes should never be collected in which of the following tubes?
   a. gold top
   b. gray top
   c. light green top
   d. red/gold top

ANSWERS AND EXPLANATIONS

1. Answer: c
   Why: A substance that prevents glycolysis, the breakdown or metabolism of glucose (blood sugar) by blood cells, is called a glycolytic inhibitor or an antiglycolytic agent. The most common antiglycolytic agent is sodium fluoride (NaF). It preserves glucose for up to 3 days and also inhibits the growth of bacteria.
   Review: Yes ☐ No ☐

2. Answer: a
   Why: Antiseptics, not disinfectants, are routinely used when performing venipuncture. Disinfectants are chemical substances or solutions that are used to remove or kill microorganisms on surfaces and instruments. They are typically corrosive and not safe for use on human skin.
   Review: Yes ☐ No ☐

3. Answer: d
   Why: SST stands for serum separator tube, a gel-barrier tube from Becton Dickinson (BD). This tube does not contain an anticoagulant, so blood collected in it will yield serum. The gel in the tube prevents glycolysis after the tube has been centrifuged. The EDTA tube and plasma preparation tube (PPT) both contain the anticoagulant EDTA. The plasma separator tube (PST) contains the anticoagulant heparin. Anticoagulants prevent the blood from clotting; consequently, they yield plasma when centrifuged.
   Review: Yes ☐ No ☐

4. Answer: d
   Why: Sodium citrate, oxalate, and EDTA are all anticoagulants that prevent blood from clotting by chelating (binding) or precipitating calcium so it is not available to the coagulation process. Sodium polyanethol sulfonate (SPS) also binds calcium, however lithium and sodium heparin prevent clotting by inhibiting the formation of thrombin needed to convert fibrinogen to fibrin in the coagulation process. Sodium fluoride (NaF) is an antiglycolytic agent, not an anticoagulant.
   Review: Yes ☐ No ☐

5. Answer: b
   Why: Evacuated tubes fill with blood automatically because there is a vacuum (negative pressure) in them. The vacuum is premeasured by the manufacturer so that the tube will draw the precise volume of blood indicated.
   Review: Yes ☐ No ☐

6. Answer: c
   Why: EDTA prevents coagulation and is primarily used to provide whole blood specimens for hematology tests because it preserves cell morphology and inhibits platelet aggregation or clumping.
   Review: Yes ☐ No ☐

7. Answer: b
   Why: The most common, efficient, and Clinical and Laboratory Standards Institute (CLSI)-preferred system for collecting blood samples is the ETS. Because it is a closed system in which the patient's blood flows directly into a collection tube, it offers many benefits. For example, blood can be collected without being exposed to air or outside contaminants or exposing the collector to the blood. Blood collected in a syringe is exposed to air and the possibility of outside contamination. In addition, the needle must be removed to attach a transfer device used to fill the tubes. This can expose the user to the patient's blood. A syringe does have the benefit of allowing the user to see when the vein has been entered, because a flash of blood appears in the hub when the vein is pierced. This does not happen when the ETS is used.
   Review: Yes ☐ No ☐

8. Answer: b
   Why: Lithium heparin causes the least interference in chemistry testing and is the most widely used anticoagulant for plasma and whole-blood chemistry tests. Heparinized plasma is often used for STAT chemistry tests and other rapid-response situations when a fast turnaround time (TAT) for chemistry test is needed.
   Review: Yes ☐ No ☐

9. Answer: b
   Why: Royal blue top tubes contain EDTA, heparin, or no additive, to meet various test requirements. Tube labels are typically color-coded to indicate the type of additive, if any, in the tube.
   Review: Yes ☐ No ☐

10. Answer: d
    Why: Royal blue top tubes are made of materials that are as free of trace element contamination as possible and are used for trace element tests, such as copper.
    Review: Yes ☐ No ☐

11. Answer: c
    Why: Some gloves come lightly dusted with powder to make them more comfortable to wear and easier to slip on and off. However, the phlebotomist should be aware that glove powder can be a source of contamination for some tests (especially those collected by skin puncture) and can also cause allergies in some users. Powder in latex gloves can help suspend latex particles in the air and pose a danger to those with latex allergy. Powder in gloves does not make them last longer.
    Review: Yes ☐ No ☐

12. Answer: d
    Why: Dermatitis is a condition that can be caused by wearing gloves. Barrier hand creams (Fig. 7-2) can help prevent skin irritation and are compatible with latex gloves.
    Review: Yes ☐ No ☐

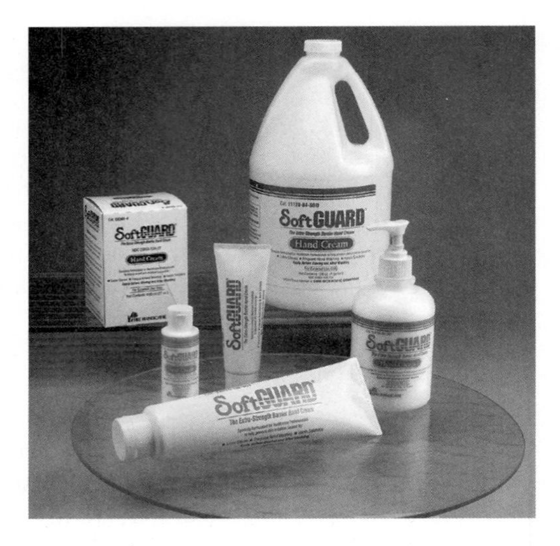

FIGURE 7-2 SoftGUARD barrier hand cream. (Courtesy Erie Scientific Co., Portsmouth, NH.)

13. Answer: a
    Why: Decontamination of hands after glove removal is essential and made very convenient, for instance, by wall-mounted hand sanitizer dispensers, such as shown in Fig. 7-3. Any type of glove may contain defects, and contamination is not always visible. Some studies suggest that vinyl gloves may not provide adequate protection to viruses. Any glove powder should be washed off because it can be a source of contamination for some tests.
    Review: Yes ☐ No ☐

14. Answer: c
    Why: Household bleach, or 5.25% sodium hypochlorite, is an effective disinfectant but is too caustic to be used as an antiseptic. Antiseptics are substances used to prevent sepsis that are safe to use on skin and are all of the solutions listed in Box 7.1 Antiseptics Used in Blood Collection.
    Review: Yes ☐ No ☐

15. Answer: d
    Why: According to CDC and HICPAC *Guidelines for Environmental Infection Control in*

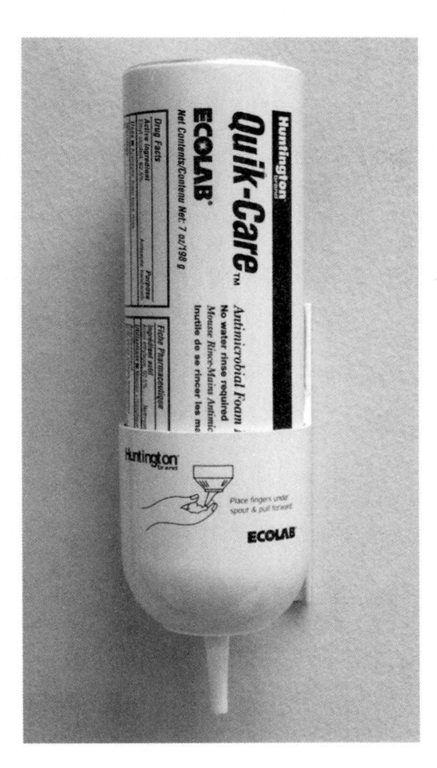

FIGURE 7-3 Wall-mounted hand sanitizer dispenser.

Healthcare Facilities, use of EPA-registered sodium hypochlorite products for disinfecting surfaces and instruments is preferred.

Review: Yes ☐ No ☐

Box 7-1 Antiseptics Used in Blood Collection

- 70% Ethyl alcohol
- 70% Isopropyl alcohol (isopropanol)
- Benzalkonium chloride (e.g., Zephiran chloride)
- Chlorhexidine gluconate
- Hydrogen peroxide
- Povidone-iodine (0.1–1% available iodine)
- Tincture of iodine

16. Answer: c

    Why: A spill involving large amounts of blood or other body fluids requires at least 10 minutes of contact time with a disinfectant for the cleanup to be considered effective.

    Review: Yes ☐ No ☐

17. Answer: b

    Why: When hands are heavily contaminated with organic material and a sink is not available, it is recommended that hands be cleaned with detergent-containing wipes followed by the use of an alcohol-based hand cleaner or sanitizer.

    Review: Yes ☐ No ☐

18. Answer: d

    Why: Transillumination is the inspection of an organ by passing light through its walls. The Venoscope II (Fig. 7-4) is a transillumination device that can be used to locate difficult veins that cannot be easily seen or felt. It works by shining a high-intensity light through the patient's subcutaneous tissue.

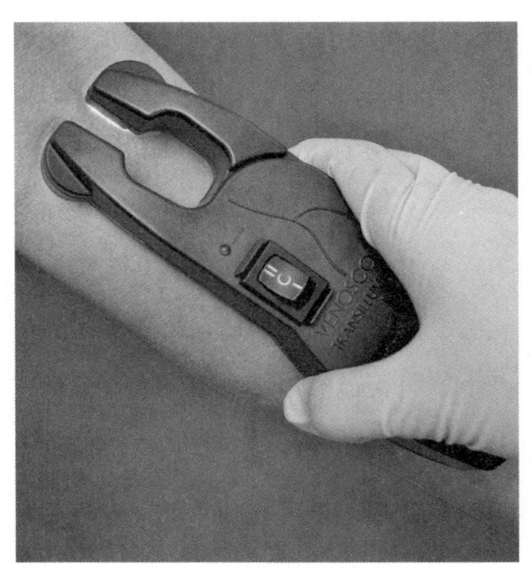

FIGURE 7-4 Venoscope II transilluminator device (Venoscope II, LLC, Lafayette, LA.)

This highlights the veins, which absorb the light rather than reflecting it and stand out as dark lines.

Review: Yes ☐ No ☐

19. Answer: c

Why: A properly applied tourniquet is tight enough to restrict venous flow out of the area, but not so tight as to restrict arterial flow into the area. Restriction of venous flow distends or inflates the veins, making them larger and easier to find and stretches the vein walls, making them thinner and easier to pierce with a needle.

Review: Yes ☐ No ☐

20. Answer: b

Why: An 18-gauge needle is used primarily as a transfer needle rather than for blood collection. Because of safety issues, the use of this practice is now discouraged. See Table 7-1: Common Venipuncture Needle Gauges With Needle Types and Typical Uses.

Review: Yes ☐ No ☐

21. Answer: b

Why: There is no needle safety feature that plugs the needle with silicon. Safety features include resheathing devices such as shields that cover the needle after use, blunting devices, and equipment with devices that retract the needle after the use.

Review: Yes ☐ No ☐

22. Answer: d

Why: OSHA regulations require that the tube holder with needle attached be disposed of as a unit in the sharps container after use. OSHA guidelines state that holders should not be reused and the needle should not be removed from the tube holder.

Review: Yes ☐ No ☐

Table 7-1 Common Venipuncture Needle Gauges with Needle Type and Typical Use

Gauge	Needle Type	Typical Use
15–17	Special needle attached to collection bag	Collection of donor units, autologous blood donation, and therapeutic phlebotomy
18	Syringe	Used primarily as a transfer needle rather than for blood collection; safety issues have diminished use
20	Multisample Syringe	Sometimes used when large-volume tubes are collected or large-volume syringes are used on patients with normal-size veins
21	Multisample Syringe	Considered the standard venipuncture needle for routine venipuncture on patients with normal veins or syringe blood culture collection
22	Multisample Syringe	Used on older children and adult patients with small veins or syringe draws on difficult veins
23	Butterfly	Veins of infants and children and difficult or hand veins of adults

23. Answer: a
Why: Evacuated tubes fill with blood automatically because there is a vacuum. The vacuum is premeasured by the manufacturer so that the tube will draw the precise volume of blood indicated. Tubes do not fill with blood all the way to the stopper. When filled properly, there is always a consistent amount of headspace between the level of blood in the tube and the tube stopper.
Review: Yes ☐ No ☐

24. Answer: b
Why: Some manufacturers offer special "short draw" tubes designed to partially fill without compromising test results. These tubes are used in situations in which it is difficult or inadvisable to draw larger quantities of blood. They are the same size as regular-fill tubes but contain adjusted amounts of additive. The "short draw" tubes can be used for any of the tests for which regular tubes are used.
Review: Yes ☐ No ☐

25. Answer: d
Why: Most ETS tubes contain some type of additive. An additive is any substance placed within a tube other than the tube stopper or the coating of the tube.
Review: Yes ☐ No ☐

26. Answer: b
Why: With the advent of plastic tubes, very few tubes are additive free anymore. Even serum tubes have an additive if they are plastic because plastic is so slick that platelet aggregation and adhesion is inhibited unless the tube contains a clot activator.
Review: Yes ☐ No ☐

27. Answer: b
Why: Improper handling or storage may affect additive integrity and tube vacuum, which can lead to compromised test results or improper filling, respectively. If plastic tubes are not stored properly, heat will cause them to melt and become disfigured. Handling the tubes improperly has not been shown to affect inert gels.
Review: Yes ☐ No ☐

28. Answer: b
Why: Citrate binds calcium. If citrate from a light blue top tube is carried over into another ETS tube used for a calcium test, the result could be affected (Table 7-2).
Review: Yes ☐ No ☐

29. Answer: c
Why: EDTA has been shown to affect creatine kinase levels. If EDTA from a lavender top tube is carried over into an ETS tube used for a creatine kinase test, the result could be affected (Table 7-2).
Review: Yes ☐ No ☐

30. Answer: c
Why: Alkaline phosphatase tests may be affected if contaminated by the additive in a light blue tube containing citrate, a gray tube that contains oxalate, or a lavender tube containing EDTA (Table 7-2). Heparin is found in the body as a naturally occurring anticoagulant and therefore does not affect alkaline phosphatase results.
Review: Yes ☐ No ☐

31. Answer: c
Why: A partial thromboplastin time result could be affected by all of the additives listed in Table 7-2, except sodium fluoride (NaF) and citrate. Results can be affected by oxalate, however, which is often combined with sodium fluoride.
Review: Yes ☐ No ☐

32. Answer: d
Why: Collection of some specimens, such as blood cultures, requires a higher degree of skin antisepsis than obtained by using

Table 7-2 Common Tests Affected by Additive Contamination

Contaminating Additive	Tests Potentially Affected
Citrate	Alkaline phosphatase Calcium Phosphorus
EDTA	Alkaline phosphatase Calcium Creatine kinase Partial thromboplasstin Potassium Protime Serum iron Sodium
Heparin (all formulations)	Activated clotting time Acid phosphatase Calcium (some test methods) Partial thromboplastin Protime Sodium (sodium formulations) Lithium (lithium formulations)
Oxalates	Acid phosphatase Alkaline phosphatase Amylase Calcium Lactate dehydrogenase Partial thromboplastin Potassium Protime Red cell morphology
Silica (clot activator)	Partial thromboplastin time Protime
Sodium fluoride	Sodium Urea nitrogen

isopropyl alcohol. Povidone-iodine, in the form of swabsticks or sponge pads, has been the traditional skin antiseptic used to collect these specimens. The use of an alcohol-based preparation for these procedures is increasing, however, because many patients are allergic to povidone-iodine. Antiseptics used in blood collection are listed in Box 7.1.

Review: Yes ☐ No ☐

33. Answer: b

Why: According to CDC and HICPAC *Guidelines for Environmental Infection Control in Healthcare Facilities*, use of EPA-registered or approved sodium hypochlorite products is preferred, but solutions made from 5.25% sodium hypochlorite (household bleach) may be used. A 1:100 dilution is recommended for decontaminating nonporous surfaces after cleaning up blood or other body fluid spills in patient care settings.

Review: Yes ☐ No ☐

34. Answer: b

Why: Disinfectants are corrosive chemical compounds that are bactericidal (kill bacteria). Some also kill viruses, such as human immunodeficiency virus and hepatitis. Disinfectants are used on surfaces and instruments to kill potential pathogens. They are *not* safe for use on human skin.

Review: Yes ☐ No ☐

35. Answer: b

Why: The most common antiseptic used for routine blood collection is 70% isopropyl alcohol (isopropanol). Bleach (5.25% sodium hypochlorite) is a disinfectant and is not safe to use on human skin. Methanol can be toxic when absorbed through the skin and is not used as a skin antiseptic. Povidone-iodine is used for collection of sterile specimens such as blood cultures.

Review: Yes ☐ No ☐

36. Answer: b

Why: Gauze or gauzelike pads are preferred for holding pressure over a venipuncture site because the fibers from cotton, Dacron, or rayon balls tend to stick to the site and re-initiate bleeding when removed.

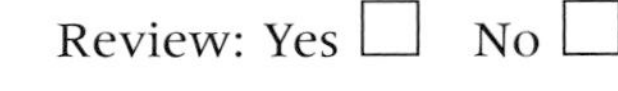

Review: Yes ☐ No ☐

37. Answer: a

Why: Adhesive bandages should not be used on infants and children younger than 2 years of age because of the danger of aspiration and suffocation if they are accidentally removed from the site.

Review: Yes ☐ No ☐

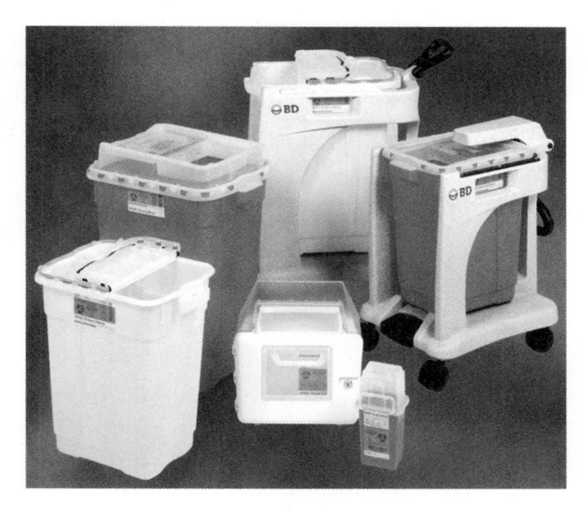

FIGURE 7-5 Several styles of sharps containers. (Courtesy Becton Dickinson, Franklin Lakes, NJ.)

38. Answer: d

Why: The Occupational Safety and Health Administration (OSHA) requires that sharps containers (Fig. 7-5) be rigid, leakproof, puncture-resistant, and disposable and have locking lids that can be easily sealed when the container is full. OSHA also requires that they be marked with a biohazard symbol, but they do not require that all of the containers be red in color.

Review: Yes ☐ No ☐

39. Answer: b

Why: Because latex and vinyl tourniquets are relatively inexpensive, they are usually discarded if soiled with blood. Autoclaving a latex or vinyl tourniquet would destroy it. Bleach disintegrates latex and makes it gummy. Alcohol is an antiseptic and would not necessarily destroy bloodborne pathogens.

Review: Yes ☐ No ☐

40. Answer: d
Why: OSHA's Bloodborne Pathogen Standard is a federal law that mandates wearing of gloves during most phlebotomy procedures. The CDC and HICPAC provide guidelines for wearing gloves, but the guidelines are not federal laws. The FDA regulates glove quality.
Review: Yes ☐ No ☐

41. Answer: b
Why: The needle gauge for venipuncture is selected according to the size and condition of the patient's vein, the type of procedure, and the equipment being used. Personal preference and the depth of the vein influence the length of needle used, rather than the gauge. The type of test being collected does not normally influence selection of the needle gauge or length.
Review: Yes ☐ No ☐

42. Answer: a
Why: The gauge of a needle is a number that is inversely related to the diameter of the lumen or internal space of the needle. It is an indication of the size of the needle; the larger the number, the smaller its diameter, and vice versa. Most needles are color-coded according to gauge; however, color-coding varies by manufacturer. Multisample needles typically have color-coded caps (Fig. 7-6 and Fig 7-7).
Review: Yes ☐ No ☐

43. Answer: a
Why: "Bore" is a term used to describe the diameter of a needle and the size of the hole it makes. There is an inverse relationship between the gauge number and the bore or diameter of the lumen of a needle. Therefore, the needle gauge with the largest bore or lumen is the one with the smallest number.
Review: Yes ☐ No ☐

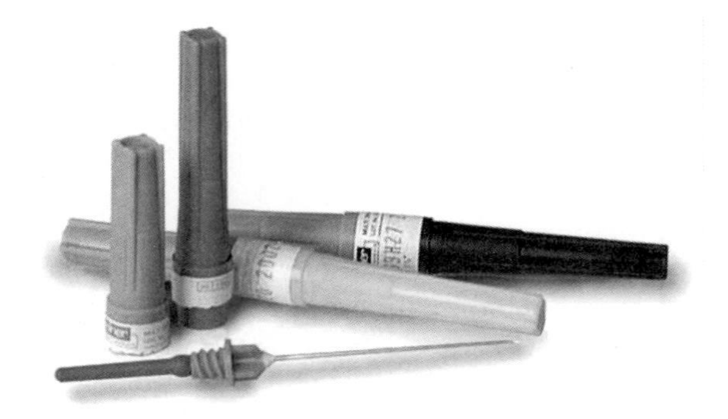

FIGURE 7-6 Multisample (traditional style) needles with color-coded caps: *Left,* green 21 gauge. *Center,* yellow 20 gauge. *Right,* black 22 gauge. (Courtesy Greiner Bio-One, Kremsmünster, Austria.)

44. Answer: c
Why: ETS multisample needles (Figs. 7-6 and 7-7) are generally available in 20-, 21-, and 22-gauge. A 21-gauge needle is considered the standard needle for routine venipuncture. Syringe needles and butterfly needles are available in smaller-size gauges for difficult draw situations.
Review: Yes ☐ No ☐

45. Answer: a
Why: The end of the needle that is inserted into the vein is called the bevel (Fig. 7-8)

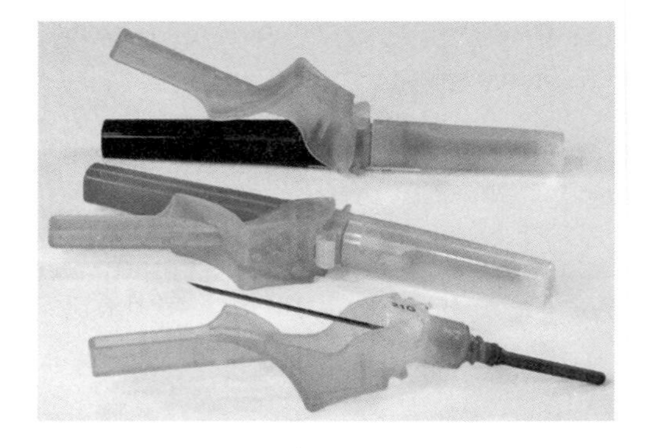

FIGURE 7-7 BD Eclipse multisample safety needles, *Top:* black 22 gauge, *Center:* green 21 gauge. (Becton Dickinson, Franklin Lakes, NJ.)

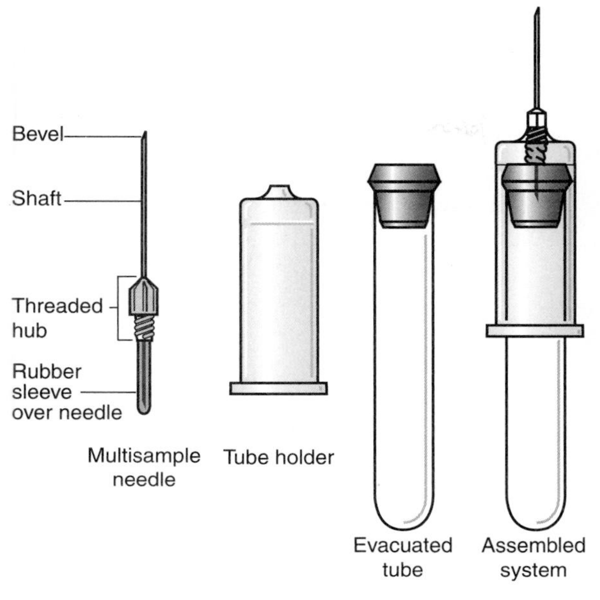

FIGURE 7-8 Traditional components of the evacuated tube system (ETS).

because it is cut on a slant or "beveled" to allow the needle to penetrate the vein easily and prevent coring (removal of a portion of the skin or vein). The hub of a needle is the end that attaches to a syringe or tube holder. The lumen of a needle is the internal space of the needle. The shaft is the long cylindrical part of the needle.

Review: Yes ☐ No ☐

46. Answer: c

Why: The rubber sleeve (Fig. 7-8) of a multiple-sample needle retracts as the needle is inserted into the tube, allowing the tube to fill with blood, and recovers the needle as the tube is removed, preventing leakage of blood into the tube holder. It is not possible to maintain a sterile sample because the sample was not collected in a sterile manner. The flanges on the holder were designed to enable smooth tube placement and removal.

Review: Yes ☐ No ☐

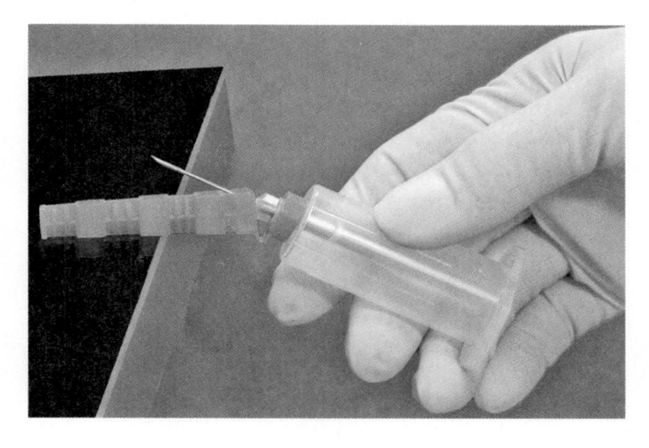

FIGURE 7-9 Venipuncture Needle-Pro with needle resheathing device. (Courtesy Retractible Technologies, Little Elm, TX.)

47. Answer: b

Why: A needle without a safety feature can be used for blood collection. However, according to OSHA regulations, it must be used with a tube holder that has a safety feature (Fig. 7-9). In addition, a needle must never be recapped or removed from its holder after use unless it has been demonstrated that it is specifically required by a medical procedure or there is no feasible alternative. In such instances, a mechanical device or some method other than a two-handed procedure must be used.

Review: Yes ☐ No ☐

48. Answer: b

Why: The size and condition of the patient's vein and sample volume required for testing play a major role when selecting the size of tubes to use for venipuncture. Age and weight play a role when drawing infants and young children so as not to deplete their blood volumes. Age is also a consideration when drawing elderly patients with fragile veins. Allergies play a role in selecting the antiseptic to use, not tube size.

Review: Yes ☐ No ☐

49. Answer: c
Why: Glass evacuated tubes are often coated on the inside with silicon to fill tiny cracks and other imperfections in the glass and create a smooth surface. The smooth surface prevents destruction of red blood cells and helps keep blood from sticking to the sides of the tube. The silicon coating also prevents activation of the clotting factors in tubes used for coagulation studies. In contrast, plastic tubes (Fig. 7-10) are so slick that platelet aggregation and adhesion are inhibited, and a clot activator must be added to the ones that are used to collect serum specimens.
Review: Yes ☐ No ☐

50. Answer: c
Why: A light blue top tube typically contains the anticoagulant sodium citrate as the additive. Sodium citrate prevents coagulation by binding calcium. It is used for coagulation specimens because it does the best job of preserving the coagulation factors, and adding calcium back to the specimen during testing easily reverses its binding effects. The most common use of green tops is to collect plasma for chemistry tests. Lavender tops are most commonly used to collect whole blood for hematology tests. Red tops are most often used for chemistry, serology, and blood bank tests.
Review: Yes ☐ No ☐

51. Answer: d
Why: There are two types of red top tubes, glass and plastic. Blood collected in either of these tubes will clot and when centrifuged, a clear fluid called serum separates from the clotted cells. Green, lavender, and light blue top tubes contain anticoagulants. Specimens that are collected in anticoagulant tubes are prevented from clotting and yield whole blood specimens. When blood in anticoagulant tubes is centrifuged, clear fluid separates from the cells and is called plasma. Green top tubes are typically centrifuged to yield plasma for certain chemistry tests.

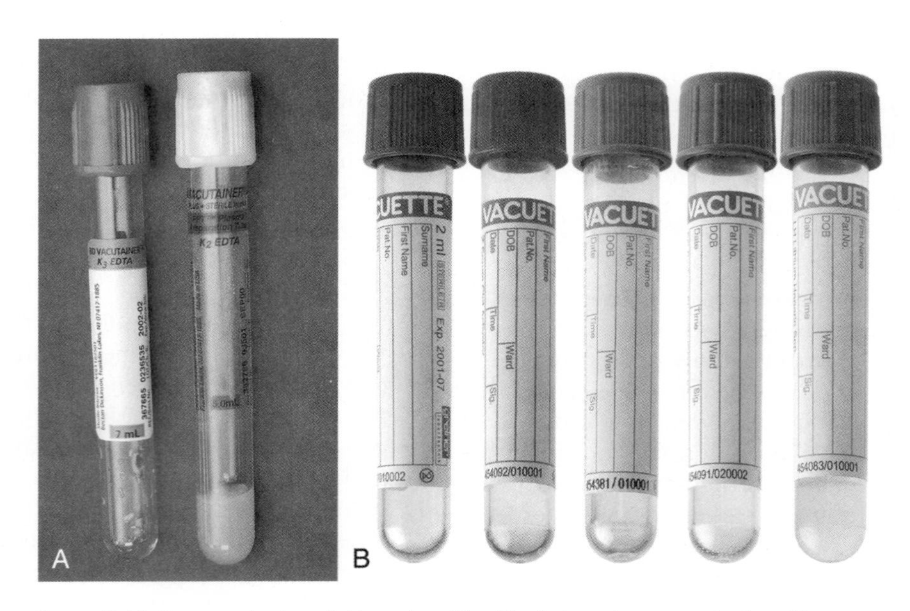

FIGURE 7-10 Evacuated tubes. **A.** Vacutainer Plus Plastic brand evacuated tubes. (Becton Dickinson, Franklin Lakes, NJ.) **B.** Vacuette evacuated tubes. (Courtesy Greiner Bio-One, Kremsmünster, Austria.)

The most common use of light blue tops is to provide plasma for coagulation tests.

Review: Yes ☐ No ☐

52. Answer: a

Why: The CDC *Guideline for Hand Hygiene in Healthcare Settings* recommends the use of alcohol-based hand sanitizers as a substitute for hand washing, provided the hands are not visibly soiled.

Review: Yes ☐ No ☐

53. Answer: d

Why: Most tube stopper colors indicate the presence (or absence) and type of additive in a tube. A green stopper indicates heparin, a lavender stopper indicates EDTA, and light blue normally indicates sodium citrate. A royal blue stopper, however, indicates that the tube and stopper are virtually trace-element–free. A royal blue top can contain no additive, potassium EDTA, or sodium heparin. Additive color-coding of a royal blue top tube is typically indicated on the label.

Review: Yes ☐ No ☐

54. Answer: d

Why: Heparin prevents coagulation by inhibiting thrombin during the coagulation process. Thrombin is necessary for the formation of fibrin from fibrinogen. Without thrombin, a fibrin clot cannot form.

Review: Yes ☐ No ☐

55. Answer: d

Why: Sodium polyanethol sulfonate (SPS) tubes are used to collect blood cultures, which are performed in the microbiology department. SPS is an anticoagulant with special properties that inhibit proteins that destroy bacteria, prevent phagocytosis of bacteria by white blood cells, and reduce the activity of some antibiotics.

Review: Yes ☐ No ☐

56. Answer: b

Why: A royal blue stopper signifies that the tube and stopper contain the lowest levels of trace elements available (i.e., they are virtually trace-element–free). Royal blue top tubes are available with EDTA, heparin, no additive (glass tube), or clot activator (plastic tube). Color-coding on the label indicates what additive, if any, is in the tube. Green color-coding on the label of a royal blue top indicates that it contains heparin.

Review: Yes ☐ No ☐

57. Answer: a

Why: Oxalate is an anticoagulant that prevents coagulation by precipitating calcium, and the form most widely used is potassium oxalate. Thromboplastin is found in tissue fluid and activates the extrinsic clotting pathway. Silica is used as a clot activator in ETS clotting tubes. Phosphate is an additive found in the special anticoagulants, ACD and CPD.

Review: Yes ☐ No ☐

58. Answer: a

Why: Excess oxalate causes hemolysis, the destruction of red blood cells and the liberation of hemoglobin into the plasma. Hemolysis will increase potassium levels, but the gray top tube containing potassium oxalate as the anticoagulant cannot be used to collect potassium specimens for obvious reasons. Microclot formation can result from too little anticoagulant, rather than too much. Hematology tests, such as evaluating stained WBCs, are collected in EDTA tubes, not oxalate.

Review: Yes ☐ No ☐

59. Answer: d

Why: Thixotropic gel is an inert (nonreacting) synthetic substance that forms a physical barrier between the cellular portion of a specimen and the serum or plasma portion after the specimen has been centrifuged.

When used in a serum tube it is called serum separator, and the tube is referred to as a serum separator tube (SST) or a gel-barrier tube. When used in a tube that contains heparin, it is called plasma separator and the tube is referred to as a plasma separator tube (PST). If it is used in a tube that contains EDTA, the tube is called a plasma preparation tube (PPT). At this time, there is no gel tube that contains sodium citrate.
Review: Yes ☐ No ☐

60. Answer: c
Why: An antiglycolytic agent is a substance that inhibits or prevents glycolysis (metabolism of glucose) by the cells of the blood. The most common glycolytic inhibitors are sodium fluoride and lithium iodoacetate.
Review: Yes ☐ No ☐

61. Answer: a
Why: Glass (silica) particles are called clot activators and are present in serum separator tubes to make the blood clot faster. Glass particles enhance or accelerate clotting by providing increased surface for platelet activation, aggregation, and adhesion. Other substances that function as clot activators in other types of tubes include inert clays, such as siliceous earth, kaolin, and Celite, and the clotting components thromboplastin and thrombin.
Review: Yes ☐ No ☐

62. Answer: a
Why: A gray top tube typically contains sodium fluoride, which prevents glycolysis. It is used for alcohol determinations and glucose tests. Alcohol values are stable because glycolysis (the metabolism of glucose or sugar in the form of alcohol) is prevented. Sodium fluoride also inhibits growth of bacteria and protects the specimen from an increase in alcohol resulting from fermentation by bacteria.
Review: Yes ☐ No ☐

63. Answer: c
Why: A CBC is a hematology test collected in a lavender top tube. A PTT is a coagulation test collected in a light blue top tube. A STAT potassium is a chemistry test collected in a green top tube. The proper order of draw for these tubes is light blue first, green next, and lavender last (Table 7-3).
Review: Yes ☐ No ☐

64. Answer: b
Why: Proper tourniquet application allows arterial blood flow into the area below the tourniquet but obstructs venous flow away from the area. This causes the veins to enlarge and makes them easier to find and pierce with a needle. However, the obstruction of blood flow can change blood components if the tourniquet is left in place for more than 1 minute.
Review: Yes ☐ No ☐

65. Answer: a
Why: Tubes or containers for specimens such as blood cultures that must be collected in a sterile manner are always collected first in the order of draw for both the syringe and ETS system of venipuncture (Table 7-3).
Review: Yes ☐ No ☐

66. Answer: c
Why: A prothrombin time (PT) is a coagulation test and is collected in a light blue top tube containing sodium citrate. The best tube for collecting a glucose specimen is a gray top containing an antiglycolytic agent such as sodium fluoride. A platelet count is sometimes ordered to assess coagulation, but it is a hematology test collected in a lavender top tube. A red blood count is a hematology test and is collected in a lavender top tube.
Review: Yes ☐ No ☐

67. Answer: c
Why: Most chemistry tests have been traditionally performed on serum, but to save

Table 7-3 Order of Draw, Stopper Colors, and Rationale for Collection Order

Order of Draw	Tube Stopper Color	Rationale for Collection Order
Blood cultures (sterile collections)	Yellow SPS Sterile media bottles	Minimizes chance of microbial contamination
Coagulation tubes	Light blue	The first additive tube in the order because all other additive tubes affect coagulation test
Glass nonadditive tubes	Red	Prevents contamination by additives in other tubes
Plastic clot activator tubes Serum separator tubes (SSTs)	Red Red & gray rubber Gold plastic	Filled after coagulation tests because silica particles activate clotting and affect coagulation tests (carryover of silica into subsequent tubes can be overridden by anticoagulant in them)
Plasma separator tubes (PSTs) Heparin tubes	Green & gray rubber Light-green plastic Green	Heparin affects coagulation tests and interferes in collection of serum specimens; causes the least interference in tests other than coagulation tests
EDTA tubes Plasma preparation tubes (PPTs)	Lavender, Pink Pearl top	Responsible for more carryover problems than any other additive: elevates Na and K levels, chelates and decreases calcium and iron levels, elevates PT and PTT results
Oxalate/fluoride tubes	Gray	Sodium fluoride and potassium oxalate affect sodium and potassium levels, respectively. After hematology tubes because oxalate damages cell membranes and causes abnormal RBC morphology. Oxalate interferes in enzyme reactions

the time it takes for a serum specimen to clot before it can be tested, STAT electrolytes and other STAT chemistry tests are often performed on plasma specimens collected in lithium heparin tubes. Sodium heparin tubes must not be used for STAT electrolytes because sodium is one of the electrolytes measured. In addition, new studies show that heparinized plasma may be the best specimen for potassium tests regardless of whether they are STAT.

Review: Yes ☐ No ☐

68. Answer: b

Why: A lavender (or purple) top indicates that the tube contains EDTA. Most hematology tests are collected in lavender top tubes. A green stopper indicates a heparin-containing tube, and a light blue stopper indicates the presence of sodium citrate unless it has a special yellow label. A royal blue stopper indicates that the tube and stopper are as free of trace elements as possible. A royal blue stopper sometimes contains EDTA, but only if it has lavender color-coding on the label or EDTA is written on the label. Fig. 7-10 shows a variety of tubes with different colors of stoppers.

Review: Yes ☐ No ☐

69. Answer: c

Why: A plasma separator tube (PST) contains heparin. Some gel-barrier tubes, such as the plasma preparation tube (PPT), contain EDTA. Serum separator tubes (SSTs) are gel-barrier tubes, but they do not contain anticoagulant. Anticoagulants are used to obtain either whole blood or plasma specimens. In the separator tubes, the plasma can be removed from the cells so that the integrity of the specimen is maintained.

Review: Yes ☐ No ☐

70. Answer: d

Why: Sodium citrate is the anticoagulant contained in light blue top tubes used to collect plasma for coagulation tests. It is used for coagulation tests because it does the best job of protecting the coagulation factors. The ratio of blood to anticoagulant is critical in coagulation testing, so it is important for sodium citrate tubes to be filled to their stated capacity.

Review: Yes ☐ No ☐

71. Answer: b

Why: The barrel of a syringe holds the fluid being aspirated or administered and is measured in cubic centimeters (cc) or milliliters (mL). The plunger is a rodlike device that fits tightly into the barrel. Pulling on the plunger creates the vacuum that allows the barrel to fill with the fluid being aspirated.

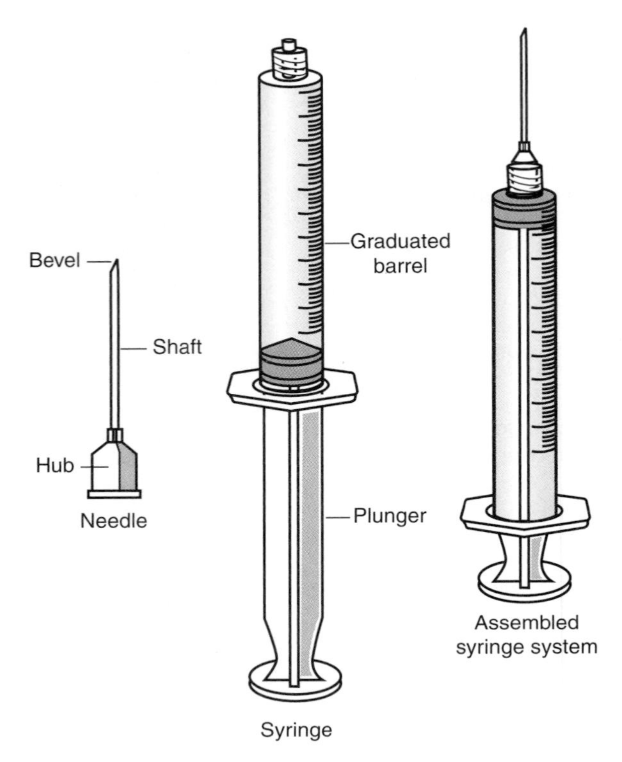

FIGURE 7-11 Traditional syringe system components.

The hub is where the needle attaches to the syringe. Traditional syringe components are shown in Fig. 7-11.

Review: Yes ☐ No ☐

72. Answer: b

Why: The flanges or extensions on the sides of the tube end of the holder are there to aid in tube placement and removal. Fig. 7-12 shows proper placement of fingers and thumb when advancing a tube in an ETS holder.

Review: Yes ☐ No ☐

73. Answer: a

Why: The butterfly needle (Fig. 7-13) is an indispensable tool for collecting blood from small or difficult veins because it allows much more flexibility and precision than either a regular needle and evacuated tube

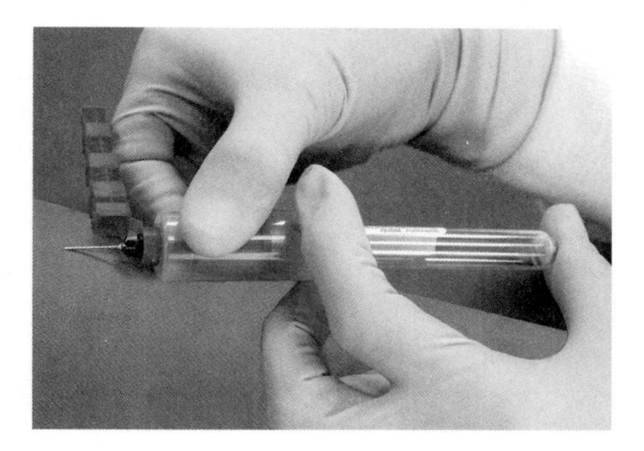

FIGURE 7-12 Proper placement of fingers and thumb when advancing a tube in an ETS holder.

holder or needle and syringe. A lancet and microtainer can be used to collect some specimens by skin puncture, but there are several tests that cannot be collected by this method.

Review: Yes ☐ No ☐

74. Answer: d

Why: Although evacuated tube collection system components from different manufacturers are similar, they are not necessarily interchangeable. Mixing components from different manufacturers can lead to problems such as improper needle fit and needles coming unscrewed, or tubes popping off of the needle during venipuncture procedures. Color-coding of tube tops is generally universal, with only a few minor variations in each company's product, so selecting the proper additive tube is not normally an issue.

Review: Yes ☐ No ☐

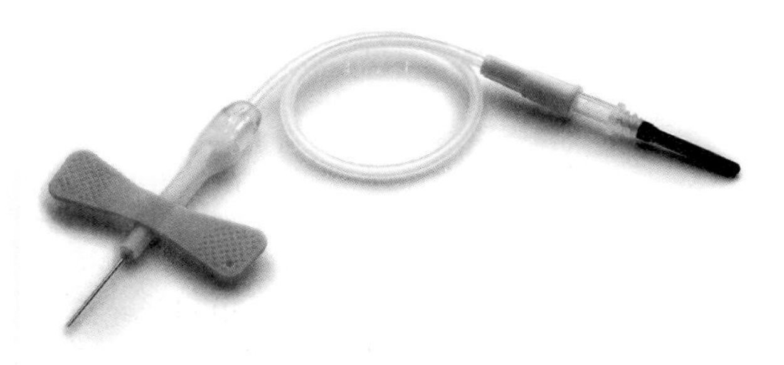

FIGURE 7-13 Vacuette safety butterfly blood collection system. (Courtesy Greiner Bio-One, Kremsmünster, Austria.)

75. Answer: d

Why: The 25-gauge butterfly needles are sometimes successfully used to collect blood specimens from infants and others with difficult veins. However, any time a needle smaller than 23g is used to collect blood, the chance of trauma to the red blood cells and resulting hemolysis is increased.

Review: Yes ☐ No ☐

76. Answer: b

Why: The purpose of a tourniquet in the venipuncture procedure is to block the venous flow, not the arterial flow, so that blood flows freely into the area but not out. This causes the veins to enlarge, making them easier to find and penetrate with a needle. The tourniquet does not redirect blood flow but does change the volume of the flow. The tourniquet must not be left on for longer than 1 minute because obstruction of blood flow changes the concentration of some analytes, leading to erroneous test results.

Review: Yes ☐ No ☐

77. Answer: a

Why: A blood pressure cuff may be used in place of a tourniquet by those familiar with its operation. The patient's blood pressure is taken, and the pressure is then maintained at 40 mm Hg or below the patient's diastolic pressure.

Review: Yes ☐ No ☐

78. Answer: b

Why: An anticoagulant prevents coagulation or clotting of the blood either by binding calcium and making it unavailable to the coagulation process, or by inhibiting thrombin formation, which is needed in the coagulation process. A specimen that is not allowed to clot because of the addition of an anticoagulant remains as it was in the body and is called a whole blood sample.

Review: Yes ☐ No ☐

79. Answer: d

Why: A needle safety device (Fig. 7-14) should allow the user's hand to remain behind the needle at all times, create a barrier between the hands of the user and the needle after use, be activated using a one-handed technique, and provide permanent (not temporary) containment of the needle. A needle safety feature should never be a temporary measure.

Review: Yes ☐ No ☐

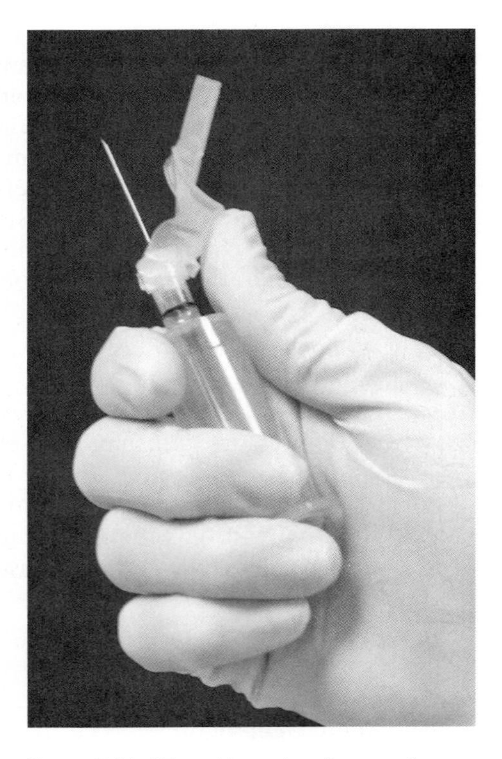

FIGURE 7-14 BD multisample safety needle attached to traditional tube holder. (Becton Dickinson, Franklin Lakes, NJ.)

80. Answer: b

Why: An EDTA tube that contains a separator gel is called a plasma preparation tube, or PPT. A plasma separator tube (PST) contains heparin and gel. A serum separator tube (SST) contains silica particles or clot activator and gel. There is no separator gel tube called an EST.

Review: Yes ☐ No ☐

81. Answer: c

Why: Sodium polyanethol sulfonate (SPS) is used in tubes for blood culture collection because in addition to being an anticoagulant, this additive is formulated to inhibit phagocytosis of bacteria by white blood cells. SPS reduces the action of a protein called complement that destroys bacteria, slows down phagocytosis (ingestion of bacteria by leukocytes), and reduces the activity of certain antibiotics. Heparin inhibits thrombin. Silica activates or enhances clotting. When a specimen is centrifuged, thixotropic gel becomes a physical barrier between the serum or plasma and the cells to prevent the cells from metabolizing substances in the serum or plasma.

Review: Yes ☐ No ☐

82. Answer: b

Why: Tissue thromboplastin affects coagulation tests the most because it is a substance found in tissue that activates the extrinsic coagulation pathway. Tissue thromboplastin is picked up by the needle as it penetrates the skin during venipuncture and is flushed into the first tube filled during ETS collection, or mixed with blood collected in a syringe. Although it is no longer considered a significant problem for prothrombin time (PT) and partial thromboplastin time (PTT) tests unless the draw is difficult or involves a lot of needle manipulation, it may compromise results of other coagulation tests. Therefore, any time a coagulation test other than PT or PTT is the first or only tube collected, a few milliliters of blood should be drawn into a "discard" tube.

Review: Yes ☐ No ☐

83. Answer: c

Why: K_2EDTA contains potassium. (K is the chemical symbol for potassium, and K_2EDTA is an abbreviation for dipotassium EDTA.) Carryover of potassium EDTA formulations into tubes for potassium testing have been known to significantly increase potassium levels in the specimen, causing erroneously elevated test results.

Review: Yes ☐ No ☐

84. Answer: c

Why: Lavender stoppers contain EDTA and are used to collect hematology specimens. In the Clinical and Laboratory Standards Institute (CLSI) order of draw for skin puncture, EDTA specimens are collected first because skin puncture blood contains tissue thromboplastin, which activates the coagulation process, causing platelet clumping and microclot formation in the specimen if it is not collected quickly. Platelet clumping and microclots cause erroneous hematology test results.

Review: Yes ☐ No ☐

85. Answer: b

Why: The intent of the alternate syringe order of draw is to fill tubes for tests that are most affected by microclot formation as soon as possible. In this order of draw, the assumption is made that blood that enters the syringe last is the freshest and least affected by microclot formation. Sterile specimens are still filled first, but are immediately followed by anticoagulant tubes because they are most affected by microclot formation. Of the anticoagulant tubes, light blue top coagulation tubes are filled first, followed by lavender tubes for hematology studies, green tops, and gray tops. Red tops, clot activator tubes, and SSTs are filled after all the anticoagulant tubes because blood in these tubes is supposed to clot. To prevent carryover when this method is used, the transfer needle must be kept above the fill level of the tube so that blood mixed with additive does not contaminate it.

Review: Yes ☐ No ☐

86. Answer: a

Why: A pink top EDTA tube typically has a special label for ID information and is used primarily for blood bank tests.

Review: Yes ☐ No ☐

87. Answer: b

Why: The S-Monovette Blood Collection system shown in Fig. 7-1 is a complete system for blood collection in which the blood collection tube and collection apparatus are combined in a single unit. The unit allows the specimen to be collected by either an evacuated tube system (ETS) or syringe system technique. The units are available with regular or butterfly-style needles. This collection system *cannot* be used as a vascular access device (VAD); it was designed for routine blood collection only.

Review: Yes ☐ No ☐

88. Answer: d

Why: A prothrombin time (PT) is collected in a light blue top tube, STAT electrolytes (lytes) require a green top or a PST, and a blood culture (BC), although usually collected in special bottles, is sometimes collected in a yellow top SPS tube. The BC (yellow) is collected first because it requires a sterile collection site. The PT (light blue) is collected next, and the lytes (green or PST) are collected last.

Review: Yes ☐ No ☐

89. Answer: c

Why: The red glass and red/light gray are used as "clear" tubes because they have no additives. The glass royal blue with red label has no additive and is designed specifically to meet test specifications for certain trace elements. Plastic red top tubes and plastic royal blue top tubes with a red label contain a clot activator because blood clots poorly in plastic tubes (Table 7-4).

Review: Yes ☐ No ☐

90. Answer: c
Why: Green stopper color means the additive in the tube is heparin. Heparin is an anticoagulant that is available in two forms, lithium heparin and sodium heparin. Each form has its own tube; however, both lithium heparin and sodium heparin tubes have green stoppers (Table 7-4). Consequently, the phlebotomist must be careful in selecting the right tube for the ordered test because the two forms of heparin are not normally interchangeable.

Review: Yes ☐ No ☐

Table 7-4 Common Stopper Colors, Additives, and Departments

Stopper Color	Additive	Department(s)
Light blue	Sodium citrate	Coagulation
Red (glass)	None	Chemistry, Blood bank, Serology/ Immunology
Red (plastic)	Clot activator	Chemistry
Red/light gray (plastic)	Nonadditive	NA (Discard tube only)
Red/black (tiger) Gold Red/gold	Clot activator and gel separator	Chemistry
Green/gray Light green	Lithium heparin and gel separator	Chemistry
Green	Lithium heparin Sodium heparin	Chemistry
Lavender Pink	EDTA	Hematology Blood bank
Gray	Sodium fluoride and potassium oxalate Sodium fluoride and ETDA Sodium fluoride	Chemistry
Orange Gray/yellow	Thrombin	Chemistry
Royal blue	None (red label) EDTA (lavender label) Sodium heparin (green label)	Chemistry
Tan (glass tube) Tan (plastic)	Sodium heparin EDTA	Chemistry
Yellow	Sodium polyanethol sulfonate (SPS)	Microbiology
Yellow	Acid citrate dextrose (ACD)	Blood bank/Immunohematology

91. Answer: a
Why: Lavender, pink, royal blue, and tan stopper tubes all contain the anticoagulant EDTA (Table 7-4).
Review: Yes ☐ No ☐

92. Answer: d
Why: The sodium polyanethol sulfonate (SPS) tube that is processed in the microbiology department has a yellow stopper, as does the tube containing acid citrate dextrose (ACD) that is used by the immunohematology department for DNA testing (Table 7-4).
Review: Yes ☐ No ☐

93. Answer: c
Why: The chemistry department uses the most tubes that have different colored stoppers. The following 12 different stopper colors can be counted from Table 7-3: red, red/black, gold, red/gold, green/gray, light green, green, gray, orange, gray/yellow, royal blue, and tan.
Review: Yes ☐ No ☐

94. Answer: c
Why: Both lithium and sodium heparin are used by the chemistry department (Table 7-4).
Review: Yes ☐ No ☐

95. Answer: c
Why: A syringe transfer device (Fig. 7-15A) is similar to an ETS tube holder but has a permanently attached needle inside the holder. The needle with sleeve is the same as you would find on a multisample ETS needle. This allows the transfer device holder to

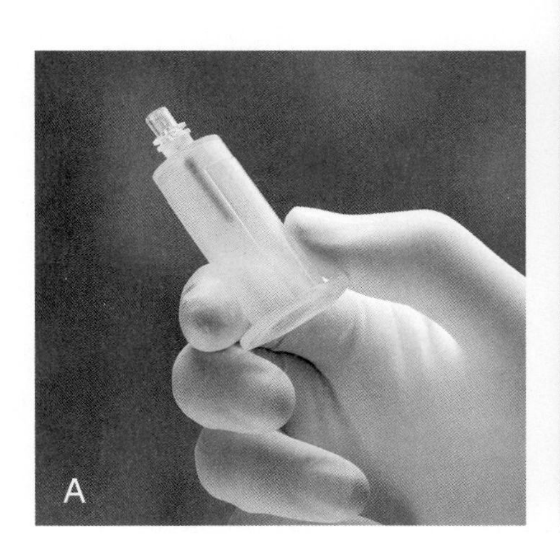

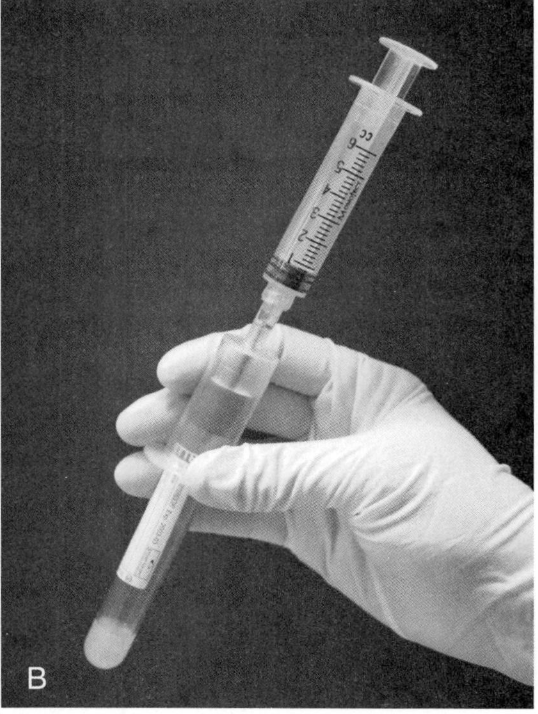

FIGURE 7-15 Syringe transfer devices. **A.** BD transfer device. (Courtesy Becton Dickinson, Franklin Lakes, NJ.) **B.** Greiner transfer device attached to a syringe.

be attached to a syringe and ETS tubes inserted, pierced by the needle inside the holder and filled from the syringe (Fig. 7-15B).

Review: Yes ☐ No ☐

96. Answer: a

Why: The first tube collected with a butterfly will underfill because of air in the tubing. If the tube contains an additive, underfilling will affect the blood-to-additive ratio. If a citrate tube is the first tube to be collected, it is important to draw a few milliliters of blood into a nonadditive tube or another additive tube of the same type, and discard it before collecting the first tube. This practice is referred to as collecting a "clear" or discard tube and is especially critical when collecting coagulation tests.

Review: Yes ☐ No ☐

97. Answer: b

Why: Tubes were drawn in the wrong order, and the position of the patient's arm during the venipuncture allowed them to fill from the stopper end first. This could cause carryover of additive from one tube to the next. Since the lab asked for three of the tests to be redrawn, it appears there was carryover of the potassium EDTA from the lavender tube for the CBC to the plasma potassium, and the anticoagulant heparin carried from that tube into the PT and PTT tube.

Review: Yes ☐ No ☐

98. Answer: d

Why: The royal blue top tubes are used for toxicology studies, which would include metal poisoning. Royal blue stoppers indicate trace-element–free tubes. These tubes are used for substances present in such small quantities that trace element contamination commonly found in glass tubes may leach into the specimen and falsely elevate test results.

Review: Yes ☐ No ☐

99. Answer: c

Why: The yellow topped tube containing ACD solution is available in two formulations (solution A and solution B) for immunohematology tests such as DNA testing used in paternity evaluation. The acid citrate prevents coagulation by binding calcium, with little effect on cells and platelets. Dextrose acts as a red blood cell nutrient and preservative by maintaining red cell viability.

Review: Yes ☐ No ☐

100. Answer: b

Why: The most common electrolytes tested are sodium and potassium. A gray top tube typically contains sodium fluoride and potassium oxalate that would greatly increase sodium and potassium results. A tube with a light green top contains lithium heparin, which is the preferred additive for electrolyte testing. Tubes with gold or red and black tops are serum separator tubes. Although recent studies suggest plasma is the preferred specimen for electrolytes testing, many labs still use serum specimens.

Review: Yes ☐ No ☐

CHAPTER 8

VENIPUNCTURE PROCEDURES

study tip

This chapter tests your ability to identify and describe venipuncture steps, including the procedure for routine evacuated tube system (ETS) and syringe venipuncture of an antecubital vein, the safe transfer of blood from a syringe into ETS tubes, and venipuncture of a hand vein using a butterfly and ETS system. Questions also test the ability to describe challenges and unique issues associated with pediatric and geriatric patients and identify appropriate equipment and procedures for venipuncture of these special populations. In addition, questions address the ability to distinguish between dialysis, long-term care, home care, and hospice patients.

overview

Venipuncture, the process of collecting or "drawing blood" from a patient's vein, is the most common way to collect blood specimens for laboratory testing. This chapter assesses knowledge of the venipuncture procedure, which includes all the steps necessary to safely obtain an appropriately identified quality blood specimen from a patient's arm, wrist, or hand vein. Phlebotomists must know the proper way to obtain a venipuncture specimen to ensure their safety and that of the patient as well as the quality of the specimen.

REVIEW QUESTIONS

Choose the BEST answer.

1. When properly anchoring a vein, the:
   a. index and middle finger are pulling the skin parallel to the arm just below the site.
   b. index finger is pulling the skin above the site and thumb is pulling toward the wrist.
   c. thumb is 1 to 2 inches below the intended site and is pulling the skin toward the wrist.
   d. thumb is next to the intended vein and pressing heavily downward into the tissue.

2. A phlebotomist can more easily gain a patient's trust if he or she does all of the following EXCEPT:
   a. act confident and assured in his or her bedside manner.
   b. arrive earlier than the assigned time of collection.
   c. be professional in dress and personal appearance.
   d. remain at ease while interacting with the patient.

3. Misidentifying a patient can lead to all of the following EXCEPT:
   a. a civil action malpractice lawsuit.
   b. grounds for dismissal from the facility.
   c. no reprimand if no one was hurt.
   d. temporary suspension of duties.

4. Needle phobia is defined as a/an:
   a. anxiety about admission to the hospital.
   b. inability to watch while others are drawn.
   c. intense fear of needles and being stuck.
   d. personal preference for smaller needles.

5. Symptoms of needle phobia include all of the following EXCEPT:
   a. arrhythmia.
   b. fainting.
   c. lightheadedness.
   d. muscle cramps.

6. A basic step that can be taken to minimize any trauma associated with a venipuncture is to:
   a. allow the patient to sit in the waiting room for half an hour before collection.
   b. choose the most skilled phlebotomist available to perform the venipuncture.
   c. have the patient wear an eye mask or close his or her eyes during the procedure.
   d. thoroughly explain every detail of the draw before doing the venipuncture.

7. All of the following are proper use of a hand sanitizer EXCEPT:
   a. allowing the alcohol to evaporate completely.
   b. performing the cleansing process at least twice.
   c. rubbing it in between and around the fingers.
   d. using a very generous amount of the sanitizer.

8. To examine by touch or feel is to:
   a. ambulate.
   b. anchor.
   c. palpate.
   d. pronate.

9. In most cases, needle insertion should be performed:
   a. at a 45° angle to the arm surface.
   b. using a smooth, steady motion forward.
   c. with a deliberate and rapid forward jab.
   d. with the bevel of the needle face down.

10. To "seat" the needle in the vein means to:
    a. anchor the vein while inserting the needle.
    b. increase the angle needed to enter the vein.
    c. redirect the needle to gain entry to the vein.
    d. thread part of the needle within the lumen.

11. Going without food or drink except water for 8–12 hours is defined as:
 a. fasting.
 b. NPO.
 c. routine.
 d. TDM.

12. The reason a test is ordered "timed" is to:
 a. assess a patient's condition after surgery.
 b. determine patient suitability for surgery.
 c. draw it at a best time for accurate results.
 d. establish a clinical diagnosis and prognosis.

13. Examples of "timed" tests are all of the following EXCEPT:
 a. basic metabolic panel.
 b. blood cultures.
 c. cardiac enzymes.
 d. lithium level.

14. A test is ordered "fasting" to:
 a. assess a patient after outpatient surgery.
 b. eliminate the effects of diet on test results.
 c. determine patient suitability for surgery.
 d. standardize test results on critical patients.

15. The practice of bending the arm up to apply pressure to the site after venipuncture can do all of the following EXCEPT:
 a. disrupt the platelet plug when the arm is eventually lowered.
 b. enable the site to quickly stop bleeding after needle withdrawal.
 c. increase the possibility of bruising and hematoma formation.
 d. keep the wound open, especially if it is at the side of the arm.

16. The unique number assigned to a specimen request is called the:
 a. accession number.
 b. health facility number.
 c. patient date of birth.
 d. patient ID number.

17. If diet restrictions have not been met before collecting a specimen, the results could lead to any of the following EXCEPT:
 a. compromised patient care and treatment.
 b. erroneous and meaningless test results.
 c. grounds for the phlebotomist's dismissal.
 d. misinterpreted test results by the physician.

18. Which of the following individuals has legal authority to authorize patient testing?
 a. laboratory director
 b. patient's nurse
 c. patient's physician
 d. phlebotomist

19. Information on a test requisition *must* include the:
 a. ordering physician.
 b. patient diagnosis.
 c. patient's location.
 d. prior draw times.

20. Which type of requisition often serves as a test request, report, and billing form?
 a. barcode
 b. computer
 c. manual
 d. verbal

21. Using information from the computer requisition (Fig. 8-1), identify the number that points to the type of tube to be drawn.
 a. 1
 b. 2
 c. 3
 d. 4

22. Using information from the computer requisition (Fig. 8-1), identify the number that points to the patient's age.
 a. 1
 b. 6
 c. 7
 d. 9

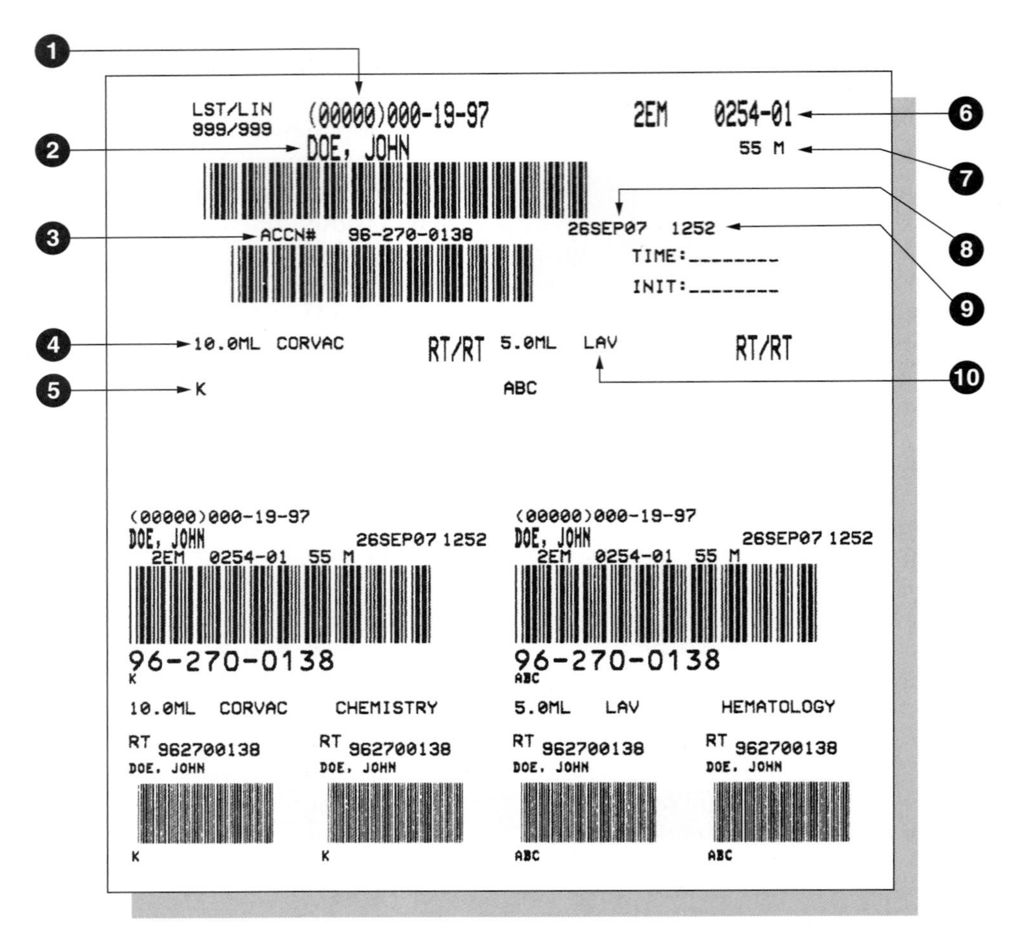

FIGURE 8-1 Computer requisition with bar code.

23. Using information from the computer requisition (Fig. 8-1), identify the number that points to the accession number.
    a. 1
    b. 3
    c. 6
    d. 7

24. A healthcare facility ID barcode can represent any of the following EXCEPT:
    a. credit information.
    b. laboratory test.
    c. patient ID number.
    d. patient's name.

25. Outpatient requisitions are typically of this type.
    a. computer
    b. e-mail
    c. manual
    d. verbal

26. When received by the laboratory, inpatient requisitions are typically sorted according to all of the following EXCEPT:
    a. alphabetically by name.
    b. collection date and time.
    c. location of the patient.
    d. priority of collection.

27. Steps taken to unmistakably connect a specimen and the accompanying paperwork to a specific individual are called:
    a. accessioning the specimen.
    b. barcoding specimen labels.
    c. collection verification.
    d. patient identification.

28. Which of the following is an example of a common timed test?
    a. cholesterol
    b. cortisol
    c. fibrinogen
    d. monospot

29. A test that is ordered STAT should be collected:
    a. as soon as it is possible to do so.
    b. immediately, without any hesitation.
    c. on the next closest scheduled sweep.
    d. within 1 hour of the test request.

30. Which of the following tests is commonly ordered STAT?
    a. creat
    b. diff
    c. lytes
    d. RAST

31. If a test is ordered STAT, it may mean that the patient is in:
    a. critical condition.
    b. fragile condition.
    c. rehabilitation.
    d. transitional state.

32. When a test is ordered ASAP, it means that the patient:
    a. is in critical condition and needs immediate attention.
    b. requires a test in which timing of collection is critical.
    c. results are needed soon for an appropriate response.
    d. results from blood work are needed for medication.

33. A pre-op patient:
    a. has been admitted to the hospital.
    b. is an ambulatory outpatient.
    c. is being assessed after surgery.
    d. will soon be going to surgery.

34. Tests are classified as routine if they are ordered:
    a. for collection at a specific time and place.
    b. in the course of establishing a diagnosis.
    c. to assess a patient's condition after surgery.
    d. to specifically eliminate the effects of diet.

35. This term means the same as STAT.
    a. fasting
    b. med emerg
    c. post-op
    d. timed

36. A patient who is NPO:
    a. cannot have any food or drink.
    b. cannot have anything but water.
    c. is in critical, but stable condition.
    d. is recovering from minor surgery.

37. An example of a test that is commonly ordered fasting is:
    a. BUN.
    b. cortisol.
    c. glucose.
    d. PTT.

38. Which liquid is acceptable to drink when fasting?
    a. black coffee
    b. diet soda
    c. plain water
    d. sugarless tea

39. Which is a common post-op test?
    a. CBC
    b. ESR
    c. H & H
    d. PTT

40. You arrive to draw a specimen on an inpatient. The patient's door is closed. What do you do?
   a. Knock lightly, open the door slowly, and verify if it is all right to enter.
   b. Knock softly and wait for someone in the room to come to the door.
   c. Leave to draw another patient in the same area and come back later.
   d. Open the door, announce yourself, and quickly proceed into the room.

41. There is a sign above the patient's bed that reads, "No blood pressures or venipuncture, right arm," as seen in Fig. 8-2. The patient has an intravenous (IV) line in the left forearm. You have a request to collect a complete blood count (CBC) on the patient. How should you proceed?
   a. Ask the patient's nurse to collect the specimen from the IV.
   b. Ask the patient's nurse what to do when the sign is posted.
   c. Collect a CBC from the right arm without using a tourniquet.
   d. Collect the specimen from the left hand by finger puncture.

NO BP OR VENIPUNCTURE

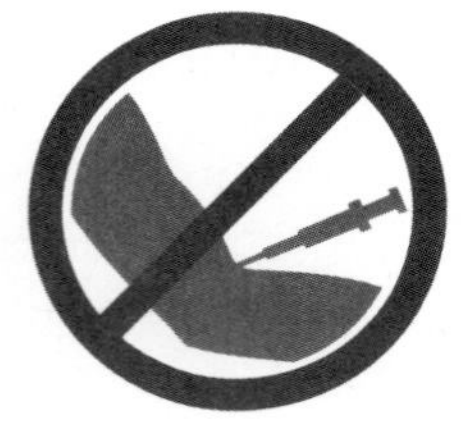

RIGHT ARM

FIGURE 8-2 Warning sign indicating "No blood pressures or venipuncture in right arm."

42. A code is a way to do all of the following EXCEPT:
   a. communicate emergency instructions from the physician.
   b. convey important information without alarming the public.
   c. transmit messages over the facility's public address system.
   d. use numbers or words to represent important information.

43. DNR means:
   a. do not alert the nurse.
   b. do not call 911.
   c. do not call relatives.
   d. do not resuscitate.

44. You greet your patient in the following manner: "Hello, my name is John and I am here to collect a blood specimen if that is all right with you." The patient responds by saying, "OK, but I would rather not." How do you proceed?
   a. Ask another phlebotomist to draw the specimen.
   b. Come back at a later time to collect the specimen.
   c. Determine what the problem is before proceeding.
   d. Go ahead and draw the specimen without comment.

45. Which one of the following tests is used to identify protein disorders that lead to nerve damage?
   a. ANA
   b. ESR
   c. PTT
   d. SPEP

46. Your inpatient is asleep when you arrive to draw blood. What do you do?
   a. Call out the patient's name softly and shake the bed gently.
   b. Cancel the test and ask the nurse to resubmit the requisition.

c. Check back every 15 minutes until the patient has awakened.
d. Fill out a form stating the specimen was not obtained and why.

47. Laboratory results can be negatively affected if the phlebotomist:
a. awakens a sleeping patient and raises the head of the patient's bed.
b. collects a specimen in dim lighting conditions in the patient's room.
c. draws a specimen from an unconscious patient without assistance.
d. startles a patient who is asleep while preparing to collect a specimen.

48. You would do all of the following when handling an unconscious patient EXCEPT:
a. have someone assist you just in case the patient moves.
b. identify yourself and inform the patient of your intent.
c. move the patient to a special phlebotomy collection area.
d. talk to the patient as you would to a patient who is alert.

49. What do you do if a physician is with the patient and the specimen is ordered STAT?
a. Ask the patient's nurse to collect the STAT specimen immediately.
b. Come back later when you know the physician is no longer there.
c. Introduce yourself and ask for permission to draw the specimen.
d. Say "excuse me" to both and proceed to collect the specimen.

50. What is the *best* thing to do if family or visitors are with a patient?
a. Ask them to wait outside of the room until you are finished.
b. Come back later to collect the specimen when they have left.
c. Have the patient's nurse tell everyone that they should leave.
d. Tell them to quietly watch from the opposite side of the bed.

51. Your patient is not in the room when you arrive to collect a timed specimen. The patient's nurse states that the patient will be unavailable for several hours. What should you do?
a. Ask the nurse to have the patient brought to the lab when the patient is available.
b. Fill out a delay slip stating you were unable to collect the specimen.
c. Report the situation to a supervisor and tell him or her to cancel the request.
d. Return to the lab and put the request in the stack for the next sweep.

52. Misidentification of a specimen for this test is *most* likely to have fatal consequences.
a. blood culture
b. cold agglutinin
c. platelet count
d. type & screen

53. You arrive to collect a specimen on a patient named John Doe in 302B. How do you verify that the patient in 302B is indeed John Doe?
a. Ask him, "Are you John Doe?" If he says yes, collect the specimen.
b. Ask him to state his name and date of birth (DOB) and match it to the requisition.
c. Check his ID band. If it matches the requisition, draw the specimen.
d. Have the nurse verify the patient's name after you check his ID band.

54. Which requisition information *must* match information on the patient's ID band?
a. medical record number
b. name of the physician
c. room and bed number
d. test collection priority

55. The medical record number on the ID band matches the number on your requisition, but the patient's name is spelled differently than the one on your requisition. What should you do?
    a. Collect the specimen and report the error to the patient's nurse.
    b. Do not collect the specimen until the difference is resolved.
    c. Draw the specimen, because the medical record number matches.
    d. Make the correction on the requisition and draw the specimen.

56. An unconscious patient does not have an ID band. The name on the door agrees with the requisition. What should you do?
    a. Ask the nurse to verify the patient's ID and collect the specimen.
    b. Complete the required procedure and then file an incident report.
    c. Do not start any procedure until the nurse attaches an ID bracelet.
    d. Make an LIS entry that will alert other phlebotomists of the issue.

57. What would be the system of choice to identify laboratory specimens from an unconscious woman in the ER?
    a. Assign a name to the patient such as Jane Doe.
    b. Assign a number to the patient until she is admitted.
    c. Use a three-part identification band with special tube labels.
    d. Wait to process the specimens until the patient can be identified.

58. Which type of inpatient is *most* likely to have more than one ID band?
    a. adult
    b. child
    c. newborn
    d. outpatient

59. What is the most critical error a phlebotomist can make?
    a. collect a timed specimen late
    b. fail to obtain the desired specimen
    c. misidentify the patient's specimen
    d. unknowingly give a patient a bruise

60. Your patient is not wearing an ID band. You see that the ID band is taped to the nightstand. The information matches your requisition. What do you do?
    a. Ask the patient to state her name; if it matches the requisition, continue.
    b. Ask the patient's nurse to attach an ID band and proceed when attached.
    c. Go to the nurse's station, get an ID bracelet, attach it, and then proceed.
    d. Tell the nurse that you will not collect the specimen and return to the lab.

61. Which one of the following types of patients is *least* likely to need their identity confirmed by the patient's nurse or a relative?
    a. a geriatric patient
    b. a very young child
    c. mentally incompetent
    d. non–English-speaking

62. The laboratory receptionist finishes checking a patient in and hands you the test request. The request is for a patient named Mary Smith. You call the name, and a woman who was just checked in responds. She is also the only patient in the waiting room. How do you verify that she is the correct patient?
    a. Ask the woman to state her complete name and date of birth to confirm her identity.
    b. Assume that you do not have to verify her identity because the receptionist already did.
    c. Conclude that she must be the right one because she is the only one in the waiting room.
    d. Decide that she must be right one because she answered you when you called the name.

63. A cheerful, pleasant bedside manner and exchange of small talk help to do all of the following EXCEPT:
    a. divert attention from any discomfort associated with the draw.
    b. increase the patient's confidence in the phlebotomist's abilities.
    c. keep the patient from fainting during the venipuncture procedure.
    d. redirect the patient's thoughts away from what is going to happen.

64. Your patient is cranky and rude to you. What do you do?
    a. Ask the patient's nurse to draw the specimen as you stand by to assist.
    b. Be as professional as you can and collect the specimen in a normal way.
    c. Do not speak to the patient; just get the necessary blood work and leave.
    d. Refuse to draw the patient and leave the request for another phlebotomist.

65. Which of the following is part of informed consent for specimen collection?
    a. advising the patient of his or her prognosis
    b. explaining what disorders the test can detect
    c. informing the patient that you are a student
    d. notifying the patient of future venipunctures

66. The patient asks if the test you are about to draw is for diabetes. How do you answer?
    a. Explain that it is best to discuss the test with the physician.
    b. If the test is for glucose say, "Yes, it is" but do not elaborate.
    c. Say, "HIPAA confidentiality rules won't let me tell you."
    d. Tell the patient that it is not for a glucose test even if it is.

67. An inpatient vehemently refuses to allow you to collect a blood specimen. What should you do?
    a. Convince the patient to cooperate and collect the sample anyway.
    b. Have the nurse physically restrain the patient and draw the specimen.
    c. Notify the patient's nurse and document the patients refusal.
    d. Return to the lab, cancel the test request and inform the physician.

68. You arrive to draw a fasting specimen. The patient is just finishing breakfast. What do you do?
    a. Check with the patient's nurse to see if it should be collected or rescheduled.
    b. Collect the specimen, but write "non-fasting" on the lab slip and the specimen.
    c. Do not draw the blood; fill out an incident slip, and leave a copy for the nurse.
    d. Proceed to collect the specimen since the patient had not quite finished eating.

69. All of the following are reasons to assemble equipment after selecting and cleaning the blood collection site EXCEPT you will:
    a. be more apt to allow sufficient time for the alcohol to dry.
    b. have a better idea of what equipment you will need to use.
    c. have time to check the other arm for a better possible site.
    d. waste less equipment by knowing exactly what is needed.

70. When performing a venipuncture, hand decontamination is required:
    a. after drawing your last patient.
    b. before and after each patient.
    c. just after removing the gloves.
    d. only before putting on gloves.

71. Proper hand washing involves all of the following EXCEPT:
    a. creating friction to dislodge surface debris and bacteria.
    b. scrubbing downward from the wrists to the fingertips.
    c. using a clean paper towel to shut off the water faucet.
    d. using a hand sanitizer just before the hands are dried.

72. You must collect a specimen on a 6-year-old. The child is a little fearful. What do you do?
   a. Explain what you are going to do to the child in simple terms.
   b. Restrain the child and draw the specimen without explanation.
   c. Tell the child that you will give him a treat if he does not cry.
   d. Tell the child to relax and not to worry because it will not hurt.

73. If the patient asks if the procedure will hurt, you should say that it:
   a. could hurt if you watch, so look the other way.
   b. is painless and will be over before you know it.
   c. might hurt just a little, but only for a short time.
   d. only hurts if the phlebotomist is inexperienced.

74. What is the proper arm position for routine venipuncture?
   a. Extended straight forward at waist height, palm facing up.
   b. In a downward position, bent at the elbow, palm facing up.
   c. Straight from shoulder to wrist with palm facing down.
   d. Straight from shoulder to wrist with the palm facing up.

75. Outpatients who have previously fainted during a blood draw should be:
   a. allowed to sit up in order to carefully watch the draw.
   b. asked to lie down, or sit in a reclining drawing chair.
   c. drawn in a separate room that has first aid equipment.
   d. permitted to sit in a chair if accompanied by an adult.

76. Which of the following acts can lead to liability issues?
   a. Asking visitors to leave the room while you draw a specimen.
   b. Drawing a patient who is lying in bed talking on a cell phone.
   c. Lowering a bedrail to make access to the patient's arm easier.
   d. Pulling the curtain between the beds while drawing a specimen.

77. Never leave a tourniquet on for more than:
   a. 30 seconds.
   b. 1 minute.
   c. 2 minutes.
   d. 3 minutes.

78. Where is the best place to apply the tourniquet?
   a. 3 to 4 inches above the venipuncture site
   b. distal to the venipuncture site on the forearm
   c. distal to the wrist bone if drawing a hand vein
   d. immediately above the venipuncture site

79. If the tourniquet is too tight, all of the following happens EXCEPT:
   a. arterial flow below it may be stopped.
   b. blood below it may hemoconcentrate.
   c. the pressure can cause the arm to ache.
   d. venous flow increases as veins expand.

80. All of the following may be used to enhance the vein selection process EXCEPT:
   a. having a patient pump his or her fist.
   b. lowering the arm alongside the chair.
   c. palpating the antecubital area firmly.
   d. using a warm towel to increase blood flow.

81. When selecting a venipuncture site, how can you tell a vein from an artery?
   a. A vein has more resilience.
   b. A vein pulses and feels larger.
   c. An artery has a distinct pulse.
   d. An artery is more superficial.

82. What does a sclerosed vein feel like?
   a. bouncy and resilient
   b. hard and cordlike
   c. pulsating and firm
   d. soft and pliable

83. It is acceptable to use an ankle vein if:
    a. coagulation tests are requested.
    b. the patient is partially paralyzed.
    c. the physician gives permission.
    d. there are no other suitable sites.

84. All of the following will help you avoid inadvertently puncturing an artery during venipuncture EXCEPT:
    a. avoid drawing the basilic vein in the antecubital area.
    b. do not select a site that is near where you feel a pulse.
    c. do not select a vein that overlies or is close to an artery.
    d. stay away from the cephalic vein when the arm is thin.

85. You must collect a light blue top tube for a special coagulation test from a patient who has an intravenous (IV) line in the left wrist area and dermatitis all over the right arm and hand. The veins on the right arm and hand are not readily visible. What is the best way to proceed?
    a. Apply a tourniquet on the right arm over a towel and do the draw.
    b. Ask the patient's nurse to collect the specimen from the IV line.
    c. Collect from the left antecubital area without using a tourniquet.
    d. Collect the specimen by capillary puncture from the left hand.

86. What is the *best* thing to do if the vein can be felt but not seen, even with the tourniquet on?
    a. Insert the needle where you think it is and probe until you find it.
    b. Keep the tourniquet on while cleaning the site and during the draw.
    c. Look for visual clues on the skin to remind you where the vein is.
    d. Mark the spot using a felt-tip pen and clean it off when finished.

87. Release the tourniquet after vein selection and before cleaning the site for all of the following reasons EXCEPT to:
    a. allow venous blood flow to return to normal.
    b. decrease hemoconcentration of the specimen.
    c. help to ensure the accuracy of the test results.
    d. increase the arterial flow to the vein selected.

88. What is the Clinical and Laboratory Standards Institute (CLSI) recommended way to clean a venipuncture site?
    a. Clean the area thoroughly with disinfectant using concentric circles.
    b. Cleanse with a circular motion from the center to the periphery.
    c. Scrub with an alcohol sponge as vigorously as you can for 1 minute.
    d. Wipe using concentric circles from the outside area to the center.

89. All of the following are reasons to wait 30 seconds for the alcohol to dry before needle insertion EXCEPT to:
    a. allow the process of evaporation to help destroy microbes.
    b. avoid a stinging sensation when the needle penetrates the skin.
    c. give the phlebotomist time to prepare equipment and supplies.
    d. prevent hemolysis of the specimen from alcohol in the needle.

90. What happens if you advance the tube past the guideline on the holder before needle insertion?
    a. The ETS tube will fail to fill with blood because of loss of tube vacuum
    b. Nothing; the line is actually a fill guideline for all evacuated tubes.
    c. The needle sleeve stops penetration of the tube until fully advanced
    d. There will be transfer of the tube additive to the needle at that point

91. It is important for the phlebotomist to visually inspect the needle tip before inserting it in a patient's vein for all of the following reasons EXCEPT to check:
   a. for imperfections that could damage a vein.
   b. for the presence of external contamination.
   c. to make sure the needle bevel is facing up.
   d. to verify that the needle is not out of date.

92. Which of the following steps are in the right order for the venipuncture procedure?
   a. clean the site, prepare equipment, put on gloves, apply tourniquet
   b. sanitize hands, select vein, release tourniquet, verify diet restrictions
   c. select the site, apply the tourniquet, prepare equipment, clean the site
   d. select vein, clean the site, position the patient, put on your gloves

93. You are about to draw blood from a patient. You touch the needle to the skin, but change your mind and pull the needle away. What do you do next?
   a. Clean the site and try again using the same needle.
   b. Stop and obtain a new needle before trying again.
   c. Try it again immediately using that same needle.
   d. Wipe the needle across an alcohol pad and retry.

94. What is the best angle to use for needle insertion during routine venipuncture?
   a. less than 15°
   b. 15° to 30°
   c. 35° to 45°
   d. 45° to 60°

95. When performing venipuncture, the needle is inserted:
   a. as you prefer.
   b. bevel facing up.
   c. bevel side down.
   d. bevel sideways.

96. How can you tell when the needle is in the vein as you insert it into the patient's arm?
   a. Blood will enter the ETS hub.
   b. The needle will start to vibrate.
   c. You will feel a slight "give".
   d. You will hear a hissing sound.

97. When is the best time to release the tourniquet during venipuncture?
   a. after the last tube has been filled completely
   b. after the needle is withdrawn and covered
   c. as soon as blood begins to flow into the tube
   d. as soon as the needle penetrates the skin

98. Prolonged tourniquet application or vigorous fist pumping can elevate all of these analytes EXCEPT:
   a. potassium.
   b. prothrombin.
   c. red cell count.
   d. total protein.

99. Proper technique for collecting specimen tubes when using the evacuated tube method includes all of the following EXCEPT:
   a. collect sterile specimens before all other specimens.
   b. draw a "clear" tube before special coagulation tests.
   c. fill each tube until the normal vacuum is exhausted.
   d. position the arm so tubes fill from stopper end first.

100. It is important to fill anticoagulant tubes to the proper level to ensure that:
   a. the specimen yields enough serum for the required tests.
   b. there is a proper ratio of blood to anticoagulant additive.

c. there is an adequate amount of blood to perform the test.
d. tissue fluid contamination of the specimen is minimized.

101. It is important to mix anticoagulant tubes immediately after filling them to:
a. avoid microclot formation.
b. encourage coagulation.
c. inhibit hemoconcentration.
d. minimize hemolysis.

102. You are in the middle of drawing a blood specimen using the evacuated tube method when you realize that you just filled an EDTA tube and still have a green top tube to collect. What do you do?
a. do not collect the green tube until the next collection sweep
b. draw several milliliters into a discard tube; then fill the green one
c. draw the green one next and hope that there is no carryover
d. it is acceptable to draw the EDTA before the green stopper

103. How many times do you mix non-additive tubes?
a. 2 or 3
b. 5–10
c. 8–12
d. none

104. What may happen if you mix tubes too vigorously?
a. hemolysis
b. jaundice
c. lipemia
d. no affect

105. Use several layers of gauze during needle removal so that:
a. blood will not contaminate your gloved hand.
b. it will not hurt when you pull out the needle.
c. pressure is adequate and bruising is prevented.
d. the patient does not see you pull out the needle.

106. It is better to use gauze and not cotton balls for pressure over the site, because cotton balls:
a. are not sufficiently porous to soak up all of the blood at the site.
b. attract more airborne contaminants and are therefore less sterile.
c. can irritate a patient's skin because they have loose cotton fibers.
d. may pull the platelets away from the puncture site upon removal.

107. Applying pressure on the gauze as the needle is removed can cause all of the following EXCEPT:
a. a painful stinging sensation.
b. bending of the needle bevel.
c. prolonged needle removal.
d. skin being slit by the bevel.

108. A needle safety feature, other than a blunting needle, should be activated:
a. after some pressure has been applied to the site.
b. as you are dropping the needle in the sharps container.
c. immediately after the needle is withdrawn.
d. while the tube is still engaged in the holder.

109. Which of these steps are in the right venipuncture procedure order?
a. establish blood flow, release tourniquet, fill and mix tubes, remove needle
b. fill and mix all the tubes, release tourniquet, remove needle, apply pressure
c. fill the tubes, remove needle, release tourniquet, mix tubes, apply pressure
d. release tourniquet, fill tubes, remove needle, apply pressure, mix all tubes

110. Proper needle disposal involves:
   a. disposing of the needle and tube holder in the sharps container as one unit.
   b. ejecting the needle from the tube holder so that the holder can be reused.
   c. removing the needle from the holder after engaging the needle safety device.
   d. unscrewing the needle from the holder by using a slot in the sharps container.

111. Labeling of routine inpatient blood specimens should take place:
   a. at the bedside immediately after collection.
   b. before the blood specimens are collected.
   c. in the lab processing area after collection.
   d. outside the patient's room after collection.

112. Mandatory information on a specimen label includes all of the following EXCEPT:
   a. patient room number and bed.
   b. patient's first and last name.
   c. phlebotomist's initials or ID.
   d. the date and time of the draw.

113. The patient's identification number is included on the specimen tube label to:
   a. avoid confusing multiple specimens from the same patient.
   b. avoid confusing specimens from patients with the same name.
   c. be used for an accession number in processing the specimen.
   d. be used for insurance identification and payment purposes.

114. All of the following precautionary information should be given to an outpatient before being allowed to leave after venipuncture EXCEPT:
   a. do not carry a heavy bag or large purse on that arm.
   b. do not drink or eat for 2 hours after collection.
   c. do not lift any heavy objects for at least 1 hour.
   d. leave the bandage on for a minimum of 15 minutes.

115. All of the following specimens require special handling EXCEPT:
   a. ammonia.
   b. bilirubin.
   c. cholesterol.
   d. cryoglobulin.

116. Which of the following is not a valid reason for failure to obtain a blood specimen?
   a. The patient adamantly refused to have blood taken.
   b. The patient was unavailable at that designated time.
   c. You attempted but were unable to obtain the blood.
   d. You did not have the right equipment on your tray.

117. You have just made two unsuccessful attempts to collect a fasting blood specimen from an outpatient. The patient rotates his arm, and you note a large vein that you had not seen before. How do you proceed?
   a. Ask another phlebotomist to collect the fasting specimen.
   b. Ask the patient to come back later so that you can try again.
   c. Call the supervisor for permission to make a third attempt.
   d. Make a third attempt on the newly discovered large vein.

118. Where is the tourniquet applied when drawing a hand vein?
   a. a tourniquet is not required
   b. above the antecubital fossa
   c. just distal to the wrist bone
   d. proximal to the wrist bone

119. A patient has difficult veins and you decide to use a butterfly for the draw. Butterfly is another name for a:
  a. hypodermic needle.
  b. multisample needle.
  c. needle safety feature.
  d. winged infusion set.

120. What is the advantage of using a butterfly?
  a. Blood flows faster than when using ETS needles.
  b. Butterflies are less expensive than other needles.
  c. Butterflies make it easier to draw difficult veins.
  d. There is a greater choice in butterfly needle size.

121. Although the evacuated tube system (ETS) is the preferred method of blood collection, it may be necessary to use a syringe when:
  a. a large amount of blood is needed.
  b. the patient's veins are very fragile.
  c. there are no butterfly needles left.
  d. you need the blood to flow faster.

122. Hemolysis of the specimen can result from all of the following EXCEPT:
  a. forcing blood from a syringe into an ETS tube.
  b. leaving the tourniquet TIED on the arm too long.
  c. mixing any of the additive tubes too vigorously.
  d. using a large-volume tube with a 23g needle.

123. How can you tell that you are in a vein when using a syringe?
  a. A "flash" of blood will appear in the hub of the needle.
  b. Blood will automatically pump into the syringe barrel.
  c. There will be a very slight vibration in the needle.
  d. You cannot tell when you are in a vein with a syringe.

124. Success of pediatric blood collection is *most* dependent on:
  a. aseptic technique.
  b. correct order of draw.
  c. patient immobilization.
  d. tourniquet application.

125. Before obtaining a blood specimen from a child, you must do all of the following EXCEPT:
  a. establish rapport with the child.
  b. greet the parents and the child.
  c. tell the child it will not hurt.
  d. tell the child what to expect.

126. A butterfly and 23g needle is the *best* choice to use for venipuncture on a young child because:
  a. children like the idea of using a butterfly.
  b. children's veins are often very sclerosed.
  c. flexible tubing allows for arm movement.
  d. it eliminates excessive bleeding tendencies.

127. When transferring blood from a syringe to evacuated tubes, which is the proper technique?
  a. Force the blood through the needle into the tubes by pushing the syringe plunger.
  b. Hold the tube steady in your hand while the syringe needle penetrates the stopper.
  c. Place the evacuated tube in a rack before penetrating stopper with the needle.
  d. Use a specially designed engineering device called a syringe transfer device.

128. Proper immobilization of the pediatric patient involves all of the following EXCEPT:
   a. allowing the child to sit with one arm bracing the other.
   b. cradling the child close to the chest of the immobilizer.
   c. grasping the child's wrist firmly in a palm-up position.
   d. using two people, an immobilizer and a blood drawer.

129. When drawing blood from an older child, the most important consideration is:
   a. assuring the child that it won't be painful.
   b. explaining all of the tests being collected.
   c. explaining the importance of holding still.
   d. offering the child a reward for not crying.

130. Dorsal hand vein procedure on infants involves all of the following EXCEPT:
   a. applying a tourniquet on the infant's forearm.
   b. cleansing the area with an isopropyl alcohol swab.
   c. identifying the infant from the patient ID band.
   d. inserting the needle in a superficial dorsal hand vein.

131. The *best* way to collect a PKU specimen from a dorsal hand vein is:
   a. Allow the blood to drip into an EDTA microcollection tube.
   b. Carefully blot the blood spot from the vein with the PKU card.
   c. Collect the blood with a syringe and 23g butterfly needle.
   d. Let the blood drip onto the PKU card by turning hand over.

132. Tremors associated with this disease can make blood collection difficult.
   a. Alzheimer's
   b. arthritis
   c. diabetes
   d. Parkinson's

133. A diabetic outpatient has had a mastectomy on her right side and cannot straighten her left arm because of arthritis. The best place to collect a blood specimen is:
   a. an ankle or foot vein on either of her legs.
   b. the left forearm or hand, using a butterfly.
   c. the right arm below the antecubital fossa.
   d. the right hand, using a capillary puncture.

134. Which of the following is proper procedure when dealing with an elderly adult patient?
   a. Address all questions to a relative or attendant if the patient is hard of hearing.
   b. Apply a pressure bandage in case the patient does not hold adequate pressure.
   c. Raise the pitch of your voice sharply to make certain you are heard properly.
   d. Refrain from drawing older adult patients if you have a cold, or else wear a mask.

135. The most common reason a patient must undergo dialysis treatment is:
   a. end stages of renal disease.
   b. Parkinson's disease effects.
   c. problems with coagulation.
   d. rheumatoid arthritis effects.

136. A type of care for patients who are terminally ill is:
   a. elder care.
   b. home care.
   c. hospice care.
   d. long-term care.

ANSWERS AND EXPLANATIONS

1. Answer: c
   Why: To anchor or pull the vein taut (Fig. 8-3), place the thumb a minimum of 1 to 2 inches below and slightly to the side of the intended venipuncture site, and pull the skin toward the wrist in line with the vein.
   Review: Yes ☐ No ☐

2. Answer: b
   Why: The manner in which you present yourself and interact with the patient sets the stage for whether or not you will gain the patient's trust. A phlebotomist with a professional bedside manner and appearance will more easily gain a patient's trust. An assured phlebotomist will convey that confidence to patients and help them feel at ease. Arriving earlier than the assigned time for collection could affect the results of the test and undermine the patient's confidence and trust in your knowledge and abilities.
   Review: Yes ☐ No ☐

3. Answer: c
   Why: Obtaining a specimen from the wrong patient can have serious, even fatal, consequences, especially specimens for type and crossmatch before blood transfusion. Misidentifying a patient or specimen can be grounds for dismissal of the person responsible and can even lead to a malpractice lawsuit (civil action) against that person. Even if no one was hurt by the misidentification, it is a serious error and would, at the least, result in a reprimand and thorough documentation of the incident.
   Review: Yes ☐ No ☐

4 Answer: c
   Why: Needle phobia is defined as intense fear of needles. The signs by the patient that suggest this phobia, such as extreme fear or apprehension in advance of venipuncture, should not be taken lightly. Although a patient may be anxious about being admitted to the hospital or have a needle preference for the venipuncture procedure, these do not constitute needle phobias.
   Review: Yes ☐ No ☐

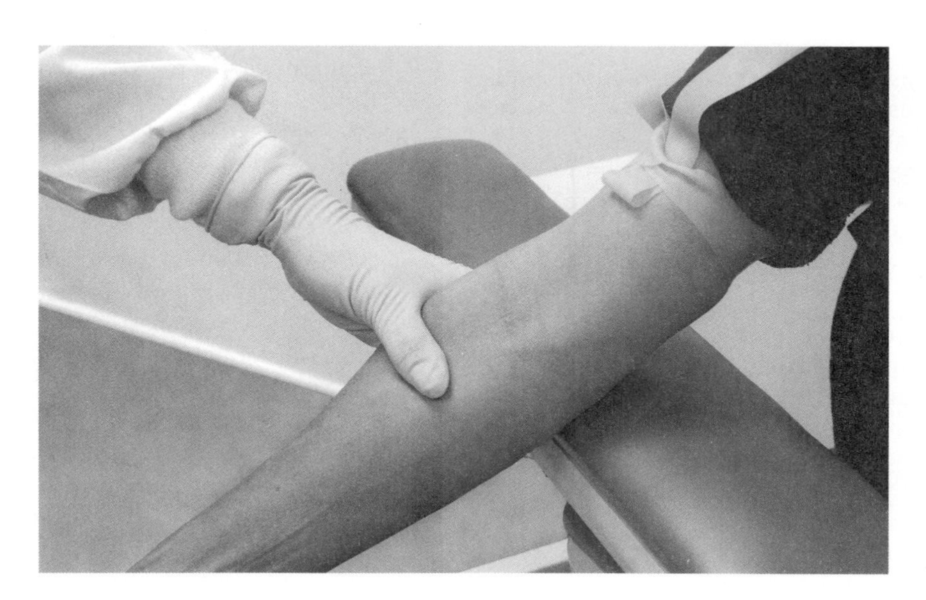

FIGURE 8-3 Proper placement of thumb and fingers when anchoring a vein.

5. Answer: d
   Why: Symptoms of needle phobia include pallor (paleness), profuse sweating, lightheadedness, nausea, and fainting. In severe cases, patients have been known to suffer arrhythmia and even cardiac arrest, but not muscle cramps.
   Review: Yes ☐ No ☐

6. Answer: b
   Why: Basic steps that can be taken to minimize any trauma associated with the venipuncture include the following: (1) having the patient lie down; (2) applying an ice pack to the site for 10 to 15 minutes before the venipuncture, and (3) having the most experienced and skilled phlebotomist perform the venipuncture. Explaining every little detail of the procedure, having patients close or cover the eyes, or having them wait outside the drawing room to calm down simply increases the trauma of this experience.
   Review: Yes ☐ No ☐

7. Answer: b
   Why: When using hand sanitizers, it is important to use a generous amount and allow the alcohol to evaporate to achieve proper antisepsis. As shown in Fig. 8-4, the sanitizer must be rubbed between and on the back of the fingers as well as the palms. If hands are not heavily soiled, it is not necessary to use a sanitizer more than once before putting on the gloves.
   Review: Yes ☐ No ☐

8. Answer: c
   Why: Some veins may be easily visible; others will have to be located entirely by feeling or palpating, as shown in Fig. 8-5. To locate a vein, examine by pushing down on the skin with the tip of the index finger. Palpating also helps determine the vein's patency, the size and depth, and the direction or the path that it follows.
   Review: Yes ☐ No ☐

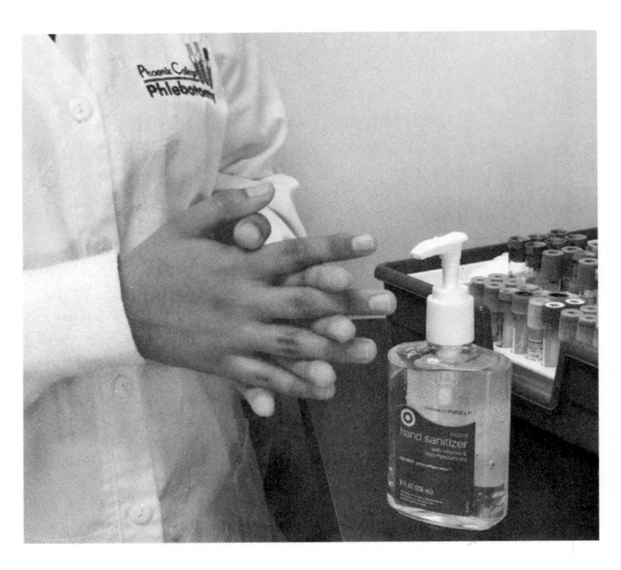

FIGURE 8-4 Phlebotomist applying hand sanitizer.

9. Answer: b
   Why: For antecubital site venipunctures, insert the needle into the skin at a 15° to 30° angle (Fig. 8-6), depending on the depth of the vein. Use one smooth, steady, forward motion to penetrate first the skin and then the vein. Advancing the needle too slowly prolongs any discomfort. A rapid jab can result in missing the vein or going all the way through it. The needle bevel should be face up, not down.
   Review: Yes ☐ No ☐

10. Answer: d
    Why: A needle is seated in a vein by carefully threading it within the lumen or the central area of the vein. This may mean changing the angle of the needle slightly to accommodate the vein's path.
    Review: Yes ☐ No ☐

11. Answer: a
    Why: Some tests are affected by the patient's diet. To eliminate the effects of diet, these tests are typically ordered fasting. This means that the patient must go

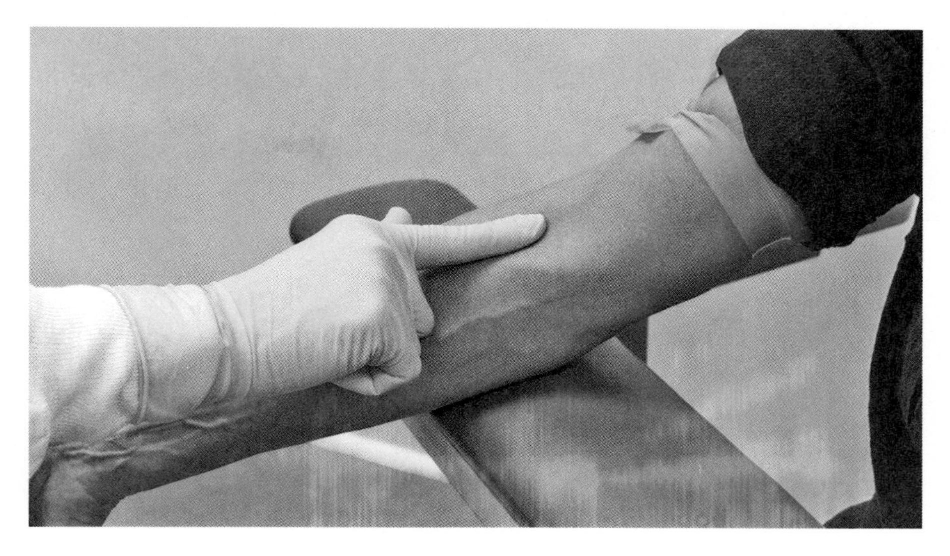

FIGURE 8-5 Phlebotomist palpating the antecubital area for a vein.

without food or drink except water for 8 to 12 hours before the specimen is to be collected. NPO (*nulla per os*) means that the patient is not allowed to have anything by mouth, including water. Patients are NPO before surgical procedures, not blood tests. See Table 8-1, Common Test Status Designations.

Review: Yes ☐ No ☐

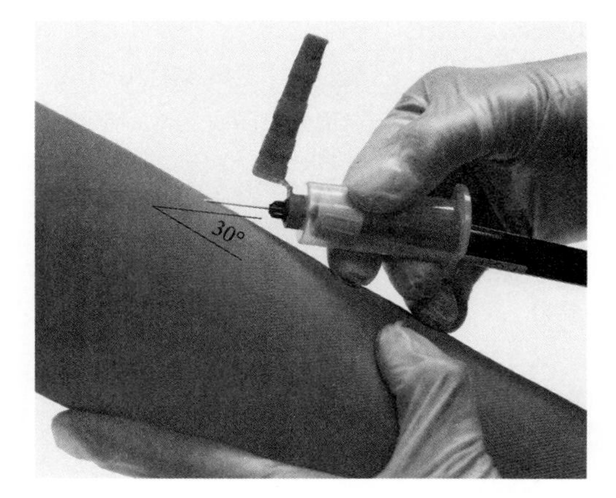

FIGURE 8-6 Illustration of a 30° angle of needle insertion.

12. Answer: c

    Why: A "timed" test means that the test is collected at a specific time because the results will be the most accurate at that specific moment. See Table 8-1.

    Review: Yes ☐ No ☐

13. Answer: a

    Why: It is critical to collect timed tests (See Table 8-1) such a as blood cultures, cardiac enzymes, and lithium levels, as close as possible to the requested time because that is when the information gained from results is most useful to the physician. Drug dosages based on results of tests that were not collected at the right time could prove to be ineffective or even toxic.

    Review: Yes ☐ No ☐

14. Answer: b

    Why: Fasting means "to go without food or drink, except water, for 8 to 12 hours." Fasting eliminates the effects food or drink may have on the results. See Table 8-1.

    Review: Yes ☐ No ☐

Table 8–1 Common Test Status Designations

Status	Meaning	When Used	Collection Conditions	Test Examples	Priority
STAT (stat)	Immediately (from Latin statim)	Test results are urgently needed on critical patients	Immediately collect, test, and report results. Alert lab staff when delivered. ER stats typically have priority over other stats	Glucose H & H Electrolytes Cardiac enzymes	First
Med Emerg	Medical Emergency (replaces STAT)	Same as STAT	Same as STAT	Same as STAT	Same as STAT
Timed	Collect at a specific time	Tests for which timing is critical for accurate results	Collect as close as possible to requested time. Record actual time collected	2-hour PP GTT, Cortisol Cardiac enzymes TDM Blood cultures	Second
ASAP	As soon as possible	Test results are needed soon to respond to a serious situation, but patient is not critical	Follow hospital protocol for type of test	Electrolytes Glucose H & H	Second or third depending on test
Fasting	No food or drink except water for 8–12 hours prior to specimen collection	To eliminate diet effects on test results	Verify patient has fasted. If patient has not fasted, check to see if specimen should still be collected	Glucose Cholesterol Triglycerides	Fourth
NPO	Nothing by mouth (from Latin nulla per os)	Prior to surgery or other anesthesia procedures	Do not give patient food or water. Refer requests to physician or nurse	N/A	N/A
Pre-op	Before an operation	To determine patient suitability for surgery	Collect before the patient goes to surgery	CBC, PTT Platelet function studies	Same as ASAP
Post-op	After an operation	Assess patient condition after surgery	Collect when patient is out of surgery	H & H	Same as ASAP
Routine	Relating to established procedure	Used to establish a diagnosis or monitor a patient's progress	Collect in a timely manner, but no urgency involved. Typically collected on morning sweeps or the next scheduled sweep	CBC Chem profile	None

15. Answer: b
 Why: Studies show that folding the arm back at the elbow to hold pressure or keep the gauze in place after a blood draw actually increases the chance of bruising by keeping the wound open. This is especially true if the puncture site is to the side of the arm. The chance of disrupting the platelet plug is also increased when the arm is lowered.
 Review: Yes ☐ No ☐

16. Answer: a
 Why: The term "accession" means "to record in the order received." To accession a specimen means "to take steps to unmistakably connect the specimen and the accompanying paperwork with a specific individual." To do this each specimen request is given a unique number called the "accession number," which is different from the patient ID number, date of birth, or the health facility's number assigned to that patient at admission.
 Review: Yes ☐ No ☐

17. Answer: c
 Why: If required diet restrictions for a test are not met before the specimen is collected, the results can be erroneous and meaningless. The test results can also be misinterpreted by the physician, which leads to compromised patient care and treatment. The phlebotomist is not responsible for supervising the patient's diet but should always verify the patient's diet status before collecting the specimen. Failing to verify diet status is not normally grounds for dismissal but does require a reprimand.
 Review: Yes ☐ No ☐

18. Answer: c
 Why: Typically, a physician or other qualified healthcare professional requests laboratory testing. Exceptions are certain rapid tests that can be purchased and performed at home by consumers, or blood specimens requested by law enforcement officials and used as evidence. A few states have legalized Direct Access Testing (DAT), in which patients are allowed to request certain blood tests themselves. So far, DAT is not widespread and the number of tests that can be requested is limited.
 Review: Yes ☐ No ☐

19. Answer: a
 Why: Test requisitions require specific information to ensure that the right patient is tested, the physician's orders are met, the correct tests are performed at the proper time under the required conditions, and the patient is billed correctly. The patient's location is generally given on inpatient requisitions only. There is no need for the patient's diagnosis, if known, to be on the request for blood work. Release of such information is limited to those with a valid need to know by the Health Insurance Portability and Accountability Act (HIPAA). Prior draw times are not normal requisition information.
 Review: Yes ☐ No ☐

20. Answer: c
 Why: The manual requisition (Fig. 8-7, p. 210) is available in many different styles and types. Some are a three-part form that serves as a request, report, and billing form. Use of manual requisitions is declining with the application of computerized systems in healthcare facilities.
 Review: Yes ☐ No ☐

21. Answer: d
 Why: On the sample requisition in Fig. 8-1 (p. 210), the type of tube to be collected appears as a mnemonic code with the volume of tube requested preceding the type of tube requested. In the example, the type of tube requested is a 10 mL Corvac (type of serum separator tube). A 5.0 mL lavender top tube is also requested.
 Review: Yes ☐ No ☐

Quest Diagnostics SmithKline Beecham Clinical Laboratories, Now a Part of Quest Diagnostics

SelecTest® HOSPITAL

85351402-2 6606516-8

REFERRED BY

BOSWELL MEMORIAL HOSPITAL
10401 W THUNDERBIRD BLVD
SUN CITY, AZ 85351-3004

PXPBROO 623-876-5381

DID YOU REMEMBER...
TO REQUEST OR MARK TEST(S)?
TO PROVIDE ORDER CODE(S) FOR HANDWRITTEN TESTS?

PATIENT INFORMATION - PLEASE PRINT
PRINT NAME (LAST, FIRST, MIDDLE) OR REGISTRATION NO

ROOM # | REGISTRATION # | LAB REFERENCE #

DOB (MM/DD/YYYY) | SEX M ☐ F ☐ | PATIENT I.D. #

REFERRING PHYSICIAN | REF. PHYSICIAN PROVIDER #

DATE COLLECTED | TIME AM PM | ☐ Fasting (Hours)

☐ Serum ☐ Plasma ☐ Blood ☐ Urine ☐ Frozen ☐ Other

☐ Call Results to:( ) ☐ Fax Results to:( )

Report Comments:

Internal Comments:

☐ STAT

☐ STAT PICK UP

F=FROZEN P=PLASMA B= LIGHT BLUE TOP TUBE L= LAVENDER TOP TUBE G= GRAY TOP TUBE R= RED TOP TUBE Y= YELLOW CAP URINE TUBE U=SCREW CAP URINE BOTTLE S= SERUM SEPARATOR TUBE

PANELS

Code	Test	
7352	☐ CARDIOLIPIN ANTIBODIES (IgG, IgA, IgM)	S
4451	☐ CK ISOENZYME PANEL (Total + Isoenzymes)	FS
7940	☐ EBV AB EVAL, COMP (anti-VCA IgM, anti-VCA IgG, anti-EA(D), anti-EA(R), anti-EBNA)	S
10306	☐ HEPATITIS PANEL, ACUTE W/REFLEX (HbsAg w/reflex confirm, HC Ab, HA Ab IgM, HbcAb, IgM)	S
7083	☐ IMMUNOGLOBULINS (IgG,IgA,IgM)	S
4411	☐ LDH ISOENZYME PANEL (Total + Isoenzymes)	S
7260	☐ THYROID AUTOANTIBODIES (Thyroglobulin + Peroxidase)	S
7065	☐ VITAMIN B12/FOLIC ACID	1

TESTS

Code	Test	
237	☐ AFP TUMOR MARKER	S
227	☐ ALDOLASE	FS
230	☐ ALDOSTERONE	S
249	☐ ANA W/REFLEX TITER	S
8431	☐ ANCA	S
683	☐ ANGIOTENSIN CONVERT ENZYME	S
4420	☐ C-REACTIVE PROTEIN	S
29256	☐ CA 125	S
5819	☐ CA 15-3	S
4698	☐ CA 19-9	FS
29493	☐ CA 27.29	S
329	☐ CARBAMAZEPINE	1
4661	☐ CARDIOLIPIN IGA AB	S
4662	☐ CARDIOLIPIN IGG AB	S
4663	☐ CARDIOLIPIN IGM AB	S
978	☐ CEA	S
377	☐ CK ISOENZYMES	FS
374	☐ CK, TOTAL	S
351	☐ COMPLEMENT C3	FS
353	☐ COMPLEMENT C4	FS
618	☐ COMPLEMENT, TOTAL (CH50)	FS
367	☐ CORTISOL	S
402	☐ DHEA SULFATE	S
255	☐ DNA AB, NATIVE	S
7849	☐ EBV ANTI-EA (D+R)	S
8564	☐ EBV ANTI-EBNA	S
8474	☐ EBV ANTI-VCA IGG	S
8426	☐ EBV ANTI-VCA IGM	S
427	☐ ERYTHROPOIETIN	S
429	☐ ESTRADIOL	S
457	☐ FERRITIN	S
467	☐ FOLIC ACID, RBC	1
466	☐ FOLIC ACID, SERUM	1
470	☐ FSH	S
4112	☐ FTA-ABS	S
478	☐ GASTRIN	FS
29407	☐ H. PYLORI IGG, QUAL	S
29408	☐ H. PYLORI IGG, QUANT	S
502	☐ HAPTOGLOBIN	S
496	☐ HEMOGLOBIN A1C	L
517	☐ HEMOGLOBIN ELECTROPHORESIS	L
508	☐ HEP A AB - TOTAL	S
512	☐ HEP A IGM AB	S
501	☐ HEP B CORE AB, TOTAL	S
4848	☐ HEP B CORE IGM AB	S
499	☐ HEP B SURFACE AB QUAL	S
8475	☐ HEP B SURFACE AB QUANT	S
498	☐ HEP B SURFACE AG W/REFLEX CONFIRM	S
8472	☐ HEP C VIRUS AB	S
6449	☐ HIV SCR-WB CONF	S
31789	☐ HOMOCYSTEINE	1
539	☐ IMMUNOGLOBULIN A	S
542	☐ IMMUNOGLOBULIN E	S
543	☐ IMMUNOGLOBULIN G	S
545	☐ IMMUNOGLOBULIN M	S
561	☐ INSULIN	FS
597	☐ LDH ISOENZYMES	S
593	☐ LDH, TOTAL	S
599	☐ LEAD (B)	1
6687	☐ LEGIONELLA PNEUMO AB 1-6	S
615	☐ LH	S
606	☐ LIPASE	S
613	☐ LITHIUM	1
7079	☐ LUPUS ANTICOAGULANT	1
6646	☐ LYME DISEASE AB-WB CONF	S
4555	☐ MICROALBUMIN (U)	1
6517	☐ MICROALB/CREAT RATIO	U
259	☐ MITOCHONDRIAL AB	S
8624	☐ MUMPS VIRUS IGG	S
659	☐ MYCO PNEUMONIAE IGG AB	S
272	☐ NORTRIPTYLINE	1
4847	☐ PREALBUMIN	1
745	☐ PROGESTERONE	S
746	☐ PROLACTIN	S
747	☐ PROTEIN ELECTROPHORESIS	S
754	☐ PROTEIN, TOTAL	S
5363	☐ PSA	S
8847	☐ PT WITH INR	1
8446	☐ PTH, INTACT W/CALCIUM	FS
8837	☐ PTH, INTACT(IRMA) W/CALCIUM	FS
787	☐ RENIN ACTIVITY	1
4418	☐ RHEUMATOID FACTOR	S
799	☐ RPR (MONITORING) W/REFLEX TITER	S
36125	☐ RPR (DX) W/REFLEX CONFIRM TP-PA	S
802	☐ RUBELLA IGG AB	S
964	☐ RUBEOLA IGG AB	S
30261	☐ STONE ANALYSIS, KIDNEY	1
30260	☐ STONE ANALYSIS, OTHER	1
34429	☐ T-3, FREE	S
859	☐ T-3, TOTAL	S
861	☐ T-3, UPTAKE	S
867	☐ T-4 (THYROXINE)	S
866	☐ T-4, FREE	S
7924	☐ T-HELPER/SUPPRESSOR RATIO	1
30741	☐ TESTOSTERONE, FREE AND TOTAL	S
873	☐ TESTOSTERONE, TOTAL	S
267	☐ THYROGLOBULIN AB	S
5081	☐ THYROID PEROXIDASE AB	S
891	☐ TRANSFERRIN	S
899	☐ TSH	S
36127	☐ TSH W/REFLEX T-4, FREE	S
916	☐ VALPROIC ACID	1
4439	☐ VARICELLA-ZOSTER IGG AB	S
4128	☐ VDRL, CSF	1
927	☐ VITAMIN B12	S
934	☐ VMA (U)	1

MICROBIOLOGY

SOURCE:

Code	Test	
8756	☐ C DIFFICILE TOXIN A	1
389	☐ CULTURE, BLOOD	1
690	☐ CULTURE, CHLAMYDIA TRACH	1
4553	☐ CULTURE, FUNGUS	1
2692	☐ CULTURE, HSV (RAPID)	1
2649	☐ CULTURE, HSV WITH TYPING	1
4554	☐ CULTURE, MYCOBACTERIUM	1
395	☐ CULTURE, URINE, RTN	1
689	☐ CULTURE, VIRUS, COMP	1
6919	☐ DNA PROBE, CHL & GC	1
8502	☐ DNA PROBE, CHLAMYDIA	1
8501	☐ DNA PROBE, GC	1
30264	☐ E. COLI SHIGA TOXINS, EIA STOOL	1
681	☐ OVA & PARASITES	1

ADDITIONAL TESTS: (MUST INCLUDE COMPLETE TEST NAME AND ORDER CODE. REFER TO SBCL DIRECTORY OF SERVICES.)

TOTAL TESTS ORDERED

REQHPLA

85351402 6606516 85351402 6606516
85351402 6606516 85351402 6606516

FOLD HERE

SB20357C- QS (2/00)

FIGURE 8-7 Newborn screening forms. A. First specimen form. B. Second specimen form. (Courtesy Brenda Romero RN, BSN, State of New Mexico Genetic and Newborn Screening program, Santa Fe, NM.)

22. Answer: c
Why: On the sample requisition in Fig. 8-1, the patient's age is signified by the number "55" followed by the letter "M," which means that the patient is a 55-year-old male.
Review: Yes ☐ No ☐

23. Answer: b
Why: A computer requisition has an accession number given to the patient's sample during the data entry phase. On the sample requisition in Fig. 8-1, arrow number 3 points to the accession number.
Review: Yes ☐ No ☐

24. Answer: a
Why: A barcode is a series of black stripes and white spaces of varying widths that correspond to letters and numbers. The stripes can be grouped together to represent identification numbers, laboratory tests, or patient names. At healthcare facilities, credit information is not found in barcode format.
Review: Yes ☐ No ☐

25. Answer: c
Why: Outpatient requisitions are typically manual forms (Fig. 8-7) that can be filled out by a physician or an office assistant and taken by the patient to the lab.
Review: Yes ☐ No ☐

26. Answer: a
Why: After the laboratory receives them, requisitions are sorted according to priority of collection, date and time of collection, and location of the patient. There is no reason to ever sort them alphabetically.
Review: Yes ☐ No ☐

27. Answer: a
Why: The steps taken to unmistakably connect a specimen and the accompanying paperwork to a specific individual is called accessioning the specimen. The accession number is automatically assigned when the request is entered into the computer.
Review: Yes ☐ No ☐

28. Answer: b
Why: Cortisol exhibits diurnal variation, with peak blood levels occurring in the morning around 8 AM. Consequently, a cortisol test is usually ordered for collection at a specific time, most commonly 8 A.M. (Table 8-1). Cholesterol, fibrinogen, and monospot tests are not typically timed tests.
Review: Yes ☐ No ☐

29. Answer: b
Why: STAT comes from the Latin word *statim,* which means "immediately." A test that is ordered STAT should be collected immediately, without hesitation. See Table 8-1.
Review: Yes ☐ No ☐

30. Answer: c
Why: Abnormal electrolyte levels can lead to death; consequently, electrolyte tests are often ordered STAT (Table 8-1).
Review: Yes ☐ No ☐

31. Answer: a
Why: When a test is ordered STAT, it means that the results are urgently needed on a patient in critical condition (Table 8-1). A patient who is in critical condition is in a life or death situation.
Review: Yes ☐ No ☐

32. Answer: c
Why: ASAP means as "soon as possible." If a test is ordered ASAP, it means that test results are needed soon to respond to a serious situation, but the patient is not in critical condition or in danger of dying (Table 8-1).
Review: Yes ☐ No ☐

33. Answer: d
Why: Pre-op means "before an operation" and indicates that the patient will soon be going to surgery (Table 8-1).
Review: Yes ☐ No ☐

34. Answer: b
Why: Routine tests are those tests that are typically ordered in the course of establishing a diagnosis or monitoring a patient's care (Table 8-1).
Review: Yes ☐ No ☐

35. Answer: b
Why: Medical emergency (med emerg) means the same as STAT (Table 8-1). It has

replaced STAT in some institutions to identify specimens whose results are needed immediately to respond to critical situations.

Review: Yes ☐ No ☐

36. Answer: a
Why: NPO comes from Latin (*non per os*) and means nothing by mouth. Patients who are NPO cannot have food or drink, not even water (Table 8-1). Patients are typically NPO before surgery, not after.
Review: Yes ☐ No ☐

37. Answer: c
Why: Glucose levels normally rise with the intake of food and return to normal fasting levels within 2 hours if no more food is eaten. Glucose levels are ordered fasting to see if glucose is being metabolized properly (Table 8-1). If glucose is not being metabolized properly, fasting levels will not be normal.
Review: Yes ☐ No ☐

38. Answer: c
Why: The only liquid that it is acceptable to drink when fasting is water (Table 8-1).
Review: Yes ☐ No ☐

39. Answer: c
Why: Post-op means "after an operation" (Table 8-1). Both hemoglobin and hematocrit are indications of the red blood cell count. H & H levels are a common post-op test to monitor blood levels after surgery.
Review: Yes ☐ No ☐

40. Answer: a
Why: If the door to the room is closed, you should knock lightly and proceed with caution. Even if the door is open, it is a good idea to knock lightly to make occupants aware that you are about to enter and to get their attention so that you can ask if it is all right to enter.
Review: Yes ☐ No ☐

41. Answer: d
Why: Because the specimen is a complete blood count (CBC), it can easily be collected by finger stick from the left hand. The right arm should not be used. Collecting the CBC from the IV is not worth the risk when it can easily be collected by capillary puncture. A competent phlebotomist should be able to decide what to do in this situation without having to ask the nurse.
Review: Yes ☐ No ☐

42. Answer: a
Why: Codes are one of the ways healthcare institutions convey important information over a public address system to those who need to know without alarming the general public. Codes use numbers or words to convey information. For example, code "blue" typically means someone has stopped breathing.
Review: Yes ☐ No ☐

43. Answer: d
Why: DNR means "do not resuscitate." It means no code should be called or heroic measures taken if the patient stops breathing. It is sometimes used when patients are terminally ill.
Review: Yes ☐ No ☐

44. Answer: c
Why: When you ask if it is all right to draw a patient's blood and the patient replies, "Yes, but I would rather not," or something similar, they have given permission and taken it back in the same breath. You should not draw the patient until you are certain that you have permission.
Review: Yes ☐ No ☐

45. Answer: d
Why: One of the tests used to identify protein or immune globulin disorders that lead to nerve damage is serum protein electrophoresis (SPEP). See Table 8-2 for more tests com-

monly ordered for geriatric patients and the indications for ordering.

Review: Yes ☐ No ☐

46. Answer: a

Why: It is acceptable procedure to wake a patient for a blood draw. If an inpatient is asleep, call out his or her name softly and shake the bed gently. Do not shake the patient because you may startle him or her. Never attempt to collect a blood specimen from a sleeping patient. Such an attempt can also startle the patient, and you or the patient may be injured. In addition, a startle reflex can affect test results and should be avoided.

Review: Yes ☐ No ☐

47. Answer: d

Why: A startle reflex can affect test results and should be avoided. Collecting the specimen in dim lighting or collecting a specimen from an unconscious patient should not affect test results, provided the specimen is collected properly. When a phlebotomist awakens a patient and elevates the head of the patient's bed before collecting the specimen, there should no negative effect to the specimen.

Review: Yes ☐ No ☐

48. Answer: c

Why: Some patients can hear what is going on around them despite being considered unconscious. Identify yourself and inform the patient of your intent, talking to him or her

Table 8-2 Tests Commonly Ordered on Geriatric Patients

Test	Typical Indications for Ordering
ANA, RA, or RF	Diagnose lupus and rheumatold arthritis, which can affect nervous system function
CBC	Determine hemoglobin levels, detect infection, and identify blood disorders
BUN/creatinine	Diagnose kidney function disorders that may be responsible for problems such as confusion, coma, seizures, and tremors
Calcium/magnesium	Identify abnormal levels associated with seizures and muscle problems
Electrolytes	Determine sodium and potassium levels, critical to proper nervous system function
ESR	Detect inflammation, identify collagen vascular diseases
Glucose	Detect and monitor diabetes; abnormal levels can cause confusion, seizures, or coma or lead to peripheral neuropathy
PT/PTT	Monitor blood-thinning medications, important in heart conditions, coagulation problems and stroke management
SPEP, IPEP	Identify protein or immune globulin disorders that lead to nerve damage
VDRL/FTA	Diagnose or rule out syphilis, which can cause nerve damage and dementia

as you would an alert patient. In addition, an unconscious patient may be able to feel pain and may move during a blood draw, so it is important to have someone assist you by holding the patient's arm still. The patient's blood may be drawn in the bed where they are. No special collection area is necessary.

Review: Yes ☐ No ☐

49. Answer: c

Why: If a physician is with the patient and the test is ordered STAT, it is generally acceptable procedure to politely introduce yourself, explain why you are there, and ask permission to collect the specimen. The physician may give you permission and may not. If no permission is given, the STAT will have to wait until the physician leaves.

Review: Yes ☐ No ☐

50. Answer: a

Why: It is acceptable and in the best interest of all to ask family or visitors to step out of the room temporarily while you collect a blood specimen. Most will be more than willing to do so.

Review: Yes ☐ No ☐

51. Answer: b

Why: All specimens and test requests must be accounted for. Generally, if a patient is unavailable for testing, a delay slip is filled out stating why you were unable to collect the specimen. The original is left at the nurse's station, and a copy goes back to the laboratory. It is then up to the patient's nurse to notify the lab when the patient is available for testing and the phlebotomist can return.

Review: Yes ☐ No ☐

52. Answer: d

Why: Misidentification of a type and screen could lead to a patient getting the wrong type of blood and a possible fatal transfusion reaction.

Review: Yes ☐ No ☐

53. Answer: b.

Why: Proper patient identification involves asking the patient to state his or her name and date of birth. This step is followed by checking the ID band and the requisition to see if they match. Verbal statement of identity from the patient is important. An ill or hard-of-hearing patient may answer "yes" to almost anything. It is not unheard of for a patient to be wearing an ID band with incorrect information.

Review: Yes ☐ No ☐

54. Answer: a

Why: It is important that certain information on the ID band match the information on the requisition exactly. The medical record number is mandatory information and should match exactly. The room number may change during a patient's stay in the hospital and should not be relied on as proper identification. In addition, the physician may change or the patient may have more than one physician ordering tests. Test status and collection priority changes with each order and is not information that is found on the ID band.

Review: Yes ☐ No ☐

55. Answer: b

Why: Any discrepancy in the patient's name, date of birth, or medical record number between the requisition and the patient's ID band should be addressed and resolved before a specimen is collected.

Review: Yes ☐ No ☐

56. Answer: c

Why: Identification should never be based on information on the patient's door. When no ID band can be found, it is necessary to ask the patient's nurse to make positive identification and attach an ID band before the specimen can be drawn.

Review: Yes ☐ No ☐

57. Answer: c

Why: It is not uncommon for an emergency room to receive an unconscious patient with no identification. Specimens should not be collected without some way to positively connect the specimen with the patient. In many institutions, a special three-part ID band will be attached to the unidentified patient's wrist. The special ID band has a unique number. The same number is on labels that are placed on specimens collected from that patient.

Review: Yes ☐ No ☐

58. Answer: c

Why: A newborn may have more than one ID band, one with the infant's information and one with the mother's.

Review: Yes ☐ No ☐

59. Answer: c

Why: The most critical error a phlebotomist can make is misidentifying a patient specimen. A misidentified specimen can have serious or even fatal consequences to the patient, especially if the specimen is for a type and screen for a blood transfusion. Misidentification of a patient's specimen can be grounds for dismissal of the person responsible and could even lead to a malpractice lawsuit against that person.

Review: Yes ☐ No ☐

60. Answer: b

Why: Identification should never be verified from an ID band that is *not* attached to the patient. An ID band on the nightstand could belong to a patient who previously occupied that bed. Even if the ID band and the requisition match, it is not adequate as proper identification of the patient. If an ID band is not attached to the patient, you must ask the patient's nurse to attach an ID band before you can collect the specimen.

Review: Yes ☐ No ☐

61. Answer: a

Why: The patient's nurse or other caregiver, or a relative, may be needed to confirm the identity of a patient who is a very young child or someone who is mentally incompetent or cannot speak English. The term "geriatric" means relating to old age; it does not mean senile or fragile. One would expect that this type of patient could identify himself or herself correctly.

Review: Yes ☐ No ☐

62. Answer: a

Why: Never make assumptions about a person's identity and do not rely on others to identify patients for you. Always verify patient identification yourself by asking the patient to state his or her name and date of birth.

Review: Yes ☐ No ☐

63. Answer: c

Why: A cheerful, pleasant bedside manner and exchange of small talk puts both you and the patient at ease, helps you gain the patient's trust and confidence, and helps divert attention from any discomfort associated with the blood draw. What it may not affect is the tendency for a patient to faint, a vasovagal response to venipuncture or needles.

Review: Yes ☐ No ☐

64. Answer: b

Why: Most patients understand that blood tests are needed in the course of their treatment. However, illness can be quite stressful and occasionally a patient who is tired of being "poked" will be cranky and rude. It is important to remain polite and professional and draw the specimen in your normal way. You may discover that the patient will actually apologize to you by the time you have finished.

Review: Yes ☐ No ☐

65. Answer: c

Why: Advising a patient of his or her prognosis or explaining what disorders the test can detect is a physician's responsibility. It is not a phlebotomist's duty and is not necessary to informed consent. Informing a patient when you are a student is important to informed consent. A patient has a right to refuse to be drawn by a student. Knowing that you are going to draw a blood specimen is necessary to informed consent. Many patients request to know the name of the test before consenting to a blood draw.

Review: Yes ☐ No ☐

66. Answer: a

Why: They are many reasons why a physician will order certain tests. Any attempt at explanation of why a test was ordered may mislead the patient. For example, a glucose test may be ordered because the patient is taking medication that can affect glucose levels, not because diabetes is suspected. Usually such inquiries are handled by explaining that the doctor has ordered the tests as part of the patient's care and that he or she will be happy to explain the tests if asked. The Health Insurance Portability and Accountability Act (HIPAA) clearly states that patient confidentiality must be protected. This does not apply to inquiries by patients about their own tests.

Review: Yes ☐ No ☐

67. Answer: c

Why: When it has been determined that a patient truly refuses to cooperate, you should write on the requisition that the patient has refused to have blood drawn. You should also notify the patient's nurse and the phlebotomy supervisor that the specimen was not obtained because of patient refusal. Some institutions have a special form on which you state that you were unable to collect the specimen and the reason why. The original form is left at the nurse's station and a copy goes to the lab.

Review: Yes ☐ No ☐

68. Answer: a

Why: If you determine that the patient has not been fasting, notify the patient's nurse so that a determination can be made regarding whether to proceed with the test. If you are told to proceed with collection, write "non-fasting" on the requisition and specimen label so that testing personnel know the status of the patient.

Review: Yes ☐ No ☐

69. Answer: c

Why: If you wait to assemble equipment after selecting the collection site, you will have a better idea of what equipment to use and will ultimately waste less equipment. For example, if you have a multisample needle and holder ready before you select the site, it will have to be thrown away if you later decide to use a butterfly instead. However, if you had waited until after selecting the site to select equipment, you would only be using the butterfly equipment. There is plenty of time to get equipment ready while you are waiting for the alcohol to dry after cleaning the site, and you will be more apt to allow sufficient time for the alcohol to dry. After cleaning, it is not the time in your procedure to check the other arm for a better site.

Review: Yes ☐ No ☐

70. Answer: c

Why: When performing a routine blood draw, the hands must be decontaminated before glove application at the beginning of the procedure and at the end after glove removal, before proceeding to the next patient.

Review: Yes ☐ No ☐

71. Answer: d
Why: Proper hand washing is an important part of the venipuncture procedure. Hands should be washed in a downward motion, scrubbing from wrists to fingertips to prevent backflow of contaminated soap and water. A circular scrubbing motion that creates plenty of friction is needed to dislodge surface debris and bacteria. If the sink does not have an automatic shut-off, a clean paper towel should be used to turn off the faucet to avoid contaminating clean hands.
Review: Yes ☐ No ☐

72. Answer: a
Why: Do everything you can to establish a rapport with the child and his or her parents. Even young children can sense when you are not being honest with them. Tell the child that the procedure may be slightly uncomfortable without being overly blunt. Never tell a child it will not hurt. Offering a child a treat is a temporary distraction but does nothing to instill trust in the phlebotomist and the procedure. In addition, any treat, sticker, or toy should be a reward just for going through the procedure, not for being brave enough to not cry.
Review: Yes ☐ No ☐

73. Answer: c
Why: You should never tell a patient that a venipuncture will not hurt, nor should you suggest that it will hurt a great deal. Some patients are more sensitive to pain than others. Tell the patient that it may hurt a little, but only for a short time. You should warn patients just before you slip the needle into the vein to help them prepare for it. You can suggest to a fearful patient that he or she look away as the needle goes in, but do not imply that looking away will keep it from hurting.
Review: Yes ☐ No ☐

74. Answer: d
Why: Proper arm position is important for successful venipuncture. An arm in proper position for routine venipuncture is supported firmly and extended downward in a straight line from shoulder to wrist. (Fig. 8-3, p. 223) with the palm up. It should not be bent at the elbow. Be aware of the angle of the arm when collecting your samples. If the arm is straight forward, the tubes will not fill from the bottom up. The hand may be turned palm down when accessing the cephalic vein or hand veins.
Review: Yes ☐ No ☐

75. Answer: b
Why: Patients rarely faint when they are lying down. An outpatient who has previously fainted during a blood draw should be asked to lie down, or the drawing chair should be reclined if possible. Sitting upright poses the danger of becoming injured if the patient faints and falls, so no exceptions should be made. In addition, a person who has fainted may be difficult to revive if not in a supine position.
Review: Yes ☐ No ☐

76. Answer: c
Why: It is acceptable to lower a bedrail to make blood collection easier; however, you can be held liable if you forget to raise it again after you are finished and the patient falls out of bed and is injured.
Review: Yes ☐ No ☐

77. Answer: b
Why: Blockage of blood flow (stasis) by the tourniquet causes hemoconcentration, which affects specimen composition and leads to erroneous test results. To minimize

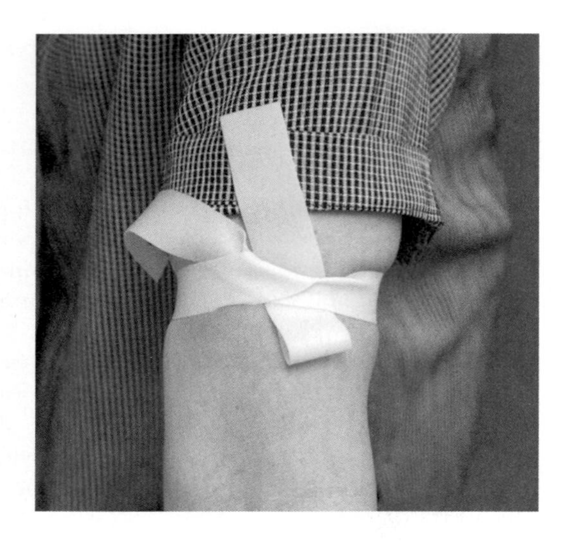

FIGURE 8-8 A properly tied tourniquet with ends pointing toward the shoulder.

these effects, the tourniquet should never be left in place longer than 1 minute.

Review: Yes ☐ No ☐

78. Answer: a
Why: The best place to apply the tourniquet is 3 to 4 inches above the intended venipuncture site (Fig. 8-8). If it is too close to the collection site, the vein may collapse as blood is withdrawn; if it is too far away, it may be ineffective. Applying a tourniquet distal or below a venipuncture site would prevent blood flow into the area and result in vein collapse and unsuccessful venipuncture. When drawing a hand vein, the tourniquet is applied proximal to the wrist bone, not distal.
Review: Yes ☐ No ☐

79. Answer: d
Why: A tourniquet that is too tight may prevent arterial blood flow into the area, resulting in failure to obtain blood. A tourniquet that is too tight increases the effects of hemoconcentration and contributes to erroneous results on the sample. A tourniquet that is too tight will pinch and hurt the patient and cause the arm to turn red or purple. A tight tourniquet will not allow for an increase in venous blood flow.
Review: Yes ☐ No ☐

80. Answer: a
Why: To enhance vein selection, you are encouraged to palpate the antecubital area, lower the arm, or use a warm towel to increase blood flow. It is not a good idea to have a patient pump (repeatedly open and close) his or her fist because it may cause erroneous results for some tests, most notably potassium levels, as a result of hemoconcentration.
Review: Yes ☐ No ☐

81. Answer: c
Why: You can easily tell an artery from a vein because an artery has a pulse; a vein does not. Veins are more superficial than arteries and may feel larger for that reason.
Review: Yes ☐ No ☐

82. Answer: b
Why: A normal vein feels bouncy and resilient; a sclerosed vein feels hard and cordlike and lacks resiliency. A sclerosed vein is difficult to penetrate, rolls easily, and should not be used for venipuncture.
Review: Yes ☐ No ☐

83. Answer: c
Why: Ankle veins are sometimes used as a last resort, but only after obtaining permission from the patient's physician.
Review: Yes ☐ No ☐

84. Answer: d
Why: To avoid inadvertently puncturing an artery, never select a vein that overlies or is close to an artery or near where you feel a pulse. Avoid drawing from the basilic vein because it is in the area of the brachial artery.
Review: Yes ☐ No ☐

85. Answer: a
Why: When a person has dermatitis and there is no other site available, it is acceptable to apply the tourniquet over a towel or washcloth placed over the patient's arm. A coagulation test should not be collected from an IV, and a coagulation tube cannot be collected by finger stick. The area above an IV must not be used regardless of whether you use a tourniquet.
Review: Yes ☐ No ☐

86. Answer: c
Why: If the vein can be felt, but not seen, try to mentally visualize its location. It often helps to note the position of the vein in reference to a mole, hair, or skin crease. Never insert the needle blindly or probe to find a vein because damage to nerves and tissue may result. Never leave the tourniquet on for more than 1 minute because hemoconcentration of the specimen may result. Marking the site with a felt-tip pen could contaminate the specimen or transfer disease from patient to patient.
Review: Yes ☐ No ☐

87. Answer: d
Why: Clinical and Laboratory Standards Institute (CLSI) guidelines recommend that if a tourniquet is used for initial vein selection, it should be released and not reapplied for a minimum of 2 minutes to allow the vein to return to normal. This avoids hemoconcentration of the specimen and helps to ensure accurate test results. Arterial flow should not be affected by the tourniquet if the pressure is correct.
Review: Yes ☐ No ☐

88. Answer: b
Why: CLSI standards recommend cleaning the site with antiseptic using a circular motion from the center to the periphery. In other words, start at the center and wipe outward in ever-increasing circles (Fig. 8-9)
Review: Yes ☐ No ☐

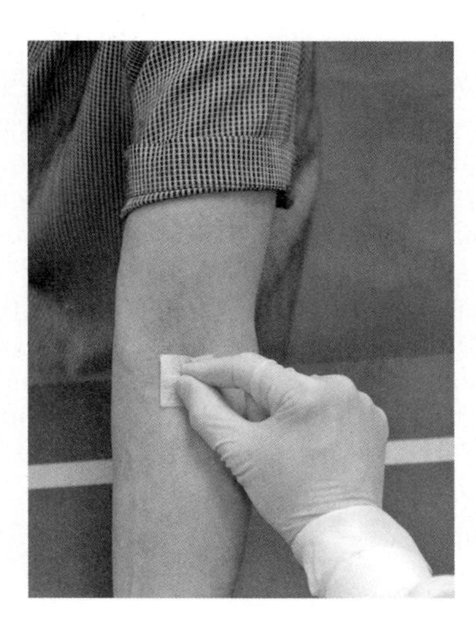

FIGURE 8-9 Cleaning a venipuncture site.

89. Answer: c
Why: Alcohol takes around 30 seconds to evaporate completely. The evaporation process helps destroy microbes. Allowing the alcohol to dry before venipuncture also prevents hemolysis of the specimen and a stinging sensation when the needle is inserted. This is a desirable time to prepare equipment, but it is not the reason you wait for the alcohol to dry.
Review: Yes ☐ No ☐

90. Answer: a
Why: When the tube is advanced past the guideline on the holder, the stopper is penetrated, causing the tube to lose its vacuum. A tube that has lost its vacuum will fail to fill with blood, which means you will have to replace it with a new tube.
Review: Yes ☐ No ☐

91. Answer: d
Why: Visually inspecting the needle tip before insertion not only ensures that you are entering bevel up but also prevents damage and unnecessary pain during the procedure should the point or beveled

edges have imperfections. Needles are sterile when first opened as long as they are not allowed to touch anything, and they should not have any external contamination. However, they should be checked nonetheless because contaminants have been observed on rare occasions. You cannot tell that a needle is outdated by inspecting the tip. The expiration date is typically printed on the label that covers the twist-apart shields or on the packaging, as in the case of butterfly needles. Outdated needles must be discarded during regular inventory of the stock.

Review: Yes ☐ No ☐

92. Answer: a

Why: The correct order for the venipuncture procedure is to clean the site and prepare equipment during the 30 seconds that it takes to dry. It is best to put on gloves before applying the tourniquet, because according to CLSI guidelines, the tourniquet should only be on the arm for 1 minute or less. It is important to remember that the tourniquet should be released as soon as blood begins to flow. Verifying diet restrictions and positioning the patient should happen before vein selection has begun.

Review: Yes ☐ No ☐

93. Answer: b

Why: If the needle touches the skin and then is withdrawn before piercing the tissue, the needle is considered contaminated and a new needle should be used for the draw to avoid a possible infection. Always be aware of any contamination to the needle before using it to penetrate the skin and possibly taking bacteria into a patient's vascular system.

Review: Yes ☐ No ☐

94. Answer: b

Why: Under normal circumstances the best angle for routine antecubital venipunctures is between 15° and 30° (see Fig. 8-6), depending on the depth of the vein. When using a butterfly, the angle will probably be less than 15°, as seen in Fig. 8-10.

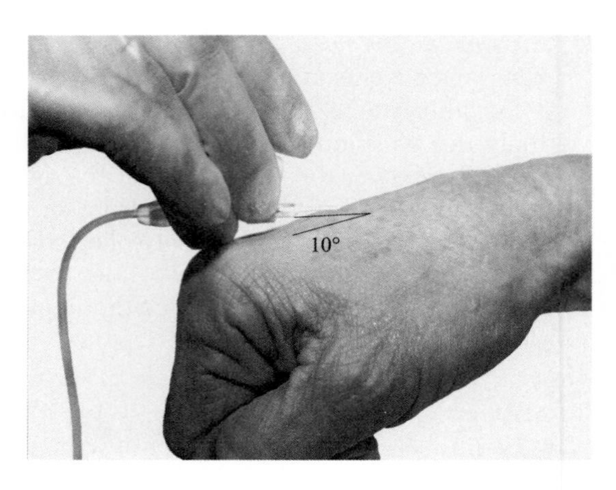

FIGURE 8-10 Illustration of 10° angle of needle insertion.

Review: Yes ☐ No ☐

95. Answer: b

Why: A venipuncture needle is always inserted bevel up.

Review: Yes ☐ No ☐

96. Answer: c

Why: When the needle enters the vein, you will feel a slight "give," or decrease in resistance. Some phlebotomists describe this as a "pop." If the needle hisses, the vacuum of the tube is drawing in air, which means that the needle bevel is partially or totally out of the vein and not completely under the skin. If you can feel the needle vibrate, the needle bevel is against the vein wall or a valve, causing flapping of tissue against the needle opening. When using the ETS, blood does not flow until the tube is fully engaged after the needle is in the vein.

Review: Yes ☐ No ☐

97. Answer: c

Why: According to CLSI guidelines, the best time to release the tourniquet is as soon as blood begins to flow into the first tube. Releasing the tourniquet as well as having the patient release the fist minimizes the effects of stasis and hemoconcentration on the specimen. A tourniquet should not remain in place longer than 1 minute.

Review: Yes ☐ No ☐

98. Answer: b
Why: Prolonged tourniquet application or vigorous fist pumping lead to hemoconcentration of the specimen notably affecting potassium, protein levels, and cell counts.
Review: Yes ☐ No ☐

99. Answer: d
Why: The arm should be in a downward position during venipuncture so that tubes fill from the bottom up and *not* from the stopper end first. This keeps blood in the tube from coming in contact with the needle, preventing reflux of tube contents into the patient's vein, and minimizing the chance of additive carryover between tubes. Collecting sterile specimens before filling tubes for other specimens, clearing for special coagulation tests, and filling tubes until the normal vacuum is exhausted are all part of proper venipuncture technique.
Review: Yes ☐ No ☐

100. Answer: b
Why: It is important to fill additive tubes to the proper fill level to ensure a proper ratio of additive to blood. The proper fill level is attained by allowing the tube to fill until the normal vacuum is exhausted and blood ceases to flow into the tube. Tubes will not fill completely because there is always dead space at the top. Blood in an anticoagulant tube does not clot. A partially filled tube would likely yield enough specimen to perform the test; however, the results would be inaccurate. Tissue thromboplastin is a problem for some tests, particularly special coagulation tests collected in tubes with light blue tops. However, contamination can be minimized by first collecting a discard tube to flush the tissue thromboplastin out of the needle.
Review: Yes ☐ No ☐

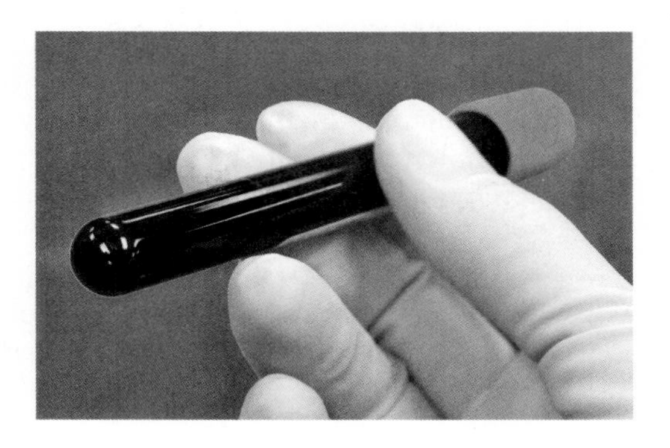

FIGURE 8-11 Phlebotomist mixing a heparin tube.

101. Answer: a
Why: Lack of or inadequate mixing immediately after filling anticoagulant tubes can lead to microclot formation. Adequate mixing requires (Fig. 8-11) inversion of the tube, as shown in. Anticoagulant tubes are not supposed to clot, so coagulation would definitely *not* be encouraged. Hemoconcentration is related to dehydration of the patient, fist pumping, and prolonged tourniquet application, not mixing of the tube. Hemolysis can be caused by mixing tubes too vigorously. Non-additive tubes do not require mixing.
Review: Yes ☐ No ☐

102. Answer: b
Why: To avoid EDTA contamination of the green top tube, draw a few milliliters of blood into a plain red top discard tube. Penetrating the stopper of the red top should help clear contamination from the outside of the needle. Drawing a few milliliters of blood into the discard tube should flush any contamination from inside the needle. If the error had been discovered after the green top tube had started to fill, that green top could be considered the discard tube and another green top collected after it.
Review: Yes ☐ No ☐

103. Answer: d
Why: Non-additive tubes should not be mixed. In fact, mixing may cause hemolysis if the sample has already begun to clot.
Review: Yes ☐ No ☐

104. Answer: a
Why: Vigorous mixing or shaking of the tube can cause hemolysis because red cells are fragile and can rupture easily.
Review: Yes ☐ No ☐

105. Answer: a
Why: Using several layers of gauze helps create adequate pressure to stop the bleeding and keeps the blood from soaking through and contaminating your glove. The purpose of using gauze as the needle is pulled out has nothing to do with whether the patient sees the needle come out or not. Whether or not it hurts when you pull the needle out depends on your technique, not the amount of gauze used. You could use several layers of gauze and still have bruising if you did not apply adequate pressure to the site.
Review: Yes ☐ No ☐

106. Answer: d
Why: Gauze pads are preferred for applying pressure to the puncture site because the loose cotton fibers of cotton balls tend to stick to the site, pulling platelets with them when the cotton ball is removed. This disrupts the platelet plug and reinitiates bleeding.
Review: Yes ☐ No ☐

107. Answer: b
Why: The gauze should be held lightly in place by the fingers until the needle exits the vein; then pressure should be applied. Applying pressure to the gauze while the needle is still in the arm can cause the needle to slit the skin, slowing down needle removal and producing pain. It should not bend the needle bevel, however.
Review: Yes ☐ No ☐

108. Answer: c
Why: An uncovered used needle is a danger to the phlebotomist. A needle safety feature should be engaged immediately after needle removal, (Fig. 8-12). Any delay increases the risk of accidental needle injury to the phlebotomist.
Review: Yes ☐ No ☐

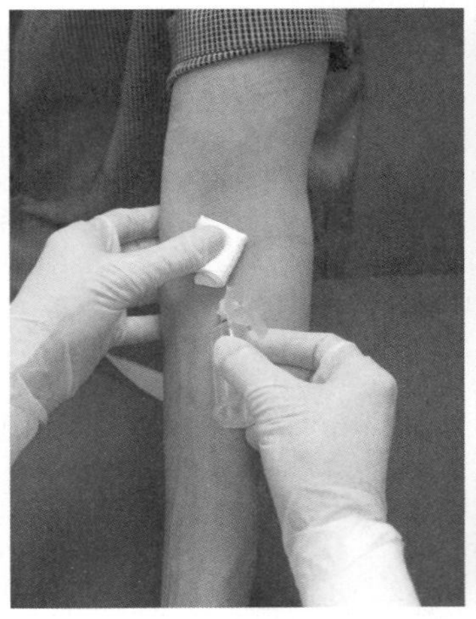
A

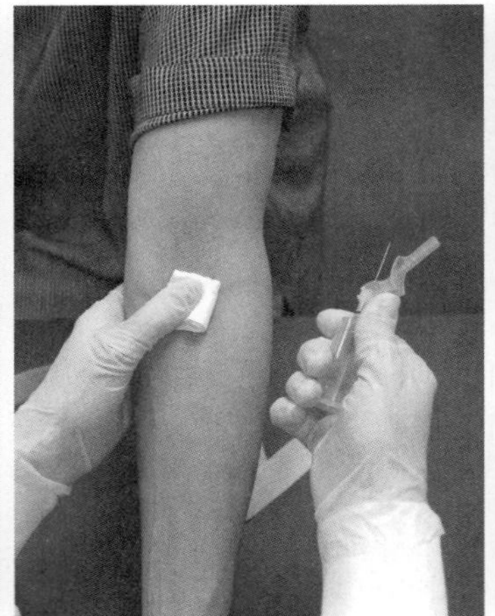
B

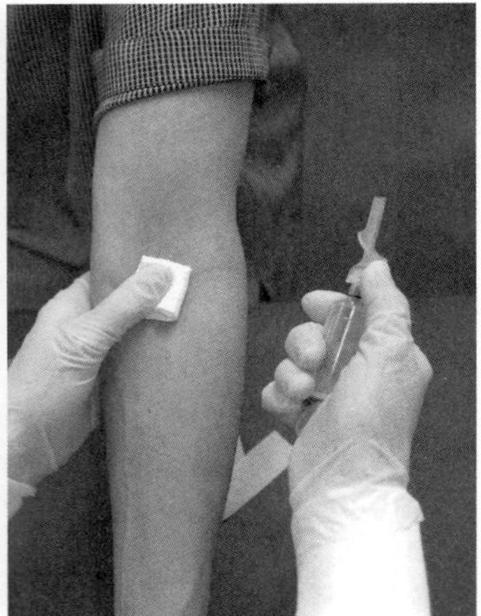
C

FIGURE 8-12 **A.** Placing gauze. **B.** Needle removed. **C.** Safety device activated.

109. Answer: a

Why: According to CLSI, the tourniquet should be released as soon as blood flow is established to minimize the effects of hemoconcentration. Additive tubes should be mixed as soon as they are removed from the tube holder for proper additive function, including the prevention of microclot formation in anticoagulant tubes. Pressure should be applied immediately after the needle is removed from the arm or hand.

Review: Yes ☐ No ☐

110. Answer: a

Why: According to the Occupational Safety and Health Administration (OSHA) regulations, a needle and holder are to be disposed of as a single unit, as shown in Fig. 8-13. Removing the needle from the holder either by ejection or unscrewing subjects the user to needlestick hazards posed by the exposed rubber sleeve end of the needle.

Review: Yes ☐ No ☐

111. Answer: a

Why: Inpatient blood specimens should be labeled at the bedside immediately following collection (Fig. 8-14). If tubes are labeled before collection and one of the tubes is not used at that time, another patient's blood could end up in that labeled tube. If tubes are labeled away from the bedside, the specimen can be misidentified.

Review: Yes ☐ No ☐

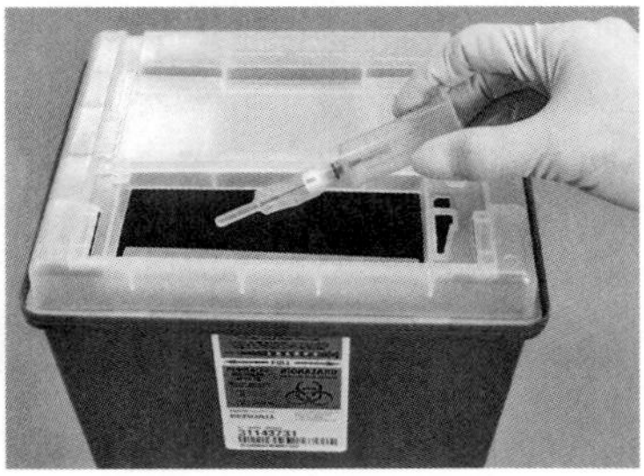

FIGURE 8-13 Discarding a needle and tube holder as a unit.

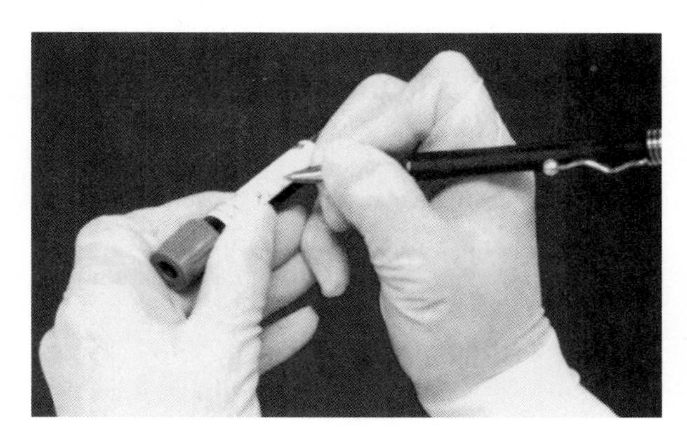

FIGURE 8-14 Labeling a tube.

112. Answer: a

Why: At a minimum, specimen labels should contain the patient's first and last name, hospital or medical record number, date of birth, date and time of the draw, and the phlebotomist's initials. The room number and bed may be found on the label if it was generated by a computer, but is not mandatory information.

Review: Yes ☐ No ☐

113. Answer: b

Why: The patient's ID number is included on the specimen label to avoid confusing samples. It is not unusual to have patients with the same or similar names in the hospital at the same time, but two patients will not have the same hospital or medical record number.

Review: Yes ☐ No ☐

114. Answer: b

Why: Carrying a bag or purse on the venipuncture arm, lifting heavy objects with that arm, or removing the bandage prematurely can all disturb the healing process, reinitiate bleeding, and lead to bruising of the site. The dietary restrictions may be necessary before the venipuncture but not afterward.

Review: Yes ☐ No ☐

115. Answer: c
Why: An ammonia specimen is transported on ice, a bilirubin specimen needs to be protected from light, and a cryoglobulin specimen must be transported at body temperature (37 °C). A cholesterol specimen, however, does not require special handling.
Review: Yes ☐ No ☐

116. Answer: d
Why: Patient refusal, unavailability, or the fact that you tried but were unsuccessful are all valid reasons for failure to obtain a specimen. Not having the right equipment to collect a specimen makes a phlebotomist appear disorganized and unprofessional, and is *not* an acceptable reason for failure to collect a specimen. You should check to see that you have the proper equipment for the test before leaving to collect the specimen.
Review: Yes ☐ No ☐

117. Answer: a
Why: After two unsuccessful attempts at blood collection, *do not* try a third time. Ask another phlebotomist to take over. Unsuccessful venipuncture attempts are frustrating to the patient and the phlebotomist. With the exception of STAT and other priority specimens, if the second phlebotomist is also unsuccessful, it is a good idea to give the patient a rest and come back at a later time. An outpatient may be given the option of returning another day, after consultation with his or her physician.
Review: Yes ☐ No ☐

118. Answer: d
Why: When drawing a hand vein, the tourniquet is applied on the forearm just proximal to the wrist bone (Fig. 8-15).
Review: Yes ☐ No ☐

119. Answer: d
Why: A winged infusion set is called a butterfly because it resembles one. A phlebotomist using a butterfly in a hand vein is shown in Figures 8-15 and 8-16.
Review: Yes ☐ No ☐

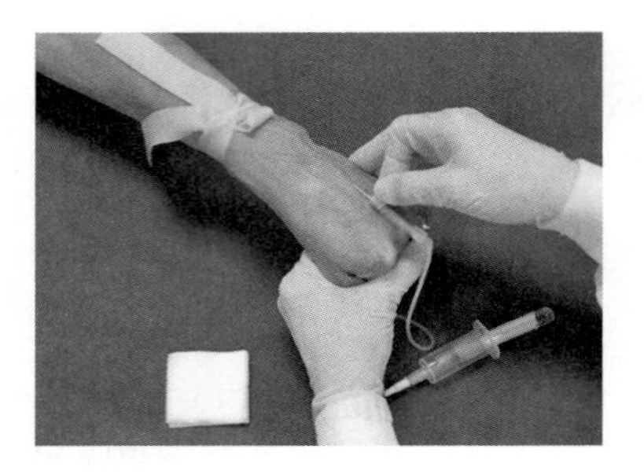

FIGURE 8-15 Phlebotomist drawing a hand vein with a tourniquet applied on the forearm just proximal to the wrist bone.

120. Answer: c
Why: The small size of the needle and flexibility afforded by the tubing makes a butterfly a good choice for drawing small, difficult, or hand veins.
Review: Yes ☐ No ☐

121. Answer: b
Why: A needle and syringe or butterfly and syringe may be used if the patient has small, fragile, or weak veins that collapse easily. The vacuum pressure of the evacuated tube may be too great for such veins. When a syringe is

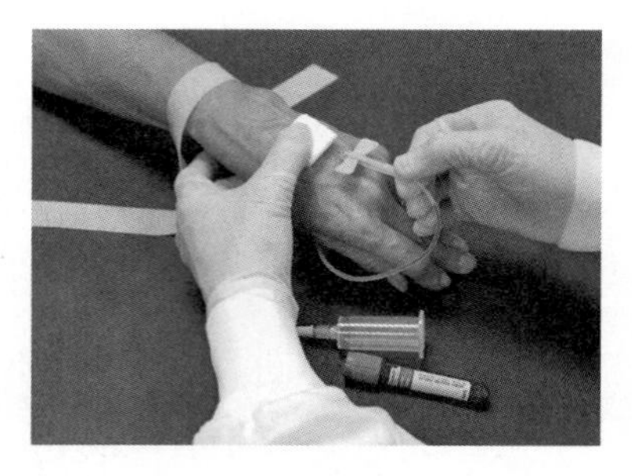

FIGURE 8-16 Phlebotomist preparing to remove a butterfly needle after using it to collect a specimen from a hand vein.

used the pressure can be controlled by pulling slowly on the syringe plunger.

Review: Yes ☐ No ☐

122. Answer: b

Why: Several things can cause specimen hemolysis, including mixing tubes too vigorously, using a large-volume tube with a small-diameter needle, and pushing on the plunger to force blood from a syringe into an evacuated tube. Leaving the tourniquet tied on the arm too long is not good for the specimen but does not cause hemolysis.

Review: Yes ☐ No ☐

123. Answer: a

Why: When a syringe needle is inserted in a vein, a "flash" of blood will usually appear in the hub of the needle.

Review: Yes ☐ No ☐

124. Answer: c

Why: A big factor in successful blood collection from pediatric patients is proper immobilization. Preventing excessive movement makes the process quicker and safer for the patient and the blood drawer.

Review: Yes ☐ No ☐

125. Answer: c

Why: It is important to greet the parents and the child and try to establish a rapport with each of them. Explain what you are going to do in terms the child can understand so that he or she knows what to expect. Answer questions honestly. *Never* tell a child it won't hurt, because chances are it will, even if just a little.

Review: Yes ☐ No ☐

126. Answer: c

Why: Small children seldom hold still for blood collection. The flexibility of the butterfly tubing enables successful blood collection despite some movement by the child. Children do like the idea of the butterfly, but it is not the reason it is used.

Review: Yes ☐ No ☐

127. Answer: d

Why: The safest and proper way to transfer blood from a syringe into evacuated tubes is to use a syringe transfer device, as shown in Fig. 8-17. If a transfer device is not available, the second best way is to place the tube in a rack before penetrating the tube stopper with the needle. Holding the tube with your hand is dangerous because the needle may slip and stick your hand. Never force the blood into the tube by pushing on the syringe plunger; let the vacuum of the tube draw the blood into it. Pushing on the plunger and forcing blood into the tube can hemolyze the specimen and can also allow blood to spurt out around the needle and contaminate you.

Review: Yes ☐ No ☐

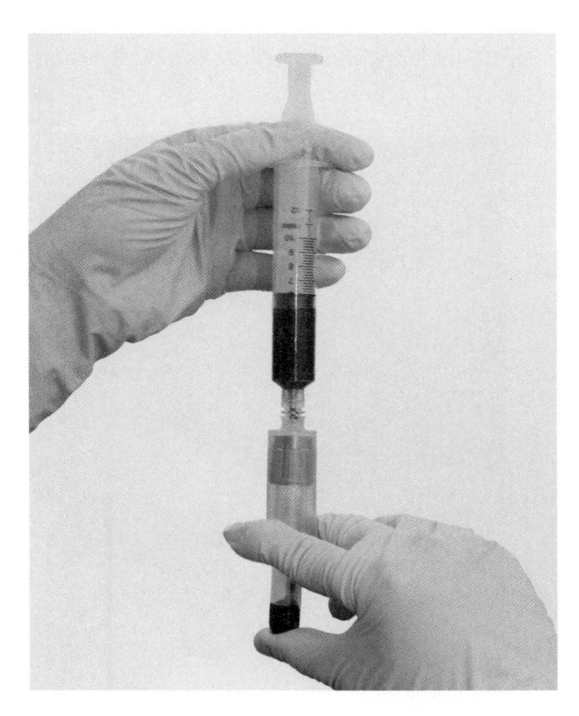

FIGURE 8-17 Filling an ETS tube using a syringe transfer device.

128. Answer: a
Why: Proper immobilization of a pediatric patient typically involves two people—the phlebotomist and someone to immobilize the child by cradling him or her and grasping the arm at the wrist, as illustrated in Fig. 8-18. Allowing a pediatric patient to brace his or her own arm is asking for trouble. Even if it appears that the child understands and will stay still, chances are that he or she will pull away as soon as the needle is seen.
Review: Yes ☐ No ☐

129. Answer: c
Why: Older children appreciate honesty and will be more cooperative if you explain what you are going to do and stress the importance of holding still. *Never* tell the child it won't hurt, because chances are it will, even if just a little. It is all right to offer the child a reward for being brave, but *do not* put conditions on receiving the reward, such as "You can only have the reward if you don't cry." Some crying is to be anticipated, and it is important to let the child know that it is all right to cry.
Review: Yes ☐ No ☐

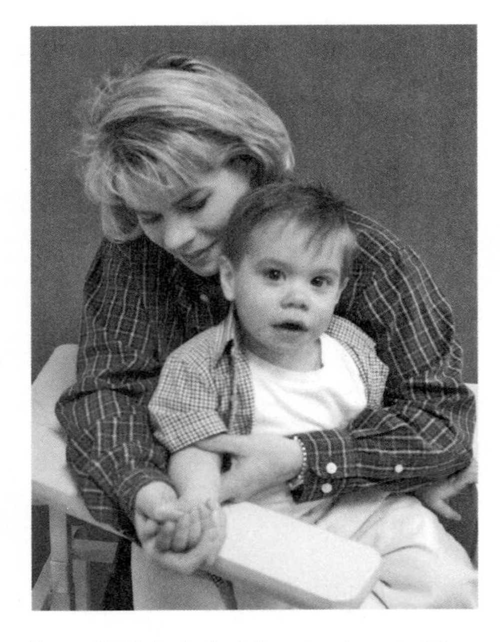

FIGURE 8-18 Seated adult restraining a toddler.

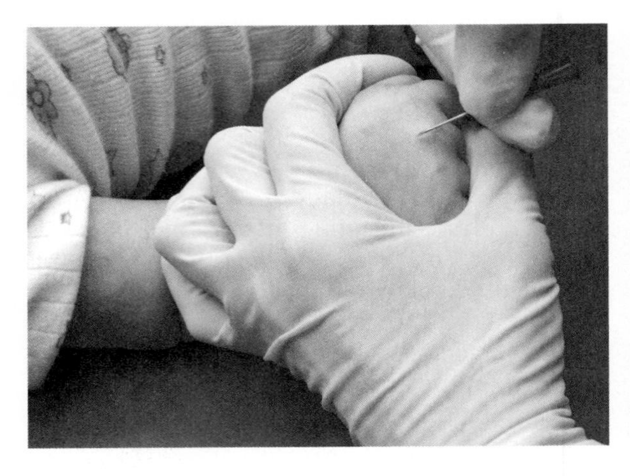

FIGURE 8-19 Venipuncture of an infant dorsal hand vein.

130. Answer: a
Why: Dorsal hand vein procedure (Fig. 8-19) on infants does not require the use of a tourniquet.
Review: Yes ☐ No ☐

131. Answer: d
Why: The *best* way to collect a PKU specimen from a dorsal hand vein is to let the blood drip directly onto the PKU filter paper. Blood collected in an EDTA microcollection tube or in a syringe may have microclots that could cause erroneous results.
Review: Yes ☐ No ☐

132. Answer: d
Why: Parkinson's disease is a neurologic disorder that causes the patient to have resting tremors. Resting tremors are involuntary rhythmic movements typically confined to the forearms and hands. They occur when the arms are relaxed. The tremors can make blood collection difficult.
Review: Yes ☐ No ☐

133. Answer: b
Why: In this scenario it is best to draw the specimen from the left arm in a position that the patient chooses. *Never* use force to extend a patient's arm. A butterfly offers the flexibility needed to access veins from an awkward angle. Diabetes can affect circulation and healing in the lower extremities and generally makes venipuncture of leg, ankle, and foot veins off limits. A blood draw should not be performed on the same side as a mastectomy without approval of the patient's physician.
Review: Yes ☐ No ☐

134. Answer: d
Why: The effects of colds and influenza are more severe in older adults. If you have a cold, refrain from drawing older adult patients if possible, or wear a mask. *Never* substitute a pressure bandage in lieu of holding pressure. You must hold pressure if the patient is unable to do so. It is discourteous to address questions to a relative or attendant as if a patient were not there. Speak clearly and distinctly, but do not raise the pitch of your voice. Raising the pitch of your voice actually makes it harder to understand.
Review: Yes ☐ No ☐

135. Answer: a
Why: The most common reason a patient must undergo dialysis is end-stage renal disease (ESRD), a serious condition in which the kidneys have deteriorated to a point at which they fail (no longer function). The most common cause of ESRD is diabetes, and the second most common cause is high blood pressure. Patients with ESRD require ongoing dialysis treatments or a kidney transplant.
Review: Yes ☐ No ☐

136. Answer: c
Why: Hospice is a type of care designed for patients who are dying. Most hospice patients have incurable forms of cancer. Hospice care allows terminally ill patients to spend their last days in a peaceful, supportive atmosphere that emphasizes pain management to help keep them comfortable.
Review: Yes ☐ No ☐

PREANALYTICAL CONSIDERATIONS

CHAPTER 9

study tip

Questions in this chapter test the ability to identify and describe physiologic variables that affect lab tests, identify problem venipuncture sites and describe what to do when they are encountered, and recognize the various types of vascular access devices (VADs) and sites and describe how and why VADs are used. Questions also test the ability to recognize and address patient complications and procedural errors and how to troubleshoot failed venipuncture attempts.

overview

This chapter assesses knowledge of the preanalytical (prior to analysis) phase of the testing process, which begins when a test is ordered and ends when testing begins. If not properly addressed, numerous factors associated with this phase of the testing process can lead to errors that can affect specimen quality, jeopardize the health and safety of the patient, and ultimately increase the cost of medical care. A phlebotomist must be able to recognize and address these factors to avoid or reduce any negative impact.

REVIEW QUESTIONS

Choose the BEST answer.

1. The preanalytical phase of the testing process begins when a:
   a. blood or body fluid specimen is collected.
   b. patient is admitted to a healthcare facility.
   c. specimen is submitted for processing.
   d. test is ordered by a patient's physician.

2. Most reference ranges are normal laboratory test values for:
   a. fasting patients.
   b. healthy people.
   c. ill individuals.
   d. treated patients.

3. Diurnal variations associated with some blood components are:
   a. abnormal changes that occur once a day.
   b. changes that follow a monthly cycle.
   c. normal fluctuations throughout the day.
   d. variations that occur on an hourly basis.

4. A patient's arm is swollen. The term used to describe this condition is:
   a. cyanotic.
   b. edematous.
   c. sclerosed.
   d. thrombosed.

5. Lipemia results from:
   a. high fat content of the blood.
   b. improper specimen handling.
   c. increased number of platelets.
   d. specimen hemoconcentration.

6. A patient with a high degree of jaundice typically has:
   a. bruising and petechiae.
   b. edematous extremities.
   c. hemolyzed specimens.
   d. yellow skin and sclera.

7. Lymphostasis is:
   a. impaired secretion of lymph fluid.
   b. obstruction of the flow of lymph.
   c. reduced lymphocyte production.
   d. stoppage of lymphoid functions.

8. This is the medical term for a nervous system response to abrupt pain, stress, or trauma.
   a. circadian response
   b. iatrogenic reflux
   c. vasovagal syncope
   d. venous stagnation

9. Small non-raised red spots appear on the patient's skin below where the tourniquet has just been tied. What are they and what causes them?
   a. a rash from tying the tourniquet too tightly
   b. bilirubin spots as a result of a diseased liver
   c. dermatitis from an allergy to the tourniquet
   d. petechiae resulting from capillary or platelet defects

10. Venous stasis is:
    a. backflow of tissue fluid into a vein.
    b. stage 1 of the coagulation process.
    c. stoppage of the normal blood flow.
    d. vein collapse from excess pressure.

11. A hematoma is a:
    a. blood clot inside of a vein.
    b. pool of fluid from an IV line.
    c. swelling or mass of blood.
    d. symptom of nerve injury.

12. Mastectomy is the medical term for breast:
    a. biopsy.
    b. reduction.
    c. removal.
    d. surgery.

13. Exsanguination is:
    a. autologous donation of blood.
    b. iatrogenic depletion of blood.
    c. life-threatening loss of blood.
    d. therapeutic removal of blood.

14. Which of the following is a product of the breakdown of red blood cells?
    a. bilirubin
    b. creatinine
    c. glucagon
    d. lipid (fat)

15. A vein that is thrombosed is:
    a. clotted.
    b. patent.
    c. scarred.
    d. swollen.

16. A vein with walls that have temporarily drawn together and shut off blood flow during venipuncture is called a:
    a. blown vessel.
    b. collapsed vein.
    c. reflux reaction.
    d. passive fistula.

17. The patient has an IV in the left arm and a large hematoma in the antecubital area of the right arm. The *best* place to collect a specimen by venipuncture is the:
    a. left arm above the IV entry point.
    b. left arm below the IV entry point.
    c. right arm distal to the hematoma.
    d. right arm in the antecubital area.

18. Fig. 9-1 shows an arm with:
    a. bruising that was most likely caused by a reflux reaction.
    b. discoloration from prolonged application of a tourniquet.
    c. evidence of partial exsanguination of the antecubital area.
    d. remains of a hematoma that formed during a blood draw.

19. Hemoconcentration from prolonged tourniquet application increases:
    a. blood plasma volume.
    b. nonfilterable analytes.
    c. pH and oxygen levels.
    d. specimen hemolysis.

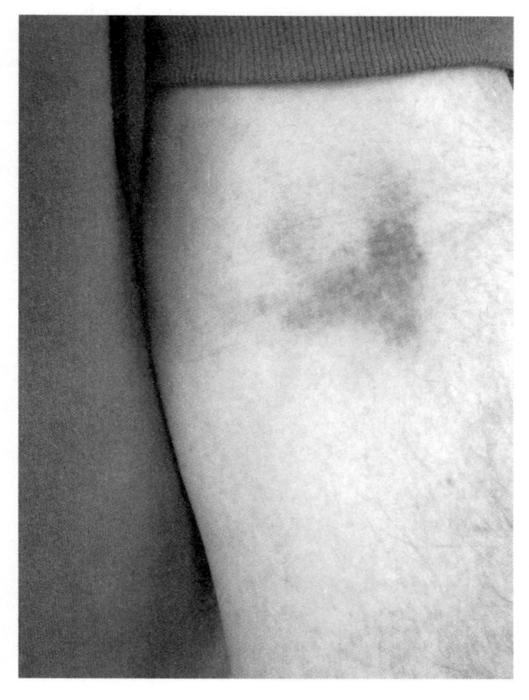

FIGURE 9-1 A patient's arm after a venipuncture.

20. Which of the following is the medical term for fainting?
    a. sclerose
    b. stasis
    c. supine
    d. syncope

21. In which instance is the patient closest to basal state? The patient who:
    a. arrived at the lab at 0800 hours and had not eaten since dinner the night before.
    b. came straight to the lab after working all night, but was fasting at work.
    c. has been awake but lying down quietly resting for the last several hours.
    d. is awakened for a blood draw at 0600 hours after fasting since 0800 hours last night.

22. The *best* specimens to use for establishing inpatient reference ranges for blood tests are:
    a. basal state specimens.
    b. steady-state specimens.
    c. fasting specimens.
    d. postprandial specimens.

23. Which of the following tests requires the patient's age when calculating results?
    a. cold agglutinin titer
    b. C-reactive protein
    c. creatine kinase MB
    d. creatinine clearance

24. Which of the following tests is most affected by altitude?
    a. cholesterol
    b. electrolytes
    c. magnesium
    d. RBC count

25. Persistent diarrhea in the absence of fluid replacement may cause:
    a. hemoconcentration.
    b. iatrogenic anemia.
    c. petechiae formation.
    d. red cell destruction.

26. The serum or plasma of a lipemic specimen appears:
    a. cloudy white.
    b. dark yellow.
    c. foamy pink.
    d. pink to red.

27. A lipemic specimen is a clue that the patient was:
    a. dehydrated.
    b. in a basal state.
    c. jaundiced.
    d. not fasting.

28. A 12-hour fast is normally required when testing for this analyte.
    a. bilirubin
    b. calcium
    c. electrolytes
    d. triglycerides

29. This blood component exhibits diurnal variation, with peak levels occurring in the morning.
    a. cortisol
    b. creatinine
    c. glucose
    d. phosphate

30. Tests influenced by diurnal variation are typically ordered:
    a. fasting.
    b. pre-op.
    c. STAT.
    d. timed.

31. A drug known to interfere with a blood test should be discontinued this many hours before the test specimen is collected.
    a. 1–3
    b. 4–24
    c. 25–30
    d. 48–72

32. A test result can be falsely decreased if:
    a. a drug competes with the test reagents for the test analyte.
    b. an analyte-detecting color reaction is enhanced by a drug.
    c. anticoagulant reflux occurred during specimen collection.
    d. SST.

33. Which of the following analytes is *most* affected by exercise prior to specimen collection?
    a. bilirubin
    b. calcium
    c. enzymes
    d. uric acid

34. All of the following hormones are affected by the presence of fever EXCEPT:
    a. cortisol.
    b. glucagon.

c. insulin.
d. melatonin.

35. Which analyte has a higher reference range for males than for females?
a. cholesterol
b. hematocrit
c. magnesium
d. potassium

36. An icteric specimen indicates all of the following EXCEPT:
a. bilirubin test results could be elevated.
b. it probably was not a fasting specimen.
c. results of some tests may be erroneous.
d. the patient might have hepatitis B or C.

37. What blood changes occur when a patient goes from supine to standing?
a. nonfilterable elements increase
b. red blood cell counts decrease
c. the level of calcium decreases
d. volume of plasma is increased

38. Why do pregnant patients have lower reference ranges for red blood cell (RBC) counts?
a. Frequent bouts of nausea lead to hemoconcentration.
b. Increased body fluids result in dilution of the RBCs.
c. Poor appetite results in a temporary form of anemia.
d. The growing fetus uses up the mother's iron reserves.

39. Which of the following analytes is typically increased in chronic smokers?
a. bicarbonate
b. hemoglobin
c. O_2 saturation
d. vitamin B_{12}

40. It is *not* a good idea to collect a complete blood count from a screaming infant because the:
a. chance of hemolysis is increased.
b. platelets are more likely to clump.
c. specimen may be hemoconcentrated.
d. WBCs may be temporarily elevated.

41. Of the following factors known to affect basal state, which is automatically accounted for when reference ranges are established?
a. diurnal variation
b. drug interferences
c. effects of exercise
d. geographic locale

42. All of the following are reasons to control temperature and humidity in a laboratory EXCEPT to:
a. ensure equipment functions properly.
b. maintain the integrity of specimens.
c. reduce any interference from drugs.
d. standardize the testing environment.

43. Scarred or burned areas should be avoided as blood collection sites for all of the following reasons EXCEPT:
a. circulation in scarred areas is typically impaired.
b. dilution of most analytes occurs in these areas.
c. newly burned sites are susceptible to infection.
d. veins may be difficult to palpate in such areas.

44. A vein that feels hard and cordlike and lacks resiliency may be:
a. an artery.
b. collapsed.
c. superficial.
d. thrombosed.

45. Drawing blood from an edematous extremity may cause:
a. erroneous specimen results.
b. hemolysis of the specimen.
c. premature specimen clotting.
d. rapid formation of petechiae.

46. If you have no choice but to collect a specimen from an arm with a hematoma, collect the specimen:
    a. above the hematoma.
    b. beside the hematoma.
    c. distal to the hematoma.
    d. through the hematoma.

47. Blood specimens should not be collected from an arm on the same side as a mastectomy without permission from the patient's physician for all of the following reasons EXCEPT:
    a. lymphostasis can affect test results.
    b. that arm is susceptible to infection.
    c. tourniquet application can injure it.
    d. veins in that arm collapse readily.

48. Of the following veins, which is often the one that is easiest to feel on obese patients?
    a. basilic
    b. brachial
    c. cephalic
    d. median

49. You must collect a protime specimen from a patient with IVs in both arms. The *best* place to collect the specimen is:
    a. above one of the IVs.
    b. below one of the IVs.
    c. from an ankle vein.
    d. from one of the IVs.

50. A phlebotomist must collect a hemoglobin specimen from a patient in the intensive care unit. There is an IV in the patient's left arm. There is no suitable antecubital vein or hand vein in the right arm. What should the phlebotomist do?
    a. ask another phlebotomist to collect it
    b. collect it from a leg, ankle, or foot vein
    c. draw it from a hand vein below the IV
    d. perform a finger stick on the right hand

51. All of the following should be avoided when selecting a venipuncture site EXCEPT:
    a. a previous IV site within 24 hours of IV removal.
    b. an arm that has a saline lock placed in the wrist.
    c. an arm that has an arteriovenous shunt or fistula.
    d. an arm used for a venipuncture just an hour ago.

52. A type of line that is commonly used to monitor blood pressure and collect blood gas specimens is:
    a. A-line
    b. CVC
    c. IV
    d. PICC

53. A vascular access pathway that is surgically created to provide access for dialysis is a(n):
    a. AV.
    b. CVC.
    c. Hep-lock.
    d. PICC.

54. When a blood specimen is collected from a heparin lock, it is important to draw:
    a. a 5-mL discard tube before the specimen tubes.
    b. coagulation specimens before other specimens.
    c. extra tubes in case other tests are ordered later.
    d. two tubes per test in case one is contaminated.

55. Central venous catheters (CVCs) include all the following EXCEPT:
    a. Broviac.
    b. Groshong.
    c. Hep-lok.
    d. Hickman.

56. This is a subcutaneous vascular access device consisting of a small chamber attached to an indwelling line that is

implanted under the skin and located by palpating the skin.
a. CVC
b. PICC line
c. saline lock
d. SVAD

57. All of the following are ways to bandage a venipuncture site when the patient is allergic to the glue in adhesive bandages EXCEPT:
a. apply a bandage that is latex-free.
b. hold pressure in lieu of a bandage.
c. place paper tape over a gauze pad.
d. wrap it with self-adhering material.

58. You may have to be careful about what type of equipment is brought into the room if a patient is severely allergic to:
a. adhesive.
b. iodine.
c. latex.
d. perfume.

59. What is the *best* thing to do if a blood collection site continues to bleed after 5 minutes?
a. Apply pressure yourself until bleeding stops.
b. Have the patient hold pressure until it stops.
c. Report it to the patient's physician or nurse.
d. Wrap the site with a tight pressure bandage.

60. Which patient should be asked to lie down during a blood draw? A patient with a:
a. central venous catheter.
b. coagulation disorder.
c. history of syncope.
d. severe latex allergy.

61. During a blood draw a patient says he feels faint. What should the phlebotomist do?
a. Ask the patient if it is all right to continue the draw.
b. Discontinue the draw and lower the patient's head.
c. Hold him up with one hand and complete the draw.
d. Wave ammonia inhalant past his nose to revive him.

62. An outpatient becomes weak and pale after a blood draw. What should the phlebotomist do?
a. Accompany the patient to his or her car.
b. Have the patient lie down until recovered.
c. Offer the patient a glass of water to drink.
d. Tell the patient to go get something to eat.

63. If an outpatient tells you before a blood draw that she is feeling nauseated, you should do all of the following EXCEPT:
a. draw the specimen, but watch her closely.
b. give her an emesis basin in case she vomits.
c. hold a cold, damp washcloth to her forehead.
d. tell her to begin breathing slowly and deeply.

64. Pain associated with venipuncture can be minimized by:
a. desensitizing the site by rubbing hard with alcohol.
b. putting the patient at ease with a little small talk.
c. tying the tourniquet tight enough to numb the arm.
d. warning the patient that the draw might hurt a lot.

65. All of the following would be reasons to eliminate a potential venipuncture site EXCEPT:
a. petechiae appear below the tourniquet.
b. scarring from a deep burn is present.
c. the arm appears slightly edematous.
d. the only vein feels hard and cordlike.

66. A patient goes into convulsions while you are drawing his blood. The last tube has just started to fill. All of the following would be appropriate actions to take EXCEPT:
    a. complete the draw as quickly as you can.
    b. immediately discontinue the blood draw.
    c. prevent the patient from injuring himself.
    d. notify the appropriate first aid personnel.

67. You are collecting a blood specimen on a patient with difficult veins. You had to redirect the needle but it is now in the vein, and you have just started to fill the first tube. The blood is filling the tube slowly. The skin around the venipuncture site starts to swell. You have several more tubes to fill. What should you do?
    a. Ask the patient if it hurts; if not, continue the draw.
    b. Continue the draw after pushing the needle in deeper.
    c. Pull back on the needle slightly and finish the draw.
    d. Stop the draw at once and apply pressure to the site.

68. All of the following can cause hematoma formation during venipuncture procedures EXCEPT:
    a. inadequate pressure application after the draw.
    b. the needle bevel entering the lumen of the vein.
    c. the needle bevel only partially inside the vein.
    d. the needle passing through the vein's back wall.

69. Which of the following is the *best* indication that you have accidentally punctured an artery?
    a. a hematoma starts to form
    b. blood obtained is dark red
    c. blood pulses into the tube
    d. there is no way to tell

70. A term used to describe anemia brought on by withdrawal of blood for testing purposes is:
    a. hemolytic.
    b. iatrogenic.
    c. icteric.
    d. neutropenic.

71. If you suspect that you have accidentally collected an arterial specimen instead of a venous specimen:
    a. apply a pressure bandage to the venipuncture site.
    b. ask another phlebotomist to recollect the specimen.
    c. discard it and collect a new one from another site.
    d. keep it, but label it as a possible arterial specimen.

72. Infection of a venipuncture site can result from:
    a. following the wrong order of draw.
    b. leaving the tourniquet on too long.
    c. touching the site after cleaning it.
    d. using an unsterile ETS tube holder.

73. Excessive or blind probing for a vein can cause all of the following EXCEPT:
    a. arterial sticks.
    b. needless pain.
    c. nerve damage.
    d. vein patency.

74. A patient complains of marked pain when you insert the needle. The pain radiates down his arm and does not subside. What should you do?
    a. Ask him if he wants you to stop the draw.
    b. Discontinue the venipuncture immediately.
    c. Collect the specimen as quickly as you can.
    d. Say "Hold on or I'll have to stick you again".

75. A stinging sensation when the needle is first inserted is *most* likely the result of:
    a. an imperfection on the bevel of the needle.
    b. having the tourniquet tied excessively tight.
    c. not allowing the alcohol to dry thoroughly.
    d. pushing down on the needle as it is inserted.

76. Which is the *best* way to avoid reflux?
    a. Draw the specimen while the patient is supine.
    b. Follow the correct order of draw when filling tubes.
    c. Keep the tourniquet on until the last tube is full.
    d. Make certain that tubes fill from the bottom up.

77. Which of the following is *least* likely to impair vein patency?
    a. drawing the same vein many times
    b. improperly redirecting the needle
    c. leaving a tourniquet on too long
    d. probing to locate a vein

78. Prolonged tourniquet application can affect blood composition because it causes:
    a. delayed hemostasis.
    b. dilution of plasma.
    c. hemoconcentration.
    d. specimen hemolysis.

79. The serum or plasma of a hemolyzed specimen appears:
    a. clear yellow.
    b. cloudy white.
    c. greenish yellow.
    d. pink or reddish.

80. Which action is *least* likely to cause hemolysis of a specimen?
    a. drawing a large tube using a small needle
    b. mixing a blood specimen too vigorously
    c. pulling back a syringe plunger too quickly
    d. transferring blood from a syringe to a tube

81. The ratio of blood to anticoagulant is *most* critical for which of the following tests?
    a. alkaline phosphatase
    b. complete blood count
    c. glycohemoglobin
    d. prothrombin time

82. A phlebotomist has tried twice to collect a light blue top tube on a patient with difficult veins. Both times the phlebotomist has been able to collect only a partial tube. What should the phlebotomist do?
    a. Collect the specimen by skin puncture.
    b. Have someone else collect the specimen.
    c. Pour the two tubes together and mix well.
    d. Send one to the lab marked "difficult draw".

83. Which of the following situations is *least* likely to cause contamination of the specimen?
    a. cleaning a finger stick site with isopropyl alcohol
    b. drawing blood cultures before the antiseptic is dry
    c. touching the filter paper while collecting a PKU
    d. using povidone-iodine to clean a heel puncture site

84. You are collecting a blood specimen. The needle is in the vein and blood flow has been established. As the tube is filling, you hear a hissing sound, there is a spurt of blood into the tube, and blood flow stops. What has *most* likely happened is the:
    a. bevel came out of the skin and the tube vacuum escaped.
    b. needle went all the way through the back wall of the vein.
    c. patient had a sudden and dramatic drop in blood pressure.
    d. tube had a crack in it and there was no more vacuum left.

85. All of the following situations could indicate that the needle has gone through the back of the vein EXCEPT:
   a. a hissing sound is heard when you first engage the tube.
   b. blood did not flow until you pulled the needle back a bit.
   c. the first tube filled with blood, but the second one did not.
   d. you felt the needle enter the vein but the tube did not fill.

86. When a vein rolls, the needle typically:
   a. ends up in the lumen of the vein.
   b. goes all the way through the vein.
   c. lands against an inside vein wall.
   d. slips beside instead of in the vein.

87. You are collecting a blood specimen. The needle is inserted but the blood is filling the tube very slowly. You see a hematoma forming very rapidly. What has *most* likely happened is the:
   a. needle is only partly in the vein.
   b. needle is up against a vein wall.
   c. patient has a clotting disorder.
   d. tube is slowly loosing vacuum.

88. You are performing a multi-tube blood draw. You collect the first tube without a problem. The second tube fails to fill with blood. You pull the needle back and nothing happens. You push the needle deeper and nothing happens. You remove the tube, pull back the needle a little, rotate the bevel, and reset the tube. Still nothing happens. Which of the following actions should you take next?
   a. discontinue the draw and try at another site
   b. let someone else take over and give it a try
   c. redirect the needle until you get blood flow
   d. try a new tube in case it is a vacuum issue

89. You insert the needle into the vein during blood collection. When you advance the tube onto the needle in the holder, you do not get blood flow. You can see that the needle is beside the vein. You redirect the needle two times and still do not get blood flow. What should you do next?
   a. anchor the vein and redirect the needle again
   b. ask a coworker to redirect the needle for you
   c. discontinue the draw and try again at a new site
   d. try pushing the needle deeper and then redirect

90. A vein may collapse for all of the following reasons EXCEPT:
   a. several large-volume tubes have been collected.
   b. the tourniquet has been applied excessively tight.
   c. the tourniquet is too close to the venipuncture site.
   d. tube vacuum is too much for the size of the vein.

ANSWERS AND EXPLANATIONS

1. Answer: d
   Why: Preanalytical means "prior to analysis." The preanalytical phase of the testing process includes all of the steps taken before a specimen is analyzed. Consequently, it begins when the test is ordered and ends when testing begins.
   Review: Yes ☐ No ☐

2. Answer: b
   Why: Most tests are performed to screen for, diagnose, or monitor disease. To be properly evaluated, test results need to be compared with test result values expected of healthy individuals. Consequently, values for most tests are established using specimens from healthy individuals. Because results vary somewhat from person to person, the results used for comparison become a range of values with high and low limits, commonly called a reference range. Some reference ranges are for fasting patients, but not all. Some tests have reference ranges for patients who are ill or are being treated for certain disorders, such as diabetes, but these reference ranges are less common.
   Review: Yes ☐ No ☐

3. Answer: c
   Why: Diurnal means "happening daily." The levels of many blood components normally exhibit diurnal variations or normal fluctuations throughout the day.
   Review: Yes ☐ No ☐

4. Answer: b
   Why: Edema is the accumulation of fluid in the tissues, characterized by swelling. An extremity with edema is described as being edematous. Cyanotic means "marked by cyanosis, or bluish in color from lack of oxygen." Sclerosed means "hardened." Thrombosed means "clotted." Sclerosed and thrombosed are terms used to describe damaged veins.
   Review: Yes ☐ No ☐

5. Answer: a
   Why: The term "lipemia" comes from the word root "lip," which means "fat." Lipemia is the presence of increased fats (lipids) in the blood that make the serum or plasma look cloudy or milky white.
   Review: Yes ☐ No ☐

6. Answer: d
   Why: Jaundice, also called icterus, is a condition characterized by increased bilirubin (a product of the breakdown of red blood cells) in the blood, leading to deposits of yellow bile pigment in the skin, mucous membranes, and sclera (whites of the eyes), giving the patient a yellow appearance.
   Review: Yes ☐ No ☐

7. Answer: b
   Why: Stasis means "stopping, controlling, or standing." Lymphostasis is defined as the obstruction or stoppage of the flow of lymph (lymph fluid).
   Review: Yes ☐ No ☐

8. Answer: c
   Why: Vasovagal means "relating to vagus nerve action on blood vessels." Syncope is the medical term for fainting. Vasovagal syncope is sudden faintness or loss of consciousness resulting from a nervous system response to abrupt pain, stress, or trauma. Circadian means "having a 24-hour cycle." Iatrogenic means "an adverse condition brought on by the effects of treatment," and reflux means "backflow," as in the backflow of blood into a patient's vein during venipuncture. Venous stasis is stagnation or stoppage of normal blood flow.
   Review: Yes ☐ No ☐

9. Answer: d
Why: Petechiae are small, non-raised red spots that appear on a patient's skin when a tourniquet is applied because of a defect in the capillary walls or the platelets.
Review: Yes ☐ No ☐

10. Answer: c
Why: Venous stasis (also called venostasis) is a condition in which the normal flow of blood through a vein is stopped or slowed. Stasis means "stopping, controlling, or standing. Venous means "relating to a vein."
Review: Yes ☐ No ☐

11. Answer: c
Why: Hematoma is the medical term for a swelling or mass of blood (usually clotted) under the skin caused by leakage of blood from a blood vessel. A hematoma can occur during or after venipuncture or arterial puncture; often as a result of poor technique. A blood clot within a vein is called a thrombus. A pool of fluid from an IV would cause localized edema. A hematoma is not a symptom of nerve injury, but pressure from the hematoma could injure a nerve.
Review: Yes ☐ No ☐

12. Answer: c
Why: The surgical removal of a breast as is sometimes done in the treatment of breast cancer, for example, is called a mastectomy. It is derived from the Greek word *mastos* which means "breast." The suffix *-tomy* means "incision or cutting."
Review: Yes ☐ No ☐

13. Answer: c
Why: Exsanguination is massive blood loss or removal of blood to a point where life cannot be sustained. Autologous donation of blood is donating blood for one's own use. Iatrogenic is an adjective used to describe an adverse condition brought on as a result of treatment. Iatrogenic blood loss can lead to exsanguination. Blood is sometimes removed for therapeutic purposes, but not in quantities that would cause exsanguination.
Review: Yes ☐ No ☐

14. Answer: a
Why: Bilirubin is a yellowish pigment that is the product of the breakdown of red blood cells by the body. High levels of bilirubin in the blood lead to deposits of the pigment in the skin, mucous membranes, and sclera (whites of the eyes), a condition called jaundice.
Review: Yes ☐ No ☐

15. Answer: a
Why: Thrombosed means "clotted." A patent vein is in a state of being freely open, not clotted. A thrombosed vein is not necessarily scarred or swollen.
Review: Yes ☐ No ☐

16. Answer: b
Why: A vein is said to be collapsed when its walls temporarily retract, cutting off blood flow. A vein can collapse if the tube being drawn has too much vacuum, a syringe is pulled back too quickly, or the tourniquet is tied too tightly or too close to the site. It can also collapse when the tourniquet is removed during the draw, especially if the tourniquet was too tight and inflated the vein excessively. A blown vein results from a small tear or enlarged hole at the site of needle entry that causes blood to escape quickly and the vein to collapse as a result. A reflux reaction is a patient reaction to the backflow of a tube additive into his or her vein during venipuncture. The type of fistula of importance to phlebotomists is the artificial connection between an artery and a vein.
Review: Yes ☐ No ☐

17. Answer: c
Why: When one arm has an IV it is best to collect the specimen from the other arm if possible. Never collect a blood specimen above an IV or a hematoma. When there is no alternative site, perform the venipuncture below or distal to the hematoma. Venipuncture or close to a hematoma is painful to the patient and can result in collection of blood from outside the vein that is hemolyzed or contaminated, and unsuitable for testing. Going below (distal) to the hematoma ensures collection of blood that is free-flowing and unaltered by the effects the coagulation process at work in the area.
Review: Yes ☐ No ☐

18. Answer: d
Why: A hematoma is a swelling or mass of blood that can be caused by blood leaking from a blood vessel during or immediately after a venipuncture. A bruise eventually spreads into the surrounding area. The bruising in Fig. 9-1 (p. 249) resulted from a hematoma that formed during a venipuncture.
Review: Yes ☐ No ☐

19. Answer: b
Why: Hemoconcentration is a condition in which plasma and filterable components of the blood pass through the walls of the blood vessels into the tissues, decreasing blood plasma volume and concentrating nonfilterable blood components such as red blood cells. Oxygen and pH are tested on arterial blood and a tourniquet is not used in collection. Prolonged tourniquet application does not cause specimen hemolysis.
Review: Yes ☐ No ☐

20. Answer: d
Why: Syncope is the temporary loss of consciousness and the ability to maintain an upright position as a result of inadequate blood flow to the brain, and is the medical term for fainting. Sclerose means "to harden." Stasis is stagnation of blood or other fluids. Supine means "lying on the back, face up"
Review: Yes ☐ No ☐

21. Answer: d
Why: Basal state refers to the condition of the body early in the morning when a patient is still at rest and fasting (approximately 12 hours after the last intake of food). The patient who has just awakened at 0600 hours (6 A.M.) and has not eaten since the previous evening meal is closest to basal state.
Review: Yes ☐ No ☐

22. Answer: a
Why: Inpatient reference ranges for laboratory tests are typically established using basal state specimens to eliminate the effects of diet, exercise, and other factors on results.
Review: Yes ☐ No ☐

23. Answer: d
Why: Some physiologic functions, such as kidney function, decrease with age. Creatinine is removed (cleared) from the blood plasma by the kidneys. The amount removed is measured by a creatinine clearance test. Since kidney function declines with age, the patient's age is required when calculating the results.
Review: Yes ☐ No ☐

24. Answer: d
Why: Red blood cells carry oxygen to the tissue cells. The oxygen content of the air decreases as the altitude increases. The decrease in oxygen content at higher altitudes causes the body to produce more red blood cells in order to fulfill the body's oxygen requirements.
Review: Yes ☐ No ☐

25. Answer: a
Why: Persistent diarrhea without fluid replacement leads to dehydration, which is a

decrease in total body fluid, including blood plasma. Blood components become concentrated in the smaller plasma volume, a condition called hemoconcentration.

Review: Yes ☐ No ☐

26. Answer: a
Why: An abnormally high concentration of lipids (fatty substances) in the blood is called *lipemia.* Lipemia can persist for 10 hours or more. Because lipids are insoluble in water they make serum or plasma look milky (cloudy white) or turbid and the specimen is described as being *lipemic.*
Review: Yes ☐ No ☐

27. Answer: d
Why: Fasting serum or plasma is normally clear yellow. The serum or plasma of a lipemic specimen is milky (cloudy white) because of high fat (lipid) content. Presence of fats is an indication that the patient was not fasting prior to specimen collection. A 12-hour fast is generally required to remove the effects of lipids from the blood.
Review: Yes ☐ No ☐

28. Answer: d
Why: Triglycerides are a type of lipid. A 12-hour fast is required to remove the effects of food ingestion on the triglyceride content of the blood (see answer to questions 26 and 27).
Review: Yes ☐ No ☐

29. Answer: a
Why: Diurnal variations are normal fluctuations throughout the day. Cortisol levels exhibit diurnal variation with highest levels occurring in the morning. Creatinine, glucose, and phosphate also exhibit diurnal variation; however, blood levels of theses analytes are lowest in the morning.
Review: Yes ☐ No ☐

30. Answer: d
Why: For consistency in evaluating or comparing results, tests that exhibit diurnal variation or fluctuations throughout the day are often ordered for a specific time of day. The requested time of collection is typically a time when the highest level of the analyte is expected.
Review: Yes ☐ No ☐

31. Answer: b
Why: According to College of American Pathologists (CAP) guidelines drugs known to interfere with blood tests should be stopped or avoided for 4–24 hours (depending on the drug) before specimens for the affected tests are collected. Drugs that interfere with urine tests should be stopped 48–72 hours before specimen collection.
Review: Yes ☐ No ☐

32. Answer: a
Why: When a drug competes with a test reagent for an analyte, the analyte is used up faster than it would be by the reagent alone. This results in a falsely low value for the analyte. A drug that enhances a color reaction during testing will falsely elevate test results. Reflux of anticoagulant during specimen collection may cause an adverse patient reaction, but does not affect the specimen being collected. Testing serum from a partially filled red top should not affect test results as long as there is enough of the specimen to perform the test.
Review: Yes ☐ No ☐

33. Answer: c
Why: Muscular activity elevates blood levels of a number of components, including enzymes. Some enzymes, such as creatine kinase and lactate dehydrogenase, may stay elevated for 24 hours or more.
Review: Yes ☐ No ☐

34. Answer: d
Why: Hypoglycemia caused by fever increases insulin levels followed by a rise in glucagon levels. Fever also increases cortisol levels and may disrupt its normal diurnal variation. Melatonin levels are affected by light, increasing at night when it is dark and decreasing during daylight hours.
Review: Yes ☐ No ☐

35. Answer: b
Why: A patient's gender has a determining effect on the concentration of a number of blood components. These differences are reflected in separate male and female reference ranges for certain analytes. For example, males tend to have greater muscle mass and normally have higher red blood cell counts to supply the muscles with oxygen. Consequently red blood cell counts and related tests such as hematocrit and hemoglobin have higher reference ranges for males. The hematocrit is a measure of the percentage of a specimen that is red blood cells.
Review: Yes ☐ No ☐

36. Answer: b
Why: An icteric specimen has no relationship to fasting. Icterus (also called jaundice) is a condition characterized by increased bilirubin in the blood and other body fluids and deposits of the yellow pigment in the skin, mucous membranes, and sclera (whites of the eyes), giving the patient a yellow appearance. A typical cause is hepatitis (liver inflammation) resulting from infection with a hepatitis virus such as hepatitis B or C. Body fluid specimens with high bilirubin levels have an abnormal deep yellow to yellow-brown color, and are described as being icteric. Abnormal specimen color can lead to erroneous results by interfering in the color reactions involved in a number of chemistry tests, including chemical reagent strip analyses on urine.
Review: Yes ☐ No ☐

37. Answer: a
Why: When a patient stands up after being supine (lying down), blood plasma filters into the tissues, *decreasing* plasma volume and *increasing* nonfilterable elements such as calcium, iron, proteins, and red blood cells.
Review: Yes ☐ No ☐

38. Answer: b
Why: Normal body fluid increases in pregnancy include an increase in blood plasma levels. The increased volume of plasma has a dilution effect on the red blood cells (RBCs), reducing red blood cell count results. Consequently, the reference ranges for red blood cell counts on pregnant women are lower than for women who are not pregnant. Hemoconcentration would elevate red blood counts. Anemia from poor appetite or inadequate iron reserves represent situations that typically result in abnormal patient results that are lower than reference ranges.
Review: Yes ☐ No ☐

39. Answer: b
Why: Chronic smokers have impaired ability to transport oxygen to the cells because as much as 10% of their hemoglobin is bound to carbon monoxide acquired from cigarette smoke. The body compensates for this by increasing the number of red blood cells. Bicarbonate, O_2 saturation, and vitamin B_{12} levels are usually decreased in chronic smokers.
Review: Yes ☐ No ☐

40. Answer: d
Why: Studies performed on crying infants have demonstrated significant increases in white blood cell (WBC) counts, which are reported as part of complete blood counts (CBCs). Counts returned to normal within 1 hour after crying stopped. For this reason, it is best if CBCs or WBC specimens are obtained after the infant has been sleeping or resting quietly for at least 30 minutes.

Because an infant usually cries during blood collection, the specimens should be collected as quickly as possible. If a specimen must be collected while an infant is crying, it should be noted on the report.

Review: Yes ☐ No ☐

41. Answer: d

Why: Reference ranges for specimens are established using basal state specimens. Environmental factors associated with geographic location do affect basal state. However, because all the specimens used to calculate reference ranges come from individuals in that particular location, geographical factors will be automatically reflected in the reference range values.

Review: Yes ☐ No ☐

42. Answer: c

Why: Temperature and humidity are known to affect test values. Closely controlling these environmental factors in a clinical laboratory standardizes the test environment, and helps ensure specimen integrity and proper functioning of equipment. Controlling temperature and humidity do not lesson drug interference in testing.

Review: Yes ☐ No ☐

43. Answer: b

Why: Scarred and burned areas should be avoided as blood collection sites because circulation in these areas is typically impaired. This can result in hemoconcentration, which can concentrate, not dilute analytes. Newly burned sites are susceptible to infection and can also be painful. Veins in scarred or burned areas can also be difficult to palpate.

Review: Yes ☐ No ☐

44. Answer: d

Why: Thrombosed means "clotted." A vein that is clotted will feel hard and cordlike and lack resiliency. An artery has a pulse that can be felt. A collapsed vein typically cannot be felt at all. Superficial simply means the vein is close to the surface of the skin.

Review: Yes ☐ No ☐

45. Answer: a

Why: Edema is swelling caused by the abnormal accumulation of fluid in the tissues. Specimens collected from edematous areas may yield erroneous test results due to contamination with tissue fluid or altered blood composition related to the swelling and impaired circulation in the area.

Review: Yes ☐ No ☐

46. Answer: c

Why: If you have no other choice, it is acceptable to collect a blood specimen distal, or below a hematoma, where blood flow is least affected by it. A venipuncture in the area of a hematoma, including above, beside, or through it, is painful to the patient, and can yield erroneous results related to the obstruction of blood flow by the hematoma. It can also result in collection of contaminated and possibly hemolyzed blood from the hematoma, instead of blood from the vein.

Review: Yes ☐ No ☐

47. Answer: d

Why: Blood should never be collected from an arm on the same side as a mastectomy (breast removal) without first consulting the patient's physician. Lymphostasis (stoppage of lymph flow) that occurs if lymph nodes have also been removed leaves the area susceptible to infection, and can change the composition of blood in the area, causing erroneous test results. Tourniquet application can also injure the arm. Veins in that arm do not necessarily collapse readily.

Review: Yes ☐ No ☐

48. Answer: c

Why: Veins on obese patients may be deep and difficult to find. The cephalic vein is sometimes the easiest vein to palpate. To locate it, rotate the patient's arm so that the hand is prone. In this position, the weight of excess tissue often pulls downward, making the cephalic vein easy to feel and penetrate with a needle.

Review: Yes ☐ No ☐

49. Answer: b

Why: It is preferred that blood specimens not be drawn from an arm with an intravenous (IV) line (Fig. 9-2). However, according to CLSI, a specimen can be drawn *below* an IV after it has been shut off for a minimum of 2 minutes. (A phlebotomist should *never* shut off an IV. It must be shut off by the patient's nurse.) It should be noted on the requisition that the specimen was drawn below an IV after it was shut off. The type of fluid in IV should also be noted. Never draw above an IV because the specimen may be contaminated with IV fluid. Drawing blood specimens from ankle veins requires permission from the patient's physician and is not recommended for protimes or other coagulation specimens or patients who have coagulation problems. Only nurses and other specially trained personnel are allowed to collect specimens from an IV.

Review: Yes ☐ No ☐

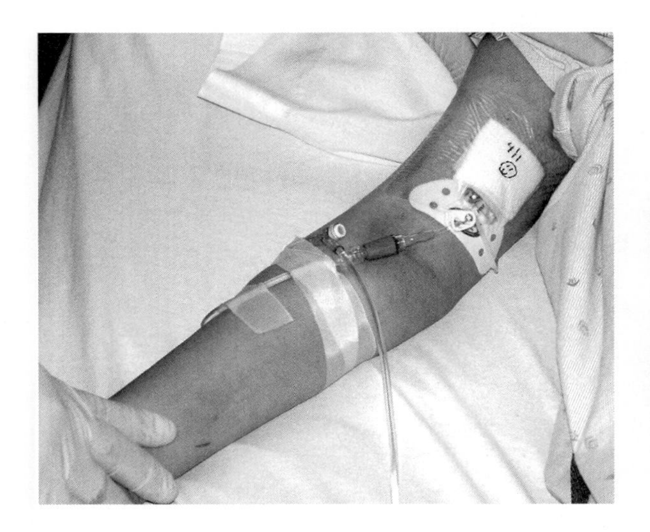

FIGURE 9-2 Patient's arm with an intravenous (IV) line.

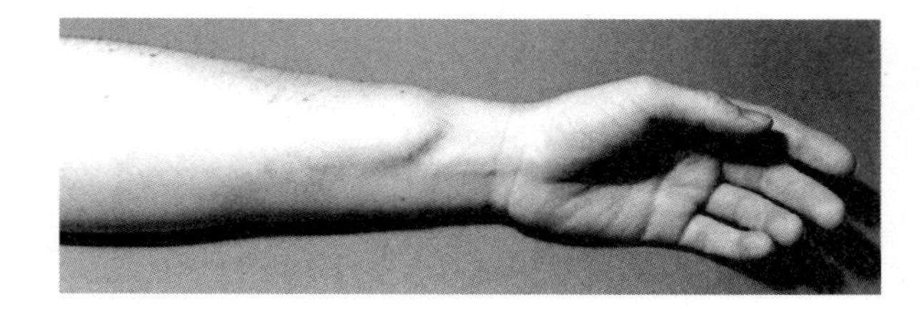

FIGURE 9-3 Arteriovenous (AV) shunt (fistula).

50. Answer: d

Why: The most expedient thing to do in this situation is to collect the specimen by finger stick. A capillary specimen can be collected and on its way to the lab in the time it would take to call another phlebotomist to come and collect the specimen, the IV to be shut off for 2 minutes to collect the specimen below it, or permission obtained to collect the specimen from a leg, ankle, or foot vein.

Review: Yes ☐ No ☐

51. Answer: d

Why: A previously active IV site within 24 hours of IV removal, an arm with an AV shunt (Fig. 9-3), or a wrist with a heparin or saline lock (Fig. 9-4) should all be avoided as current blood collection sites. An

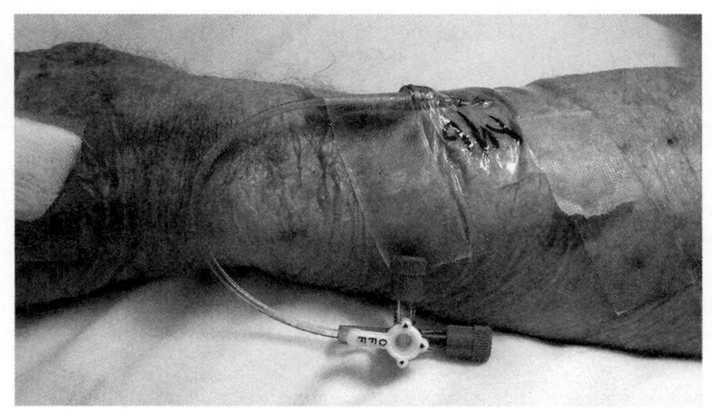

FIGURE 9-4 Saline lock with needleless entry stopcock.

arm where venipuncture was performed an hour ago is not ruled out as a current venipuncture site, although it is best to alternate arms if possible, when venipuncture times are close together.

Review: Yes ☐ No ☐

52. Answer: a

Why: An arterial line (A-line) or catheter is most commonly located in the radial artery and is used to provide continuous measurement of a patient's blood pressure. It is also commonly used for collection of blood gas specimens.

Review: Yes ☐ No ☐

53. Answer: a

Why: A surgically created graft or connection of an artery and a vein in the forearm is called an AV shunt or fistula (Fig. 9-3) and is most commonly created to provide access for dialysis. A CVC is a line inserted into a large vein and advanced into the superior vena cava proximal to the right atrium (Fig. 9-5). It is used to administer medications and sometimes draw blood specimens. A heparin lock (Hep-lok) is a special winged needle set or cannula that can be left in a patient's arm for up to 48 hours and used to administer medications and draw blood. A peripherally inserted

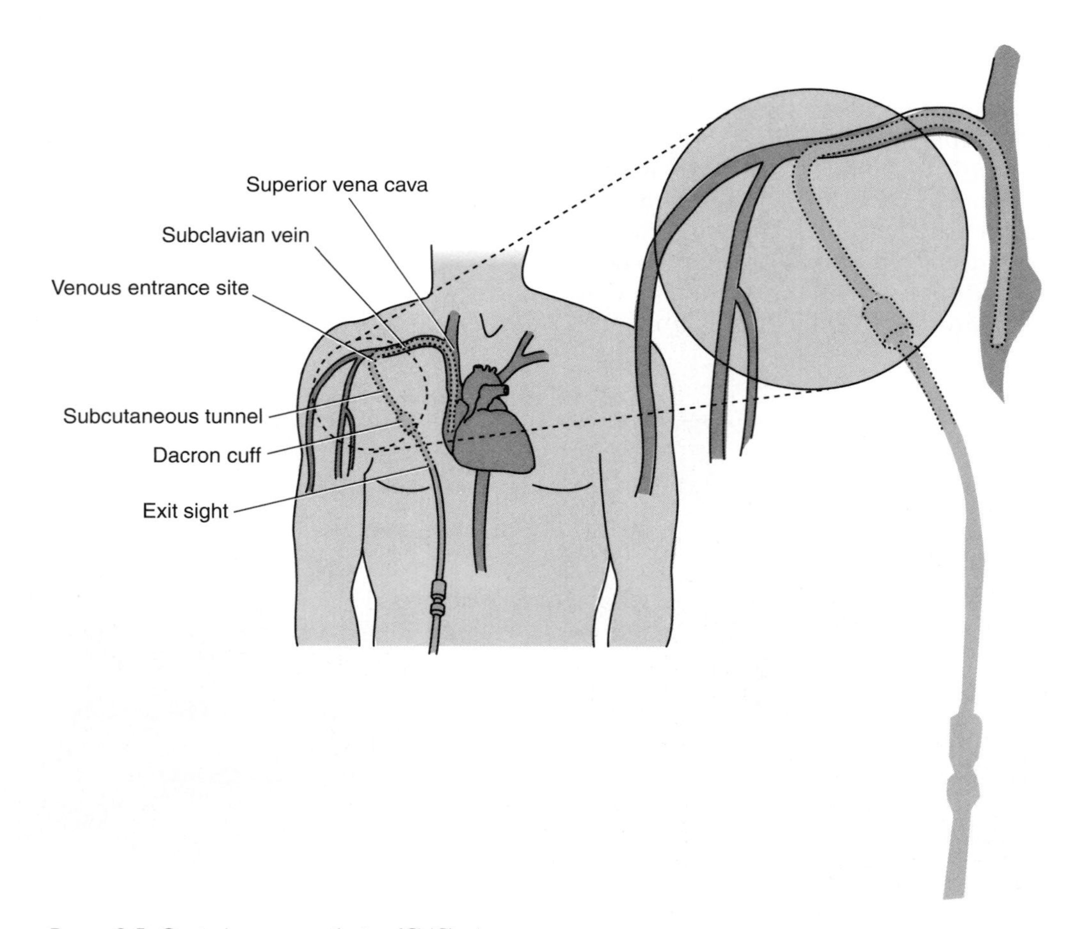

FIGURE 9-5 Central venous catheter (CVC) placement.

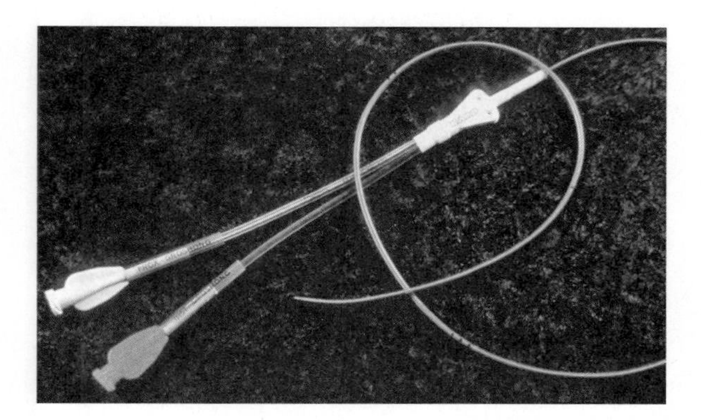

FIGURE 9-6 Groshong peripherally inserted central catheter. (Courtesy Bard Access System, Inc., Salt Lake City, UT.)

central catheter (PICC) (Fig. 9-6) is inserted into the peripheral venous system (veins of the extremities) and threaded into the central venous system (main veins leading to the heart).

Review: Yes ☐ No ☐

54. Answer: a

Why: When a blood specimen is collected from a heparin lock, a 5-mL discard tube must be drawn first to eliminate residual heparin used to flush the device and keep it from clotting. The only extra tube collected is the clear tube. Drawing coagulation specimens from a heparin lock is not recommended.

Review: Yes ☐ No ☐

55. Answer: c

Why: A CVC (Fig. 9-5) is an indwelling line inserted into a main vein, such as the subclavian, and advanced into the vena cava. Broviac, Groshong, and Hickman are all types of CVCs. Examples of Groshong and Hickman CVCs are shown in Fig. 9-7. A heparin lock (Hep-lok) is a special winged needle set or cannula that is typically inserted into a vein in the lower arm above the wrist area.

Review: Yes ☐ No ☐

56. Answer: d

Why: A subcutaneous vascular access device (SVAD), also called an implanted port (Fig. 9-8), is a small chamber that is attached to an indwelling line. The chamber is surgically implanted under the skin in the upper chest or arm. It is located by palpating the skin, and access is gained by inserting a special non-coring needle through the skin into the self-sealing septum (wall) of the chamber. (See explanation of question 55 for a description of a CVC.) A peripherally inserted central catheter (PICC) (Fig. 9-6) is a type of line

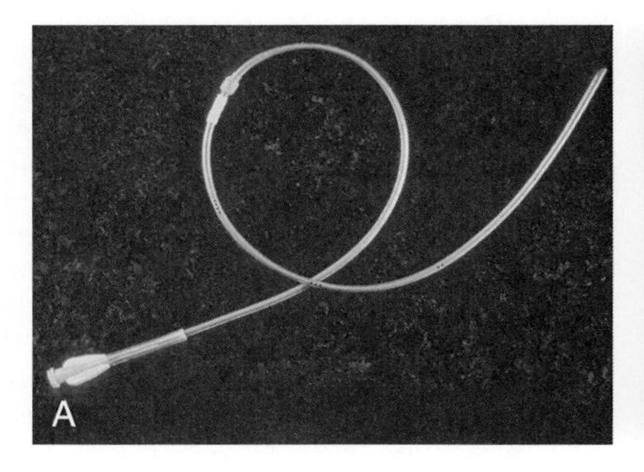

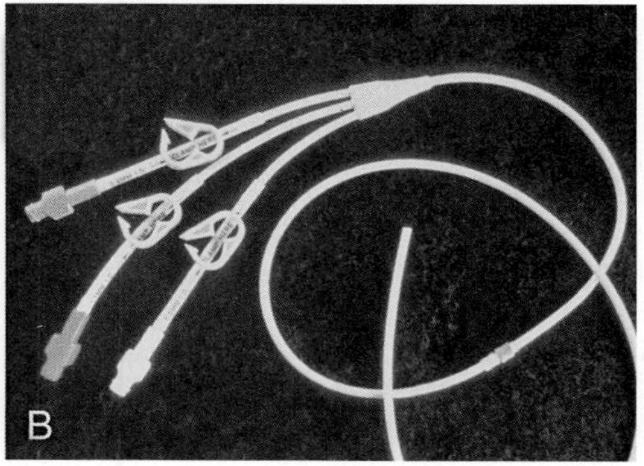

FIGURE 9-7 Central venous catheters. **A.** Groshong. **B.** Hickman. (Courtesy Bard Access Systems, Inc., Salt Lake City, UT.)

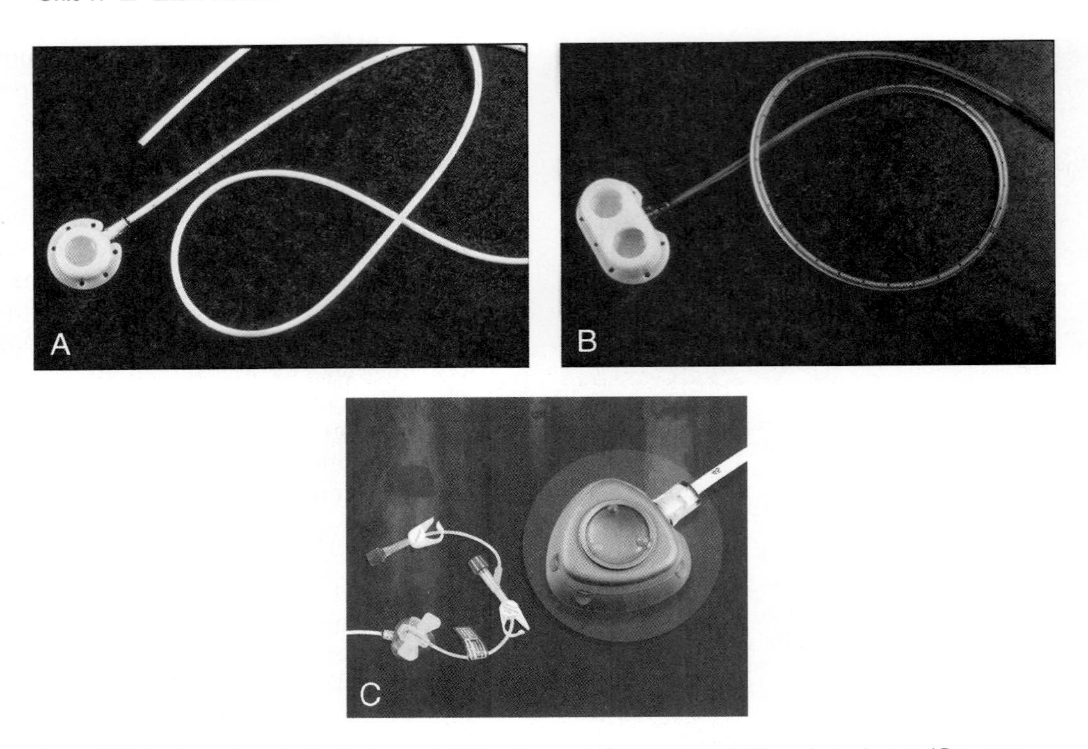

FIGURE 9-8 Implanted ports. **A.** Single port. **B.** Double port. **C.** POWERPORT implanted port. (Courtesy Bard Access Systems, Inc., Salt Lake City, UT.)

inserted into the peripheral venous system (veins of the extremities) and threaded into the central venous system (main veins leading to the heart). A saline lock is similar to a heparin lock, which is explained in the answer to question 53.

Review: Yes ☐ No ☐

57. Answer: a

Why: Some patients are allergic to the glue used in adhesive bandages. Paper tape placed over a folded gauze square can usually be used instead. If the patient is also allergic to paper tape, the area can be wrapped with bandaging material such as Coban that sticks to itself, eliminating the need for tape. The patient may also be asked to hold pressure until bleeding stops in lieu of bandaging the site. Using a latex-free bandage is not an option because the patient is allergic to the adhesive used for the bandage, not latex.

Review: Yes ☐ No ☐

58. Answer: c

Why: Increasing numbers of individuals are developing allergies to latex. Some allergies are so severe that being in the same room where latex materials are used can set off a life-threatening reaction. If a patient is known to have a severe allergy to latex, there is typically a warning sign on the door to his or her room. It is important that no items made of latex be brought into the room. This means the phlebotomist must wear non-latex gloves, use a non-latex tourniquet, use non-latex bandages, and make sure all other equipment is latex-free, when collecting blood from the patient or the patient's roommate.

Review: Yes ☐ No ☐

59. Answer: c
    Why: A site that continues to bleed five minutes after venipuncture is not normal. The patient's nurse or physician should be notified so the situation can be addressed. Do not bandage a site until you are certain that bleeding has stopped. Never wrap a pressure bandage around a site in lieu of holding pressure.
    Review: Yes ☐ No ☐

60. Answer: c
    Why: Syncope means "fainting." A patient with a history of fainting during blood collection should be asked to lie down during a blood draw.
    Review: Yes ☐ No ☐

61. Answer: b
    Why: If an outpatient feels faint during blood collection, discontinue the draw immediately and lower his or her head. Do not continue the draw, even if the patient wants you to. The use of ammonia inhalants can have adverse side effects such as respiratory distress in asthmatic individuals.
    Review: Yes ☐ No ☐

62. Answer: b
    Why: An outpatient who becomes weak and pale following a draw may faint and should be encouraged to lie down until he or she recovers. The patient should not drive for at least 30 minutes.
    Review: Yes ☐ No ☐

63. Answer: a
    Why: A feeling of nausea often precedes vomiting, so it is a good idea to give the patient an emesis basin to hold as a precaution. Apply a cold, damp washcloth or other cold compress to the patient's forehead and ask him or her to breathe slowly and deeply. Do not attempt blood collection until the nausea subsides.
    Review: Yes ☐ No ☐

64. Answer: b
    Why: Engaging in small talk before venipuncture can put patients at ease and help them relax. A relaxed patient is less likely to feel as much pain associated with the draw as someone who is anxious and tense. Rubbing with alcohol can abrade the skin and can be painful rather than desensitizing. Tying the tourniquet too tight can make the arm feel numb, but it is a sign of nerve compression and is never recommended. It also increases the chance of hemoconcentration, which can cause erroneous test results. Telling patients that the draw might hurt a lot can increase their anxiety and actually make it hurt more. The patient should be warned just before the needle enters the arm, however, to prevent a startle reflex.
    Review: Yes ☐ No ☐

65. Answer: a
    Why: Petechiae (Fig. 9-9) are small, red, non-raised spots that appear with tourniquet application on some patients with platelet or capillary defects. They do not compromise test results and may not be avoidable because they will probably occur at any site that is chosen. Sites with massive scarring, edema, or veins that feel hard and cordlike should be avoided.
    Review: Yes ☐ No ☐

66. Answer: a
    Why: Do not attempt to complete the draw on a patient who goes into convulsions during venipuncture. Continuing the draw is dangerous and could result in injury to the patient. In addition, you could receive an accidental needlestick. Discontinue the draw immediately and remove, shield, and discard the needle as soon as possible. Try to prevent

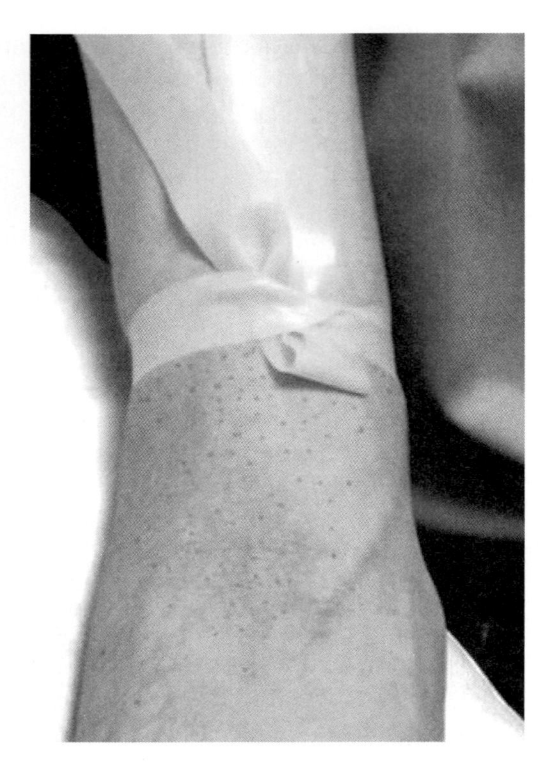

FIGURE 9-9 Petechiae. (Photo courtesy medtraining.org. Used with permission).

the patient from injuring himself or herself and notify the appropriate first aid personnel as soon as possible.

Review: Yes ☐ No ☐

67. Answer: d

Why: A hematoma caused by blood leaking into the tissues and identified by swelling at or near the venipuncture site is the most common complication of venipuncture. It is painful to the patient, results in unsightly bruising (Fig. 9-1, p. 249), and can cause compression injuries to nerves, which lead to lawsuits. If a hematoma starts to form during blood collection, immediately release the tourniquet, withdraw the needle, and hold pressure over the site for a minimum of 2 minutes.

Review: Yes ☐ No ☐

68. Answer: b

Why: Hematoma formation can be caused by several different errors in phlebotomy technique, including failure to apply adequate pressure to the site after a blood draw, leakage of blood from a vein because the needle is only partly inserted in the vein, and leakage of blood from a hole made by a needle that penetrated through the back wall of the vein during needle entry or the collection process. A needle bevel that is in the lumen of the vein is right where it should be and would not be the cause of hematoma formation.

Review: Yes ☐ No ☐

69. Answer: c

Why: Blood pulsing or spurting into the tube is an indication that you may have accidentally hit an artery. A hematoma can start to form if you hit an artery, but there are several other reasons for hematoma formation. Color is not a good way to identify arterial blood. Normal venous blood is typically dark red. Arterial blood in normal individuals is bright red, but it may look as dark as venous blood if the patient has a pulmonary problem.

Review: Yes ☐ No ☐

70. Answer: b

Why: Iatrogenic is an adjective used to describe an adverse condition brought on by the effects of treatment. Blood loss as a result of removal for testing purposes is called iatrogenic blood loss. Removal of blood on a regular basis or in large quantities can lead to anemia in some patients, especially infants.

Review: Yes ☐ No ☐

71. Answer: d

Why: An inadvertently collected arterial specimen can usually be submitted for testing, rather than redrawing the patient. However, the specimen should be labeled as arterial because some test values are different for arterial specimens. If you suspect that you have accidentally punctured an artery, you must hold pressure over the site for 3 to 5 minutes. Do not have the patient hold pressure or apply a pressure bandage in lieu of holding pressure.

Review: Yes ☐ No ☐

72. Answer: c
Why: Infection at the site following venipuncture is rare but not unheard of. Using proper aseptic technique, including not touching the site after it has been cleaned, minimizing the time between removing the needle cap and venipuncture, not opening adhesive bandages ahead of time, and reminding the patient to keep the bandage on for at least 15 minutes after specimen collection, should minimize the risk of infection. The wrong order of draw and leaving a tourniquet on too long can affect the specimen but do not cause infection of the site. ETS tube holders are not normally sterile.
Review: Yes ☐ No ☐

73. Answer: d
Why: Excessive or blind probing during venipuncture is usually painful and can result in the accidental piercing of nerves and arteries and the possibility of permanent damage. Lawsuits have been filed over permanent nerve injuries caused directly by needles or indirectly by compression of the nerves by hematomas that resulted from inadvertent arterial sticks. Patency is the state of being freely open. Rather than causing vein patency, probing can damage veins and make them less patent.
Review: Yes ☐ No ☐

74. Answer: c
Why: Marked (extreme or significant) pain, numbness of the arm, and pain that radiates up or down the arm are signs of nerve involvement and any one of them requires immediate removal of the needle. A patient may not understand the significance of the symptoms or may be stoic in an effort to not appear weak. It is up to the phlebotomist to recognize the signs of nerve injury and discontinue the venipuncture immediately. Continuing the draw can worsen the damage.
Review: Yes ☐ No ☐

75. Answer: c
Why: Performing venipuncture before the alcohol has dried completely is the most common cause of a stinging sensation to the patient and can also cause slight hemolysis of the specimen. Blood collection needles are used only once and are not likely to be dull or flawed, but they should be examined when first opened to detect defects that could cause pain or injure the patient. Pushing down on the needle as it is inserted can be painful but does not normally produce a stinging sensation. A tourniquet that is tied too tightly is typically described as a pinching sensation.
Review: Yes ☐ No ☐

76. Answer: d
Why: "Reflux" is a term used to describe the backflow of blood from a collection tube into a patient's vein during venipuncture. Reflux can happen if there is a pressure change in the vein that occurs normally or when the tourniquet is released. It can only occur if blood in the tube is in contact with the needle during venipuncture. Reflux of blood mixed with an additive such as EDTA can cause an adverse patient reaction. Keeping the arm in a downward position so that tubes fill from the bottom up, and avoiding back-and-forth movement of tube contents during blood collection, prevent blood from being in contact with the needle and therefore prevent reflux.
Review: Yes ☐ No ☐

77. Answer: c
Why: Leaving the tourniquet on for 2 minutes is not likely to impair vein patency (state of being freely open). It may, however, lead to erroneous test results caused by hemoconcentration brought on by prolonged blockage of blood flow. Improperly redirecting the needle, probing for deep veins, and performing numerous venipunctures in the same area are all actions that can damage veins and impair vein patency.
Review: Yes ☐ No ☐

78. Answer: c
Why: Prolonged tourniquet application causes stagnation of blood flow (venous stasis), which causes the plasma portion of the blood to filter into the tissues. This decreases blood plasma volume and increases nonfilterable blood components, a condition called hemoconcentration. To minimize the effects of hemoconcentration, the tourniquet should be released within 1 minute of application and the patient should not be allowed to continuously make and release a fist.
Review: Yes ☐ No ☐

79. Answer: d
Why: Hemolysis is the destruction of red blood cells and the liberation of hemoglobin into the serum or plasma portion of the specimen, causing it to appear pink to reddish depending on the degree of hemolysis. The specimen is described as being hemolyzed.
Review: Yes ☐ No ☐

80. Answer: d
Why: Mixing tubes vigorously instead of gently inverting them, pulling blood into a syringe too quickly, and using a small-bore needle to collect blood into a large-volume tube can all result in hemolysis of the specimen. Transferring blood from a syringe to a tube should *not* cause hemolysis if done correctly.
Review: Yes ☐ No ☐

81. Answer: d
Why: A prothrombin time is a coagulation test. The ratio of blood to anticoagulant is *most* critical for coagulation tests because a ratio of nine parts blood to one part anticoagulant must be maintained for accurate test results. The excess anticoagulant in a short draw dilutes the plasma portion of the specimen used for testing, causing falsely prolonged test results.
Review: Yes ☐ No ☐

82. Answer: b
Why: There is no skin puncture container for collecting plasma specimens for coagulation tests because, except for those that can be performed with special point-of-care instruments, coagulation tests cannot be performed by skin puncture. Partially filled coagulation tubes have an incorrect blood-to-additive ratio and are unacceptable for testing. Pouring two partially filled tubes together still results in an improper ratio of blood to additive and is also unacceptable. A phlebotomist should never make more than two attempts at venipuncture on a patient at one time. After the second attempt, another phlebotomist should be asked to collect the specimen.
Review: Yes ☐ No ☐

83. Answer: a
Why: Cleaning a skin puncture site with isopropyl alcohol is accepted technique. Drawing a blood culture while the povidone-iodine is still damp can contaminate the specimen with povidone-iodine residue, which can inhibit growth of microorganisms and lead to false-negative results. Touching the filter paper while collecting a phenylketonuria (PKU) specimen can be a

source of contamination that leads to erroneous results. Povidone-iodine should not be used to clean skin puncture sites because it interferes with phosphorus, potassium, and uric acid.

Review: Yes ☐ No ☐

84. Answer: a

Why: When the vacuum escapes from an evacuated tube during blood collection, it typically makes a hissing sound. This can happen if the needle backs out of the skin slightly, allowing the tube to draw air instead of blood. If the needle penetrates all the way through a vein, the tube will not draw blood but the vacuum will be still intact because the bevel is under the skin. A drop in a patient's blood pressure would not cause a hissing sound. A tube with a crack in it and no vacuum would not draw blood or make a hissing sound because the vacuum was gone before the draw was even started.

Review: Yes ☐ No ☐

85. Answer: a

Why: A hissing sound indicates that the vacuum escaped from the tube, which can happen if the needle backs out of the skin slightly, not when it goes through the vein. If you fail to get blood flow until you pull back on the needle, the needle most likely went too deep and through the back of the vein. Being certain that the needle entered the vein but failing to get blood flow could also indicate that the needle has gone through the vein, and you will need to pull back on the needle. In addition, if you fill one tube but the second does not fill, it is possible that the needle pushed through the vein as you pushed the second tube onto the needle, and you will have to pull the needle back to get blood flow.

Review: Yes ☐ No ☐

86. Answer: d

Why: Vein walls are fairly tough. If a vein is not anchored well, it may roll (move away) slightly and the needle may slip beside the vein (Fig. 9-10F) instead of going into it. A needle is supposed to end up in the lumen of the vein during venipuncture (Fig. 9-10A). A needle can go through a vein (Fig. 9-10D) if it is inserted too quickly or deeply and if the tube holder is not held securely during the draw (i.e., when pushing a tube onto the needle). The needle can end up against an inside wall of the vein if it enters it at an angle that is too shallow, if there is a bend in the vein (Fig. 9-10B), or if the bevel is down (Fig. 9-10C) instead of up when it enters the vein.

Review: Yes ☐ No ☐

87. Answer: a

Why: If the needle is only partially inserted in the vein during blood collection (Fig. 9-10E), the tube will fill very slowly and blood will leak into the tissue around the vein, causing a hematoma.

Review: Yes ☐ No ☐

88. Answer: d

Why: Failure to achieve blood flow in a second tube after the first tube filled without a problem initially suggests that the needle position could have changed slightly when the tube was removed and replaced. If this had been the case, however, blood flow would have been re-established with slight manipulation of the needle. This suggests there could be a problem with the tube. Always try a new tube before giving up on a blood draw. Further redirections of the needle amount to probing and should not be done.

Review: Yes ☐ No ☐

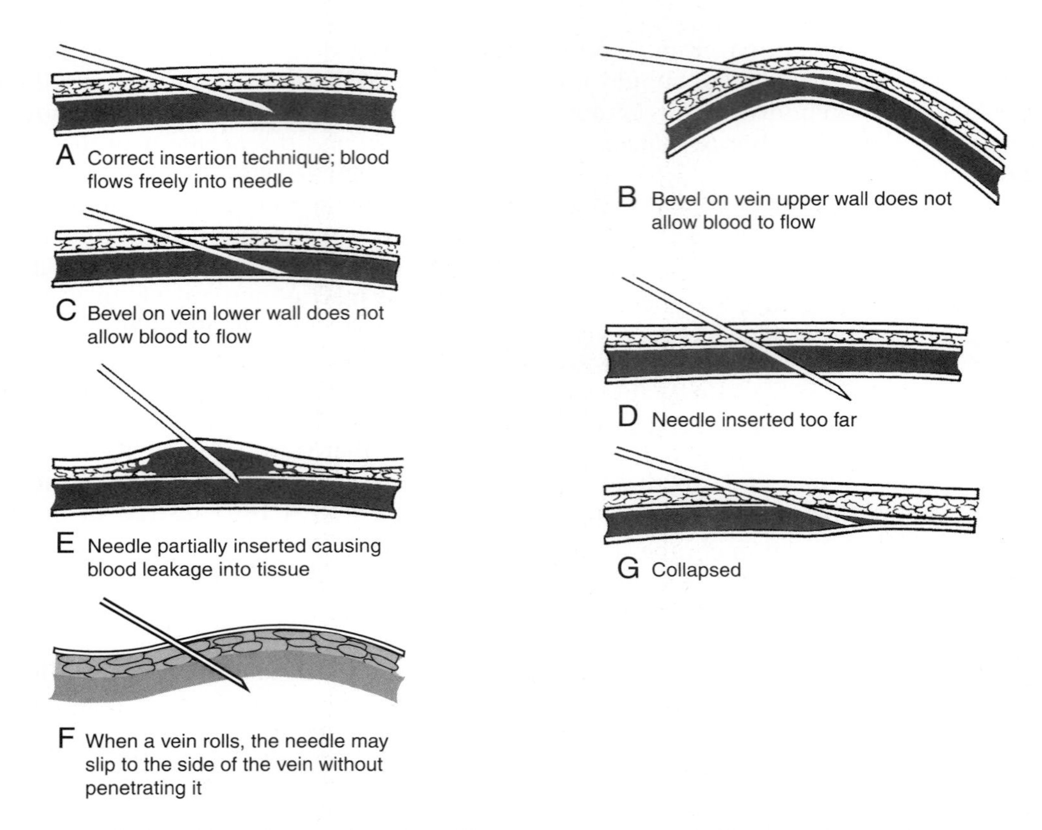

FIGURE 9-10 **A.** Correct needle insertion. **B.** Bevel on upper vein wall. **C.** Bevel on lower vein wall. **D.** Needle inserted too far. **E.** Partially inserted needle causes blood leakage into tissue. **F.** Needle slipped beside a vein that rolled. **G.** Collapsed vein.

89. Answer: c

Why: Multiple redirections of the needle while attempting venipuncture amount to probing, which is dangerous and should not be done, even if a second phlebotomist takes over the draw for you. If you cannot obtain blood flow with one or two redirections of the needle, discontinue the draw and try again at a new site.

Review: Yes ☐ No ☐

90. Answer: a

Why: A vein may collapse (Fig. 9-10G) if the tourniquet is applied too tightly or too close to the venipuncture site, or if the tube has too much vacuum for the size of the vein. Filling multiple large volume tubes should not cause vein collapse if proper procedures were followed for equipment selection, vein selection, and tourniquet application.

Review: Yes ☐ No ☐

CHAPTER 10

CAPILLARY PUNCTURE EQUIPMENT AND PROCEDURES

study tip

Questions in this chapter test the ability to identify capillary puncture equipment and describe the principles of capillary puncture, including how reference values differ from venous specimens, when capillary puncture is indicated and when it is not, tests that cannot be collected by capillary puncture, order of draw, and issues involved in proper site selection. Questions also test the ability to identify and describe each step in finger puncture and heel puncture and describe special procedures that include capillary blood gases, neonatal bilirubin, newborn screening, and blood smear preparation.

overview

Capillary puncture, in which drops of blood for testing are collected from the capillary dermis of the skin, is especially practical for pediatric patients in whom removal of larger quantities of blood can have serious consequences. This chapter assesses knowledge of routine and special capillary puncture procedures, including required equipment, principles of capillary specimens, and the steps necessary to safely obtain an appropriately identified quality blood specimen. Phlebotomists must know the proper way to obtain capillary specimens to ensure their safety and that of the patient as well as the quality of the specimen.

REVIEW QUESTIONS

Choose the BEST answer.

1. "Arterialized" means:
   a. arterial content has been increased.
   b. composition is the same as arterial.
   c. oxygen levels equal arterial levels.
   d. venous blood flow was increased.

2. A blood smear is all of the following EXCEPT:
   a. blood collected on a special filter paper.
   b. blood spread out on a microscope slide.
   c. made from a fresh or EDTA specimen.
   d. used to identify the types of blood cells.

3. The calcaneus is a bone located in the:
   a. earlobe.
   b. finger.
   c. heel.
   d. thumb.

4. This is the abbreviation for a pulmonary function test.
   a. AFP
   b. CBG
   c. PKU
   d. TSH

5. A cyanotic extremity would:
   a. appear jaundiced.
   b. be bluish in color.
   c. exhibit erythema.
   d. look pale yellow.

6. A differential is a test that determines all of the following EXCEPT:
   a. a platelet estimate.
   b. packed cell volume.
   c. red cell morphology.
   d. WBC characteristics.

7. "Feather" is a term used to describe the appearance of:
   a. a newborn screening blood spot.
   b. blood in a thick malaria smear.
   c. lipemia in a bilirubin specimen.
   d. the thinnest area of a blood film.

8. Fluid in the spaces between the cells is called:
   a. interstitial fluid.
   b. intracellular fluid.
   c. lymphatic fluid.
   d. peritoneal fluid.

9. This is a sharp-pointed device used to make capillary punctures.
   a. bullet
   b. lancet
   c. laser
   d. scalpel

10. Which of the following statements most accurately describes capillary puncture blood?
    a. a mix of venous, arterial, and capillary blood
    b. mostly tissue fluid mixed with arterial blood
    c. mostly venous blood mixed with tissue fluid
    d. nearly identical to a venous blood specimen

11. Microhematocrit tubes are all of the following EXCEPT:
    a. coated with lithium heparin.
    b. filled using capillary action.
    c. narrow-bore capillary tubes.
    d. used for PCV determination.

12. Referring to Fig. 10-1, identify the letters of the fingers that are recommended as sites for capillary puncture.
    a. A and B
    b. B and C
    c. C and D
    d. D and E

13. Osteochondritis is:
    a. abnormal bone formation and growth.
    b. an inherited bone metabolism disorder.
    c. infection of the bone and bone marrow.
    d. inflammation of the bone and cartilage.

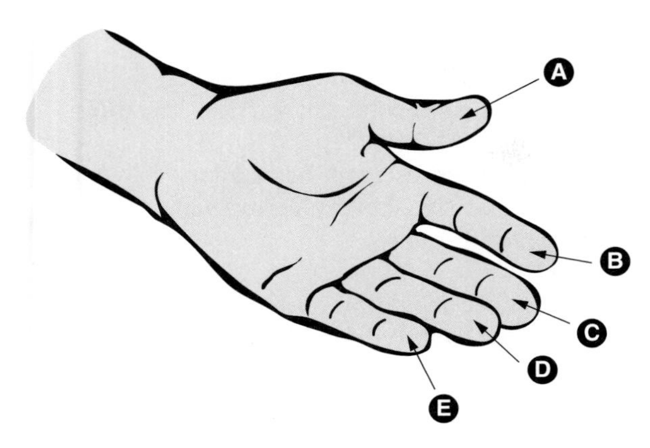

FIGURE 10-1 Adult hand.

14. This is a term for the bottom surface of the heel.
    a. distal
    b. dorsal
    c. lateral
    d. plantar

15. Whorls as related to capillary puncture are:
    a. blebs created during skin tests.
    b. formations seen in blood films.
    c. newborn screening blood spots.
    d. spiral patterns of fingerprints.

16. The temperature of heel warming devices should not exceed:
    a. 37°C.
    b. 42°C.
    c. 98°F.
    d. 112°F.

17. Which of the following is the medical term for a finger bone?
    a. calcaneus
    b. clavicle
    c. patella
    d. phalanx

18. CBG specimens are collected in:
    a. amber syringe-style devices.
    b. bullets with heparin in them.
    c. circles on special filter paper.
    d. narrow-bore capillary tubes.

19. Capillary specimens contain all of the following EXCEPT:
    a. arterial blood.
    b. serous fluids.
    c. tissue fluids.
    d. venous blood.

20. Which numbered arrows on the diagram of an infant's foot in Fig. 10-2 point toward the safest areas for capillary puncture?
    a. 1 and 4
    b. 2 and 3
    c. 3 and 5
    d. 4 and 5

21. All of the following are required characteristics of capillary puncture lancets EXCEPT:
    a. a controlled depth of puncture.
    b. blades or points that are sterile.
    c. color-coding by width of blade.
    d. permanently retractable blades.

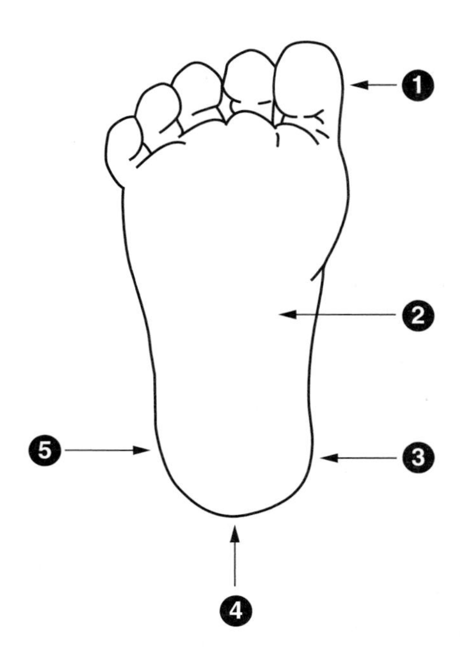

FIGURE 10-2 Infant foot.

22. Which of the following equipment is used to collect a manual packed cell volume test?
    a. circles on filter paper
    b. glass microscope slide
    c. microhematocrit tube
    d. mixing bar and magnet

23. All of the following equipment may be required to collect capillary blood gases EXCEPT:
    a. caps for both tube ends.
    b. filter paper for blotting.
    c. magnet and iron filings.
    d. long, thin capillary tube.

24. An example of a microcollection container that contains a fluid for direct dilution of the specimen is a:
    a. bullet.
    b. microtube.
    c. CBG tube.
    d. Unopette

25. A microcollection container is sometimes called a:
    a. bullet.
    b. flea.
    c. fleam.
    d. pipet.

26. The composition of blood obtained by capillary puncture more closely resembles:
    a. arterial blood.
    b. lymph fluid.
    c. tissue fluid.
    d. venous blood.

27. If venous blood is placed in a bullet, it is important to:
    a. label it as a venous specimen.
    b. shield the specimen from light.
    c. transport it to the lab ASAP.
    d. vigorously mix the specimen.

28. A laboratory report form should state that a specimen has been collected by capillary puncture:
    a. for equipment inventory control purposes.
    b. because results can vary by specimen source.
    c. so other tests will be capillary collections.
    d. to satisfy liability insurance requirements.

29. Blood collected by puncturing the skin is called capillary blood because:
    a. it is collected with capillary tubes.
    b. it is from the dermal capillary bed.
    c. microtubes fill by capillary action.
    d. small drops of blood are collected.

30. This test is typically performed on capillary blood.
    a. CBC
    b. GTT
    c. PKU
    d. PTT

31. Reference values for this test are higher for capillary specimens:
    a. calcium.
    b. glucose.
    c. phosphorus.
    d. total protein.

32. You need to collect blood cultures, and green, light blue, and purple top tubes on an adult with difficult veins. Which of them can be collected by skin puncture?
    a. blood cultures and green top
    b. blood cultures and purple top
    c. green top and purple top
    d. light blue and purple top

33. If collected by capillary puncture, which of the following specimens should be collected in an amber microtube (Fig. 10-3)?
    a. bilirubin
    b. glucose
    c. lead
    d. PKU

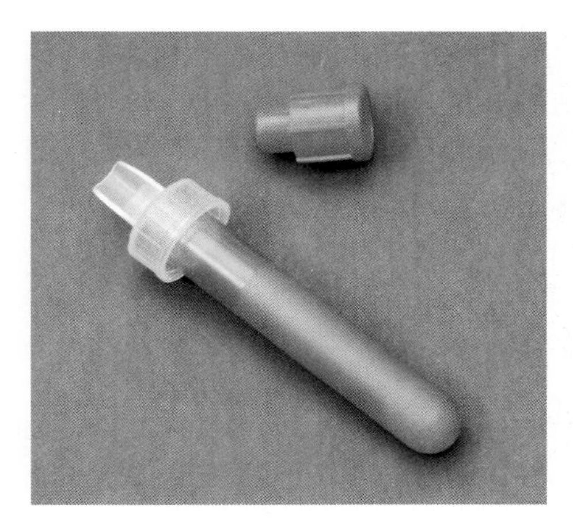

FIGURE 10-3 Amber microcollection tube.

34. A capillary puncture can be done in all of the following situations EXCEPT when:
    a. a child is younger than 2 years old.
    b. a light blue top tube has been ordered.
    c. an adult has veins that are difficult.
    d. veins must be saved for chemotherapy.

35. All of the following patient conditions would make capillary puncture a poor choice for specimen collection EXCEPT:
    a. acute dehydration.
    b. iatrogenic anemia.
    c. poor circulation.
    d. state of shock.

36. Which of the following is normally a proper site for finger puncture on an adult?
    a. distal segment of the middle finger
    b. end segment of either of the thumbs
    c. medial segment of the index finger
    d. proximal phalanx of the ring finger

37. Capillary puncture is the preferred method to obtain blood from infants and children for all of the following reasons EXCEPT:
    a. restraining used for venipuncture can cause injury.
    b. results on capillary specimens are more accurate.
    c. infants and children have small blood volumes compared to adults.
    d. venipuncture can damage their veins and tissues.

38. Which of the following sites would normally be eliminated as a capillary puncture site?
    a. index finger of a woman
    b. infant lateral plantar heel
    c. middle finger of an adult
    d. ring finger on an IV arm

39. It is necessary to control the depth of lancet insertion during heel puncture to avoid:
    a. damage to the tendons.
    b. injuring the calcaneus.
    c. puncturing an artery.
    d. unnecessary bleeding.

40. According to the Clinical and Laboratory Standards Institute (CLSI), depth of heel puncture should not exceed:
    a. 1.5 mm.
    b. 2.0 mm.
    c. 2.4 mm.
    d. 4.9 mm.

41. Which of the following can be a complication of a heel puncture that is too deep?
    a. osteoarthritis
    b. osteoporosis
    c. osteomyelitis
    d. osteosarcoma

42. Which of the following is the safest area of an infant's foot for capillary puncture?
    a. any area of the arch
    b. center of the big toe
    c. medial plantar heel
    d. posterior curvature

43. A recommended capillary puncture site on children 2 years of age or older is on the:
    a. bottom of an earlobe.
    b. fleshy side of a thumb.
    c. pad of a middle finger.
    d. medial or lateral heel.

44. In which of the following areas does capillary specimen collection differ from routine venipuncture for tests that can be collected either way?
    a. additives used
    b. antiseptic used
    c. ID procedures
    d. order of draw

45. The distance between the skin surface and the bone in the end segment of a finger is:
    a. shortest at the side and the tip.
    b. equal throughout the fingertip.
    c. thickest of all in fifth fingers.
    d. thinnest in the middle finger.

46. The major blood vessels of the skin are located:
    a. at the dermal-subcutaneous junction.
    b. between the epidermis and the dermis.
    c. in the epidermis and the subcutaneous.
    d. within the epidermis and the dermis.

47. A capillary puncture that parallels the whorls of the fingerprint will:
    a. allow blood to run down the finger.
    b. cause blood to form in round drops.
    c. continue to bleed for a lot longer.
    d. make specimen collection easier.

48. Capillary puncture equipment includes all of the following EXCEPT:
    a. blood culture bottles.
    b. various lancet types.
    c. microcollection tubes.
    d. skin warming devices.

49. Which color-coded bullet would be used to collect a CBC?
    a. gray
    b. green
    c. lavender
    d. yellow

50. If the following tests are collected from a patient by capillary puncture, which test specimen is collected first?
    a. bilirubin
    b. CBC
    c. lytes
    d. glucose

51. What is the purpose of warming the site before capillary puncture?
    a. enhance visibility of veins
    b. increase the flow of blood
    c. prevent sample hemolysis
    d. relax and comfort patients

52. For accurate results, the heel *must* be warmed before collecting a capillary specimen for this test.
    a. CBG
    b. lytes
    c. PKU
    d. WBC

53. The recommended antiseptic for cleaning capillary puncture sites is:
    a. 70% isopropanol.
    b. povidone-iodine.
    c. soap and water.
    d. tincture of iodine.

54. The antiseptic must be completely dried before performing capillary puncture to avoid:
    a. hematoma formation.
    b. hemoconcentration.
    c. premature clotting.
    d. specimen hemolysis.

55. Povidone-iodine contamination of a capillary specimen notably interferes in all of following tests EXCEPT:
    a. magnesium.
    b. phosphorus.
    c. potassium.
    d. uric acid.

56. Errors in capillary glucose results have been attributed to:
    a. excessive depth of the capillary puncture.
    b. failure to collect the initial drop of blood.
    c. isopropanol contamination of the specimen.
    d. warming of the site prior to capillary puncture.

57. Proper finger puncture technique includes all of the following EXCEPT:
    a. choosing a middle or ring finger site.
    b. puncturing parallel to the fingerprint.
    c. trying not to squeeze or milk the site.
    d. wiping away the first drop of blood.

58. Hemolysis of a capillary specimen can erroneously elevate results for this test.
    a. cholesterol
    b. hemoglobin
    c. potassium
    d. RBC count

59. The purpose of wiping away the first drop of blood (Fig. 10-4) during capillary specimen collection is to:
    a. avoid contamination with bacteria.
    b. reduce tissue fluid contamination.
    c. improve blood flow to the site.
    d. minimize platelet aggregation.

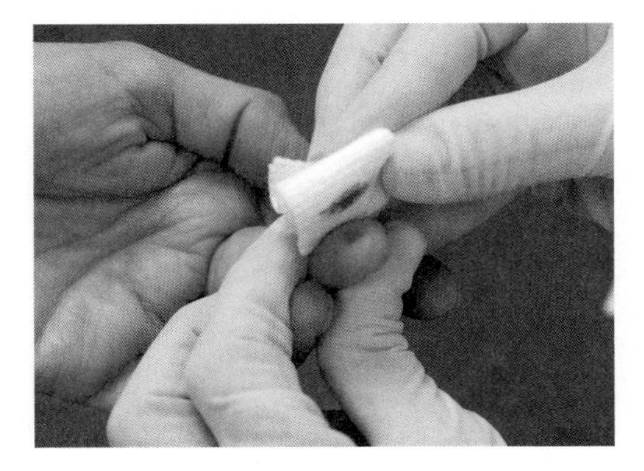

FIGURE 10-4 Wiping the first blood drop with gauze.

60. Proper technique for filling microcollection tubes includes all of the following EXCEPT:
    a. letting blood run down the tube's inside wall.
    b. scooping up blood as it runs down the finger.
    c. tapping the tube gently to settle the specimen.
    d. touching the tube's scoop to each blood drop.

61. Which of the following would be *least* likely to introduce excess tissue fluid into a capillary puncture specimen?
    a. collecting the first drop
    b. pressing hard on the site
    c. squeezing the puncture
    d. wiping the alcohol dry

62. Which of the following can result in microclot formation in a specimen collected in an anticoagulant microtube?
    a. mixing it too soon
    b. mixing it forcefully
    c. overfilling the tube
    d. underfilling the tube

63. During multisample capillary specimen collection, blood smears and EDTA specimens are obtained before other specimens to minimize:
    a. effects of platelet aggregation.
    b. hemolysis of red blood cells.
    c. specimen hemoconcentration.
    d. tissue fluid contamination.

64. A blood smear is required for this test.
    a. manual differential
    b. neonatal bilirubin
    c. newborn screening
    d. packed cell volume

65. An acceptable routine blood smear:
    a. covers the entire slide.
    b. forms a bullet shape.
    c. has a feathered edge.
    d. looks short and thick.

66. A blood smear prepared from an EDTA specimen should be made:
a. after the blood cells settle in the tube.
b. at the time the specimen is collected.
c. before the specimen has been mixed.
d. within 1 hour of specimen collection.

67. When making a blood smear by hand using two glass slides, the typical angle required of the spreader slide is:
a. 15°.
b. 20°.
c. 30°.
d. 45°.

68. If the phlebotomist makes a blood smear that is too short, he or she should try again and:
a. decrease the angle of the spreader slide.
b. increase the angle of the spreader slide.
c. place a smaller blood drop on the slide.
d. put more pressure on the spreader slide.

69. Holes in a blood smear can be caused by all of the following EXCEPT:
a. low hemoglobin.
b. dirt on the slide.
c. high lipid level.
d. smudged slide.

70. Collection of a thick blood smear may be requested to detect:
a. elevated bilirubin.
b. hypothyroidism.
c. malaria microbes.
d. phenylketonuria.

71. Iron fillings used in capillary blood gas collection:
a. help mix the anticoagulant.
b. prevent platelet adhesion.
c. stabilize the oxygen levels.
d. stop air bubble formation.

72. All of the following statements are true of capillary blood gases EXCEPT:
a. they are less dangerous to collect than ABGs.
b. results are much more accurate than ABGs.
c. specimens contain venous and arterial blood.
d. collection exposes the blood specimen to air.

73. An infant may require a blood transfusion if blood levels of this substance exceed 18 mg/dL.
a. bilirubin
b. carnitine
c. galactose
d. thyroxine

74. Phenylketonuria is a:
a. disorder caused by excessive phenylalanine ingestion.
b. contagious condition caused by lack of phenylalanine.
c. genetic disorder involving phenylalanine metabolism.
d. temporary condition caused by lack of phenylalanine.

75. Which of the following is a newborn screening test?
a. bilirubin
b. GALT
c. H & H
d. WBC

76. Falsely decreased bilirubin results can be caused by:
a. collecting the specimen 5 minutes late.
b. failing to protect the specimen from light.
c. puncturing the heel close to the calcaneus.
d. using isopropyl alcohol to clean the site.

77. A PKU test can be contaminated by all of the following EXCEPT:
a. neglecting to discard the first blood drop.
b. touching the inside of a filter paper circle.
c. stacking specimen slips while wet or dry.
d. using isopropyl alcohol to clean the site.

78. Erroneous newborn screening results can be caused by all of the following EXCEPT:
    a. applying blood drops to both sides of the filter paper.
    b. hanging a specimen slip to dry in a vertical position.
    c. layering successive blood drops in a collection circle.
    d. using one large drop to entirely fill a collection circle.

79. Neonatal screening for this disorder is required by law in the United States.
    a. diabetes
    b. HDN
    c. HBV
    d. PKU

80. Jaundice in a newborn is associated with high levels of:
    a. bilirubin.
    b. glucose.
    c. ketones
    d. thyroxine.

81. It is inappropriate to apply a bandage to a capillary puncture site on an infant or child younger than 2 years of age for all of the following reasons EXCEPT that it can:
    a. irritate an infant's tender skin.
    b. pull off and be a choking hazard.
    c. tear delicate skin when removed.
    d. turn into a contamination source.

82. Which of the following action words associated with capillary puncture procedure steps are in the correct order?
    a. clean, puncture, warm, wipe, collect
    b. clean, warm, puncture, collect, wipe
    c. warm, clean, puncture, wipe, collect
    d. warm, puncture, clean, wipe, collect

83. The best way to mix blood in an additive bullet is to:
    a. invert it gently.
    b. shake it briskly.
    c. roll it in the hands.
    d. tap it sharply.

84. Strong repetitive pressure, such as squeezing or milking a site during capillary specimen collection:
    a. is necessary to obtain adequate blood flow.
    b. can hemolyze and contaminate specimens.
    c. improves the accuracy of complete blood count (CBC) test results.
    d. increases venous blood flow into the area.

85. Which of the following collection devices fill by capillary action?
    a. amber microtubes
    b. filter paper circles
    c. hematocrit tubes
    d. lavender bullets

86. Which of the following equipment is reusable?
    a. heel warmer
    b. laser lancet
    c. metal flea
    d. microtube

87. Lancets with permanently retractable blades are disposed of in the:
    a. autoclave waste.
    b. biohazard trash.
    c. sharps container.
    d. regular trash can.

88. Capillary puncture is *not* a good choice for specimen collection if the patient is:
    a. comatose.
    b. dehydrated.
    c. jaundiced.
    d. nauseated.

89. Which of the following steps should be omitted from infant heel puncture?
    a. Apply bandage.
    b. Clean the site.
    c. ID the patient.
    d. Warm the site.

90. After making a blood smear:
    a. blow on it until dry.
    b. let it dry naturally.
    c. place it in alcohol.
    d. wave it until dry.

91. Which test *cannot* be collected by capillary puncture?
    a. blood culture
    b. electrolytes
    c. hemoglobin
    d. lithium level

92. Neonatal screening is the testing of:
    a. babies for contagious diseases.
    b. infants with certain symptoms.
    c. newborns for certain disorders.
    d. pregnant women for diseases.

93. Microhematocrit tubes with a red band on one end contain:
    a. EDTA.
    b. heparin.
    c. nothing.
    d. silica.

94. In an infant's heel, the area of the vascular bed that is rich in capillary loops is located:
    a. between 0.35 and 0.82 mm deep.
    b. from 1.00 mm to 2.00 mm deep.
    c. in the top layer of the epidermis.
    d. starting at around 2.4 mm deep.

95. Which of the following is *not* a correct capillary puncture technique?
    a. Discard equipment packaging in the regular trash.
    b. Position the site downward to promote blood flow.
    c. Press the lancet down into the skin so it does not slip.
    d. Tap microtubes gently to settle blood to the bottom.

ANSWERS AND EXPLANATIONS

1. Answer: a
Why: "Arterialized" is a term used to describe a capillary blood specimen in which the arterial content has been increased by warming the site prior to collection. Warming increases arterial composition of a specimen because it increases arterial blood flow into the area. Although an arterialized specimen more closely resembles an arterial specimen than one that has not been arterialized, oxygen levels and other components would not be exactly the same. Venous blood flows away from the area, not into it.
Review: Yes ☐ No ☐

2. Answer: a
Why: A blood smear or film is a drop of blood spread on a glass microscope slide. Blood smears can be made from fresh blood or blood collected in EDTA, depending on the test requested. A manual differential is the most common reason a blood smear is made. A differential is used to identify and count the different types of cells in a blood smear. Blood collected on a special type of filter paper is required for most newborn screening tests.
Review: Yes ☐ No ☐

3. Answer: c
Why: "Calcaneus" is the medical term for the heel bone. Finger bones, including the thumb, are called phalanges (singular, phalanx). The earlobe is cartilage, not bone.
Review: Yes ☐ No ☐

4. Answer: b
Why: Capillary blood gases (CBGs) are collected to assess levels of blood components such as oxygen, carbon dioxide, and pH, which are measures of pulmonary function.
Review: Yes ☐ No ☐

5. Answer: b
Why: Cyanotic means "marked by cyanosis or bluish in color from lack of oxygen"; consequently, a cyanotic extremity looks bluish in color. Jaundiced skin would be a deep yellow color. Erythema is redness.
Review: Yes ☐ No ☐

6. Answer: b
Why: A differential determines the type and characteristics of WBCs, RBC morphology, and an estimate of the platelet count. Packed cell volume (PCV) is another name for hematocrit (HCT), which is part of a complete blood count (CBC), but not part of a differential.
Review: Yes ☐ No ☐

7. Answer: d
Why: A properly made routine blood film or smear shows a smooth transition from thick to thin. The thinnest area of the film is only one cell thick and is called the feather because of its appearance when held up to the light. The feather is the area where a manual differential is performed.
Review: Yes ☐ No ☐

8. Answer: a
Why: Interstitial means "pertaining to spaces between tissues." Consequently, fluid in the spaces between the cells is called interstitial fluid. Intracellular fluid is the fluid within cells. The fluid in the lymphatic system is called lymph. Lymph is derived from excess tissue fluid, and is similar to, but not the same as, interstitial fluid. Peritoneal fluid is found in the abdominal cavity.
Review: Yes ☐ No ☐

9. Answer: b
Why: The typical lancet is a sterile, disposable, sharp-pointed or bladed device used to puncture or make an incision in the skin to obtain

a capillary blood specimen. A laser lancet, which does not have a sharp point or blade, vaporizes water in the skin to make a small hole in the capillary bed. A scalpel should never be used for capillary puncture because puncture depth cannot be controlled. A microcollection container is sometimes called a bullet because it resembles one.

Review: Yes ☐ No ☐

10. Answer: a

Why: Capillary puncture blood is a mixture of arterial blood (from arterioles), venous blood (from venules), and capillary blood, along with interstitial and intracellular fluids from the surrounding tissues.

Review: Yes ☐ No ☐

11. Answer: a

Why: Microhematocrit tubes are thin, narrow-bore, disposable plastic or plastic-clad glass tubes that fill by capillary action. They are most commonly used to collect and perform manual hematocrit (HCT) tests. An HCT is also called a packed cell volume (PCV) test. Some microhematocrit tubes are coated with ammonium heparin, not lithium heparin.

Review: Yes ☐ No ☐

12. Answer: c

Why: The fingers identified by letters C and D in Fig. 10-1 are the middle and ring fingers, which are the recommended fingers to use for capillary puncture (See Fig. 10-5).

Review: Yes ☐ No ☐

13. Answer: d

Why: Osteochondritis means "inflammation of the bone and cartilage." It can be the result of capillary punctures that are too deep.

Review: Yes ☐ No ☐

14. Answer: d

Why: Plantar means "concerning the sole or bottom of the foot." Distal means "farthest from the center of the body, origin, or point of attachment." Dorsal means "to the back of the body." Lateral means "toward the side of the body."

Review: Yes ☐ No ☐

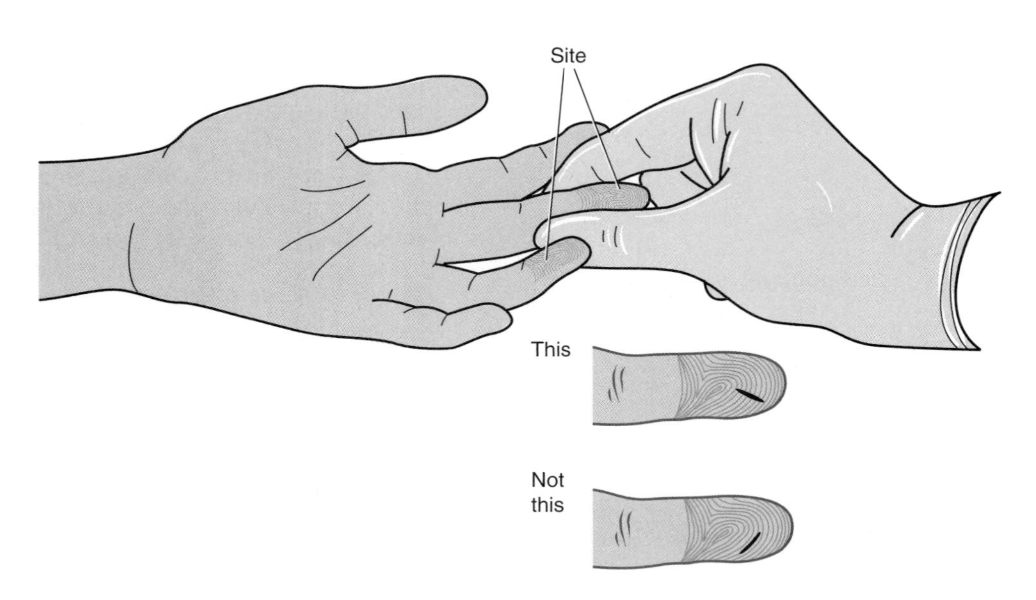

FIGURE 10-5 Recommended site and direction of finger puncture.

15. Answer: d
    Why: Whorls are circular or spiral patterns formed by the lines of the fingerprint.
    Review: Yes ☐ No ☐

16. Answer: b
    Why: To prevent burning the patient, heel warmers and other material used to warm the collection site prior to capillary puncture should provide a uniform temperature that does not exceed 42°C.
    Review: Yes ☐ No ☐

17. Answer: d
    Why: The medical term for a finger or toe bone is phalanx (plural, phalanges). "Calcaneus" is the medical term for heel bone. "Clavicle" is the medical term for the shoulder bone. "Patella" is the medical term for the kneecap.
    Review: Yes ☐ No ☐

18. Answer: d
    Why: Capillary blood gas (CBG) specimens are collected in special long, thin narrow-bore plastic capillary tubes. They are generally 100 mm long with a capacity of 100 µL. They typically contain sodium heparin and are color-coded with a green band. Other equipment required includes a device to warm the site, stirrers and a magnet for mixing the specimen, and caps for both ends of the capillary tube so that the anaerobic condition of the specimen can be maintained. Capillary blood gas equipment is shown in Fig. 10-6.
    Review: Yes ☐ No ☐

19. Answer: b
    Why: Capillary specimens are a mixture of arterial and venous blood and tissue fluids that include interstitial fluid from the tissue spaces between the cells and intracellular fluid from within the cells. Serous fluids are pale yellow, watery fluids similar to serum that are found between double-layered membranes that line the pleural, pericardial, and peritoneal cavities.
    Review: Yes ☐ No ☐

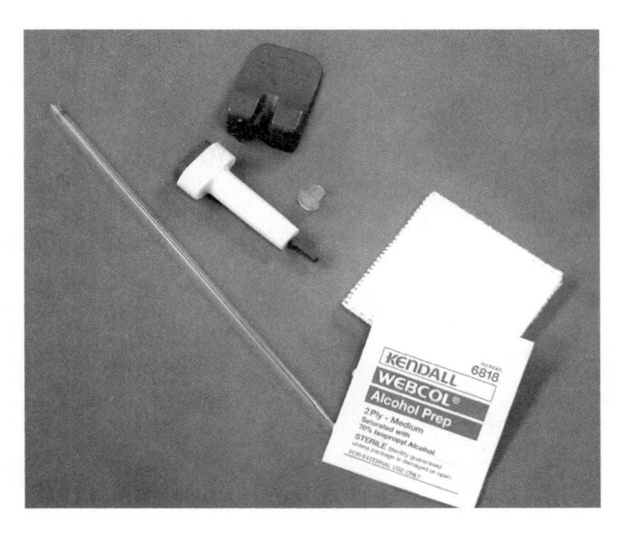

FIGURE 10-6 Capillary blood gas collection equipment.

20. Answer: c
    Why: According to Clinical and Laboratory Standards Institute (CLSI) standards, the safest areas for heel puncture are on the plantar surface of the heel, medial to an imaginary line extending from the middle of the great toe to the heel, or lateral to an imaginary line extending from between the fourth and fifth toes to the heel (Fig. 10-7). Punctures in other areas of an infant's foot risk bone, nerve, tendon, and cartilage injury.
    Review: Yes ☐ No ☐

21. Answer: c
    Why: Capillary puncture lancets should be sterile and disposable after a single use. They should also have puncture depths that are controlled, and blades or points that are permanently retractable for safety. Lancets are *not* color-coded by blade width.
    Review: Yes ☐ No ☐

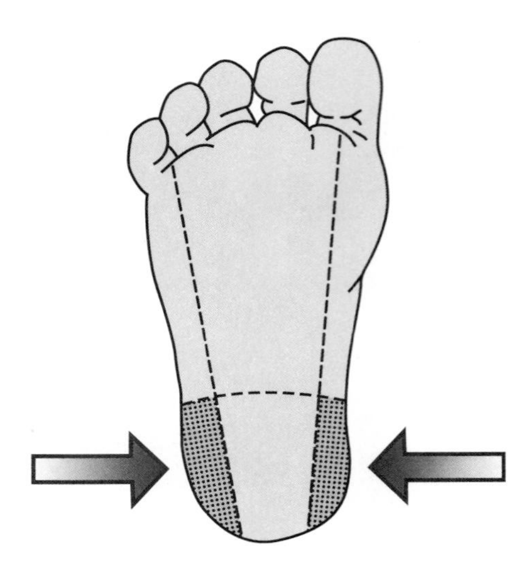

FIGURE 10-7 Infant foot. Shaded areas indicated by arrows represent recommended safe areas for heel puncture.

22. Answer: c
 Why: A plastic or plastic-clad glass microhematocrit tube (Fig. 10-8) is used to collect and perform a manual hematocrit (packed cell volume) test.
 Review: Yes ☐ No ☐

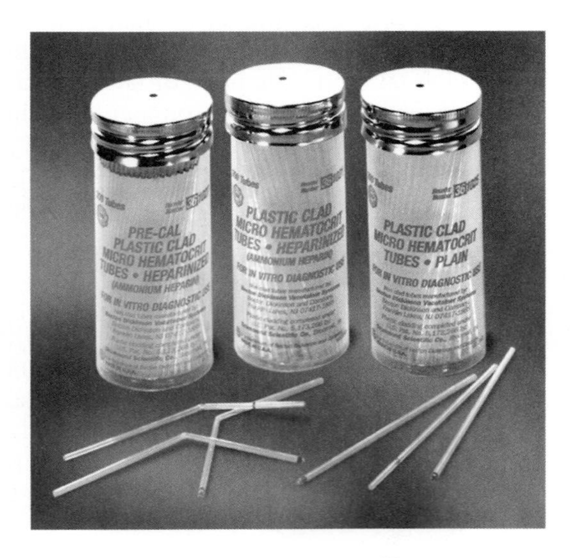

FIGURE 10-8 Microhematocrit tubes. (Courtesy Becton-Dickinson, Franklin Lakes, NJ.)

23. Answer: b
 Why: Capillary blood gas equipment (Fig. 10-6) typically includes a special long, thin capillary tube, a magnet and iron fillings (referred to as fleas) or metal bar to aid in mixing the specimen, and caps for sealing both ends of the tube.
 Review: Yes ☐ No ☐

24. Answer: d
 Why: The Becton Dickinson Unopette is an example of a micropipet dilution system. The system consists of a sealed plastic reservoir that contains a premeasured amount of diluting fluid; a detachable glass, self-filling capillary pipet; and a pipet shield, which also serves as a device to puncture the reservoir covering or diaphragm before adding the sample.
 Review: Yes ☐ No ☐

25. Answer: a
 Why: A microcollection container (microtube) is sometimes called a bullet because it resembles one. A flea is another name for a metal filing used to aid in mixing capillary blood gas specimens. Fleam is an old term for a type of lancet. A pipet is a special long narrow tube used to draw up fluid by suction.
 Review: Yes ☐ No ☐

26. Answer: a
 Why: Capillaries contain both venous and arterial blood. The percentage of arterial blood is higher, however, because arterial blood enters the capillaries under pressure. Consequently, the composition of blood obtained by capillary puncture more closely resembles arterial blood than venous blood. This is especially true if the area has been warmed, because warming increases arterial flow into the area.
 Review: Yes ☐ No ☐

27. Answer: a
 Why: Sometimes venous blood obtained by syringe during difficult draw situations is put into microcollection containers. When

this is done, it is important to label the specimen as venous. Otherwise, it will be assumed to be a skin puncture specimen, which may have different normal values.

Review: Yes ☐ No ☐

28. Answer: b
Why: Test results can vary depending on the source of the specimen. A laboratory report form should indicate that a specimen was collected by skin puncture, because skin puncture blood differs in composition from venous blood and may have different reference ranges for some tests.
Review: Yes ☐ No ☐

29. Answer: b
Why: Blood obtained by puncturing the skin with a lancet is called capillary blood because it comes from the area of the dermis that is rich in capillaries and referred to as the vascular or capillary bed.
Review: Yes ☐ No ☐

30. Answer: c
Why: Phenylketonuria (PKU) is a newborn screening test. PKU and most other newborn screening tests were designed to be performed on capillary blood and are typically performed on capillary specimens collected by heel puncture. CBCs can be performed on capillary specimens but are most commonly performed on venipuncture specimens. glucose tolerance tests (GTTs) are rarely performed on capillary specimens. PTTs are typically performed on venous specimens and are only performed on capillary specimens by using point-of-care testing equipment.
Review: Yes ☐ No ☐

31. Answer: b
Why: Reference values for glucose tests are higher for capillary puncture specimens. They are lower for calcium, phosphorus, and total protein.
Review: Yes ☐ No ☐

32. Answer: c
Why: Blood cultures cannot be collected by capillary puncture because of the volume of blood required for testing and contamination issues. The light blue top tube cannot be collected by capillary puncture because coagulation tests are greatly affected by tissue thromboplastin. Green top and purple top microtubes are available.
Review: Yes ☐ No ☐

33. Answer: a
Why: Infant bilirubin specimens are collected in amber microcollection containers (Fig. 10-3) to help protect them from light. Light breaks down bilirubin and leads to false low values.
Review: Yes ☐ No ☐

34. Answer: b
Why: Light blue top tubes cannot be collected by capillary puncture for coagulation tests that are performed later in the laboratory; consequently, there is no microcollection container that corresponds to a light blue top tube. There are, however, some point-of-care instruments that directly perform coagulation tests from capillary blood that is immediately placed in the instrument and tested.
Review: Yes ☐ No ☐

35. Answer: b
Why: Capillary puncture is generally *not* appropriate for patients who are dehydrated or have poor circulation to the extremities from other causes, such as a state of shock, because specimens may be hard to obtain and may not be representative of blood elsewhere in the body. Capillary puncture is actually a good choice for a patient with iatrogenic anemia, so that as little blood as possible is removed.
Review: Yes ☐ No ☐

36. Answer: a
    Why: The palmar surface of the distal or end segment of the middle or ring finger (Fig. 10-5) is the recommended site for routine skin puncture on an adult.
    Review: Yes ☐ No ☐

37. Answer: b
    Why: Capillary puncture is the preferred method to obtain blood from infants and children for several reasons. Restraining methods used during venipuncture can injure infants and children. They have such small blood volumes that removing larger quantities of blood typical of venipuncture can lead to anemia. Removal of more than 10% of an infant's blood volume at one time can lead to cardiac arrest. In addition, venipuncture in infants and children is difficult and may damage veins and surrounding tissues. Test results on capillary specimens are not more accurate than results on venous specimens.
    Review: Yes ☐ No ☐

38. Answer: a
    Why: Under normal circumstances, capillary puncture is not performed on an index finger. Like venipuncture, a capillary puncture can be performed below an IV. The lateral plantar surface of an infant's heel and the middle or ring finger of an adult are recommended capillary puncture sites.
    Review: Yes ☐ No ☐

39. Answer: b
    Why: The depth of lancet insertion must be controlled to avoid injuring the heel bone. The medical term for the heel bone is "calcaneus." Puncturing an artery or damaging tendons is avoided by puncturing in a recommended area. A deep puncture does not necessarily produce more bleeding.
    Review: Yes ☐ No ☐

40. Answer: b
    Why: Studies have shown that heel punctures deeper than 2.0 mm risk injuring the calcaneus, or heel bone. For this reason, the latest Clinical and Laboratory Standards Institute (CLSI) capillary puncture standard states that heel puncture depth should not exceed 2.0 mm.
    Review: Yes ☐ No ☐

41. Answer: c
    Why: A deep heel puncture can penetrate the calcaneus (heel bone), leading to painful osteomyelitis (inflammation of the bone including the marrow) or osteochondritis (inflammation of the bone and cartilage).
    Review: Yes ☐ No ☐

42. Answer: c
    Why: According to the Clinical and Laboratory Standards Institute (CLSI), the safest areas for performing heel puncture are on the plantar surface of the heel, medial to an imaginary line extending from the middle of the great (big) toe to the heel, or lateral to an imaginary line extending from between the fourth and fifth toes to the heel (Fig. 10-7). In other words, safe areas are on the medial or lateral plantar surface of the heel. Punctures should not be performed in the central portion of the heel or the posterior curvature of the heel because bone and cartilage injury can occur. All areas of the arch should be avoided because nerves and tendons can be injured. The big toe should not be punctured because it has an artery that could inadvertently be punctured.
    Review: Yes ☐ No ☐

43. Answer: c
    Why: The recommended site for capillary puncture on older children and adults (Fig. 10-5) is the pad (fleshy portion) of the

palmar surface of the distal or end segment of a middle or ring finger.

Review: Yes ☐ No ☐

44. Answer: d

Why: Capillary puncture releases tissue thromboplastin, which activates the coagulation process and leads to platelet clumping and microclot formation in specimens that are not collected quickly. This affects hematology specimens the most; consequently, they are collected first. Serum specimens are collected last because they are supposed to clot. In the order of draw for venipuncture, which was designed to minimize problems caused by additive carryover between tubes, serum specimens are collected before hematology specimens. Carryover is not an issue with capillary collection. Isopropyl alcohol is the recommended antiseptic for capillary puncture and routine venipuncture. Patient identification is the same regardless of specimen collection method. Additives in microcollection tubes and stopper colors correspond to those of evacuated tubes.

Review: Yes ☐ No ☐

45. Answer: a

Why: The distance between the skin surface and the bone in the end segment of the finger varies. It is less at the side and tip of the finger than at the center. It is thinnest in the fifth, or little, finger.

Review: Yes ☐ No ☐

46. Answer: a

Why: The major blood vessels of the skin are located at the dermal-subcutaneous junction, which in a newborn's heel is located between 0.35 and 1.6 mm below the surface of the skin (Fig. 10-9).

Review: Yes ☐ No ☐

47. Answer: a

Why: If a capillary puncture is made parallel to the whorls of the fingerprint (Fig. 10-5), blood will run down the grooves of the fingerprint rather than form round drops that are easy to collect. It will not bleed longer.

Review: Yes ☐ No ☐

48. Answer: a

Why: Blood cultures cannot be collected by capillary puncture because of the large volume of blood required. In addition, capillary blood is exposed to air during collection, which increases the possibility of contamination.

Review: Yes ☐ No ☐

49. Answer: c

Why: A bullet with a lavender stopper contains EDTA, which is the additive used to collect complete blood counts (CBCs).

Review: Yes ☐ No ☐

50. Answer: b

Why: A complete blood count (CBC) is a hematology test. When collected by capillary puncture, slides, platelet counts, and other hematology tests are collected first to avoid the effects of platelet aggregation (clumping) and microclot formation. Other anticoagulant containers are collected next, and serum specimens are collected last.

Review: Yes ☐ No ☐

51. Answer: b

Why: Warming the site before capillary puncture increases blood flow up to seven times. Warming is said to *arterialize* the specimen because it increases arterial blood flow into the area. Enhancing visibility of veins is *not* necessary for capillary puncture. Hemolysis is mainly caused by squeezing the site, puncturing before the alcohol is dry, or using the first drop of blood instead of wiping it away;

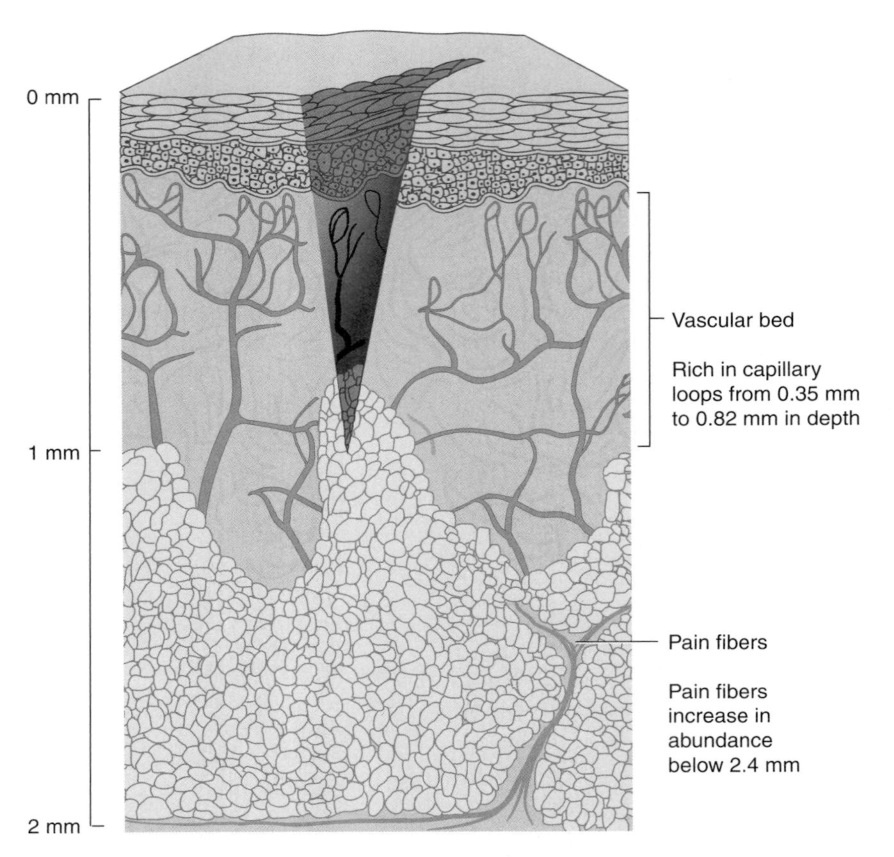

FIGURE 10-9 Cross-section of full-term infant's heel showing lancet penetration depth needed to access the capillary bed.

it and can happen regardless of whether or not the site was warmed.

Review: Yes ☐ No ☐

52. Answer: a

Why: Warming the site for 5 to 10 minutes to increase arterial blood flow into the area is an important step in the collection of capillary blood gas (CBG) specimens. This arterializes the specimen, which means it increases the arterial content and makes it more similar to arterial blood. A towel or diaper dampened with warm tap water can be used to warm the site; however, care must be taken not to get the water too hot, or the patient may be scalded. Special warming devices (Fig. 10-10) that provide a uniform temperature that does not exceed 42°C are available. Warming the site before collecting other specimens is done to make collection easier, not for accuracy of results.

Review: Yes ☐ No ☐

53. Answer: a

Why: The Clinical and Laboratory Standards Institute (CLSI) recommends using 70% isopropyl alcohol (isopropanol or ETOH) to cleaning capillary puncture sites.

Review: Yes ☐ No ☐

54. Answer: d

Why: The antiseptic used to clean a capillary puncture site is isopropyl alcohol. If the site is

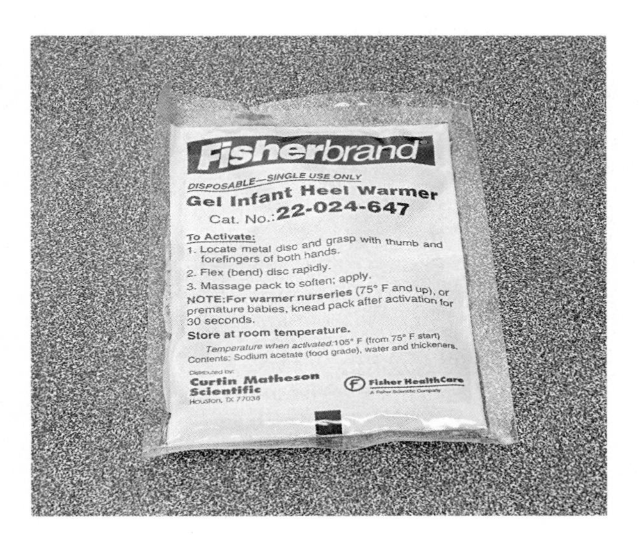

FIGURE 10-10 Infant heel warmer.

not completely dry before capillary puncture, alcohol residue can cause hemolysis of the specimen and lead to erroneous test results.

Review: Yes ☐ No ☐

55. Answer: a

Why: Povidone-iodine contamination of capillary puncture blood has been shown to cause erroneous results for uric acid, phosphorus, and potassium tests.

Review: Yes ☐ No ☐

56. Answer: c

Why: Errors in glucose results have been attributed to isopropyl alcohol (isopropanol) contamination of the specimen. Deep punctures can injure bone but do not affect test results. The first drop of blood should be wiped away (Fig. 10-4) to eliminate alcohol residue and tissue fluid contamination. Errors in glucose results have not been attributed to warming the site.

Review: Yes ☐ No ☐

57. Answer: b

Why: Finger sticks should be made perpendicular to the whorls or grooves of the fingerprint (Fig. 10-5) so that the blood forms round drops (Fig. 10-11) that can be collected easily. A puncture parallel to the whorls allows the blood to run down the finger and makes collection difficult.

Review: Yes ☐ No ☐

58. Answer: c

Why: Blood cells contain potassium. Residual alcohol can hemolyze blood cells, releasing potassium into the liquid portion of the specimen, erroneously elevating potassium results.

Review: Yes ☐ No ☐

59. Answer: b

Why: It is important to wipe away the first drop of blood during capillary puncture (Fig. 10-4) because excess tissue fluid that is typically found in the first drop can affect test results. Omitting the first drop from the sample also eliminates alcohol residue that can keep the blood from forming well-rounded drops, and also hemolyze the specimen.

Review: Yes ☐ No ☐

60. Answer: b

Why: Scooping or scraping up blood that runs down the finger is *not* proper technique because it introduces contamination, activates platelets, and can cause hemolysis of the specimen. Correct technique includes touching the tube's scoop to the drop of

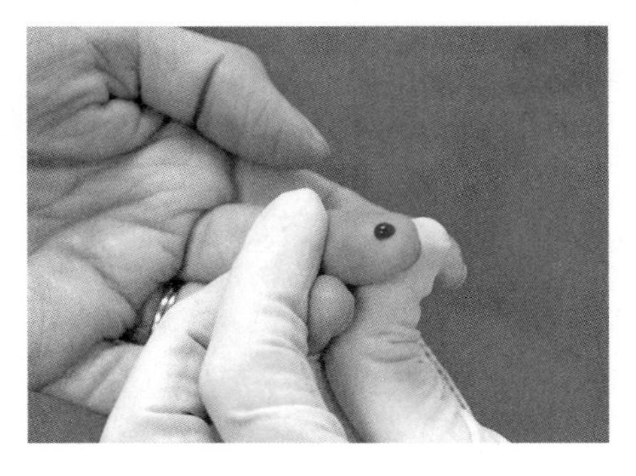

FIGURE 10-11 Round blood drop forming at the puncture site.

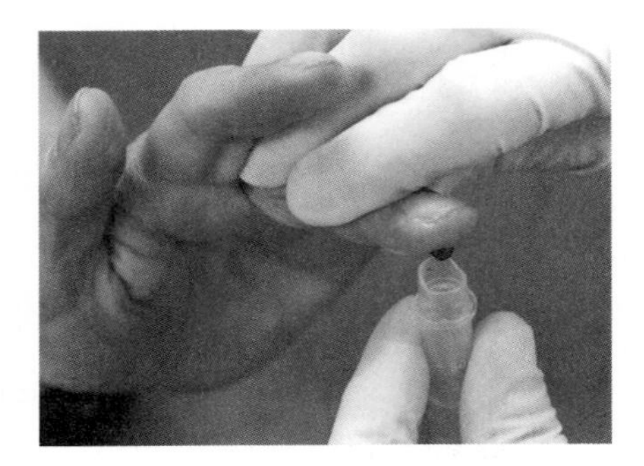

FIGURE 10-12 Touching the scoop of a microtube to a drop of blood.

blood (Fig.10-12) and letting the blood run down the inside of the tube. An occasional tap of the tube may be necessary to settle the blood to the bottom of the tube.

Review: Yes ☐ No ☐

61. Answer: d
Why: Collecting the first drop instead of wiping it away, pressing hard on the site, and squeezing the site can all introduce excess tissue fluid into the specimen and affect test results, and can also cause hemolysis. Wiping the alcohol dry can contaminate the site and is *not* recommended technique but does *not* affect the tissue fluid level in the specimen.
Review: Yes ☐ No ☐

62. Answer: c
Why: Microtubes contain a proper amount of anticoagulant for the recommended fill level. If a microtube is overfilled, there is not enough anticoagulant for the increased volume of blood, which can result in the formation of microclots, or complete clotting of the specimen. A specimen should be mixed as soon as possible after collection. Mixing a specimen forcefully can cause hemolysis. Underfilling a tube can result in excess anticoagulant for the volume of blood, which can cause distortion of the cells.
Review: Yes ☐ No ☐

63. Answer: a
Why: Blood smears and EDTA specimens are obtained before other specimens to minimize the effects of platelet aggregation (clumping). When tissue is disrupted by skin puncture, the coagulation process is set in motion and platelets start to aggregate (stick or clump together) and adhere to the site to seal off the injury. This can lead to erroneously low platelet counts. Platelets are evaluated and their numbers estimated as part of a differential performed on a blood smear. A platelet count is part of a complete blood count performed on an EDTA specimen.
Review: Yes ☐ No ☐

64. Answer: a
Why: A manual differential is performed on a stained blood smear. A neonatal bilirubin test is typically performed on serum collected in an amber microtube or bullet. Most newborn screening tests involve the collection of blood in circles on special filter paper. A manual packed cell volume (PCV) or hematocrit (HCT) is collected in a microhematocrit tube.
Review: Yes ☐ No ☐

65. Answer: c
Why: An acceptable smear (Fig. 10-13) will cover about one half to three fourths of the surface of the slide and have the appearance of a feather, in that there will be a smooth gradient from thick to thin when held up to the light. The thinnest area of a properly made smear, often referred to as the "feather," is one cell thick and is the most important area because that is where a differential is performed.
Review: Yes ☐ No ☐

66. Answer: d
Why: A blood smear prepared from an EDTA specimen should be made within 1 hour of collection to prevent cell distortion caused by prolonged contact with the anticoagulant.
Review: Yes ☐ No ☐

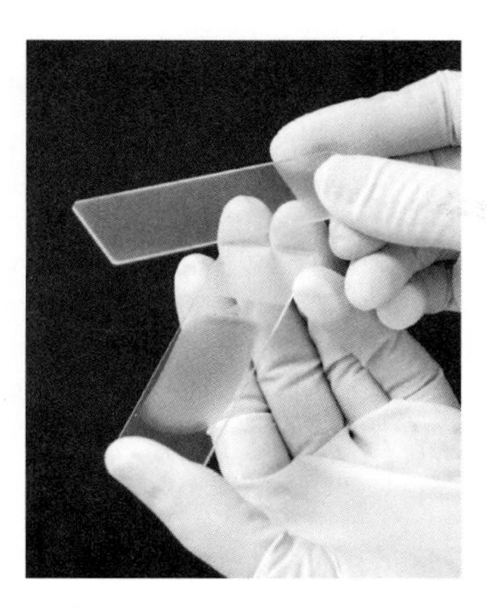

FIGURE 10-13 Completed blood smear.

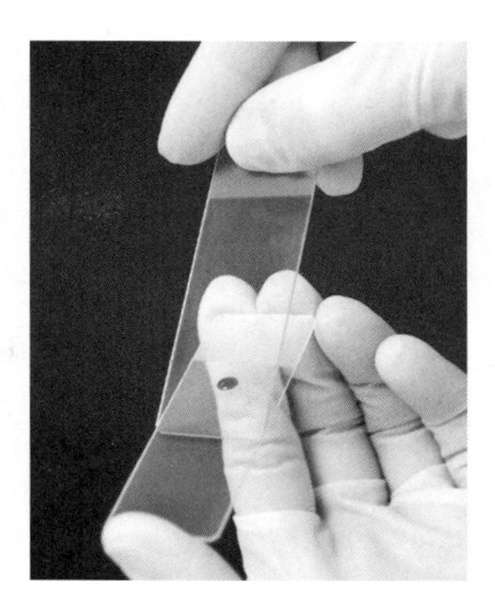

FIGURE 10-14 Drop of blood on slide with pusher slide placed in front.

67. Answer: c
    Why: When a blood smear is prepared using the two-slide method, one slide holds the drop used to make the smear and a second slide, placed on the first slide at an angle of approximately 30° (Fig. 10-14), is used to spread the drop of blood across the slide and create the blood film.
    Review: Yes ☐ No ☐

68. Answer: a
    Why: Blood smears that are too long or too short are not acceptable. The length of a blood smear can be controlled by adjusting the angle of the spreader slide or the size of the drop of blood. If a smear is too short, decreasing the angle of the spreader slide or using a larger drop of blood on the next attempt should result in a longer smear. Exerting more pressure will only distort the smear. Increasing the angle of the spreader slide or using a smaller drop will make an even shorter smear.
    Review: Yes ☐ No ☐

69. Answer: a
    Why: Dirt or fingerprints on the slide and fat globules or lipids in the specimen can result in holes in a blood smear. Blood with a low hemoglobin level may be thin and require a smaller drop or adjustment of the pusher slide to create a proper smear, but it will *not* cause holes in a blood smear.
    Review: Yes ☐ No ☐

70. Answer: c
    Why: Malaria can be caused by any of four different species of microorganisms called plasmodia. It is diagnosed by detecting the presence of plasmodia organisms in a peripheral blood smear. Diagnosis typically requires the evaluation of both regular and thick blood smears. Presence of the organism is observed most frequently in a thick smear; however, identification of the species requires evaluation of a regular blood smear.
    Review: Yes ☐ No ☐

71. Answer: a
    Why: Capillary blood gases are commonly collected in a heparinized capillary tube. After the specimen is collected, one end of the tube is immediately sealed and iron filings, often called "fleas," or a metal bar are inserted into the specimen. The other end of the tube is then quickly sealed to prevent

posure to air. Next the specimen is mixed y running a magnet along the outside of the tube. The magnet drags the fleas or metal bar back and forth, mixing the specimen with the heparin to prevent clotting.

Review: Yes ☐ No ☐

72. Answer: b
Why: Capillary blood gases (CBGs) are less dangerous to collect than arterial blood gases (ABGs). However, CBG results are *not* as accurate as ABG results because of the partial arterial composition of capillary blood and because the open system of collection temporarily exposes the specimen to air, which can affect test results.
Review: Yes ☐ No ☐

73. Answer: a
Why: Bilirubin can cross the blood–brain barrier in infants, accumulating to toxic levels that can cause permanent brain damage or even death. A transfusion may be needed if levels increase at a rate equal to or greater than 5 mg/dL per hour or when levels exceed 18 mg/dL.
Review: Yes ☐ No ☐

74. Answer: c
Why: Phenylketonuria (PKU) is a hereditary disorder caused by an inability to metabolize the amino acid phenylalanine. Patients with PKU lack the enzyme necessary to convert phenylalanine to tyrosine. Phenylalanine accumulates in the blood and can rise to toxic levels. PKU cannot be cured, but it can normally be treated with a diet low in phenylalanine. If left untreated or if not treated early on, PKU can lead to brain damage and mental deficiences.
Review: Yes ☐ No ☐

75. Answer: b
Why: Newborn screening is the term used to describe testing of newborns for the presence of genetic, or inherited, diseases such as galactosemia (GALT), congenital hypothyroidism (CH), homocystinuria (HCY), maple syrup urine disease (MSUD), phenylketonuria (PKU), and sickle cell disease (Hb SS). The March of Dimes recommends the screening of all newborns for 29 specific disorders, including hearing loss (Table 10-1). Bilirubin, hemoglobin and hematocrit (H & H), and white blood cell (WBC) counts may be performed on newborns but are not screening tests.
Review: Yes ☐ No ☐

76. Answer: b
Why: Bilirubin is broken down in the presence of light. Collecting the specimen too slowly or failing to protect the specimen from light after collection allows the specimen to be exposed to light for longer than necessary and leads to falsely decreased results.
Review: Yes ☐ No ☐

77. Answer: d
Why: Isopropyl alcohol is the recommended antiseptic for cleaning prior to capillary puncture, including heel punctures performed to collect PKU specimens. PKU specimens are collected by placing large drops of blood within circles on special filter paper that is typically part of the test requisition (Fig. 10-15). Using the first drop of blood can contaminate an entire blood spot with tissue fluid and lead to erroneous results. Blood spots can also be contaminated by touching the circles with hands (with or without gloves) before, during, or after specimen collection. Stacking filter paper requisitions together after collection can lead to cross-contamination between different patient specimens.
Review: Yes ☐ No ☐

78. Answer: d
Why: Newborn screening blood spots must be collected properly to prevent erroneous results. Applying blood to both sides of the

Table 10-1 March of Dimes Recommended Newborn Screening Tests by Category

Disorder Category	Description	Consequence if Untreated	Screening Tests
Organic acid metabolism disorders	Inherited disorders resulting from inactivity of an enzyme involved in the breakdown of amino acids and other body substances such as lipids, sugars, and steroids	Toxic acids build up in the body and can lead to coma and death within the first month of life,	IVA (isovaleric-acidemia) GA I (glutaric acidemia) HMG (3-OH3-CH_3-glutaric aciduria) MCD (multiple carboxylase deficiency) MUT (methylmalonic acidemia from mutase deficiency) Cbl A, B (methylmalonic acidemia) 3MCC (3-methylcrotonyl-CoA carboxylase deficiency) PROP (propionic acidemia) BKT (beta-ketothiolase deficiency)
Fatty acid oxidation disorders	Disorders involving inherited defects in enzymes that are needed to convert fat into energy	The body is unable to produce alternate fuel when it runs out of glucose as can happen with illness or skipping meals. Glucose deprivation negatively affects the brain and other organs, and can lead to coma and death,	MCAD (medium-chain acyl-CoA dehydrogenase deficiency) VLCAD (very long-chain acyl-CoA dehydrogenase deficiency) LCHAD (long-chain L-3-OH-acyl-CoA dehydrogenase deficiency) TFP (trifunctional protein deficiency) CUD (carnitine uptake defect)
Amino acid metabolism disorders	A diverse group of disorders. Some involve lack of an enzyme needed to breakdown an amino acid. Others involve deficiencies of enzymes that aid in the elimination of nitrogen from amino acid molecules	Toxic levels of amino acids of ammonia can build up in the body, causing a variety of symptoms and even death. Severity of symptoms varies by disorder,	PKU (phenylketonuria) MSUD (maple syrup urine disease) HCY (homocystinuria) CIT (citrullinemia) ASA (argininosuccinic acidemia) TYR (tyrosinemia type I)
Hemoglo-binopathies	Inherited disorders of the red blood cells that result in varying degrees of anemia and other health problems	Anemias that vary in severity by disorder and by individual,	Hb SS (sickle cell anemia) Hb S/Th (hemoglobin S/beta thalassemia) Hb S/C (hemoglobin S/C disease)

Newborn Screening SPECIMEN NM
1067723014
DO NOT WRITE IN THIS SPACE

Baby's Last Name: | Baby's First Name: | PCP Name: | CODE:
PCP Phone Number:
( ) Single Birth, or ( ) Multi-Birth A B C D E F Circle One
Birth Date: (_ _/_ _/_ _) | Time of Day: (:) 24 hr am pm | Birth Wt.: Lbs. oz ____ gms
Sex: M F | ID Chart #:
Food Source Last 24 Hours: (Check all that apply) 4 Breast 3 Soy Formula 5 NPO 6 Lactose Formula 7 Tube Feeding 0 Other ______
Specimen Date: (_ _/_ _/_ _) | Time of Day: (:) 24 hr am pm | Present Wt.: Lbs. oz ____ gms
Baby's Race: 1 White 2 Black 3 Amer. Ind./Alaskan Native 9 Unknown/Other 0 Asian/Pacific Islander | Hispanic? No Yes
Other Factors: ☐ Hyperalimentation ☐ Transfused | Last RBC Transfusion Date / /
Mother's Last Name: | First Name: | Mother's Birth Date: / /
Hosp. or Hosp. CODE:
Mother's Address-Number & Street:
City: | State: | Zip Code:
Specimen Collected by: ______
Telephone Number: | 2nd Telephone Contact: Name: ______ Number: ______
Mother's Maiden Name:

AVOID HANDLING COLLECTION AREA
EXPIRES 1-1-2011
Whatman 903®
LOT # W-051
NM1067723014
COMPLETELY FILL IN ALL CIRCLES WITH BLOOD.
BE SURE THAT BLOOD SOAKS COMPLETELY THROUGH FILTER PAPER.

2nd Newborn Screening SPECIMEN NM
2067723014
DO NOT WRITE IN THIS SPACE

Baby's Last Name: | Baby's First Name: | PCP Name: | CODE:
Address:
( ) Single Birth, or ( ) Multi-Birth A B C D E F Circle One
PCP Phone Number:
Sex: M F | ID Chart #:
Birth Date: (_ _/_ _/_ _) | Time of Day: (:) 24 hr am pm | Birth Wt.: Lbs. oz ____ gms
Food Source Last 24 Hours: (Check all that apply) 4 Breast 3 Soy Formula 5 NPO 6 Lactose Formula 7 Tube Feeding 0 Other ______
Specimen Date: (_ _/_ _/_ _) | Time of Day: (:) 24 hr am pm | Present Wt.: Lbs. oz ____ gms
Other Factors: ☐ Hyperalimentation ☐ Transfused | Last RBC Transfusion Date / /
Mother's Last Name: | Mother's First Name:
Hosp. or Hosp. CODE:
Mother's Maiden Name:
2nd Telephone Contact: Name: ______
Specimen Collected by: ______ | Number: ______

AVOID HANDLING COLLECTION AREA
EXPIRES 1-1-2011
Whatman 903®
LOT # W-051
NM2067723014
COMPLETELY FILL IN ALL CIRCLES WITH BLOOD
BE SURE THAT BLOOD SOAKS COMPLETELY THROUGH FILTER PAPER.

FIGURE 10-15 Newborn screening forms. A. First specimen form. B. Second specimen form. (Courtesy Brenda Romero RN, BSN, State of New Mexico Genetic and Newborn Screening program, Santa Fe, NM.)

filter paper or layering successive drops in the same circle increase the amount of blood in the test area and can lead to erroneously increases results. Hanging specimens to dry can cause the blood to migrate and concentrate toward the lower end of the filter paper. This leaves the upper areas of the circle with less blood and the lower areas with more blood than required for testing. In this case, the results will be erroneous on any area that is used for testing. Letting one large drop of blood entirely fill a circle is correct procedure.

Review: Yes ☐ No ☐

79. Answer: d

Why: Newborn screening to detect PKU, galactosemia (GALT), and hypothyroidism is required by law in all 50 states in the United States.

Review: Yes ☐ No ☐

80. Answer: a
Why: High levels of bilirubin in the blood result in jaundice, a condition characterized by yellow color of the skin, whites of the eyes, mucous membranes, and body fluids.
Review: Yes ☐ No ☐

81. Answer: d
Why: Adhesive bandages can irritate the tender skin of infants, come off and become a choking hazard, or tear the skin when removed. Consequently, they should not be used on infants or children younger than 2 years of age. Adhesive bandages are not likely to become a source of contamination.
Review: Yes ☐ No ☐

82. Answer: c
Why: Heel puncture includes the following steps: (1) *warm* the site; (2) *clean* the site; (3) *puncture* the site, (4) *wipe* away the first blood drop, and (5) *collect* the specimen.
Review: Yes ☐ No ☐

83. Answer: a
Why: Capillary specimens should be handled gently, just like venous blood specimens. After capping, gentle inversions are required to adequately mix an anticoagulant bullet without hemolyzing red blood cells. Tapping the tube gently on a hard surface can be used to settle blood to the bottom of the tube during collection but is not adequate to mix the specimen. Tapping sharply can hemolyze the specimen. Rolling the specimen in the hands may not mix the specimen adequately.
Review: Yes ☐ No ☐

84. Answer: a
Why: Strong repetitive pressure such as squeezing or milking the site can contaminate a capillary specimen with excess tissue fluid and can also hemolyze the red blood cells and compromise test results. If adequate blood flow cannot be obtained without such action, a new puncture should be made at a different site. Venous blood flows out of the area, not into it.
Review: Yes ☐ No ☐

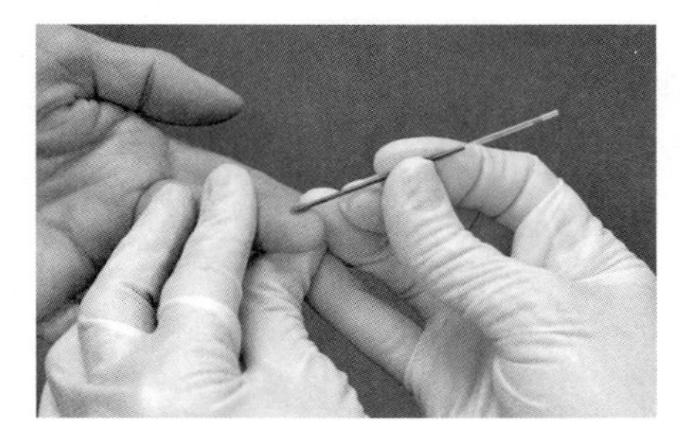

FIGURE 10-16 Filling an hematocrit tube by capillary action.

85. Answer: c
Why: Hematocrit tubes fill automatically when they come in contact with a drop of blood (Fig. 10-16) by a force called capillary action or attraction. Blood drops must be dripped onto filter paper circles for newborn screening tests and into microtubes or bullets regardless of the type or stopper color.
Review: Yes ☐ No ☐

86. Answer: b
Why: A laser lancet is a reusable device that vaporizes water in the skin to make a small hole in the capillary bed. Because no sharp instrument is involved, there is no risk of accidental injury and no sharp to discard. Although the device is reusable, single-use disposable inserts are used with it to prevent cross-contamination between patients. Heel warmers, metal fleas used in CBG specimens, and microtubes are not reusable.
Review: Yes ☐ No ☐

87. Answer: c
Why: Used lancets must be disposed of in a sharps container even though the blades are permanently retractable.
Review: Yes ☐ No ☐

88. Answer: b
Why: Capillary puncture is generally not appropriate for patients who are dehydrated because specimens may be hard to obtain and results may not be representative of blood elsewhere in the body.
Review: Yes ☐ No ☐

89. Answer: a
Why: A bandage should not be applied to an infant or child younger than 2 years old because it can pose a choking hazard. In addition, bandage adhesive can stick to the paper thin skin of newborns and tear it when removed.
Review: Yes ☐ No ☐

90. Answer: b
Why: A blood smear must be allowed to air dry naturally. Blowing on it or waving it dries it too quickly, which can distort red blood cells and also introduce contaminants. A blood smear should not be placed in alcohol before it is stained.
Review: Yes ☐ No ☐

91. Answer: a
Why: Blood cultures cannot be collected by capillary puncture because the volume of blood required for the tests is too large and the open collection method increases the possibility of contamination. Electrolytes, hemoglobin, and lithium levels can all be collected by capillary puncture.
Review: Yes ☐ No ☐

92. Answer: c
Why: Newborn screening is the routine testing of newborns (neonates) for the presence of certain genetic (inherited), metabolic, hormonal, and functional disorders that can cause severe mental handicaps or other serious abnormalities if not detected and treated early. The disorders are not contagious and do not normally show symptoms at birth.
Review: Yes ☐ No ☐

93. Answer: b
Why: Most microhematocrit tubes are either plain, meaning they have no additive, or are coated with ammonium heparin. Color-coding does not correspond to ETS tubes or microtubes. Non-additive microhematocrit tubes have a blue band on one end; those containing heparin have a red band on one end.
Review: Yes ☐ No ☐

94. Answer: a
Why: The area of an infant's heel that is richest in capillary loop is located in the dermis between 0.35 and 0.82 mm deep (Fig. 10-9). Pain fibers increase in abundance below 2.4 mm.
Review: Yes ☐ No ☐

95. Answer: c
Why: Use only enough pressure to keep the lancet firmly against the skin. Pressing down hard on the lancet compresses the skin and can result in a deeper puncture than intended.
Review: Yes ☐ No ☐

CHAPTER 11

SPECIAL COLLECTIONS AND POINT-OF-CARE TESTING

➤ study tip

This chapter tests the ability to identify and describe special procedures and point-of-care testing (POCT), including the principle behind each test, steps and any timing involved, and any special supplies or equipment needed. Special procedures covered include collection of specimens for blood bank tests, blood cultures, coagulation tests, postprandial glucose tolerance tests, paternity testing, therapeutic drug monitoring, therapeutic phlebotomy, toxicology tests, and trace element tests. POCT covered includes bleeding time tests, coagulation monitoring, arterial blood gas and chemistry panels, cardiac tests, glucose and glycosylated hemoglobin, H & H, occult blood, pregnancy tests, skin tests, strep tests, and urinalysis.

overview

Most laboratory tests require blood specimens collected using routine venipuncture. Some tests, however, require special collection procedures. This chapter assesses knowledge of special procedures, including special preparation, equipment, handling, or timing. Phlebotomists must be able to identify special procedures and perform them correctly for accurate test results.

REVIEW QUESTIONS

Choose the BEST answer.

1. Forsenic toxicology is concerned with:
   a. deliberate, not accidental, toxin contact.
   b. legal consequences of toxin exposure.
   c. toxin contamination in water resources.
   d. treatment for the effects of the toxins.

2. TB test administration involves:
   a. applying pressure right after injection.
   b. checking for a reaction in 12 to 24 hours.
   c. cleaning the site with povidone-iodine.
   d. injecting the antigen just under the skin.

3. All of the following are urine drug screen patient collection requirements as defined by the NIDA EXCEPT:
   a. a proctor is required to be present at the collection time to verify the sample.
   b. appropriate labeling is not required because chain of custody is not needed.
   c. documentation must be carefully maintained from courier to receiver.
   d. specimen must be sealed and placed in a locked container during transport.

4. The correct order when collecting a blood culture is:
   a. cleanse bottle tops, select equipment, perform friction scrub, perform venipuncture.
   b. perform friction scrub, select equipment, perform venipuncture, cleanse bottle tops.
   c. select equipment, cleanse bottle tops, perform friction scrub, perform venipuncture.
   d. select equipment, perform friction scrub cleanse bottle tops, perform venipuncture.

5. False-positive results of lactose tolerance tests have been found in all of the following EXCEPT:
   a. congenital cystic fibrosis.
   b. male multiple myeloma.
   c. patients with flat glucose tolerance test GTTs.
   d. slow gastric emptying.

6. If an assumed parent in a paternity case is *not* excluded by ABO grouping, any of the following testing may be required EXCEPT:
   a. buccal sample for DNA.
   b. human leukocyte antigen.
   c. red blood cell indices.
   d. white blood cell enzymes.

7. All of the following are allowed to order paternity testing EXCEPT a:
   a. child support agent.
   b. child who is a minor.
   c. defense attorney.
   d. family physician.

8. What is the recommended blood culture site disinfectant for infants 2 months and older?
   a. isopropyl alcohol swab
   b. chlorhexidine gluconate
   c. benzalkonium chloride
   d. Povidone-iodine swab

9. All of the following statements about autologous donations are true EXCEPT:
   a. blood can be collected up to 72 hours before surgery.
   b. patients must have a written order from their physician.
   c. unused autologous units may be used by other patients.
   d. using the patient's own blood eliminates many risks.

10. The CPD additive in a donor unit of blood serves to do all of the following EXCEPT:
    a. control bacterial contamination.
    b. prevent the blood from clotting.
    c. provide nutrition for the cells.
    d. stabilize the pH of the plasma.

11. A transfusion of incompatible blood is often fatal because it:
    a. causes a major allergic reaction, releasing too much histamine.
    b. causes lysis, or rupturing, of red cells within the vascular system.
    c. overwhelms the patient's lungs with nonfunctioning red cells.
    d. results in hemochromatosis in the patient's circulatory system.

12. When using a cell salvaging procedure during surgery, what analyte must be evaluated before the patient's blood can be re-infused?
    a. chemical toxins
    b. free hemoglobulin
    c. plasma glucose
    d. white cell count

13. All of the following are donor unit collection principles EXCEPT the:
    a. additives EDTA and sodium fluoride are contained in the collection bag.
    b. collection bag is placed on a mixing unit while the blood is being drawn.
    c. collection unit is a closed system connected to a tube and 16–18g needle.
    d. unit is filled by weight, which normally corresponds to 450 mL when full.

14. You are asked to collect the blood specimen on a patient undergoing a D-xylose test. What type of tube would most likely be required?
    a. gray top
    b. green top
    c. white top
    d. yellow top

15. Some individuals lack the necessary mucosal enzyme to convert which of the following sugars so that it can be digested?
    a. glucose
    b. glucagon
    c. lactose
    d. pentose

16. All of the following instructions are given to a patient when preparing for D-xylose testing EXCEPT:
    a. do not eat any kind of fruit for 3 days prior.
    b. drink 1 gallon of water per day for 3 days prior.
    c. fast after midnight the day of the procedure.
    d. remain fasting for 5 hours until the test is finished.

17. Which of the following sample types is used in D-xylose testing?
    a. feces
    b. saliva
    c. sweat
    d. urine

18. Potassium plays a major role in all of the following EXCEPT:
    a. muscle function.
    b. nerve conduction.
    c. osmotic pressure.
    d. transporting Hgb.

19. Which test is used to diagnose failure of the small intestine to absorb nutrients?
    a. 2-hour postprandial
    b. D-xylose absorpton
    c. glucose tolerance
    d. lactose tolerance

20. ARD or FAN blood culture bottles:
    a. detect problems in carbohydrate metabolism.
    b. eliminate vital interference from blood cells.
    c. remove any antibiotics that are in the blood.
    d. treat bloodborne pathogens in the circulation.

21. Septicemia is:
    a. a positive test for transmissible disease.
    b. bacteria measurement in whole blood.
    c. fever in which the cause is not known.
    d. microorganisms found in the blood.

22. The MedPoint Transfusion System is a:
    a. management system for IV therapy during transfusions.
    b. plasma/low hemoglobin point-of-care analyzer system.
    c. portable bedside barcode scanning system and printer.
    d. special ID bracelet having a self-carbon adhesive label.

23. Eligibility requirements for donating blood include:
    a. age 17–66 years, 110 lb or more.
    b. age 18–75 years, 110 lb or more.
    c. 21–65 years old, at least 100 lb.
    d. minimum of 21 years old, 100 lb.

24. Identify the condition in which a unit of blood is withdrawn from a patient as a treatment.
    a. ABO incompatibility
    b. autologous donation
    c. hemochromatosis
    d. hemolytic anemia

25. Which specimen requires especially strict identification and labeling procedures?
    a. aldosterone
    b. crossmatch
    c. plasminogen
    d. valproic acid

26. All of the following are classified as drugs of abuse EXCEPT:
    a. amphetamines.
    b. cannabinoids.
    c. crack and ice.
    d. phenobarbital.

27. Donor units of blood are typically collected using needles that are:
    a. 16–18 gauge.
    b. 18–28 gauge.
    c. 20–22 gauge.
    d. 23–25 gauge.

28. A typical unit of donated blood contains approximately:
    a. 250 mL.
    b. 450 mL.
    c. 750 mL.
    d. 1.00 L.

29. Which of the following tests is collected from patients with FUO to rule out septicemia?
    a. blood cultures times two
    b. nasopharyngeal culture
    c. urine culture and sensitivity
    d. wound and skin culture

30. All of the following types of tubes can be used to collect blood for a type and screen EXCEPT:
    a. large gel-barrier tube.
    b. lavender colored top.
    c. non-additive red top.
    d. pink stopper EDTA.

31. Which of the following tests is collected using special skin decontamination procedures?
    a. blood urea nitrogen
    b. complete blood count
    c. set of blood cultures
    d. type and crossmatch

32. Which type of test is performed to determine the probability that a specific individual was the father of a particular child?
    a. coagulation
    b. crossmatch
    c. paternity
    d. RBC indices

33. Why would blood cultures be collected with an antimicrobial adsorbing resin?
    a. the patient has fever spikes
    b. the patient is taking a broad-spectrum antibiotic

c. to eliminate contaminating normal flora
d. to remove bacteria-caused contamination

34. Which specimen tubes must contain a 9:1 ratio of blood to anticoagulant to be accepted for testing?
a. blood bank
b. chemistry
c. coagulation
d. hematology

35. What type of additive is best for collecting an ethanol specimen?
a. CPD + adenine
b. potassium EDTA
c. sodium citrate
d. sodium fluoride

36. Which blood culture container is inoculated first when the specimen has been collected by syringe?
a. aerobic media
b. anaerobic vial
c. ARD container
d. it does not matter

37. The most critical aspect of blood culture collection is:
a. needle gauge.
b. skin antisepsis.
c. specimen handling.
d. volume collected.

38. A blood culture collection site can typically be cleaned with any of the following EXCEPT:
a. chlorhexidene gluconate.
b. povidone-iodine.
c. sodium hypochlorite.
d. tincture of iodine.

39. Which of the following additives is sometimes used to collect blood culture specimens?
a. ACD
b. CPD
c. EDTA
d. SPS

40. Which type of specimen may require collection of a discard tube before the test specimen is collected?
a. blood culture
b. coagulation
c. drug testing
d. paternity

41. This is an abbreviation for a test that evaluates platelet plug formation in the capillaries.
a. ACT
b. BT
c. CBC
d. PT

42. Which test is used as a screening test for glucose metabolism problems?
a. 2-hour PP
b. GTT
c. lactose
d. WBG

43. All of the following activities can affect glucose tolerance test (GTT) results EXCEPT:
a. chewing sugarless gum.
b. drinking tea without sugar.
c. lying down during the test.
d. smoking low-tar cigarettes.

44. When does the timing of specimen collection begin during a glucose tolerance test (GTT)?
a. after the fasting blood specimen has been collected
b. as soon as the patient begins to drink the beverage
c. before the fasting blood specimen is to be collected
d. when the patient has finished the glucose beverage

45. A phlebotomist arrives to collect a 2-hour postprandial glucose specimen on an inpatient and discovers that 2 hours have not elapsed since the patient's meal. What should the phlebotomist do?
    a. Ask the patient's nurse to verify the correct collection time.
    b. Come back later at the time the patient tells you is correct.
    c. Draw the specimen and write the time collected on the label.
    d. Fill out an incident report form and return to the laboratory.

46. A patient undergoing a glucose tolerance test (GTT) vomits within 30 minutes of drinking the glucose beverage. What action should the phlebotomist take?
    a. Continue the test and note on the lab slip that the patient vomited and at what time.
    b. Discontinue the test and write on the requisition that the patient vomited the drink.
    c. Give the patient another dose of the glucose beverage and continue with the test.
    d. Notify the nurse or physician immediately to see if the test should be rescheduled.

47. Increased blood glucose is called:
    a. hyperglycemia.
    b. hyperinsulinism.
    c. hyperkalemia.
    d. hypernatremia.

48. When does a blood glucose level in normal individuals typically peak after glucose ingestion?
    a. 15 to 20 minutes
    b. $^1/_2$ hour to 1 hour
    c. 1 to $1^1/_2$ hours
    d. roughly 2 hours

49. Which of the following must remain consistent throughout an oral glucose tolerance test (OGTT)?
    a. arm used for the draw
    b. blood specimen source
    c. position of the patient
    d. size of ETS tubes used

50. Patient preparation before a GTT involves all of the following EXCEPT:
    a. a prescribed amount of exercise for 3 days prior.
    b. eating meals with measured carbohydrate 3 days prior.
    c. fasting for at least 12 hours before beginning the test.
    d. no smoking or chewing gum before or during the test.

51. Which of the following can be used to clean a site before blood alcohol specimen collection?
    a. diluted methanol
    b. isopropyl alcohol
    c. tincture of iodine
    d. Zephiran chloride

52. Which of the following may require "chain of custody" documentation when collected?
    a. blood culture
    b. crossmatch
    c. drug screen
    d. trace elements

53. The purpose of TDM is to:
    a. determine and maintain a beneficial drug dosage.
    b. maintain peak levels of drug in a patient's system.
    c. prevent trough levels of drug in a patient's system.
    d. screen for illegal drug use using multiple samples.

54. Which of the following tests would not be subject to therapeutic drug monitoring?
    a. digitoxin
    b. gentamicin
    c. phenylalanine
    d. theophylline

55. A peak drug level has been ordered for 0900 hours. You draw the specimen 10 minutes late because of unavoidable circumstances. What additional action does this necessitate?
    a. Draw two tubes for duplicate drug screening.
    b. Establish the last dosage time from the chart.
    c. Fill out a delay slip and leave with the desk clerk.
    d. Record the actual time of specimen collection.

56. A trough drug level is collected:
    a. 30 minutes after administration of the drug intravenously.
    b. immediately before the next scheduled drug dose is given.
    c. immediately after administration of the drug by the nurse.
    d. when the highest serum concentration of drug is expected.

57. Which test requires the collection of multiple specimens?
    a. ACT
    b. GTT
    c. HCT
    d. PTT

58. Timing of collection is most critical for drugs with short half-lives such as:
    a. digitoxin.
    b. gentamicin.
    c. methotrexate.
    d. phenobarbital.

59. A bleeding time (BT) test assesses the functioning of which of the following cellular elements?
    a. erythrocytes
    b. leukocytes
    c. neutrophils
    d. thrombocytes

60. The most common reason for glucose monitoring through point-of-care testing (POCT) is to:
    a. check for sporadic glucose in the urine.
    b. diagnose glucose metabolism problems.
    c. monitor glucose levels for diabetic care.
    d. control medication-induced mood swings.

61. A trace-element–free tube is the best choice for collecting a specimen for all of the following EXCEPT:
    a. copper.
    b. lead.
    c. sodium.
    d. zinc.

62. The definition of toxicology is:
    a. protocol for drug trafficking.
    b. scientific study of poisons.
    c. study of drug therapy levels.
    d. tracking of illicit drug trade.

63. Which test typically has the shortest TAT if performed by point-of-care testing (POCT)?
    a. BUN
    b. DNA
    c. GTT
    d. PSA

64. Which of the following is not a POCT analyzer?
    a. CoaguChek
    b. Hemochron Jr.
    c. IRMA system
    d. BactALERT

65. Monitoring blood coagulation through point-of-care testing may be performed during all of the following EXCEPT:
    a. cardiac bypass.
    b. coumadin therapy.
    c. heparin therapy.
    d. lithium therapy.

66. Which of the following is one of the most common bedside or POCT tests?
 a. bilirubin
 b. cholesterol
 c. glucose
 d. troponin

67. Which of the following tests is used to monitor heparin therapy?
 a. ACT
 b. BNP
 c. BT
 d. PT

68. Which of the following equipment is *not* needed for a bleeding time test?
 a. butterfly bandage
 b. incision template
 c. small stopwatch
 d. vinyl tourniquet

69. At what intervals is the blood blotted during a bleeding time test?
 a. 10 seconds
 b. 20 seconds
 c. 30 seconds
 d. 60 seconds

70. When performing the bleeding time test, a sphygmomanometer is inflated to:
 a. 20 mm Hg.
 b. 40 mm Hg.
 c. 60 mm Hg.
 d. 100 mm Hg.

71. All of the following will prolong a bleeding time test EXCEPT:
 a. allowing the pressure on a BP cuff to drop.
 b. an abnormally low post-op platelet count.
 c. recent ingestion of aspirin by the patient.
 d. touching the wound with the filter paper.

72. This test can determine if an individual has developed antibodies to a particular antigen.
 a. hematocrit
 b. skin test
 c. strep test
 d. troponin T

73. Ionized calcium plays a critical role in all of the following EXCEPT:
 a. blood clotting.
 b. cardiac function.
 c. glycosylation.
 d. nerve impulses.

74. Below-normal blood pH is referred to as:
 a. blood acidosis.
 b. blood alkalosis.
 c. hypokalemia.
 d. hyponatremia.

75. Which of the following is a protein that is specific to heart muscle?
 a. ALT
 b. BNP
 c. LDL
 d. TnT

76. B-type natriuretic peptide is a cardiac:
 a. antibody.
 b. enzyme.
 c. hormone.
 d. protein.

77. This test is used to evaluate long-term effectiveness of diabetes therapy.
 a. 2-hour postprandial
 b. glucose tolerance
 c. hemoglobin A1c
 d. random glucose

78. This test is also referred to as packed cell volume.
 a. ESR
 b. HCT
 c. Hgb
 d. HMT

79. This test detects occult blood.
 a. D-xylose
 b. guaiac

c. lactose
d. skin test

80. Which of the following is a skin test for tuberculosis exposure?
a. cocci
b. histo
c. PPD
d. Schick

81. The hormone detected in urine pregnancy testing is:
a. ACT
b. HCG
c. PPD
d. TSH

82. Which point-of-care blood glucose analyzer uses a microcuvette instead of a test strip?
a. Advantage HQ®
b. HemoCue 201®
c. I-STAT System®
d. ONE TOUCH®

83. An uncorrected imbalance of this analyte in a patient can quickly lead to death.
a. hemoglobin
b. potassium
c. prothrombin
d. troponin T

84. What type of specimen is needed for a guaiac test?
a. saliva
b. blood
c. feces
d. urine

85. How much diluted antigen is injected when performing a PPD test?
a. 0.01 mL
b. 0.1 mL
c. 0.5 mL
d. 1.0 mL

86. "Erythema" means:
a. hardness.
b. inflamed.
c. redness.
d. swollen.

87. When reading a patient's tuberculin (TB) test, there is an area of induration and erythema that measures 7 mm in diameter. The result of the test is:
a. doubtful.
b. negative.
c. positive.
d. unreadable.

88. Point-of-care detection of Group A strep normally requires a:
a. blood sample.
b. nasal collection.
c. throat swab.
d. urine specimen.

89. Which of the following *cannot* be detected in urine on a special reagent strip that is dipped in the urine specimen and then compared visually against color codes on the reagent strip container?
a. bilirubin
b. glucose
c. leukocytes
d. thrombin

90. Which point-of-care test helps a physician differentiate chronic obstructive pulmonary disease (COPD) and congestive heart failure (CHF)?
a. ALT
b. BNP
c. Hgb
d. Tn I

ANSWERS AND EXPLANATIONS

1. Answer: b
   Why: Toxicology is the scientific study of toxins (poisons). Forensic toxicology is concerned with the legal consequences of toxin exposure, both intentional and accidental. Clinical toxicology is concerned with the detection of toxins and treatment for the effects they produce. Toxicology tests examine blood, hair, urine, and other body substances for the presence of toxins, often present in very small amounts.
   Review: Yes ☐ No ☐

2. Answer: d
   Why: When one is administering a tuberculin (TB) skin test, the antigen must be injected just beneath the skin for accurate interpretation of the results. Appearance of the bleb, or wheal, is a sign that the antigen has been injected properly (Fig. 11-1). Applying pressure after injection of the antigen could force it out of the site. The injection site should be cleaned with alcohol and allowed to dry before injection. The site should be checked for a reaction in 48 to 72 hours.
   Review: Yes ☐ No ☐

3. Answer: c
   Why: The National Institute on Drug Abuse (NIDA) has defined patient preparation and collection requirements for drug screening for healthcare organizations, sports associations, and major companies requiring pre-employment drug screening. There are legal implications to drug screening, and chain of custody protocol is required whether it is performed for legal reasons or not. Consequently, appropriate labeling is required. NIDA requirements include documentation from courier to receiver; presence of a proctor to verify collection, and placement of the specimen in a sealed and locked container during transport.
   Review: Yes ☐ No ☐

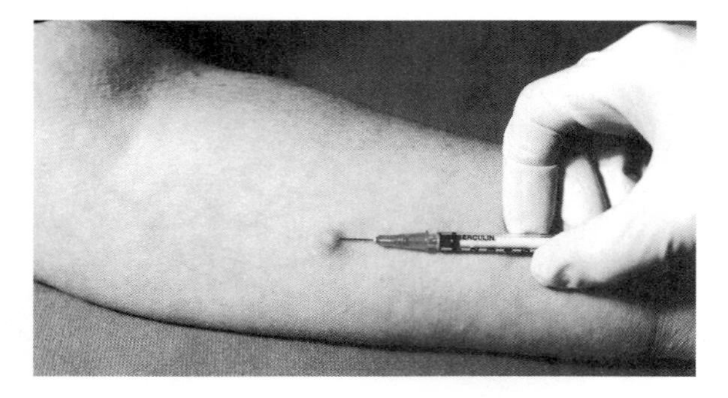

FIGURE 11-1 Wheal (bleb) formed by intradermal injection of antigen during skin test procedure.

4. Answer: d
   Why: Blood culture procedure steps in correct order are as follows: aseptically select and assemble the equipment, perform the friction scrub for 30 to 60 seconds, and allow the site to dry because antisepsis does not occur instantly. Next cleanse the culture bottle stopper while the site is drying, and then perform the venipuncture without touching or repalpating the site.
   Review: Yes ☐ No ☐

5. Answer: b
   Why: False-positive results for the lactose tolerance test have been demonstrated in patients with disorders such as slow gastric emptying and cystic fibrosis but not multiple myeloma. If the patient is lactose intolerant, the glucose curve will be flat. Some individuals normally have a flat GTT curve, and it is suggested that they have a 2-hour GTT performed the day before the lactose tolerance so results can be evaluated adequately.
   Review: Yes ☐ No ☐

6. Answer: c
   Why: If the putative or alleged parent is not excluded by basic red cell antigen testing (ABO grouping), further testing is performed until the individual is excluded or the likelihood of parentage is established. Further testing includes identifying extended red cell

antigens, red cell enzymes and serum proteins, white cell enzymes, and HLA (human leukocyte antigen) or white cell antigens. Red cell indices provide information about the RBC size, hemoglobin content, and concentration of hemoglobin in the red blood cells, which does not provide definitive information for paternity issues.

Review: Yes ☐ No ☐

7. Answer: b

Why: Paternity testing is performed to determine the probability that a specific individual fathered a particular child. Unlike routine clinical tests, which require an order from a physician, paternity testing can be requested by lawyers, child support enforcement bureaus, physicians, and individuals, with the exception of minor children.

Review: Yes ☐ No ☐

8. Answer: b

Why: According to the Clinical and Laboratory Standards Institute (CLSI), chlorhexidine gluconate is the recommended blood culture site disinfectant for infants 2 months and older.

Review: Yes ☐ No ☐

9. Answer: c

Why: An autologous donation is the process by which a person donates blood for his or her own use. This is done for elective surgeries when it is anticipated that a transfusion will be needed, because using one's own blood eliminates many risks associated with transfusions. Although blood is normally collected several weeks prior to the scheduled surgery, the minimum time between donation and surgery can be as little as 72 hours. To be eligible to make an autologous donation, a person must have a written order from a physician. If autologous units of blood are not used by the person who donated them, they must be discarded.

Review: Yes ☐ No ☐

10. Answer: a

Why: Citrate phosphate dextrose (CPD) is an anticoagulant and preservative that is typically used in collecting units of blood for transfusion purposes. The citrate prevents clotting by chelating (removing) calcium. A phosphate compound stabilizes the pH, and the dextrose provides energy to the cells and helps keep them alive. There is nothing in CPD that serves to control bacterial contamination.

Review: Yes ☐ No ☐

11. Answer: b

Why: A transfusion of donor blood that is not compatible with the patient's blood can be fatal because it causes agglutination (clumping) and lysis (rupturing) of the red blood cells within the patient's circulatory system. This massive destruction of red blood cells can overwhelm the patient's liver and kidneys, causing death.

Review: Yes ☐ No ☐

12. Answer: b

Why: When patients request reinfusion of their own blood lost during surgery, the blood must be salvaged and washed before being reinfused. Prior to reinfusion, it is recommended that the salvaged blood be tested for residual free hemoglobin. A high free hemoglobin level indicates that too many red cells were destroyed during the salvage process, and renal dysfunction could result if the blood were reinfused. Free hemoglobin can be detected using point-of-care instruments such as the HemoCue Plasma/Low Hemoglobin analyzer, as seen in Fig. 11-2.

Review: Yes ☐ No ☐

13. Answer: a

Why: The collection unit is a sterile, closed system consisting of a blood bag connected by a length of tubing to a sterile 16- to 18-gauge needle. The collection bag contains an anticoagulant and preservative solution and is placed on a mixing unit while the blood is

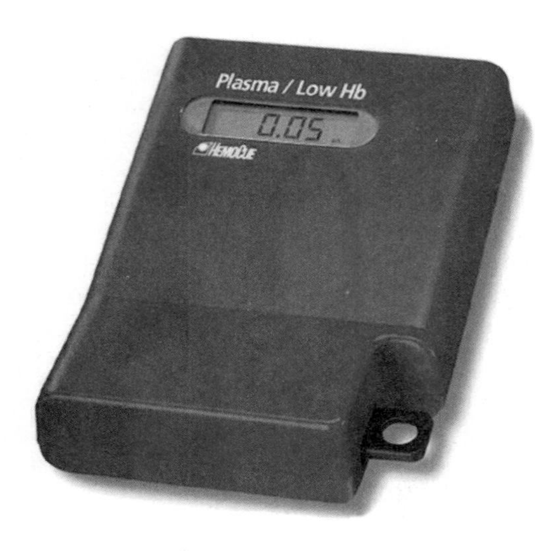

FIGURE 11-2 HemoCue Plasma/Low Hb. (HemoCue, Inc., Lake Forest, CA.)

being drawn. The unit is normally filled by weight but typically contains around 450 mL of blood when full. The additive in a unit of blood is CPD (citrate phosphate dextrose) or CPD plus adenine (CPDA).

Review: Yes ☐ No ☐

14. Answer: a
Why: D-xylose is a type of carbohydrate that is classified as a simple sugar called a pentose. The gray top tube is preferred when testing for sugars of any type because it has an antiglycolytic agent that prevents carbohydrate metabolism.
Review: Yes ☐ No ☐

15. Answer: c
Why: The milk sugar lactose is converted by the body into glucose and galactose by the action of an enzyme called mucosal lactase. A person lacking this enzyme has gastrointestinal distress and diarrhea when milk and other lactose-containing foods are consumed. Symptoms are relieved by eliminating milk from the diet.
Review: Yes ☐ No ☐

16. Answer: b
Why: The patient is instructed not to eat fruit or other foods containing D-xylose for 3 days before the test, to fast after midnight the day of the test, and to remain fasting until the test is completed 5 hours later. There are no special requirements for water consumption prior to the test.
Review: Yes ☐ No ☐

17. Answer: d
Why: The patient is instructed to void and discard the urine prior to the start of the test. All urine voided by the patient is collected, pooled, and refrigerated for the duration of the test. A blood specimen is collected 1 hour after the start of the procedure and tested for D-xylose. A final urine specimen is collected at the end of the 5 hours and added to the pooled specimen, which is then tested for D-xylose.
Review: Yes ☐ No ☐

18. Answer: d
Why: Potassium plays a major role in nerve conduction, muscle function, acid-base balance, and osmotic pressure. It has no role in transporting hemoglobin (Hgb).
Review: Yes ☐ No ☐

19. Answer: b
Why: The D-xylose absorption test is a noninvasive way to help diagnose malabsorption, or failure of the small intestine to absorb nutrients. D-xylose is a simple sugar that is not normally present in blood or urine unless foods containing it are eaten. The patient is asked to avoid all fruits and other foods containing D-xylose for 3 days prior to the test. On test day the patient is given a drink containing 25 g of D-xylose. Urine and blood samples are taken throughout a 5 hour period.
Review: Yes ☐ No ☐

20. Answer: c
    Why: It is not unusual for patients to be on antimicrobial (antibiotic) therapy at the time blood culture specimens are collected. Presence of the antimicrobial agent in the patient's blood can inhibit any growth of microorganisms in the blood culture bottle. Antimicrobial removal device (ARD) or fastidious antimicrobial neutralization (FAN) blood culture bottles contain, respectively, resins or activated charcoal that neutralize antibiotics.
    Review: Yes ☐ No ☐

21. Answer: d
    Why: Septicemia is defined as microorganisms or their toxin in the blood. Bacteremia is a type of septicemia, but more specific to bacteria in the bloodstream.
    Review: Yes ☐ No ☐

22. Answer: c
    Why: The MedPoint Transfusion System, as seen in Fig. 11-3, is an example of an electronic blood bank ID system. It is a portable bedside barcode scanning system that provides electronic verification and tracing of the blood transfusion process. The hardware includes a portable data terminal and printer.

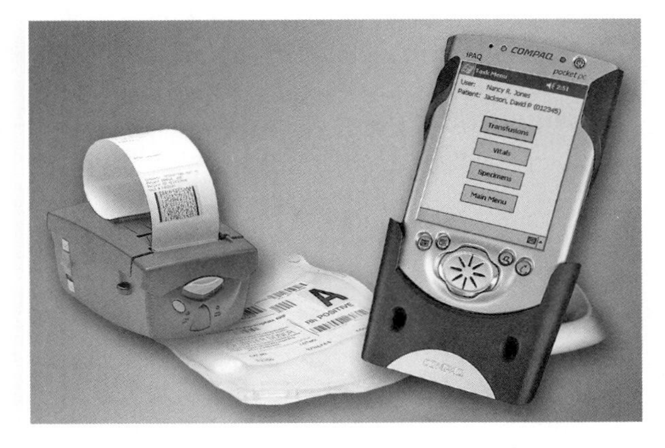

FIGURE 11-3 Bridge Medical MedPoint transfusion system. (Bridge Medical Inc., Solana Beach, CA.)

At the time of specimen collection, the phlebotomist scans his or her ID badge and then the patient's barcoded wristband. The barcoded data are used throughout the transfusion process and appear on the unit of blood prepared for transfusion.
    Review: Yes ☐ No ☐

23. Answer: a
    Why: To donate blood, an individual must normally be between the ages of 17 and 66 and weigh at least 110 lb.
    Review: Yes ☐ No ☐

24. Answer: c
    Why: Hemochromatosis is a disease characterized by excess iron deposits in the tissues. Periodic removal of single units of blood gradually depletes excess iron stores because the body uses iron to make new red blood cells to replace those removed.
    Review: Yes ☐ No ☐

25. Answer: b
    Why: Specimens for crossmatch testing require especially strict identification and labeling procedures. Misidentification of a specimen for crossmatch can lead to a patient receiving an incompatible unit of blood and having a serious and possibly fatal transfusion reaction. Special blood bank specimen identification systems intended to reduce errors are available. Fig. 11-4 shows a phlebotomist comparing information on a blood bank tube containing a label peeled from a special blood bank ID bracelet, with the carbon copy of the label on the bracelet attached to the patient's arm.
    Review: Yes ☐ No ☐

26. Answer: d
    Why: Amphetamines (ice) and cocaine (crack) are classified as drugs of abuse, as are cannabinoids (marijuana compounds). Phenobarbital is a drug that is prescribed for

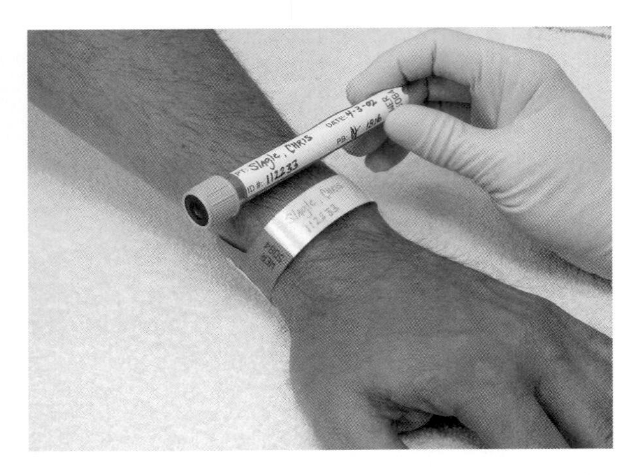

FIGURE 11-4 A phlebotomist compares labeled blood bank tube with blood bank ID bracelet.

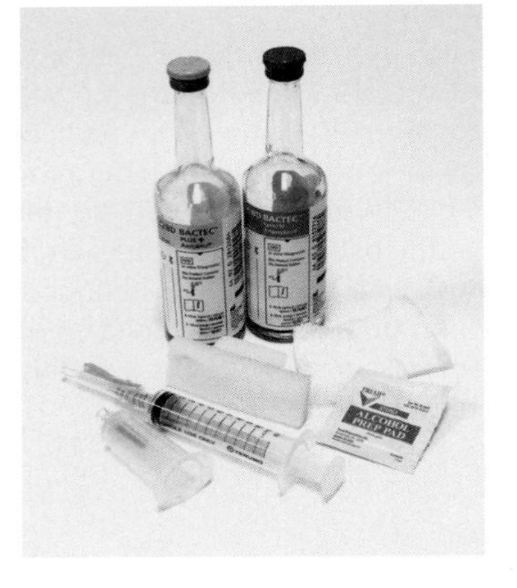

FIGURE 11-5 Blood culture equipment.

epilepsy, seizure prevention, and mood stabilization and typically requires therapeutic monitoring.

Review: Yes ☐ No ☐

27. Answer: a

Why: Large-bore (16–18 gauge) needles are used to collect donor units. The large bore helps keep the blood flowing freely and minimizes hemolysis of red blood cells during collection.

Review: Yes ☐ No ☐

28. Answer: b

Why: A donor unit is filled by weight, but typically contains around 450 mL blood.

Review: Yes ☐ No ☐

29. Answer: a

Why: The response of the body to septicemia is to raise body temperature to kill the microorganisms. When a patient experiences fever with no known cause (referred to as fever of unknown origin, or FUO), a physician may suspect septicemia and order blood cultures. Fig. 11-5 shows equipment necessary for collection of a blood culture. Blood cultures are typically ordered immediately before or after anticipated fever spikes when bacteria are most likely to be present. When more than one set is ordered for collection at the same time, the second set should be obtained from a separately prepared site on the opposite arm. However, in some cases, "second-site" blood cultures are more useful when drawn 30 minutes apart.

Review: Yes ☐ No ☐

30. Answer: a

Why: A type and screen can be performed on a specimen collected in a non-additive red top, lavender top EDTA, or special pink top EDTA tube, depending on laboratory preference. Blood bank specimens are never collected in gel-barrier tubes because the gel and clot activator could affect antigen and antibody testing and cause erroneous results.

Review: Yes ☐ No ☐

31. Answer: c

Why: Special skin decontamination procedures are used to collect blood cultures to prevent contamination of the specimen with normal flora from the patient's skin. Fig. 11-6 shows examples of several types of blood culture site cleaning supplies.

Review: Yes ☐ No ☐

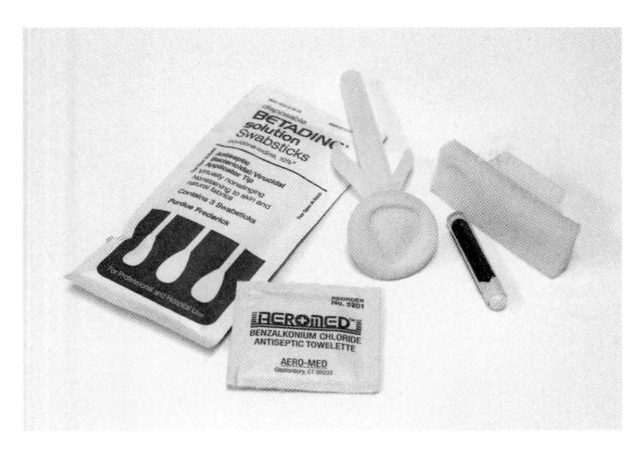

FIGURE 11-6 Four types of blood culture cleaning supplies. **Left to right,** Betadine swabsticks (The Purdue Frederick Co., Norwalk, CT); **center,** Benzalkonium Chloride (Aero-Med, Glastonbury, CT); Chloroprep (Medi-Flex Hospital Products, Inc., Overland Park, KS); Frepp/Sepp II (MediFlex Inc., Overland Park, KS).

32. Answer: c
    Why: A paternity test can determine the probability that a specific individual was the father of a particular child. Results of paternity tests can exclude an individual as the father rather than prove that he is the father.
    Review: Yes ☐ No ☐

33. Answer: b
    Why: It is not unusual for patients to be on antibiotics when a blood culture is collected. Antibiotic present in the blood specimen can inhibit the growth of microorganisms and lead to a false-negative blood culture. The special resin removes or neutralizes antibiotics. The blood is then cultured by conventional techniques.
    Review: Yes ☐ No ☐

34. Answer: c
    Why: Coagulation specimens must have a 9:1 ratio of blood to anticoagulant, or test results on the specimen will not be accurate. If a coagulation tube is not filled completely, this ratio is altered and the lab will not accept the specimen for testing.
    Review: Yes ☐ No ☐

35. Answer: d
    Why: The recommended additive for collecting blood alcohol (ethanol) specimens is the antiglycolytic agent sodium fluoride, which prevents the breakdown of alcohol and also inhibits the growth of bacteria. Fermentation by bacteria can increase alcohol concentration.
    Review: Yes ☐ No ☐

36. Answer: b
    Why: If both aerobic and anaerobic cultures are collected at one time, the anaerobic bottle is inoculated first when filled from a syringe. If a butterfly with tubing is used and blood is collected directly into the bottles, the aerobic bottle is filled first because air from the tubing will be drawn into the bottle ahead of the blood. The antimicrobial removal device (ARD) is resin that is typically found in the bottles of aerobic and anaerobic media. Therefore, inoculation into a separate container would not be required.
    Review: Yes ☐ No ☐

37. Answer: b
    Why: Skin antisepsis, the destruction of microorganisms on the skin, is a critical part of the blood culture collection procedure, as seen in Fig. 11-7. Failure to follow proper antiseptic technique can result in contamination of the blood culture by skin surface bacteria

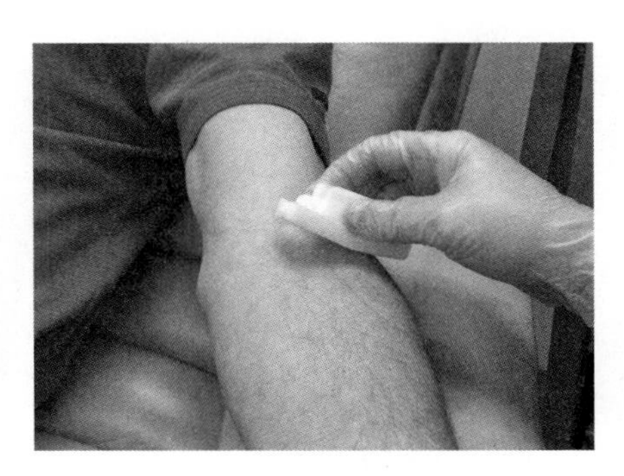

FIGURE 11-7 Performing a friction scrub.

or other microorganisms and interfere with interpretation of results. The laboratory must report all microorganisms detected, so it is up to the patient's physician to determine whether the organism is clinically significant or merely a contaminant.

Review: Yes ☐ No ☐

38. Answer: b

Why: Antiseptic or sterile technique for blood culture collection site varies slightly from one laboratory to another. Traditionally, 10% povidone or 1–2% tincture of iodine compounds in the form of swabsticks, or special cleaning pad kits containing benzalkonium chloride (BZK), shown in Fig. 11-6, have been used to clean the collection site. When using a povidone-iodine swabstick (Fig. 11-8), the swab should be placed at the site of the needle insertion and moved outward in concentric circles without going over any area more than once, as shown in Fig. 11-9. The area should be 3 to 4 inches in diameter.

Review: Yes ☐ No ☐

39. Answer: d

Why: Blood is sometimes collected in an intermediate collection tube rather than blood culture bottles. A yellow top sodium polyanethol sulfonate (SPS) tube is acceptable for this purpose. Other anticoagulants are toxic to bacteria and are not recommended.

Review: Yes ☐ No ☐

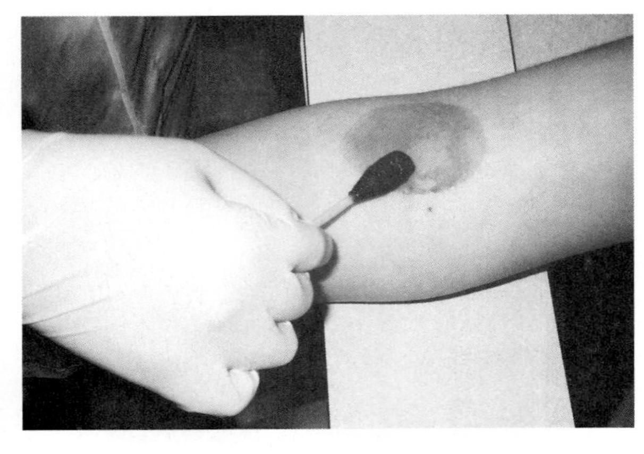

FIGURE 11-8 Cleaning a blood culture site using a povidone-iodine swabstick.

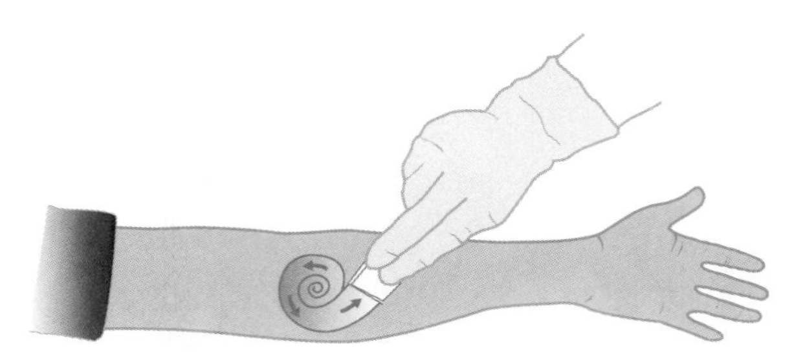

FIGURE 11-9 Pattern of concentric circles used when cleaning a blood culture site.

40. Answer: b

Why: At one time it was customary to draw a "clear" or discard tube prior to drawing a tube for a coagulation testing. A few milliliters of blood were collected into a plain red top tube to clear the needle of tissue thromboplastin contamination picked up as the needle penetrated the skin. The "clear" tube was discarded if it was not needed for other tests. New studies have shown that a "clear" tube is not necessary when collecting a PT or PTT. A clear tube is required for all other coagulation tests (e.g., factor VIII) because the Clinical and Laboratory Standards Institute (CLSI) still recommends that they be the second or third tube drawn.

Review: Yes ☐ No ☐

41. Answer: b

Why: The bleeding time (BT) test (Fig. 11-10) evaluates platelet plug formation in the capillaries to detect platelet function disorders and capillary integrity problems.

Review: Yes ☐ No ☐

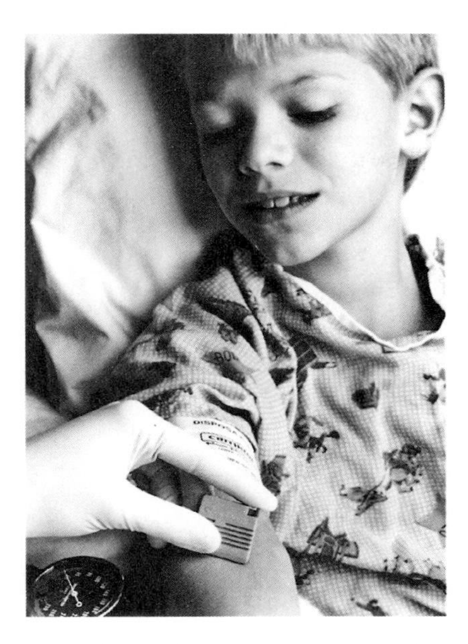

FIGURE 11-10 A bleeding time test being performed photo? (Courtesy ITC, Edison, NJ.)

42. Answer: a
Why: Postprandial (PP) means "after a meal." Glucose levels in blood specimens obtained 2 hours after a meal are rarely elevated in normal individuals but may be significantly increased in diabetic patients. Therefore, a glucose test on a specimen collected 2 hours after a meal (2-hour PP) is an excellent screening test for diabetes and other metabolism problems.
Review: Yes ☐ No ☐

43. Answer: c
Why: Chewing sugarless gum, drinking sugarless tea, and smoking cigarettes stimulate the digestive process and therefore can affect glucose tolerance test (GTT) results. A person may feel nauseated during the testing and need to lie down, which is perfectly acceptable and does not affect the test results.
Review: Yes ☐ No ☐

44. Answer: d
Why: The timing of specimen collection during a GTT begins as soon as the patient finishes the glucose beverage, as seen in Fig. 11-11. For example, if a patient finishes the glucose beverage at 0805 hours, the $^1/_2$-hour specimen is collected at 0835 hours, the 1-hour specimen is collected at 0905 hours, and so on. Timing of specimen collection is critical for computation of the GTT curve and correct interpretation of results.
Review: Yes ☐ No ☐

45. Answer: a
Why: If there is a discrepancy concerning the timing of a 2-hour postprandial specimen, the patient's nurse should be consulted to establish the correct time to draw the specimen. It is not a good idea to ask the patient because he or she may not know the correct time or understand the importance of exact timing. The specimen should not be collected

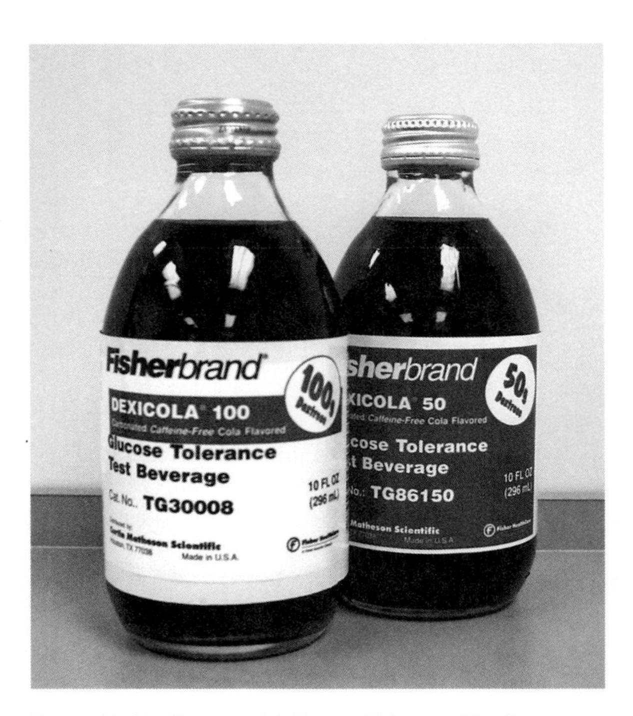

FIGURE 11-11 Commercial Glucose Tolerance Test Beverage, 50-g and 100-g doses.

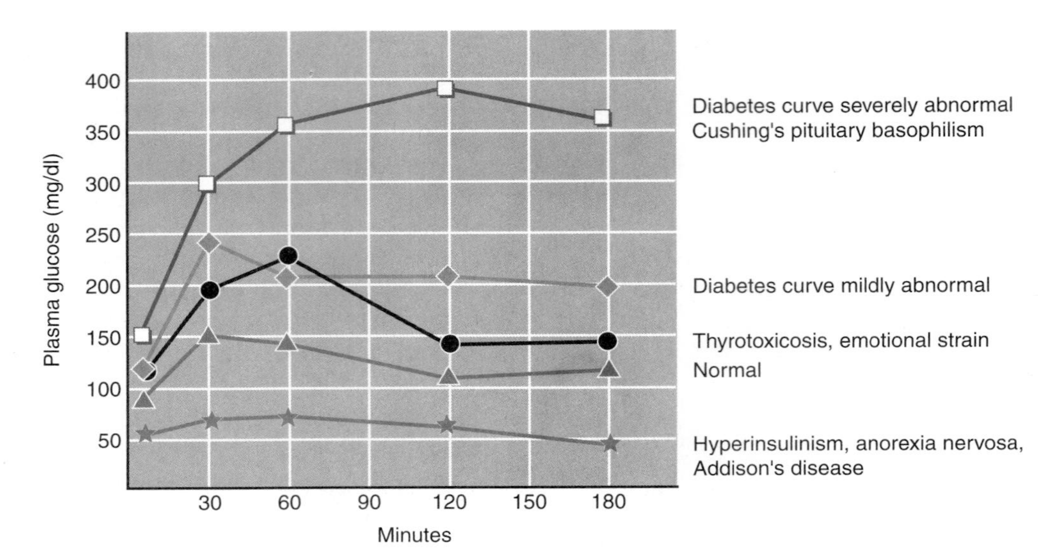

FIGURE 11-12 Glucose tolerance test (GTT) curves.

early because glucose levels may still be elevated and lead to misinterpretation of results. Filling out an incident report and returning to the lab may cause the correct collection time to be missed.

Review: Yes ☐ No ☐

46. Answer: d

Why: If a patient undergoing a GTT vomits within 30 minutes of drinking the glucose beverage, his or her nurse or physician should be notified immediately to determine if the test should be continued or rescheduled.

Review: Yes ☐ No ☐

47. Answer: a

Why: Increased blood glucose (sugar) is called hyperglycemia. Hyperinsulinism is excessive blood insulin levels, hyperkalemia is excessive blood potassium levels, and hypernatremia is excess sodium in the blood.

Review: Yes ☐ No ☐

48. Answer: b

Why: Blood glucose levels in normal individuals typically peak within 30 minutes to 1 hour of glucose ingestion and return to normal fasting levels within 2 hours. GTT specimen results are plotted on a graph to create what is referred to as a GTT curve. Fig. 11-12 shows a graph with examples of normal and abnormal GTT curves.

Review: Yes ☐ No ☐

49. Answer: c

Why: OGTT is another name for a glucose tolerance test. Blood glucose vary according to the source of the specimen. It is important that the specimen source be consistent for the duration of the test for proper interpretation of results. Consequently, GTT blood specimens can be collected by capillary puncture or venipuncture, but not a combination of the two methods, if at all possible.

Review: Yes ☐ No ☐

50. Answer: a

Why: Proper patient preparation before a GTT involves eating balanced meals containing 150 g of carbohydrate for 3 days prior to the test, fasting for at least 12 hours before the test, and avoiding smoking or chewing gum before or during the test. There is no exercise requirement.

Review: Yes ☐ No ☐

51. Answer: d

Why: Zephiran chloride (benzalkonium chloride) and povidone-iodine are if the preferred antiseptics, for blood alcohol collection. Isopropyl alcohol (isopropanol) and methanol are types of alcohol. Alcohol solutions or alcohol-based antiseptics can cause interference in blood alcohol testing and should not be used to clean a site prior to blood alcohol specimen collection. Tincture of iodine cannot be used because tinctures contain alcohol.

Review: Yes ☐ No ☐

52. Answer: c

Why: "Chain of custody" documentation is required for legal or forensic specimens. Whether performed for legal reasons or not, drug screening has legal implications that require use of "chain of custody" protocol. Fig. 11-13 shows an example of a chain of custody requisition form.

Review: Yes ☐ No ☐

53. Answer: a

Why: Therapeutic drug monitoring (TDM) is performed to determine and maintain a beneficial drug dosage for a patient. Peak drug levels represent the highest serum concentrations of a drug and are collected during TDM to screen for drug toxicity. Trough drug levels are monitored during TDM to ensure drug levels stay within the therapeutic or effective range. TDM has nothing to do with screening for illegal drug use.

Review: Yes ☐ No ☐

54. Answer: c

Why: Digitoxin, gentamicin, and theophylline are drugs. Phenylalanine is an amino acid, not a drug.

Review: Yes ☐ No ☐

55. Answer: d

Why: Timing of TDM specimens is extremely important. A pharmacist calculates drug dosages based on blood levels of the drug at specific times. If a specimen is collected late, it is important that the actual time of collection be recorded so that the pharmacist is aware of the time change and can calculate values accordingly. It is not the phlebotomist's responsibility to establish the collection time. Not collecting the specimen and leaving a notification with the desk clerk or at the nursing station could cause an unnecessary and expensive delay.

Review: Yes ☐ No ☐

56. Answer: b

Why: A trough, or minimum drug level, is collected when the lowest serum concentration of the drug is expected. A trough drug level is easiest to obtain because it is collected immediately before administration of the next scheduled drug dose.

Review: Yes ☐ No ☐

57. Answer: b

Why: A glucose tolerance test (GTT) involves the collection of multiple blood specimens. Blood specimens are serially collected at specific times throughout the duration of the test. Urine specimens are sometimes collected at the same times as the blood specimens.

Review: Yes ☐ No ☐

58. Answer: b

Why: A half-life is the time required for the body to metabolize half the amount of the drug. Timing of collection is most critical for aminoglycoside drugs with short half-lives, such as gentamicin, amikacin, and tobramycin. Timing is less critical for drugs such as phenobarbital, methotrexate, and digoxin, which have longer half-lives.

Review: Yes ☐ No ☐

ORDERING PHYSICIAN/COMPANY OR FACILITY

SPECIMEN ID NO. 0000000

VARIABLE BARCODE

Sonora Quest Laboratories
A Subsidiary of Laboratory Sciences of Arizona

1255 West Washington Street
Tempe, Arizona 85281
602.685.5000 • 800.766.6721

LAB ACCESSION NO.

CHAIN OF CUSTODY REQUISITION FORM

STEP 1: COMPLETED BY COLLECTOR OR EMPLOYER REPRESENTATIVE

Donor SSN or Employee I.D. No.

Donor Name: Last: First:

Donor ID Verified: ☐ Photo ID ☐ Emp. Rep. ______

Reason for Test: ☐ Pre-employment ☐ Random ☐ Reasonable Suspicion/Cause ☐ Post-Accident ☐ Promotion
☐ Return to Duty ☐ Follow-up ☐ Other (specify) ______

Drug Tests to be Performed:

STEP 2: COMPLETED BY COLLECTOR (Collector Instructions)

Read specimen temperature within 4 minutes. Is temperature between 90° and 100° F? ☐ Yes ☐ No, Enter Remark	Specimen Collection: ☐ Split ☐ Single ☐ None Provided (Enter Remark)	☐ Observed (Enter Remark)
REMARKS		

Collection Site Address/Site Code:

Collector Phone No. ______

Collector Fax No. ______

STEP 3: Collector affixes bottle seal(s) to bottle(s). Collector dates seal(s). Donor initials seal(s). Donor completes STEP 5

STEP 4: CHAIN OF CUSTODY - INITIATED BY COLLECTOR AND COMPLETED BY LABORATORY

I certify that the specimen given to me by the donor identified in step 1 of this form was collected, labeled, sealed and released to the Delivery Service noted.

X ______ Signature of Collector — ______ AM/PM Time of Collection ► **SPECIMEN BOTTLE(S) RELEASED TO:**

______ (PRINT) Collector's Name (First, MI, Last) — __/__/__ Date (Mo./Day/Yr.) ► ______ Name of Delivery Service Transferring Specimen to Lab

RECEIVED AT LAB:
X ______ Signature of Accessioner ►

______ (PRINT) Accessioner's Name (First, MI, Last) — __/__/__ Date (Mo./Day/Yr.) ►

Primary Specimen Bottle Seal Intact
☐ Yes
☐ No, Enter Remark Below

SPECIMEN BOTTLE(S) RELEASED TO:

STEP 5: COMPLETED BY DONOR

I certify that I provided my urine specimen to the collector; that I have not adulterated it in any manner; each specimen bottle used was sealed with a tamper-evident seal in my presence; and that the information numbers provided on this form and on the label affixed to each specimen bottle is correct.

X ______ Signature of Donor — ______ (PRINT) Donor's Name (First, MI, Last) — __/__/__ Date (Mo./Day/Yr.)

Daytime Phone No. ( ) ______ Evening Phone No. ( ) ______ Date of Birth __/__/__ Mo. Day Yr.

Q7230 (Rev. 9/07) Sonora Quest Laboratories

COPY 1 - LABORATORY COPY 2 - COLLECTOR COPY COPY 3 - COMPANY/MRO COPY COPY 4 - LABORATORY-CONFIDENTIAL DONOR

FIGURE 11-13 Chain of custody requisition form. (Courtesy of Sonora Quest Laboratories, Tempe, AZ.)

59. Answer: d
Why: "Thrombocyte" is the medical term for platelet. A bleeding time (BT) test evaluates platelet plug formation in the capillaries to detect platelet function disorders and capillary integrity problems. Platelet plug formation at the site of a standardized incision is evaluated. Blood is wicked away from the site to determine the end point. The "wicking" technique is critical in getting the correct end point of the test.
Review: Yes ☐ No ☐

60. Answer: c
Why: Glucose monitoring in diabetics (people with diabetes mellitus) is the most common reason for performing glucose testing through point-of-care testing (POCT). An example of a POCT glucose analyzer is seen in Fig. 11-14.
Review: Yes ☐ No ☐

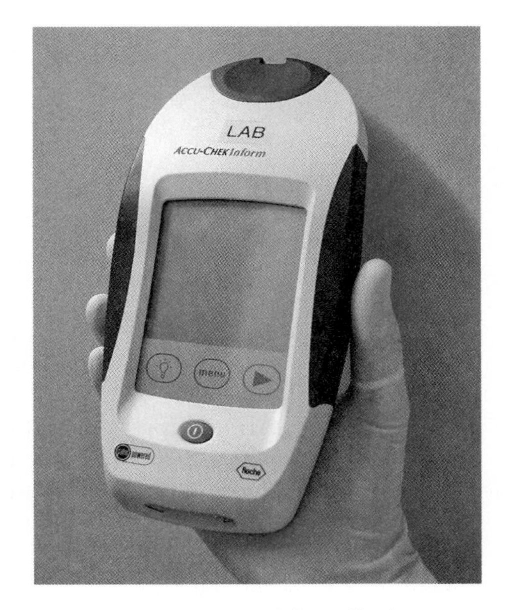

FIGURE 11-14 Advantage Inform. (Roche Diagnostics, Indianapolis, IN.)

61. Answer: c
Why: Traces of elements or minerals such as copper, lead, and zinc can be contaminants in glass and other materials used to make blood collection tubes and stoppers and can leach from the tube into the specimen. Trace-element–free tubes have the lowest possible contaminating amounts of these elements. Iron, lead, and zinc are all elements or minerals measured in such small quantities that it is best if they are collected in trace-element–free tubes. Sodium is not considered a trace element.
Review: Yes ☐ No ☐

62. Answer: b
Why: Toxicology is defined as the scientific study of poisons or toxins. There are two types: clinical toxicology and forensic toxicology. Clinical toxicology is involved with detection of the toxins and the treatment of their effects. Forensic toxicology is concerned with the legal consequences of both intentional and accidental exposure to toxins.
Review: Yes ☐ No ☐

63. Answer: a
Why: Turnaround time (TAT) in laboratory testing is the amount of time that elapses between when a test is ordered and when the results are returned. BUN results are part of a panel that can be performed on the small, portable hand-held instruments, such as the I-STAT or IRMA. Once the instrument's cartridge is injected with blood, the BUN test results are available in less than 2 minutes, but calibration of the instrument, which must be done first to ensure quality results, takes several minutes to perform. A GTT is a timed test involving collection of serial specimens over a period of 1 to 6 hours depending on how it is ordered by the physician. A DNA profile can be performed on buccal samples, which are collected by rubbing a swab against the inside of the cheek to collect loose cells. DNA results are not immediate; TAT may be

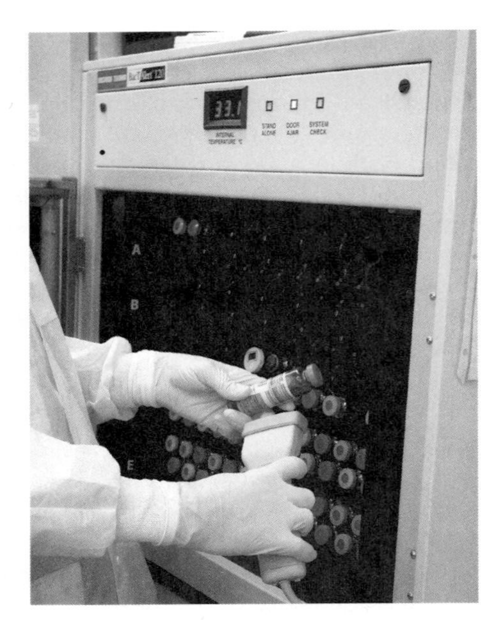

FIGURE 11-15 Microbiologist reviews blood cultures processed by the BactALERT 3D.

several days. PSA is not a POCT test and must be collected by venipuncture, processed in the laboratory, and delivered for testing, which makes TAT several hours at least.

Review: Yes ☐ No ☐

64. Answer: d

Why: CoaguChek, Hemochron Jr., and IRMA system are all POCT analyzers. BactALERT, as shown in Fig. 11-15, is a blood culture collection system.

Review: Yes ☐ No ☐

65. Answer: d

Why: Lithium levels are used for drug evaluation therapy, and do not involve the coagulation process. Coumadin and heparin are anticoagulants, the effects of which can be closely monitored through point-of-care testing (POCT). See Fig. 11-16 for an example of a coagulation monitoring instrument for

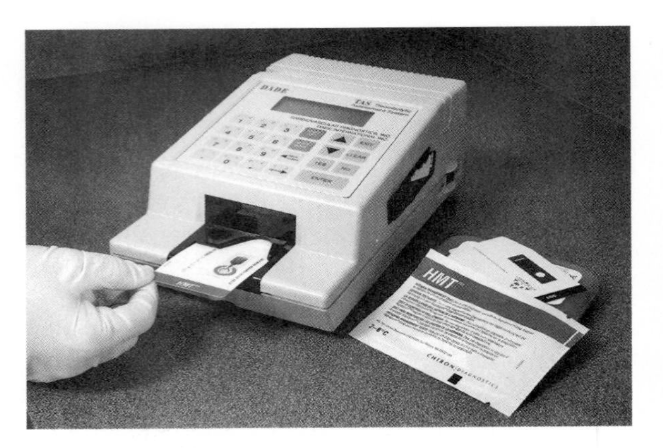

FIGURE 11-16 Rapid Point Coag used for HMT (Bayer, Tarrytown, NY).

POCT. High-dose heparin use during certain surgeries, such as cardiac bypass surgery.

Review: Yes ☐ No ☐

66. Answer: c

Why: Whole blood glucose or bedside glucose monitoring is one of the most common point-of-care tests. Troponin and cholesterol are point-of-care tests but are not performed nearly as often. Bilirubin testing is not commonly performed at the bedside.

Review: Yes ☐ No ☐

67. Answer: a

Why: The activated clotting time (ACT) test is used to monitor heparin therapy. The Hemochron Jr. Signature analyzer (Fig. 11-17) is an example of a POCT instrument used to perform ACT tests. The prothrombin time (PT) is used to monitor coumadin therapy. The bleeding time test (BT) evaluates platelet function. B-type natriuretic peptide (BNP) is a cardiac hormone produced by the heart. BNP levels help physicians differentiate chronic obstructive pulmonary disease (COPD) and congestive heart failure (CHF).

Review: Yes ☐ No ☐

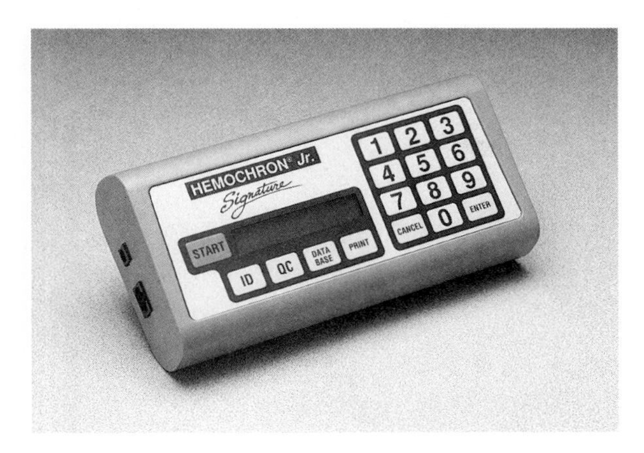

FIGURE 11-17 Hemochron Jr. Signature analyzer for ACT determinations. (Courtesy International Technidyne Corp., Edison, NJ.)

68. Answer: d
Why: A butterfly bandage, standardized incision device or lancet, and a stopwatch are all bleeding time (BT) test equipment (Fig. 11-18). A tourniquet is not used during a BT. A blood pressure cuff is used to provide a standard pressure of 40 mm Hg.
Review: Yes ☐ No ☐

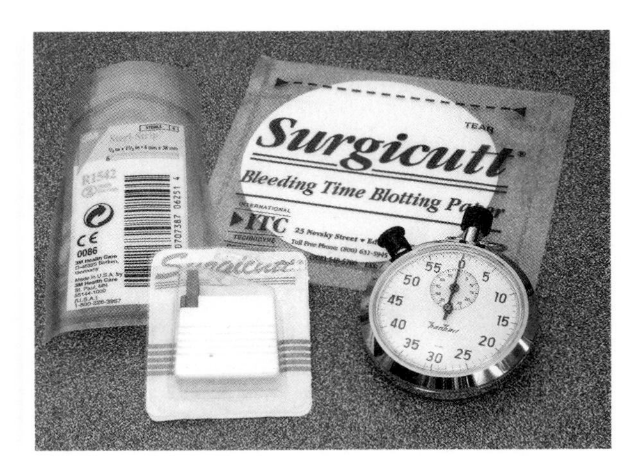

FIGURE 11-18 Equipment for bleeding time test, including Surgicutt automated bleeding time device, blotting paper, stopwatch, and Steri-Strips. (ITC, Edison, NJ.)

69. Answer: c
Why: During a bleeding time test, special filter paper is brought close to the incision every 30 seconds to carefully wick or absorb the blood away. Care must be taken not to touch the incision site, or the platelet plug will be disturbed and the BT will be falsely prolonged.
Review: Yes ☐ No ☐

70. Answer: b
Why: When one is performing a bleeding time (BT) test, a blood pressure cuff is used to provide a uniform pressure of 40 mm Hg.
Review: Yes ☐ No ☐

71. Answer: a
Why: A bleeding time (BT) tests platelet plug formation in the capillaries. During the performance of the test, it is important to maintain consistent BP cuff pressure for standardization purposes, thus resulting in a reproducible bleeding time. Allowing the pressure of the cuff to drop would shorten the bleeding time. If the patient has an abnormally low platelet count, it will take longer for the platelet plug to form, resulting in a prolonged BT. Aspirin inhibits platelet function for the life of the platelet. Consequently, if the patient has taken aspirin within 2 weeks of the test, the BT will be prolonged. Touching the incision site or wound disturbs platelet plug formation and also prolongs the test.
Review: Yes ☐ No ☐

72. Answer: b
Why: Skin tests involve intradermal injection of an antigenic substance that causes an allergic response if the patient has an antibody directed against it, but does not cause the disease. For example, to perform a tuberculin (TB) skin test, a modified TB antigen is injected just under the skin on a patient's forearm. (Properly injected antigen forms a temporary wheal, or bleb). If the patient has TB antibodies, they will combine with the

antigen to cause a visible reaction on the surface of the skin within 48 to 72 hours.

Review: Yes ☐ No ☐

73. Answer: c
Why: Ionized calcium makes up approximately 45% of the calcium in the blood. The rest is bound to protein and other substances. Only ionized calcium can be used for critical functions such as blood clotting, cardiac function, and nerve impulses. Glycosylation is the forming of links between glucose and hemoglobin. Ionized calcium does not play a critical role in this process.
Review: Yes ☐ No ☐

74. Answer: a
Why: Normal arterial blood pH is 7.35 to 7.45. Below-normal blood pH is called acidosis. Above-normal pH is called alkalosis. Hyponatremia is reduced sodium in the blood. Hypokalemia is reduced potassium in the blood.
Review: Yes ☐ No ☐

75. Answer: d
Why: Troponin T (TnT) is a protein that is specific to heart muscle. It is measured in the diagnosis of acute myocardial infarction (MI) or heart attack.
Review: Yes ☐ No ☐

76. Answer: c
Why: B-type natriuretic peptide (BNP) is a cardiac hormone produced by the heart in response to ventricular volume expansion and pressure overload.
Review: Yes ☐ No ☐

77. Answer: c
Why: Hemoglobin A1c is a type of hemoglobin formed by glycosylation (the reaction of glucose with hemoglobin). Fig. 11-19 shows a POCT meter used for hemoglobin A1c measurement. Glycosylated Hgb levels reflect the average blood glucose level during the preceding 4 to 6 weeks and therefore can be used to evaluate long-term effectiveness of diabetes therapy.
Review: Yes ☐ No ☐

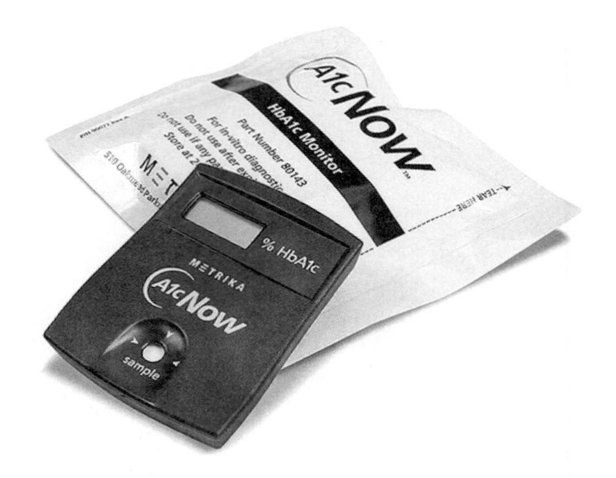

FIGURE 11-19 A1c NOW meter. (Metrika Inc., Sunnyvale, CA.)

78. Answer: b
Why: The hematocrit (HCT) test is a measure of the volume of RBCs in a patient's blood. It is also called packed cell volume (PCV) because it can be calculated by centrifuging a specific volume of anticoagulated blood to separate the cells from the plasma to determine the proportion of red blood cells to plasma.
Review: Yes ☐ No ☐

79. Answer: b
Why: Occult blood is blood that is hidden, or present in such small amounts that it is not apparent on visual examination. The guaiac test detects hidden blood in feces using

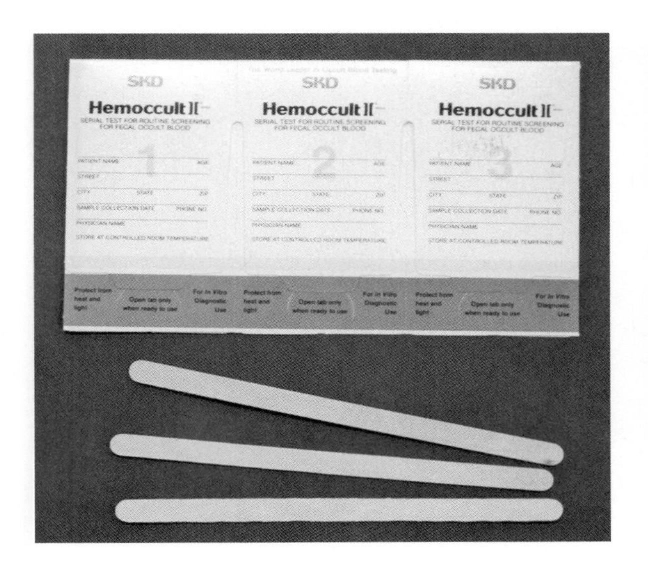

FIGURE 11-20 Hemoccult II occult blood collection cards. (Beckman Coulter, Fullerton, CA.)

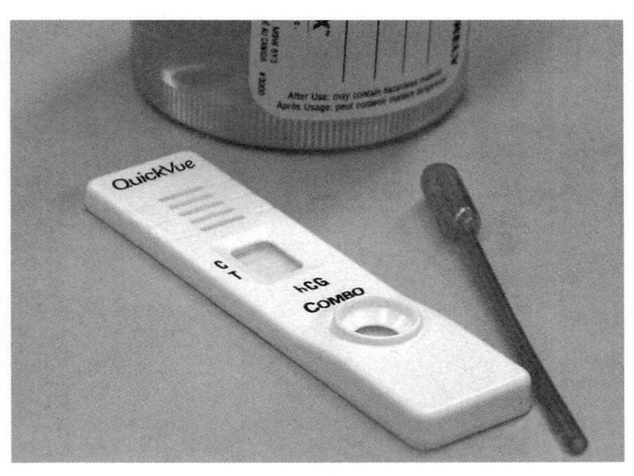

FIGURE 11-21 Quick Vue pregnancy test kit. (Quidel Corp., San Diego, CA.)

an alcoholic solution of a tree resin called guaiac. Detection of occult blood in stool (feces) is an important tool in diagnosing gastric ulcer and screening for colon cancer. Several different companies make occult blood kits containing special cards (Fig. 11-20) on which feces samples are collected and tested.

Review: Yes ☐ No ☐

80. Answer: c

Why: The test for tuberculosis exposure, the tuberculin (TB) test, is also called a PPD test because of the purified protein derivative (PPD) used in testing. The Cocci test is for an infectious fungus disease caused by *Coccidioides immitus;* the Histo test detects present or past infection with the fungus *Histoplasma capsulatum;* and the Schick test is for susceptibility to diphtheria.

Review: Yes ☐ No ☐

81. Answer: b

Why: Most rapid urine pregnancy tests detect human chorionic gonadotropin (HCG), a hormone produced by the placenta that appears in both urine and serum beginning approximately 10 days after conception. Peak urine levels of HCG occur at approximately 10 weeks of gestation. An example of a urine pregnancy testing kit is Quidel Quick Vue One Step (Fig. 11-21).

Review: Yes ☐ No ☐

82. Answer: b

Why: HemoCue® blood glucose analyzer (Fig. 11-22) uses a microcuvette instead of a test strip. The Advantage HQ® and ONE TOUCH® use a reagent strip for testing. The I-STAT® uses a special cartridge for testing.

Review: Yes ☐ No ☐

83. Answer: b

Why: Potassium is an electrolyte. The body maintains electrolytes in specific proportions within narrow ranges, and any uncorrected

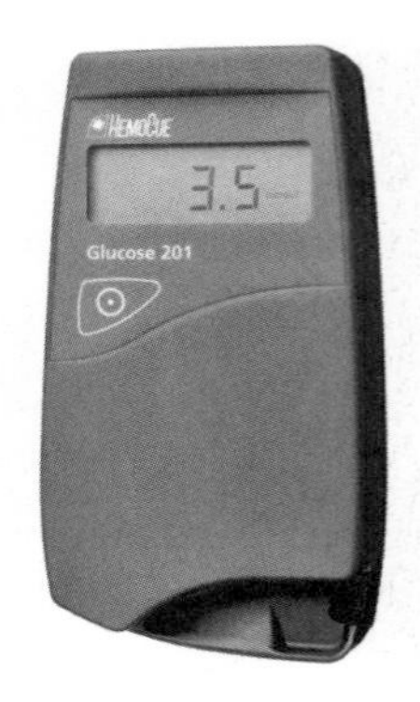

FIGURE 11-22 Glucose 201 system from HemoCue. (HemoCue, Inc., Lake Forest, CA.)

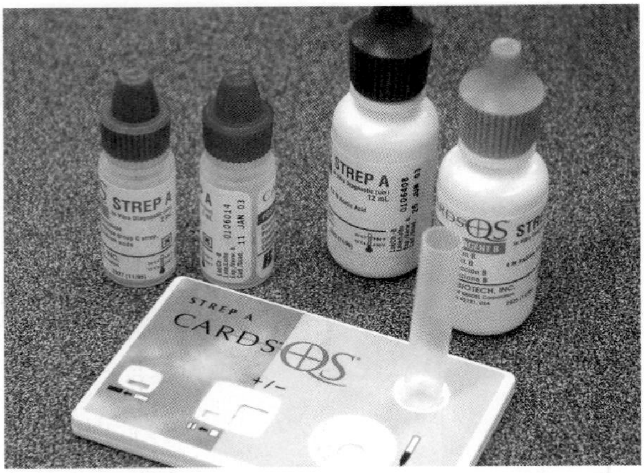

FIGURE 11-23 Cards QS Strep A test kit. (Quidel Corp., San Diego, CA.)

imbalance can lead to death. Potassium plays a major role in nerve conduction, muscle function, acid-base balance, and osmotic pressure. It influences cardiac output by helping to control the rate and force of heart contraction.

Review: Yes ☐ No ☐

84. Answer: c

Why: The guaiac test detects occult or hidden blood in feces.

Review: Yes ☐ No ☐

85. Answer: b

Why: When one is performing a PPD or tuberculin (TB) test, 0.1 mL of diluted antigen is injected under the skin. The antigen injected is purified protein derivative, or PPD (Fig. 11-1).

Review: Yes ☐ No ☐

86. Answer: c

Why: Erythema means "redness."

Review: Yes ☐ No ☐

87. Answer: a

Why: Skin test reactions often produce erythema (redness) or induration (hardness), or both, around the injection site. Interpretation of a TB skin test is based on the presence or absence of induration, or a firm raised area of swelling around the injection site. A positive test results when the area of induration measures 10 mm or greater in diameter. An area between 5 and 9 mm is considered doubtful. An area less than 5 mm is considered negative.

Review: Yes ☐ No ☐

88. Answer: c

Why: Point-of-care detection of Group A strep normally requires a throat swab specimen. Secretions from the swab are tested for the presence of strep A antigen. Several different companies make special test kits (Fig. 11-23) for rapid detection of strep A.

Review: Yes ☐ No ☐

89. Answer: d

Why: Bilirubin, glucose, and leukocytes are all commonly detected in urine by reagent

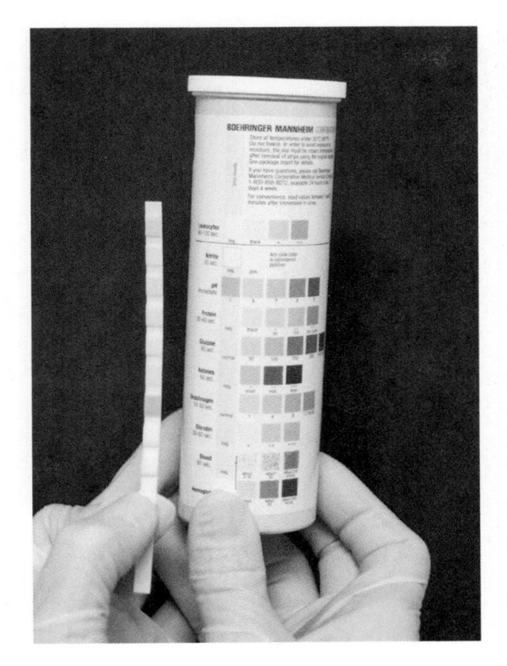

FIGURE 11-24 Technician comparing a urine reagent strip with the chart on a reagent strip container.

strip methods. Reagent strips also typically detect bacteria, blood, pH, protein, specific gravity, and urobilinogen. A chemical reaction resulting in color changes to the strip takes place when the strip is dipped in a urine specimen. Results are determined by visually comparing color changes on the strip with a chart of color codes on the reagent strip container (Fig. 11-24).

Review: Yes ☐ No ☐

90. Answer: b

Why: B-type natriuretic peptide (BNP) is a cardiac hormone and is the first objective measurement for congestive heart failure (CHF). BNP levels help physicians differentiate between COPD and CHF.

Review: Yes ☐ No ☐

ARTERIAL PUNCTURE PROCEDURES

CHAPTER 12

study tip

Questions in this chapter test the ability to describe ABG procedures, including the primary reason for the test, commonly measured ABG parameters, supplies and equipment needed, and radial ABG procedure steps. Questions also test the ability to describe patient assessment and preparation procedures including steady state requirements, the modified Allen test, optional administration of anesthetic, and site selection criteria, including the advantages and disadvantages of each collection site. Questions also test the ability to identify hazards, complications, sampling errors associated with ABG collection, and the criteria for specimen rejection.

overview

The primary reason arterial puncture is performed is to collect arterial blood gas (ABG) specimens. ABG evaluation is used in the diagnosis and management of respiratory disease to provide valuable information about a patient's oxygenation and ventilation status, and acid-base balance. It is also used in the management of electrolyte and acid-base balance in patients with other disorders.

This chapter assesses knowledge of ABG collection procedures from initial patient assessment through specimen handling and transportation. Hazards, complications, and sampling errors associated with arterial puncture are also covered. Phlebotomists must have a thorough understanding of all aspects of ABG collection to ensure accurate results and the safety of the patient.

REVIEW QUESTIONS

Choose the BEST answer.

1. Arteriospasm is defined as:
   a. a tingling feeling in the fingertips when a needle enters an artery.
   b. artery contraction resulting from pain, irritation by a needle, or anxiety.
   c. fainting related to hypotension caused by a nervous response.
   d. pain that shoots up the side of the arm after needle penetration.

2. Formation of a thrombus can result in all of the following EXCEPT:
   a. entire blockage of the lumen.
   b. impairment of the circulation.
   c. injury to the inner arterial wall.
   d. obstruction of the blood flow.

3. Significantly inaccurate arterial blood gas values can result from all of the following EXCEPT:
   a. delay of the blood gas analysis.
   b. improper use of anticoagulant.
   c. microclots that are undetected.
   d. puncture of the femoral artery.

4. All of the following can affect the integrity of a blood gas sample EXCEPT:
   a. improper mixing of the sample.
   b. increased vagus nerve activity.
   c. too much or too little heparin.
   d use of the wrong anticoagulant.

5. Blood gas specimen rejection criteria include all of the following EXCEPT:
   a. improper labeling or missing label.
   b. inadequate volume of the specimen.
   c. unexpected replacement of the syringe.
   d. visible hemolysis of the specimen.

6. Patient complications associated with arterial puncture include all of the following EXCEPT:
   a. hematoma.
   b. infection.
   c. numbness.
   d. venostasis.

7. Which of the following actions associated with arterial blood gas procedure are in the correct order?
   a. assess, position, clean, puncture, fill, expel, label
   b. clean, position, assess, puncture, fill, label, expel
   c. label, clean, position, puncture, fill, assess, expel
   d. position, clean, assess, puncture, fill, expel, label

8. Why is arterial blood better for blood gas determination than a venous sample?
   a. Analytes in venous blood specimens are not as stable.
   b. Arterial analytes are consistent throughout the body.
   c. It is technically easier to perform arterial puncture.
   d. Venous blood is more subject to preanalytical error.

9. The blood gas parameter HCO_3 measures the amount of:
   a. bicarbonate circulating in the blood.
   b. carbon dioxide dissolved in the blood.
   c. oxygen dissolved in the bloodstream.
   d. oxygen that is bound to hemoglobin.

10. Which of the following tests requires an arterial specimen?
    a. blood culture
    b. blood gases
    c. blood glucose
    d. blood typing

11. Which of the following is *not* a blood gas component?
    a. pCO_2
    b. pH
    c. PO_2
    d. PO_4

12. Arterial blood gas evaluation would *most* likely be performed on a patient with:
a. chronic hepatitis.
b. hypothyroidism.
c. osteochondritis.
d. pulmonary disease.

13. All of the following are typically used in arterial puncture instruction EXCEPT:
a. diagnosis of the condition at bedside.
b. extensive training involving theory.
c. observation of the actual procedure.
d. supervised arterial puncture practice.

14. Arterial puncture site selection is based on all of the following EXCEPT:
a. available equipment in the room.
b. presence of collateral circulation.
c. size and accessibility of the artery.
d. type of tissue surrounding the site.

15. All of the following conditions would be reasons to avoid a site as a choice for arterial puncture EXCEPT:
a. a pulse that is especially strong.
b. inflammation of the extremity.
c. presence of a fistula or a shunt.
d. recent arterial puncture at the site.

16. The preferred and most common site for arterial puncture is the:
a. brachial artery.
b. femoral artery.
c. radial artery.
d. ulnar artery.

17. Which artery is generally easiest to access during low cardiac output?
a. brachial
b. femoral
c. radial
d. ulnar

18. The *biggest* advantage of choosing the radial artery for arterial blood gas collection is:
a. good collateral circulation is present.
b. it is easier to locate when there is low blood pressure.
c. it is easy to compress to stop bleeding.
d. it is the largest artery and the most easily palpated.

19. Which of the following is a disadvantage of using the radial artery for ABG collection?
a. It is not easy to fully compress.
b. It is small and difficult to feel.
c. There is a risk of hematoma formation.
d. There is no collateral circulation.

20. Which of the following is an advantage of using the brachial artery for arterial blood collection?
a. It is large and much easier to palpate.
b. It is not as deep as the radial artery.
c. Risk of hematoma formation is lower.
d. The artery is easy to compress.

21. Disadvantages of puncturing the brachial artery include all of the following EXCEPT that it:
a. has erratic blood pressure.
b. is deep and harder to feel.
c. lies close to the basilic vein.
d. lies near the median nerve.

22. Which arterial site poses the greatest risk of infection?
a. brachial
b. femoral
c. radial
d. ulnar

23. Other sites where arterial specimens may be obtained include all of the following EXCEPT:
a. common carotid artery in the neck.
b. dorsal pedis FOOT arteries of adults.
c. indwelling arterial lines in the arm.
d. infant scalp and umbilical arteries.

24. In addition to normal patient identification information, an arterial blood gas requisition typically includes all of the following EXCEPT:
    a. age at onset of respiratory disease.
    b. method of ventilation or delivery.
    c. patient activity and body position.
    d. temperature and respiration rate.

25. Which of the following equipment is *not* necessary for blood gas collection?
    a. 1- to 5-mL self-filling syringe
    b. antiseptic cleaning solution
    c. disposable tourniquet strap
    d. self-adhering gauze bandage

26. Arterial blood gas specimens are collected in syringes rather than tubes because:
    a. a syringe holds the right amount of blood.
    b. anaerobic conditions are easier to maintain.
    c. evacuated tube pressure can change results.
    d. the sterility of the specimen is guaranteed.

27. PPE required when collecting arterial specimens includes all of the following EXCEPT:
    a. boots.
    b. gloves.
    c. lab coat.
    d. mask.

28. Commercially prepared arterial sampling kits typically contain all of the following EXCEPT:
    a. 1% lidocaine-filled syringe.
    b. cover for the syringe hub.
    c. needle with safety device.
    d. special heparinized syringe.

29. Heparin is used in arterial sample collection to:
    a. increase blood flow in the area.
    b. numb the area around the site.
    c. prevent clotting of the specimen.
    d. stabilize the oxygen content.

30. Lidocaine is sometimes used during arterial puncture to:
    a. anesthetize the site prior to the puncture.
    b. help dissolve air bubbles in the specimen.
    c. keep clots from forming in the specimen.
    d. maintain specimen in an anaerobic state.

31. Prior to collection of arterial blood gases, a patient should have been in a steady state for at least:
    a. 5 to 10 minutes.
    b. 10 to 15 minutes.
    c. 15 to 20 minutes.
    d. 20 to 30 minutes.

32. Steady state means that the patient has:
    a. been fasting for at least 8 hours.
    b. been sleeping for at least 1 hour.
    c. had no O_2 therapy for 12 hours.
    d. had no suction or respirator changes.

33. The purpose of performing the modified Allen test prior to arterial specimen collection is to:
    a. assess patient ventilation status.
    b. determine collateral circulation.
    c. locate the pulse in the ulnar artery.
    d. measure the radial artery pressure.

34. When performing the modified Allen test, which artery is released first?
    a. brachial
    b. femoral
    c. radial
    d. ulnar

35. What constitutes a positive modified Allen test? The:
    a. blood pressure increases in the radial artery.
    b. color drains from the hand in at least 30 seconds.
    c. hand color returns to normal in 15 seconds.
    d. pulse in the ulnar artery becomes irregular.

36. Which of the following is proper procedure if a patient *does not* have collateral circulation?
    a. Check for collateral circulation in the other arm.
    b. Perform arterial puncture on the femoral artery.
    c. Perform arterial puncture on the radial artery.
    d. Perform arterial puncture on the ulnar artery.

37. A patient who has collateral circulation:
    a. does not need respiratory therapy or assessment.
    b. does not need to undergo radial artery puncture.
    c. has multiple arteries supplying blood to an area.
    d. has normal arterial pressure in both wrist areas.

38. Which one of the following radial arterial blood gas specimen collection steps is optional?
    a. administration of local anesthetic
    b. collateral circulation assessment
    c. current steady state determination
    d. verification of required conditions

39. Positioning of the arm for radial arterial blood gas specimen collection includes all of the following EXCEPT:
    a. 30° wrist angle.
    b. arm adducted.
    c. palm facing up.
    d. supported wrist.

40. The radial artery is located in the:
    a. antecubital fossa.
    b. crease of the groin.
    c. pinky side of the wrist.
    d. thumb side of the wrist.

41. The thumb should not be used to feel for an artery because it:
    a. has a pulse.
    b. is insensitive.
    c. is too large.
    d. is too strong.

42. Proper antisepsis prior to arterial specimen collection includes all of the following EXCEPT:
    a. allowing the site to air dry before puncturing.
    b. cleaning the phlebotomist's dominant hand.
    c. maintaining antisepsis at the puncture site.
    d. prepping with isopropyl alcohol, three times.

43. When performing arterial puncture, direct the needle:
    a. away from the hand, facing the blood flow.
    b. bevel down to prevent reflux of the blood.
    c. perpendicular to the wrist and lower arm.
    d. toward the hand, against the blood flow.

44. Which of the following is an acceptable angle of needle insertion for drawing radial arterial blood gases?
    a. 15°
    b. 20°
    c. 45°
    d. 90°

45. The proper angle of needle insertion for drawing femoral arterial blood gas is:
    a. 15°.
    b. 30°.
    c. 45°.
    d. 90°.

46. The typical needle used to collect blood from a radial artery is:
    a. 18-gauge 1 inch.
    b. 22-gauge 1 inch.
    c. 23-gauge 1 ½ inch.
    d. 25-gauge 1 ½ inch.

47. How do you know when you have "hit" an artery during arterial blood gas collection?
    a. A flash of blood appears in the syringe hub.
    b. Blood immediately seeps around the needle.
    c. The pulse in the artery becomes erratic.
    d. The syringe needle bends because of resistance.

48. Which of the following is the *best* way to tell if a specimen is arterial? As the specimen is collected, the blood will:
    a. appear bright cherry red.
    b. contain some air bubbles.
    c. look dark bluish-red in color.
    d. pump into the collection syringe.

49. As soon as the needle is withdrawn following arterial blood gas specimen collection, the:
    a. nurse should apply a special arterial puncture bandage.
    b. patient should apply pressure to the site for 3 to 5 minutes.
    c. phlebotomist should apply a pressure bandage to the site.
    d. phlebotomist should apply site pressure for 3 to 5 minutes.

50. Proper specimen handling immediately following specimen collection includes all of the following EXCEPT:
    a. mix the specimen to prevent clotting.
    b. place the specimen in a pink top tube.
    c. remove air bubbles from the specimen.
    d. remove and discard the safety needle.

51. After performing arterial puncture, check the pulse:
    a. distal to the puncture site.
    b. in the ulnar artery in the wrist.
    c. medial to the puncture site.
    d. proximal to the puncture site.

52. What should the phlebotomist do if the pulse is absent or faint following arterial blood gas collection?
    a. Apply a pressure bandage to the site immediately.
    b. Gently massage the patient's wrist and hand.
    c. Nothing, because an arteriospasm is expected.
    d. Notify the patient's nurse or the lab supervisor.

53. An arterial specimen collected in an appropriate plastic syringe is typically transported:
    a. at room temperature.
    b. in a small heat block.
    c. in an ice slurry cup.
    d. vertically in a syringe.

54. Specimens for electrolyte testing in addition to arterial blood gas analysis should be:
    a. kept in a heat block during delivery.
    b. placed in a cup of ice slurry ASAP.
    c. transferred to a red top test tube.
    d. transported at room temperature.

55. If the patient has an elevated white blood count, the arterial blood gas specimen should be:
    a. analyzed ASAP.
    b. collected in EDTA.
    c. kept in a heat block.
    d. mixed continually.

56. Which of the following is the most common arterial puncture complication even when proper procedure is used?
    a. arteriospasm
    b. bacteremia
    c. clot formation
    d. hematoma

57. Which of the following would be a reason to terminate arterial puncture?
    a. Bright red-colored blood spurts into the syringe.
    b. The artery is missed and needle redirection is required.
    c. The patient complains of extreme pain and discomfort.
    d. The specimen appears dark reddish blue.

58. Sudden fainting during arterial puncture is all of the following EXCEPT:
    a. called vasovagal syncope.
    b. caused by extreme pain.
    c. related to hypoglycemia.
    d. triggered by hypotension.

59. Which of the following should *not* be a cause of erroneous arterial blood gas results?
    a. 45-minute delay in processing
    b. air bubbles in the specimen
    c. failure to place the syringe on ice
    d. microclots found in the specimen

60. All of the following would cause an arterial blood gas specimen to be rejected EXCEPT:
    a. improper specimen labeling.
    b. insufficient specimen amount.
    c. obvious microclot formation.
    d. unavoidable delay in collection.

ANSWERS AND EXPLANATIONS

1. Answer: b
   Why: Pain or irritation caused by needle penetration of the artery muscle and even patient anxiety can cause a reflex (involuntary) contraction of the artery referred to as an arteriospasm. The condition is transitory but can make it difficult to obtain a specimen.
   Review: Yes ☐ No ☐

2. Answer: c
   Why: Injury to the intima, or inner wall of the artery, can lead to thrombus, or clot formation. A thrombus may grow until it blocks the entire lumen of the artery, obstructing blood flow and impairing circulation. Even though a thrombus may attach temporarily to a vessel, it does not injure the inner arterial wall.
   Review: Yes ☐ No ☐

3. Answer: d
   Why: Blood cells continue to metabolize at room temperature, so processing the specimen as soon as possible after it is collected helps ensure the most accurate results. Anticoagulants other than heparin can alter results, especially pH. Undetected microclots can lead to erroneous results. All acceptable sites for arterial puncture will result in accurate values if the procedure is performed correctly.
   Review: Yes ☐ No ☐

4. Answer: b
   Why: Improper mixing of the sample, use of the wrong anticoagulant, and too much or too little of the anticoagulant heparin can affect the integrity of the blood gas sample. Vasovagal syncope (faintness or fainting resulting from increased vagus nerve activity on the artery) can occur during arterial puncture but will not affect the integrity of the sample.
   Review: Yes ☐ No ☐

5. Answer: c
   Why: Blood gas rejection criteria include improper labeling and inadequate volume and hemolysis of the specimen. If for some reason the syringe in the prepackaged kit is faulty, replacement of that syringe with one from another kit would be the appropriate action to take and would not be a reason for rejection of the sample.
   Review: Yes ☐ No ☐

6. Answer: d
   Why: Complications or hazards associated with arterial puncture include infection, hematoma, and numbness. Venostasis is defined as trapping of blood in an extremity by compression of the veins and is usually the result of tying the tourniquet too tight and leaving it in place for too long. When one is performing an arterial puncture, a tourniquet is not used.
   Review: Yes ☐ No ☐

7. Answer: a
   Why: The ABG procedure includes the following steps: (1) *assess* steady state; (2) *position* arm; (3) *clean* the site; (4) *puncture* at a 30° to 45° angle; (5) *fill* the syringe to a proper level; (6) *expel* air bubbles; and (7) *label* the specimen.
   Review: Yes ☐ No ☐

8. Answer: b
   Why: Arterial blood is the ideal specimen for many analyses because its composition is fairly consistent throughout the body, whereas the composition of venous blood varies relative to the metabolic needs of the area of the body it serves.
   Review: Yes ☐ No ☐

9. Answer: a
   Why: HCO_3 is bicarbonate. This ABG component is a measure of the amount of bicarbonate in the blood and is used to evaluate the

bicarbonate buffer system of the kidneys. Metabolic disturbances alter HCO_3 levels.

Review: Yes ☐ No ☐

10. Answer: b
Why: The primary reason for performing arterial puncture is to obtain blood for evaluation of arterial blood gases (ABGs). Blood bank specimens for typing, blood cultures, and blood glucoses are performed on venous specimens.
Review: Yes ☐ No ☐

11. Answer: d
Why: Arterial blood gas components commonly measured include pCO_2, pH, and PO_2. PO_4 is the designation for phosphate and is not a blood gas component.
Review: Yes ☐ No ☐

12. Answer: d
Why: Arterial blood gas evaluation is used in the diagnosis and management of respiratory or pulmonary disease to provide information about a patient's oxygenation, ventilation, and acid-base balance.
Review: Yes ☐ No ☐

13. Answer: a
Why: Personnel who perform ABG procedures are normally certified by their healthcare institutions after successfully completing extensive training involving theory, demonstration of technique, observation of the actual procedure, and performance of arterial puncture under the supervision of qualified personnel. Diagnosis is not part of the phlebotomist's training or duties.
Review: Yes ☐ No ☐

14. Answer: a
Why: Several different sites can be used for arterial puncture, and the choice of site is never based on what equipment is available in the room or on the phlebotomist's tray. The criteria for site selection include the presence of collateral circulation, how large and accessible the artery is, and the type of tissue surrounding the puncture site.
Review: Yes ☐ No ☐

15. Answer: a
Why: The presence of inflammation or edema, a fistula or shunt in the extremity, or a recent previous arterial puncture in the same site are all reasons to avoid a site as a choice for arterial puncture. A pulse that is especially strong would be of benefit to the phlebotomist in locating the artery and is not a reason to avoid the area as a site for ABG collection.
Review: Yes ☐ No ☐

16. Answer: c
Why: The radial artery (Fig. 12-1) located in the thumb side of the wrist is the preferred and therefore the first choice and most common site used for arterial puncture. The brachial artery is the second choice. Puncture of the femoral artery (Fig. 12-2) is typically performed only in emergency situations by physicians and specially trained emergency room personnel. The ulnar artery is reserved to provide collateral circulation to the hand in the event the radial artery is damaged and is never used for arterial puncture.
Review: Yes ☐ No ☐

17. Answer: b
Why: The femoral artery is large and easily located and punctured. It is sometimes the only site where arterial sampling is possible on patients with low cardiac output.
Review: Yes ☐ No ☐

18. Answer: a
Why: The biggest advantage of choosing the radial artery for ABG collection is the presence of good collateral circulation. Collateral circulation means that more than one artery

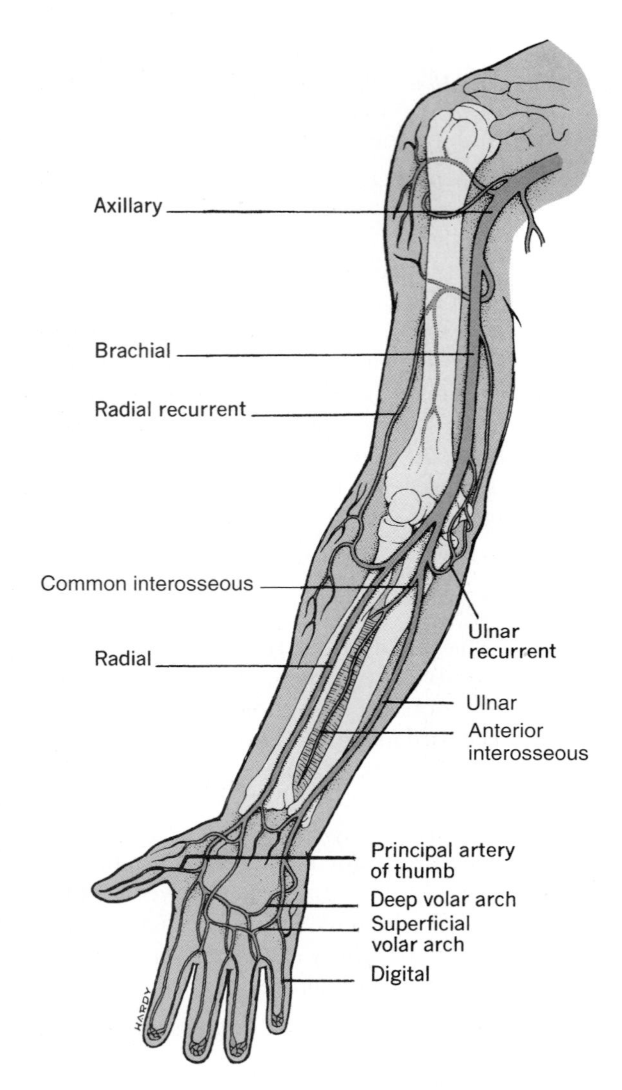

FIGURE 12-1 Arteries of the arm and hand.

supplies blood to the area. If the radial artery were to be inadvertently damaged, the ulnar artery would still supply blood to the area.
Review: Yes ☐ No ☐

19. Answer: b
Why: One disadvantage of collecting ABGs from the radial artery is the considerable skill it takes to successfully puncture since it is so small. The presence of ligaments and bone in the area to aid in compression *decreases* the chance of hematoma formation, which is an advantage. The presence of collateral circulation via the ulnar artery is also an advantage.
Review: Yes ☐ No ☐

20. Answer: a
Why: One advantage of using the brachial artery is it is large and easily palpated. However, it is located deeper than the radial artery, rather than not as deep, which is a disadvantage. In addition, there is increased risk of hematoma formation, not less, because lack of underlying ligaments or bones to support compression makes it harder to compress.
Review: Yes ☐ No ☐

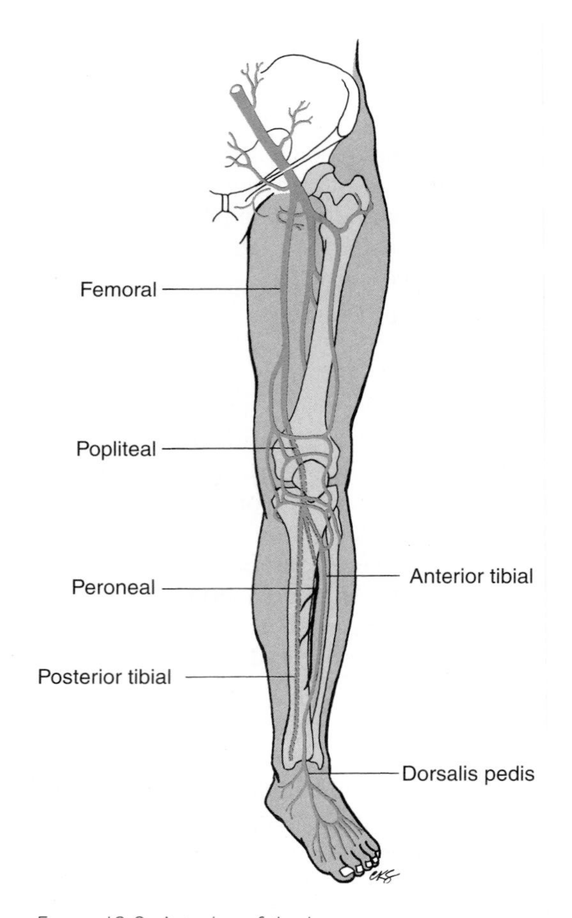

FIGURE 12-2 Arteries of the leg.

21. Answer: a
Why: Disadvantages of puncturing the brachial artery are that it is deeper and harder to palpate than the radial artery and that it lies close to the basilic vein and the median nerve, both of which could be inadvertently punctured. Blood pressure in the brachial artery should be consistent with the arterial system throughout the body and would not be significantly different than that of the radial artery.
Review: Yes ☐ No ☐

22. Answer: b
Why: The femoral artery (Fig. 12-2) is located superficially in the groin lateral to the pubis bone. This area poses the greatest risk of infection because the presence of pubic hair makes it difficult to achieve an aseptic site.
Review: Yes ☐ No ☐

23. Answer: a
Why: In addition to the radial, brachial, and femoral arteries, arterial specimens may be obtained from the dorsal pedis foot arteries of adults, scalp and umbilical arteries in infants, and indwelling lines. The phlebotomist is not normally trained to perform arterial punctures at these additional sites or from indwelling lines. Arterial specimens are not normally collected from the carotid artery.
Review: Yes ☐ No ☐

24. Answer: a
Why: An ABG requisition typically includes the patient's body temperature and respiratory rate, method of ventilation or delivery, and patient activity and body position in addition to normal patient identification information. The patient's age at onset of respiratory disease is not found on the requisition.
Review: Yes ☐ No ☐

25. Answer: c
Why: A tourniquet is not necessary to find the artery and not used when collecting an arterial specimen. To locate an artery, the phlebotomist feels for the pulse. Arterial blood gas equipment is shown in Fig. 12-3.
Review: Yes ☐ No ☐

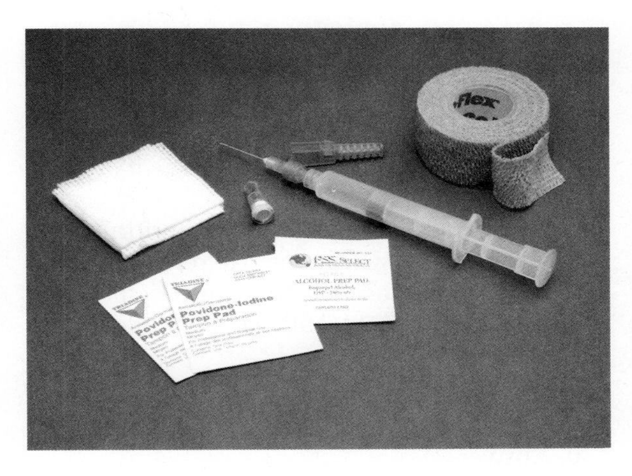

FIGURE 12-3 ABG equipment.

26. Answer: c
Why: Arterial blood gas specimens are not collected in evacuated tubes, because the tube pressure or vacuum would alter test results.
Review: Yes ☐ No ☐

27. Answer: a
Why: Personal protective equipment (PPE) required when collecting arterial specimens includes a fluid-resistant lab coat, gloves, and face protection. Wearing boots is not required.
Review: Yes ☐ No ☐

28. Answer: a
Why: Commercially prepared arterial sampling kits are available from several manufacturers. A kit typically contains a safety needle, a heparinized syringe with a filter that removes residual air, and a cap or other device to plug or cover the syringe hub after specimen collection to maintain anaerobic conditions. Use of local anesthetic is optional;

consequently, equipment to administer local anesthetic (i.e., a lidocaine-filled syringe) is *not* normally part of a prepared ABG kit.

Review: Yes ☐ No ☐

29. Answer: c
Why: Arterial blood gases are performed on whole blood specimens. Therefore, an anticoagulant is needed to keep the specimen from clotting. The anticoagulant of choice is heparin.
Review: Yes ☐ No ☐

30. Answer: a
Why: Lidocaine is sometimes used to numb the site before arterial puncture. Although once part of standard arterial puncture procedure, use of local anesthetic is now optional. The advent of improved thin-wall needles that make arterial puncture less painful has made the routine administration of anesthetic prior to arterial puncture unnecessary.
Review: Yes ☐ No ☐

31. Answer: d
Why: Current body temperature, breathing pattern, and the concentration of oxygen inhaled all affect arterial blood gas results. Consequently, it is best if a patient has been in a steady state (i.e., no exercise, suctioning, or respirator changes) for 20 to 30 minutes before blood gases are obtained.
Review: Yes ☐ No ☐

32. Answer: d
Why: Steady state, which is required prior to ABG collection, means that the patient has had no exercise, suctioning, or respirator changes during the 20 to 30 minutes immediately preceding specimen collection.
Review: Yes ☐ No ☐

33. Answer: b
Why: The modified Allen test, as shown in Fig. 12-4, is performed to determine the presence of collateral circulation. Collateral circulation means that the area of the body receives blood from more than one artery. Collateral circulation is necessary in the event that damage to the artery occurs during arterial puncture. If the patient has circulation through an alternate artery, the area of the body that is normally fed by the damaged artery will receive blood from the alternate artery.
Review: Yes ☐ No ☐

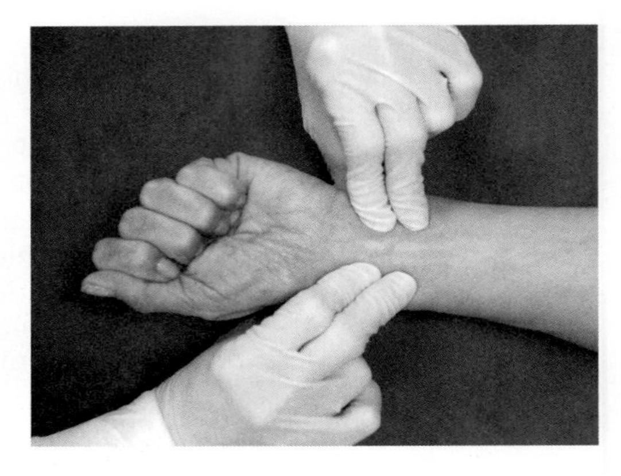

FIGURE 12-4 Obstruction of radial and ulnar arteries in initial step of Allen's test.

34. Answer: d
Why: The modified Allen test checks for the presence of collateral circulation to the hand via the ulnar artery. Circulation via the ulnar artery is important in the event that the radial artery is damaged during arterial puncture. Consequently, when one is performing the modified Allen test, the ulnar artery is released first (Fig. 12-5).
Review: Yes ☐ No ☐

35. Answer: c
Why: When one is performing the modified Allen test, both the ulnar and radial arteries are compressed to stop arterial flow to the hand. With both arteries compressed, the hand should appear blanched, or drained of color. If the patient has collateral circulation, the hand will flush pink or normal color when the ulnar artery is released even though the radial artery is still compressed.

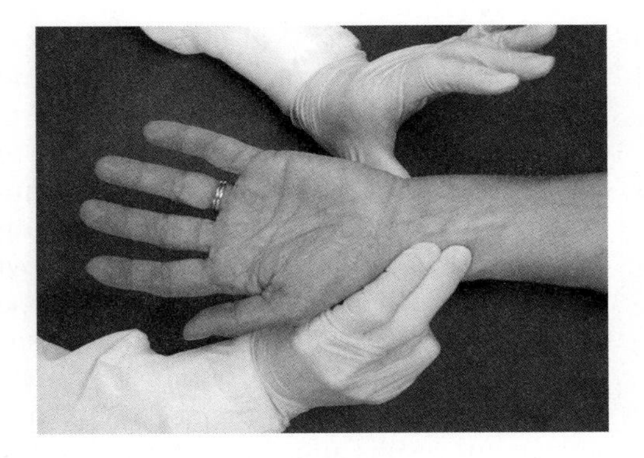

FIGURE 12-5 Ulnar artery released to allow return of blood to the hand.

The presence of collateral circulation constitutes a positive modified Allen test.

Review: Yes ☐ No ☐

36. Answer: a
    Why: If the modified Allen test result is negative, the patient does not have collateral circulation and arterial puncture cannot be performed on the radial artery of that arm. At this point, the phlebotomist should check for collateral circulation in the other arm. Arterial puncture should never be performed on the ulnar artery. Phlebotomists are not normally trained to perform femoral punctures.
    Review: Yes ☐ No ☐

37. Answer: c
    Why: A patient who has collateral circulation has more than one artery supplying blood to that area of the body.
    Review: Yes ☐ No ☐

38. Answer: a
    Why: Administration of local anesthetic to numb the site before arterial puncture is optional. Verification of required conditions, assessment of steady state, and determination of the presence of collateral circulation are mandatory steps of the procedure.
    Review: Yes ☐ No ☐

39. Answer: b
    Why: Proper arm positioning before puncture of the radial artery includes having the patient's arm abducted (out to the side), not adducted (toward the midline of the body), with the palm up and the wrist extended at approximately 30° and supported (e.g., by a rolled towel placed under it).
    Review: Yes ☐ No ☐

40. Answer: d
    Why: The radial artery is located in the thumb side of the wrist. The brachial artery is located in the antecubital area. The femoral artery is located in the groin. The ulnar artery is located in the little finger (pinky) side of the wrist.
    Review: Yes ☐ No ☐

41. Answer: a
    Why: The thumb should never be used to feel for an artery because it has a pulse that could be misleading when locating an artery.
    Review: Yes ☐ No ☐

42. Answer: d
    Why: Proper antisepsis before arterial specimen collection is important. The site must be cleaned using a suitable antiseptic such as povidone-iodine and allowed to air dry. The phlebotomist's nondominant index finger should be prepped in the same manner because it will be used to relocate the artery. Antisepsis of the site must be maintained. No nonsterile object should touch the site before puncture.
    Review: Yes ☐ No ☐

43. Answer: a
    Why: During puncture of the radial artery, the needle with the bevel up is directed away from the hand, facing the arterial blood flow.
    Review: Yes ☐ No ☐

44. Answer: c
Why: An acceptable angle of needle insertion during radial arterial blood gas collection is between 30° and 45° (Fig. 12-6).
Review: Yes ☐ No ☐

45. Answer: d
Why: The proper angle of needle insertion when collecting femoral arterial blood gases is 90° owing to the location of the femoral artery.
Review: Yes ☐ No ☐

46. Answer: b
Why: The 20- to 23-gauge and 25-gauge needles can be used for arterial puncture, depending on the collection site. However, a 22-gauge 1-inch needle is most commonly used for radial artery puncture.
Review: Yes ☐ No ☐

47. Answer: a
Why: Under normal circumstances, a flash of blood appears in the hub of the syringe when an artery is entered and blood will continue to pump into the syringe under its own power.
Review: Yes ☐ No ☐

48. Answer: d
Why: Blood pumping into the syringe under its own power is the best way to be certain that a specimen is arterial. Color is not a reliable indicator of successful arterial puncture. Although normal arterial blood is bright cherry red, arterial blood of patients with abnormal pulmonary function may appear almost as dark as venous blood. Arterial specimens do not normally contain air bubbles. Introduction of air into the specimen causes erroneous results and should be avoided.
Review: Yes ☐ No ☐

49. Answer: d
Why: The phlebotomist should manually apply pressure (Fig. 12-7) to the site for 3 to 5 minutes as soon as the needle is withdrawn following arterial puncture. The patient should never be allowed to hold pressure because he or she may not apply it firmly enough. A pressure bandage should never be used in place of manual pressure over the site. A pressure bandage can be applied after manual pressure has been held for the appropriate amount of time and bleeding has stopped.
Review: Yes ☐ No ☐

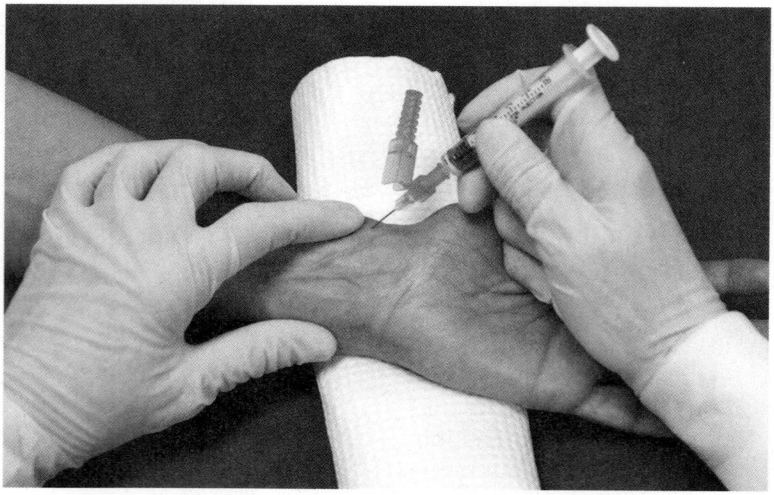

FIGURE 12-6 Needle insertion in radial artery at a 30 to 45 degree angle.

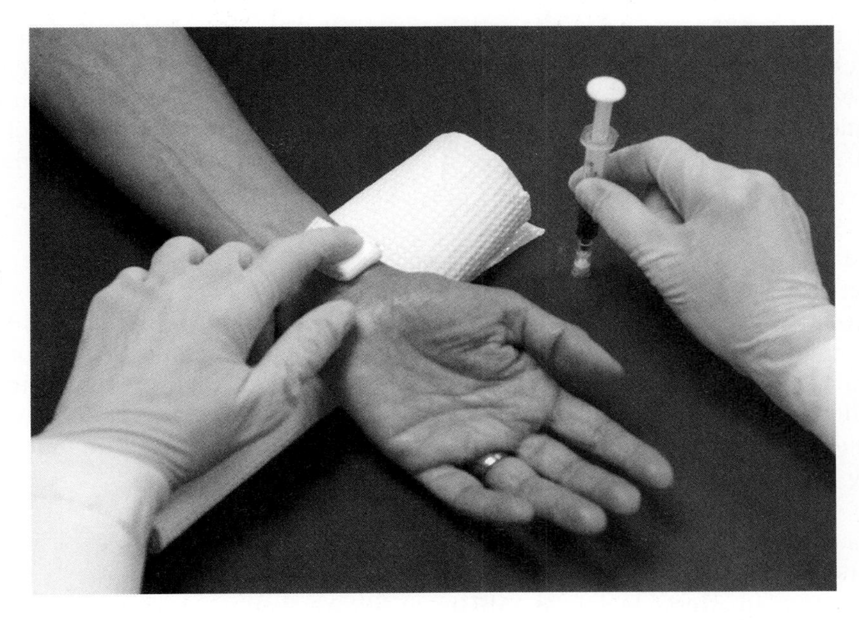

FIGURE 12-7 Clean, folded gauze firmly held on site 3 to 5 minutes after needle removal.

50. Answer: b
    Why: As soon as the arterial blood gas needle is removed from the arm, the needle safety feature is activated. The needle is then removed from the syringe, air bubbles are ejected from the specimen, and the syringe is capped with a device to prevent exposing the specimen to air (Fig. 12-7). The specimen is mixed as soon as possible to prevent clotting and transported to the lab in the syringe. An arterial blood gas must be maintained in anaerobic condition and consequently cannot be transferred to an evacuated tube at any time.
    Review: Yes ☐ No ☐

51. Answer: a
    Why: After performing arterial puncture, the pulse is checked distal or below the puncture site to ensure that blood flow is normal and no damage has occurred during the draw. If the pulse is faint or absent, a blood clot, or thrombus, may be obstructing blood flow, and the patient's nurse or physician must be notified immediately so that steps can be taken to restore proper circulation.
    Review: Yes ☐ No ☐

52. Answer: d
    Why: An absent or faint pulse following arterial puncture is not normal and indicates blood flow may be partially or completely blocked by a blood clot, or thrombus. The patient's nurse or physician, or lab supervisor in the case of an outpatient, must be notified immediately so that steps can be taken to restore proper circulation.
    Review: Yes ☐ No ☐

53. Answer: a
    Why: An arterial specimen should be transported ASAP according to laboratory protocol. At one time it was standard procedure to transport arterial blood gas (ABG) specimens on ice. The Clinical and Laboratory Standards Institute (CLSI) guidelines now call for transporting ABG specimens at room temperature

provided they are to be analyzed within 30 minutes of collection. If the patient has an elevated white blood cell count, the specimen should be analyzed within 5 minutes of collection.

Review: Yes ☐ No ☐

54. Answer: d
Why: Specimens for electrolyte testing in addition to arterial blood gas (ABG) analysis should be transported at room temperature. They should never be placed on ice because cooling affects potassium levels. ABG specimens should never be placed in a heat block.
Review: Yes ☐ No ☐

55. Answer: a
Why: If the patient has an elevated white blood cell count, an arterial blood gas (ABG) specimen should be transported at room temperature and analyzed within 5 minutes of collection. ABG specimens should never be placed in a heat block or collected in EDTA. An ABG specimen should not be mixed continually because hemolysis may result.
Review: Yes ☐ No ☐

56. Answer: a
Why: Arteriospasm is a reflex constriction of the artery that can occur even when proper technique is used. It can be caused by patient anxiety, pain during the procedure, or irritation caused by needle penetration of the artery muscle. Although this common complication is transitory, it may make it difficult to obtain a specimen. Hematoma, thrombus formation, and infection are less common complications.
Review: Yes ☐ No ☐

57. Answer: c
Why: Arterial puncture is typically more painful than venipuncture but should not cause the patient extreme pain. Extreme or significant pain indicates nerve involvement and requires immediate termination of the procedure. It is not unusual for arterial blood to spurt into the syringe during collection. Arterial blood from a patient with pulmonary function problems may be dark reddish blue (because of reduced oxygen content) rather than the typical bright red of normal arterial blood. Slight redirection of the needle to successfully access the artery is acceptable.
Review: Yes ☐ No ☐

58. Answer: c
Why: Vasovagal syncope is sudden fainting related to hypotension (not hypoglycemia) caused by a nervous system response to abrupt pain or trauma. Hypoglycemia can make a person feel faint but is associated with a low glucose level, not a nervous system response.
Review: Yes ☐ No ☐

59. Answer: c
Why: Air bubbles or microclots in the specimen, or a delay in processing longer than 30 minutes following collection, can all cause erroneous arterial blood gas (ABG) results. The Clinical and Laboratory Standards Institute (CLSI) guidelines no longer recommend transporting ABG specimens on ice provided they are processed within 30 minutes of collection.
Review: Yes ☐ No ☐

60. Answer: d
Why: If for some reason there is unavoidable delay in collection, this does not mean that the specimen would automatically be rejected. A delay in collecting the specimen could mean that the draw would have to be rescheduled if the timing was critical, however. A specimen with improper labeling would be rejected because it could result in misidentification of the specimen. A specimen would also be rejected if there is not enough specimen to perform the test. A specimen with microclots would be rejected because ABGs are performed on whole blood samples, and microclots cause erroneous results.
Review: Yes ☐ No ☐

NONBLOOD SPECIMENS AND TESTS

CHAPTER 13

study tip

Questions in this chapter test the ability to name the various types of nonblood specimens and tests, identify the source of each type of specimen, and list reasons why these specimens are collected. Questions also test the ability to describe collection procedures, including applicable patient collection instructions; preferred specimen types; specimen components tested; how results are reported, if applicable; and any special handling and transportation requirements.

overview

Although blood is the type of specimen most frequently analyzed in a medical laboratory, various other body substances are also analyzed. The phlebotomist may be involved in obtaining these specimens (e.g., throat swab collection) or in test administration (e.g., sweat chloride collection); instruction (e.g., urine collection); processing (accessioning and preparing the specimen for testing); or merely in the labeling or transporting of specimens. This chapter assesses knowledge of routine and special nonblood specimen procedures, including the collection and handling of urine specimens and other nonblood body fluids and substances. A phlebotomist with a thorough understanding of all aspects of nonblood specimen collection helps ensure the quality of the specimen and the accuracy of test results.

REVIEW QUESTIONS

Choose the BEST answer.

1. An antibiotic susceptibility test determines which antibiotics:
   a. are effective against a particular microbe.
   b. cause an allergic reaction in the patient.
   c. cause the fewest side effects in the patient.
   d. reduce a patient's infection susceptibility.

2. Body fluids can be all of the following EXCEPT:
   a. buccal material for DNA tests.
   b. found in intracellular spaces.
   c. liquid or semiliquid material.
   d. produced by some body organs.

3. A catheterized urine specimen is collected:
   a. after stimulating urine production with intravenous histamine.
   b. by aspirating it with a sterile syringe inserted into the bladder.
   c. following midstream, clean-catch urine collection procedures.
   d. from a sterile tube passed through the urethra into the bladder.

4. CSF is the abbreviation for fluid that comes from the:
   a. joint cavities.
   b. lung cavity.
   c. pelvic cavity.
   d. spinal cavity.

5. Clean-catch refers to a urine specimen that is collected:
   a. after cleaning the genital area.
   b. from a catheter in the bladder.
   c. in a container that is sterile.
   d. the first thing in the morning.

6. A test that identifies bacteria and the antibiotics that can be used against them is:
   a. AFP
   b. C & S
   c. guaiac.
   d. O & P

7. Which of the following types of infections would be classified as a UTI?
   a. bladder
   b. lung
   c. nasal
   d. throat

8. Fluid aspirated from the sac that surrounds the heart is:
   a. amniotic fluid.
   b. pericardial fluid.
   c. peritoneal fluid.
   d. synovial fluid.

9. This test includes a physical, chemical, and microscopic analysis of the specimen.
   a. AFP
   b. C & S
   c. GTT
   d. UA

10. A technician is aspirating a specimen from a flexible tube coming out of a patient's nose. What type of test was most likely ordered?
    a. gastric analysis
    b. *H. pylori* culture
    c. sputum culture
    d. stomach biopsy

11. This type of specimen is obtained by inserting a flexible swab through the nose.
    a. AFP
    b. buccal
    c. gastric
    d. NP

12. This test can be used to evaluate stomach acid production.
    a. C-urea breath
    b. gastric analysis
    c. hydrogen breath
    d. sweat chloride

13. A technician collects a specimen from a child's mouth by rubbing a swab on the inside of the cheek. What type of specimen is most likely being collected?
 a. breath
 b. buccal
 c. sputum
 d. throat

14. A type of bacteria that can damage the stomach lining is:
 a. *Bordetella pertussis.*
 b. *Helicobacter pylori.*
 c. *Neisseria meningitidis.*
 d. *Staphylococcus aureus.*

15. An exocrine gland disorder that primarily affects the lungs, upper respiratory tract, liver, and pancreas is:
 a. cystic fibrosis.
 b. emphysema.
 c. herpes zoster.
 d. tuberculosis.

16. A term used to describe blood that cannot be seen with the naked eye is:
 a. guaiac.
 b. micro.
 c. occult.
 d. serous.

17. What special information in addition to routine identification information is required when labeling a nonblood specimen?
 a. any special handling needs
 b. biohazard warning sticker
 c. ordering physician's name
 d. type and source of specimen

18. Which type of specimen must be handled and analyzed STAT?
 a. buccal swab
 b. gastric fluid
 c. spinal fluid
 d. throat swab

19. The most frequently analyzed nonblood specimen is:
 a. feces.
 b. saliva.
 c. CSF.
 d. urine.

20. All of the following can occur in urine specimens that are not processed in a timely fashion EXCEPT:
 a. breakdown of bilirubin.
 b. decomposition of cells.
 c. increased ketone levels.
 d. overgrowth of bacteria.

21. Which specimen is ideal for most urine tests?
 a. 8-hour
 b. 24-hour
 c. fasting
 d. random

22. Routine urinalysis specimens that cannot be analyzed within 2 hours require:
 a. 25° C storage.
 b. a preservative.
 c. recollection.
 d. refrigeration.

23. A routine urinalysis typically includes all of the following EXCEPT:
 a. chemical analysis.
 b. cytological analysis.
 c. microscopic analysis.
 d. physical analysis.

24. A urine C & S is typically ordered to:
 a. check for glucose in the urine.
 b. diagnose urinary tract infection.
 c. evaluate function of the kidneys.
 d. monitor urinary protein levels.

25. Urine cytology studies look for the presence of:
 a. abnormal cells.
 b. heavy metals.
 c. illegal drugs.
 d. microbe toxins.

26. Urine drug screening can be used to do all of the following EXCEPT:
    a. detect prescription drug abuse.
    b. detect the use of illegal drugs.
    c. identify a deliberate overdose.
    d. monitor therapeutic drug use.

27. Suspected pregnancy is typically confirmed by testing urine for the presence of:
    a. ADH
    b. FSH
    c. HCG
    d. TSH

28. Which type of urine specimen is best for pregnancy testing?
    a. 24-hour
    b. clean-catch
    c. first voided
    d. random

29. Which type of specimen is typically used for routine urinalysis?
    a. 24-hour
    b. double-voided
    c. first morning
    d. random

30. Which urine specimen is normally the most concentrated?
    a. 24-hour
    b. first morning
    c. random
    d. timed

31. This test typically requires serial urine specimens collected at specific times.
    a. creatinine clearance
    b. glucose tolerance test
    c. urine drug screening
    d. urine pregnancy test

32. What is the recommended procedure for collecting a 24-hour urine specimen?
    a. Collect the first morning specimen and all other urine for 24 hours except the first specimen the following morning.
    b. Collect the first morning specimen and all urine for 24 hours, including the first specimen the following morning.
    c. Discard the first morning specimen; start timing; collect all urine for 24 hours including the next morning specimen.
    d. Start the timing and collect and preserve every urine specimen that is voided in any consecutive 24-hour period.

33. All of the following statements are true of a urine creatinine clearance test EXCEPT:
    a. a 24-hour urine specimen is required.
    b. a blood specimen is also collected.
    c. all urine needs to be double-voided.
    d. refrigeration of the urine is needed.

34. This type of specimen is sometimes used to compare urine concentrations of glucose and ketones to blood concentrations.
    a. 8-hour
    b. 24-hour
    c. double-voided
    d. pooled timed

35. Which urine test requires a midstream clean-catch specimen?
    a. creatinine clearance
    b. culture and sensitivity
    c. glucose tolerance test
    d. routine urinalysis

36. Which of the following midstream urine collection steps are in the proper order?
    a. void into container; void into second container; void last urine into toilet
    b. void into container; void into toilet; void remaining urine into container
    c. void into toilet; void into container; void any remaining urine into toilet
    d. void into toilet; void into container; void into toilet; void into container

37. Midstream clean-catch urine specimens require all of the following EXCEPT:
    a. a preservative in the container.
    b. collection in a sterile container.

c. prompt processing of the urine.
d. site cleaning prior to collection.

38. Which urine specimen is obtained by inserting a sterile needle directly into the urinary bladder and aspirating a sample of urine?
a. catheterized
b. double-void
c. pediatric
d. suprapubic

39. Which of the following tests is sometimes performed on amniotic fluid?
a. alkaline phosphatase
b. alpha-fetoprotein
c. lactic dehydrogenase
d. reticulocyte count

40. Amniotic fluid comes from the:
a. cavity surrounding the spinal cord.
b. membranes that enclose the lungs.
c. sac containing a fetus in the womb.
d. spaces within the moveable joints.

41. CSF analysis is used in the diagnosis of:
a. meningitis.
b. osteoporosis.
c. pneumonia.
d. renal failure.

42. Tests commonly performed on CSF include all the following EXCEPT:
a. cell counts.
b. glucose.
c. hemoglobin.
d. total protein.

43. This test requires intravenous administration of histamine or pentagastrin.
a. alpha-fetoprotein
b. gastric analysis
c. sweat chloride
d. urine porphyrins

44. An NP culture swab is sometimes collected to detect the presence of organisms that cause:
a. inflamed throats.
b. stomach ulcers.
c. urinary infection.
d. whooping cough.

45. Saliva can be tested for all of the following reasons EXCEPT to:
a. check hormone levels.
b. confirm alcohol abuse.
c. detect recent drug use.
d. diagnose tuberculosis.

46. Semen analysis can be performed to:
a. detect bladder infection.
b. evaluate fertility status.
c. identify cancerous cells.
d. monitor prostate growth.

47. A semen specimen is unlikely to be accepted for testing if it is:
a. collected in a condom.
b. collected on site.
c. in a sterile container.
d. kept at 37°C.

48. Which of the following fluids is obtained through lumbar puncture?
a. amniotic
b. gastric
c. pleural
d. spinal

49. Which of the following is a type of serous fluid?
a. gastric
b. pleural
c. seminal
d. synovial

50. Peritoneal fluid comes from the:
a. abdominal cavity.
b. lung cavities.
c. pericardial sac.
d. spinal cavity.

51. Fluid from joint cavities is called:
a. pericardial fluid.
b. peritoneal fluid.
c. pleural fluid.
d. synovial fluid.

52. Pleural fluid is aspirated from the:
    a. lungs.
    b. joints.
    c. pine
    d. stomach

53. Accumulation of excess fluid in the peritoneal cavity is called:
    a. ascites.
    b. edema.
    c. peritonitis.
    d. septicemia.

54. What is sputum?
    a. gastric fluid
    b. nasal fluid
    c. phlegm
    d. saliva

55. Sputum specimens are collected in the diagnosis of:
    a. genetic defects.
    b. lung maturity.
    c. strep throat.
    d. tuberculosis.

56. This test is used to diagnose cystic fibrosis.
    a. C-urea breath
    b. CSF analysis
    c. gastric studies
    d. sweat chloride

57. Which of the following types of ETS tubes are used for synovial fluid specimens?
    a. ACD, CPD, and serum separator
    b. citrate, EDTA, and gel separator
    c. EDTA, heparin, and non-additive
    d. sodium fluoride, CPD, and heparin

58. Synovial fluid can be tested to identify:
    a. arthritis and gout.
    b. *H. pylori* and TB.
    c. hemolytic anemia.
    d. lactose intolerance.

59. A process called iontophoresis is used to collect:
    a. breath.
    b. semen.
    c. sweat.
    d. tears.

60. Bone marrow is typically aspirated from the:
    a. iliac crest.
    b. left femur.
    c. vertebrae.
    d. wrist bone.

61. Bone marrow is studied to identify:
    a. arthritic disease.
    b. blood disorders.
    c. diabetes mellitus.
    d. osteochondritis.

62. A breath specimen can be used to detect:
    a. bacterial meningitis.
    b. *H. pylori bacteria.*
    c. pertussis microbes.
    d. whooping cough.

63. Which of the following tests may require a 72-hour stool specimen?
    a. fecal fat analysis
    b. fecal occult blood
    c. ova and parasites
    d. stool culture

64. A refrigerated stool specimen would be acceptable for all of the following EXCEPT:
    a. fecal fat analysis.
    b. fecal occult blood.
    c. guaiac testing.
    d. ova and parasites.

65. The guaiac test detects:
    a. cystic fibrosis.
    b. lung maturity.
    c. occult blood.
    d. tuberculosis.

66. Which type of sample can be tested to detect chronic drug abuse?
    a. blood
    b. hair
    c. saliva
    d. urine

67. What type of specimen is required for a "rapid strep" test?
    a. buccal swab
    b. stool sample
    c. throat swab
    d. urine sample

68. What type of specimen is collected during for a biopsy?
    a. blood
    b. stool
    c. sweat
    d. tissue

69. Which site is typically used when performing a sweat chloride test on a toddler?
    a. arm
    b. hand
    c. thigh
    d. wrist

70. The first tube of cerebrospinal fluid (CSF) collected is typically used for:
    a. chemistry studies.
    b. counting the cells.
    c. immunology tests.
    d. microbiology tests.

71. A minimally invasive way of obtaining cells for DNA analysis is to collect a:
    a. breath sample.
    b. buccal swab.
    c. stool sample.
    d. throat swab.

72. This fluid comes from the male reproductive system.
    a. pleural
    b. seminal
    c. serous
    d. synovial

73. This type of sample is sometimes collected for drug testing because it is not easily tampered with or altered.
    a. bone marrow
    b. buccal swab
    c. hair sample
    d. urine sample

74. This test detects parasites and their eggs in feces.
    a. C & S
    b. FOBT
    c. HCG
    d. O & P

75. The hydrogen breath test detects:
    a. *H. pylori bacteria.*
    b. lactose intolerance.
    c. respiratory disease.
    d. whooping cough.

ANSWERS AND EXPLANATIONS

1. Answer: a
   Why: An antibiotic susceptibility test is the sensitivity part of a culture and sensitivity test. If a microorganism is identified by culture, a sensitivity test is performed to determine which antibiotics will be effective against the microorganism—in other words, which antibiotics the microorganism is susceptible to and can be used to treat the patient.
   Review: Yes ☐ No ☐

2. Answer: a
   Why: Body fluids include blood and other liquid or semiliquid substances produced by the body and found in the intracellular and interstitial spaces and within various organs such as the bladder and body spaces such as joints. Cellular material, not fluid, from buccal swabs is used for DNA analysis.
   Review: Yes ☐ No ☐

3. Answer: d
   Why: A urine catheter is a narrow, flexible tube inserted through the urethra directly into the bladder. A catheterized urine specimen is collected when a patient is having trouble urinating or is already catheterized for other reasons. Catheterized specimens are sometimes collected on infants to obtain C & S specimens, on female patients to prevent vaginal contamination of the specimen, and on bedridden patients when serial urine specimens are needed.
   Review: Yes ☐ No ☐

4. Answer: d
   Cerebrospinal fluid (CSF) is the normally clear, colorless fluid that circulates within the cavities surrounding the brain and spinal cord.
   Review: Yes ☐ No ☐

5. Answer: a
   Why: Clean catch refers to a urine specimen collected after following a special cleaning procedure used to ensure that the specimen is free of contaminating material from the external genital area. A catheterized specimen is collected from a catheter inserted into the bladder. A urine specimen collected in a sterile container is not necessarily a clean-catch specimen, although a clean-catch specimen *is* collected in a sterile container. Urine collected first thing in the morning is called an 8-hour or first voided specimen and is not necessarily collected by clean-catch procedures.
   Review: Yes ☐ No ☐

6. Answer: b
   Why: A urine culture and sensitivity (C & S) is a test that is sometimes ordered on patients with symptoms of urinary tract infection (UTI). In the culture portion of the test, urine is placed on nutrient media that encourage the growth of bacteria. If any grow, they are identified and a sensitivity test is performed. A sensitivity test identifies antibiotics that will be effective against the bacteria.
   Review: Yes ☐ No ☐

7. Answer: a
   Why: A urinary tract infection (UTI) is an infection anywhere in the urinary system. The bladder is part of the urinary tract.
   Review: Yes ☐ No ☐

8. Answer: b
   Why: The sac that surrounds the heart is called the pericardium. Fluid found in this sac is called pericardial fluid.
   Review: Yes ☐ No ☐

9. Answer: d
   Why: A urinalysis (UA) test typically includes the physical, chemical, and microscopic analysis of a urine specimen. The physical analysis includes macroscopic observations of color, clarity, and odor and measurements of volume and specific gravity. Chemical

analysis detects the presence of substances such as bacteria, blood, white blood cells, protein, and glucose. The microscopic analysis identifies components in the urine such as cells, crystals, and microorganisms.

Review: Yes ☐ No ☐

10. Answer: a
Why: A gastric analysis test examines stomach contents for abnormal substances and measures gastric acid concentration to evaluate stomach acid production. A gastric analysis specimen is aspirated through a tube passed through the mouth or nose and the throat into the stomach.
Review: Yes ☐ No ☐

11. Answer: d
Why: A nasopharynx (NP) specimen is collected using a special flexible swab inserted gently through the nose into the nasopharynx. Alpha-fetoprotein (AFP) is a type of test that can be performed on amniotic fluid to assess fetal development. Buccal (cheek) specimens for DNA analysis are collected by swabbing the inside of the cheek. DNA is later extracted from cells on the swab. Gastric specimens are collected by passing flexible tubing through the mouth and throat (oropharynx) or nose and throat (nasopharynx) into the stomach and aspirating stomach (gastric) fluid through the tubing.
Review: Yes ☐ No ☐

12. Answer: b
Why: Gastric means "stomach." A gastric analysis test examines fluid material from the stomach for abnormal substances and measures the acid concentration in it to evaluate stomach acid production. To perform the test, a sample of gastric material is aspirated through a flexible tube passed through the mouth and throat (oropharynx) or nose and throat (nasopharynx) into the stomach following a period of fasting. This sample is tested to determine acidity. A gastric stimulant, most commonly histamine or pentagastrin, is then administered intravenously and several more samples are collected at timed intervals. The C-urea breath test detects *Helicobacter pylori (H. pylori)* bacteria. A hydrogen breath test detects lactose intolerance. A sweat chloride test is used in the diagnosis of cystic fibrosis.
Review: Yes ☐ No ☐

13. Answer: b
Why: The specimen being collected is most likely a buccal (cheek) specimen for DNA analysis. A buccal specimen is collected by swabbing the inside of the cheek. DNA is later extracted from cells on the swab.
Review: Yes ☐ No ☐

14. Answer: b
Why: H. pylori is a bacteria found in the stomach that secretes substances that damage the lining of the stomach, causing chronic gastritis that can lead to peptic ulcer disease.
Review: Yes ☐ No ☐

15. Answer: a
Why: Cystic fibrosis is a disorder of the exocrine glands that affects many body systems, but primarily the lungs, upper respiratory tract, liver, and pancreas. Emphysema and tuberculosis affect the respiratory system but are not exocrine gland disorders. Herpes zoster (shingles) is an infection caused by varicella zoster virus that results in a painful eruption of blisters along the course of a nerve.
Review: Yes ☐ No ☐

16. Answer: c
Why: Occult means "hidden or concealed." Occult blood is blood in feces that is present in such tiny amounts that it cannot be seen with the naked eye. Guaiac is a type of tree resin that contains a chemical that can detect blood.

Occult blood tests that use this chemical are called guaiac tests.

Review: Yes ☐ No ☐

17. Answer: d

Why: As minimum, nonblood specimens should be labeled with the same identification information as blood specimens. However, because many nonblood specimens are similar in appearance, most institutions also require information on the type and source of the specimen.

Review: Yes ☐ No ☐

18. Answer: c

Why: Spinal fluid (cerebrospinal fluid, or CSF) is obtained by a physician through lumbar puncture. It should be delivered to the lab STAT and analysis started immediately so that the specimen is not compromised.

Review: Yes ☐ No ☐

19. Answer: d

Why: Urine is fairly easy to obtain and provides valuable information in several circumstances, including monitoring wellness, diagnosing and treating urinary tract infections, detecting and monitoring metabolic disease, and drug screening applications. Consequently, it is the most frequently analyzed nonblood specimen.

Review: Yes ☐ No ☐

20. Answer: c

Why: Some components in a urine sample are not stable. If a urine specimen is not processed in a timely fashion, any bilirubin in the sample can break down to biliverdin, cellular elements can decompose, and bacteria can multiply.

Review: Yes ☐ No ☐

21. Answer: a

Why: Although not always required, a first morning (also called first voided or 8-hour) specimen is the ideal specimen for most urine studies because it is the most concentrated.

Review: Yes ☐ No ☐

22. Answer: d

Why: Specimens for routine urinalysis that cannot be transported or analyzed promptly can be held at room temperature if protected from light for up to 2 hours. Specimens held longer should be refrigerated.

Review: Yes ☐ No ☐

23. Answer: b

Why: A routine urinalysis typically includes a physical, chemical, and microscopic analysis. Physical analysis notes the color, odor, transparency, and specific gravity of the specimen. Chemical analysis typically involves dipping a reagent strip (Fig. 11-24) into the specimen to detect the presence of bacteria, blood, white blood cells, protein, glucose, and other substances. A microscopic analysis of urine sediment identifies urine components such as casts, cells, and crystals. Cytological analysis of urine is performed to detect cancer, cytomegalovirus, and other viral and inflammatory diseases of the bladder and other structures of the urinary system but is not part of a routine urinalysis.

Review: Yes ☐ No ☐

24. Answer: b

Why: The most common reason for ordering a culture and sensitivity (C & S) on a urine specimen is to diagnose urinary tract infection (UTI). Urine C & S testing can detect the presence of UTI by culturing (growing) and identifying microorganisms present in the urine. When microorganisms are identified, an antibiotic susceptibility test is performed to determine which antibiotics are effective against the microorganism.

Review: Yes ☐ No ☐

25. Answer: a

Why: Urine cytology studies look for the presence of abnormal cells that have been shed from the urinary tract into the urine. Cytological analysis of urine can detect cancer, cytomegalovirus, and other viral and inflammatory diseases of the bladder and other structures of the urinary system.

Review: Yes ☐ No ☐

26. Answer: c
Why: Urine drug screening can be used to detect illegal drug use, abuse or unwarranted use of prescription drugs, and use of performance-enhancing steroids as well as to monitor therapeutic drug use to minimize withdrawal symptoms or confirm drug overdose. Drug screening identifies drugs in urine but cannot prove whether or not a drug overdose was intentional.
Review: Yes ☐ No ☐

27. Answer: c
Why: Pregnancy can be confirmed by testing urine for the presence of human chorionic gonadotropin (HCG), a hormone produced by cells within a developing placenta that appears in serum and urine approximately 8 to 10 days after conception or fertilization.
Review: Yes ☐ No ☐

28. Answer: c
Why: Although a random urine specimen can be used for testing, the first morning (also called first voided or 8-hour) specimen is preferred because it is normally the most concentrated and therefore would have the highest HCG concentration if the patient is pregnant.
Review: Yes ☐ No ☐

29. Answer: d
Why: Random urine specimens are typically used for routine urinalysis. Random refers only to the timing of the specimen and not the method of collection.
Review: Yes ☐ No ☐

30. Answer: b
Why: The first morning specimen is the usually the most concentrated.
Review: Yes ☐ No ☐

31. Answer: b
Why: The standard glucose tolerance test requires individual urine specimens collected serially at specific times that correspond with the timing of blood collection, such as fasting, 0.5 hour, 1 hour, and so on. A creatinine clearance test requires a 24-hour urine specimen. A pregnancy test requires a single concentrated urine specimen. A urine culture and sensitivity test requires a midstream clean-catch specimen collected in a sterile container.
Review: Yes ☐ No ☐

32. Answer: c
Why: A 24-hour urine specimen is collected to allow quantitative analysis of a urine analyte. Collection of all urine voided in the 24-hour period is critical. A special large collection container (Fig. 13-1) is required. The best time to begin a 24-hour collection is when the patient wakes in the morning, typically between 6 and 8 A.M. The first morning

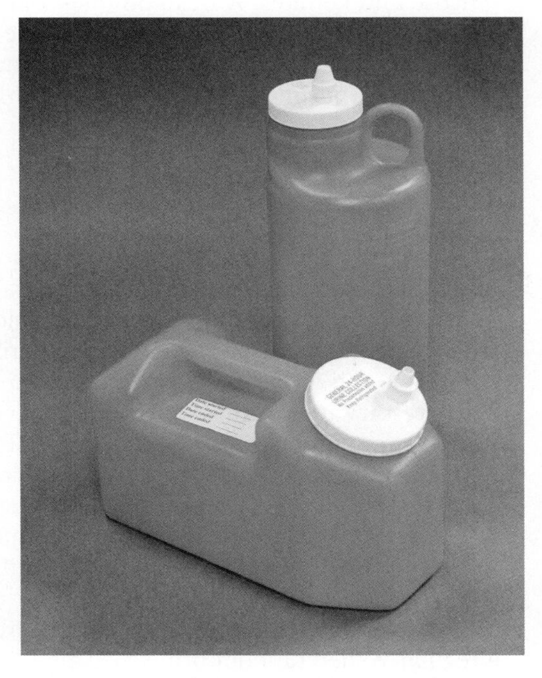

FIGURE 13-1 Two styles of 24-hour urine specimen collection containers.

specimen is from the previous 24 hours and must be voided and discarded before timing is started. All urine voided over the next 24 hours is collected, including the next morning's specimen.

Review: Yes ☐ No ☐

33. Answer: c

Why: A urine creatinine clearance requires collection of a 24-hour urine, which is kept refrigerated, and a blood creatinine specimen. A double-voided specimen is collected to compare the urine concentrations of an analyte to its concentration in the blood. It is most commonly used to test urine for glucose and ketones.

Review: Yes ☐ No ☐

34. Answer: c

Why: A double-voided specimen is collected to compare the urine concentrations of an analyte to its concentration in the blood. It is most commonly used to test urine for glucose and ketones. A fresh double-voided specimen is thought to more accurately reflect the blood concentration of an analyte than a specimen that has been held in the bladder for some time.

Review: Yes ☐ No ☐

35. Answer: b

Why: A urine culture and sensitivity test is most often ordered to detect urinary tract infection. It requires collection of a midstream clean-catch specimen into a sterile container. Midstream clean-catch procedures are necessary to ensure that the specimen is free of contamination by microorganisms from the external genital area. A creatinine clearance requires a 24-hour urine specimen. A glucose tolerance test requires individual urine specimens collected serially at specific times that correspond with the timing of blood collection. A routine urinalysis requires a regular voided random urine specimen.

Review: Yes ☐ No ☐

36. Answer: c

Why: A midstream urine collection is performed to obtain a specimen that is free of genital secretions, pubic hair, and bacteria from the area around the urinary opening. To collect a midstream urine specimen, void initial urine into the toilet; bring the container into the urine stream and collect a sufficient amount of urine; void any excess urine into the toilet.

Review: Yes ☐ No ☐

37. Answer: a

Why: A midstream clean-catch urine collection is typically performed to obtain a specimen for culture and sensitivity testing to detect urinary tract infection. It is important that the specimen be free of genital secretions, pubic hair, and bacteria that surround the urinary opening. This requires cleaning of the genital area before collecting a midstream specimen into a sterile container (Fig. 13-2), and prompt processing to prevent overgrowth of any microorganisms present, decomposition of the specimen, and misinterpretation of results. A preservative is not normally required.

Review: Yes ☐ No ☐

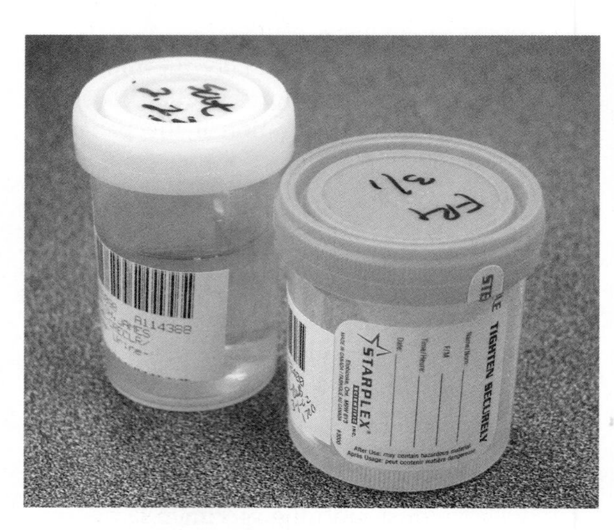

FIGURE 13-2 Urine specimens collected in sterile containers for C & S testing.

38. Answer: d
Why: A suprapubic urine specimen is collected in a sterile syringe by inserting the needle directly into the urinary bladder and aspirating urine directly from the bladder. Suprapubic collection is used for samples for microbial analysis or cytology studies.
Review: Yes ☐ No ☐

39. Answer: b
Why: Alpha-fetoprotein (AFP) is an antigen normally present in the human fetus that is also found in amniotic fluid and maternal serum. Abnormal AFP levels may indicate problems in fetal development, such as neural tube defects. AFP testing is initially performed on maternal serum, and abnormal results are confirmed by AFP testing on amniotic fluid.
Review: Yes ☐ No ☐

40. Answer: c
Why: Amniotic fluid is the clear, almost colorless-to-pale yellow fluid that fills the membrane (amnion or amniotic sac) that contains a fetus within the uterus. It is obtained by transabdominal amniocentesis, a procedure that involves inserting a needle through the mother's abdominal wall into the uterus and aspirating approximately 10 mL of fluid from the amniotic sac.
Review: Yes ☐ No ☐

41. Answer: a
Why: The primary reason for collecting cerebrospinal fluid (CSF) is to diagnose meningitis. An increased white blood cell count in spinal fluid is most often associated with bacterial or viral meningitis.
Review: Yes ☐ No ☐

42. Answer: c
Why: Routine tests performed on spinal fluid include cell counts, glucose, chloride, and total protein. Other tests are performed if indicated. Hemoglobin (Hgb), the iron-containing pigment of red blood cells, is not normally found in spinal fluid because red blood cells are not found in spinal fluid unless there is a "traumatic tap" in which blood enters as the lumbar puncture is performed.
Review: Yes ☐ No ☐

43. Answer: b
Why: A typical gastric analysis called a basal gastric analysis involves aspirating a sample of gastric secretions by means of a tube passed through the mouth and throat (oropharynx) or nose and throat (nasopharynx) into the stomach following a period of fasting. This sample is tested to determine acidity. After the basal sample has been collected, a gastric stimulant, most commonly histamine or pentagastrin, is administered intravenously and several more samples are collected at timed intervals. Serum gastrin levels may also be collected.
Review: Yes ☐ No ☐

44. Answer: d
Why: Nasopharyngeal (NP) secretions can be collected on a special swab and cultured to detect the presence of microorganisms that cause diphtheria, meningitis, pneumonia, and whooping cough (pertussis).
Review: Yes ☐ No ☐

45. Answer: d
Why: Saliva specimens are increasingly being used to detect or confirm alcohol and drug abuse and monitor hormone levels because they can be collected quickly and easily in a noninvasive manner. Detection of drugs in saliva is a sign of recent drug use. Sputum, not saliva, is cultured to diagnose and monitor lower respiratory infections such as tuberculosis (TB).
Review: Yes ☐ No ☐

46. Answer: b
Why: Semen is the sperm-containing thick fluid discharged during male ejaculation.

Analysis of semen is primarily ordered to assess fertility or determine the effectiveness of sterilization after vasectomy.

Review: Yes ☐ No ☐

47. Answer: a

Why: Semen specimens should be collected in sterile containers, kept warm at or near body temperature of 37° C, and delivered to the lab immediately, which means an on-site collection is ideal. Semen specimens should *never* be collected in a condom. Condoms often contain spermicides (substances that kill sperm), which invalidate test results.

Review: Yes ☐ No ☐

48. Answer: d

Why: Spinal fluid is obtained from the spinal cavity through lumbar puncture. Amniotic fluid is aspirated from the sac that surrounds a fetus in the womb. Gastric fluid is aspirated from the stomach via a tube passed through the mouth or nose and the throat into the stomach. Pleural fluid is aspirated from the pleural (lung) cavity.

Review: Yes ☐ No ☐

49. Answer: b

Why: Serous fluid is a pale yellow, watery fluid resembling serum that is found between the double-layered membranes that enclose the pleural, pericardial, and peritoneal cavities and is identified according to the cavity of origin. Gastric fluid is liquid material from the stomach. Seminal fluid (semen) is a thick, yellowish white fluid. Synovial fluid is a clear, viscous, pale yellow fluid that comes from movable joints.

Review: Yes ☐ No ☐

50. Answer: a

Why: Peritoneal fluid is aspirated from within the membranes lining the abdominal cavity. Fluid from the lung cavity is called pleural fluid. Fluid from the pericardial sac surrounding the heart is called pericardial fluid. Fluid from the cavities surrounding the brain and spinal cord is called cerebrospinal fluid (CSF), or spinal fluid for short.

Review: Yes ☐ No ☐

51. Answer: d

Why: The clear, pale yellow, viscous fluid found in movable joint cavities is called synovial fluid. The fluid lubricates the joints and decreases friction in them. It is normally present in small amounts but increases when inflammation is present. It can be tested to identify or differentiate arthritis, gout, and other inflammatory conditions. Pleural fluid comes from the lungs. Pericardial fluid comes from the pericardial sac surrounding the heart. Peritoneal fluid comes from within the membranes that line the abdominal cavity.

Review: Yes ☐ No ☐

52. Answer: a

Why: Pleural fluid is aspirated from within the pleural membranes in the lungs. Peritoneal fluid is aspirated from within the membranes that line the abdominal cavity. Synovial fluid is aspirated from joint cavities. Fluid from the spinal cavity is called cerebrospinal fluid (CSF) or simply spinal fluid.

Review: Yes ☐ No ☐

53. Answer: a

Why: Ascites (a-si′-tez) is the accumulation of excess serous fluid in the peritoneal cavity. Edema is the accumulation of excess fluid in the tissues. Peritonitis is inflammation of the peritoneum, the membranes lining the abdominal cavity. Septicemia is the presence of pathogenic microbes or their toxins in the bloodstream.

Review: Yes ☐ No ☐

54. Answer: c
Why: Sputum is mucus or phlegm that is ejected from the trachea, bronchi, and lungs through deep coughing.
Review: Yes ☐ No ☐

55. Answer: d
Why: Sputum specimens are sometimes collected and cultured to detect the presence of microorganisms in the diagnosis or monitoring of lower respiratory tract infections such as tuberculosis (TB). The sputum test for TB is called an acid-fast bacillus (AFB) culture.
Review: Yes ☐ No ☐

56. Answer: d
Why: A sweat chloride test analyzes a sweat specimen for chloride content in the diagnosis of cystic fibrosis in children and adolescents. Patients with cystic fibrosis have abnormally high (2 to 5 times normal) levels of chloride in their sweat.
Review: Yes ☐ No ☐

57. Answer: c
Why: Synovial fluid is typically collected in an EDTA or heparin tube for cell counts, identification of crystals, and smear preparations; a non-additive tube for macroscopic appearance, chemistry, and immunology tests and to observe clot formation; and a sterile tube or container for culture and sensitivity testing.
Review: Yes ☐ No ☐

58. Answer: a
Why: Synovial fluid is normally present in small amounts but levels increase when inflammation is present. Synovial fluid specimens can be aspirated from joints and tested to identify or differentiate arthritis, gout, and other inflammatory conditions.
Review: Yes ☐ No ☐

59. Answer: c
Why: A sweat chloride test involves producing measurable quantities of sweat by transporting pilocarpine (a sweat-stimulating drug) into the skin by means of electrical stimulation (iontophoresis) from electrodes placed on the skin. Sweat is then collected, weighed to determine the volume, and analyzed for chloride content.
Review: Yes ☐ No ☐

60. Answer: a
Why: A physician obtains a bone marrow specimen by inserting a special large-gauge needle into the iliac crest (hip bone) or sternum (breast bone) and aspirating some of the marrow into a syringe.
Review: Yes ☐ No ☐

61. Answer: b
Why: Because it is the site of blood cell production, bone marrow may be obtained and examined to detect and identify blood disorders.
Review: Yes ☐ No ☐

62. Answer: b
Why: Breath specimens are collected and analyzed in the detection of *H. pylori,* a type of bacteria that secretes substances that damage the lining of the stomach, causing chronic gastritis and leading to peptic ulcer disease.
Review: Yes ☐ No ☐

63. Answer: a
Why: A fecal fat analysis sometimes requires a 72-hour refrigerated stool specimen. Fecal occult blood testing (FOBT) typically requires small amounts of feces collected on special test cards on 3 separate days. Ova and parasite testing typically requires small amounts of feces from a fresh stool specimen that are placed in special vials containing preservative. A stool culture requires a single fresh specimen.
Review: Yes ☐ No ☐

64. Answer: d
Why: Stool specimens for detection of parasites or their eggs should be kept at body temperature (37° C). Twenty-four-, 48-, or 72-hour stool collections for fecal fat are refrigerated throughout the collection period. Refrigeration will not affect fecal occult blood (FOBT) or guaiac testing.
Review: Yes ☐ No ☐

65. Answer: c
Why: Occult blood is blood that is in such tiny amounts that it is invisible to the naked eye. Guaiac is a type of tree resin that contains a chemical that can detect small amounts of blood. Tests that use this chemical to detect blood in feces are called guaiac tests. An example of an occult blood test called the Hemoccult II is shown in Chapter 11, Fig. 11-20.
Review: Yes ☐ No ☐

66. Answer: b
Why: Samples of hair are sometimes analyzed to detect drugs of abuse. Hair can show evidence of chronic drug use rather than recent use. Use of hair samples for drug testing is advantageous because hair cannot easily be altered.
Review: Yes ☐ No ☐

67. Answer: c
Why: A throat swab (Fig. 13-3) is used for a "rapid strep" test. Results are typically ready in minutes.
Review: Yes ☐ No ☐

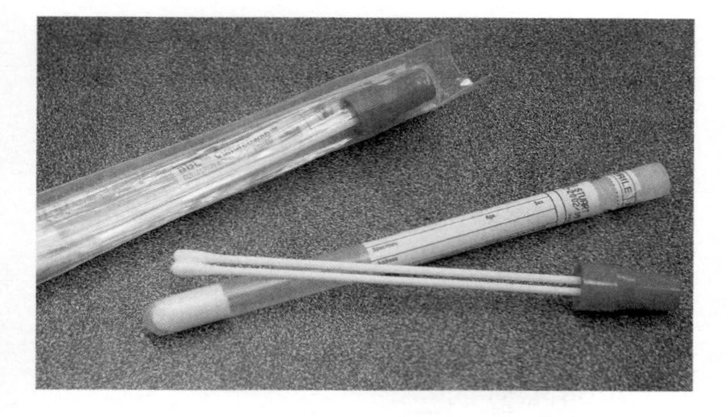

FIGURE 13-3 Throat swab and transport tube.

68. Answer: d
Why: A biopsy involves collection of a tissue sample from the area in question.
Review: Yes ☐ No ☐

69. Answer: c
The forearm is the preferred site for sweat chloride testing on adults, but the leg or thigh is often used on infants or toddlers.
Review: Yes ☐ No ☐

70. Answer: a
Why: CSF is generally collected in three special sterile tubes numbered in order of collection. Laboratory protocol dictates which tests are to be performed on each particular tube, unless indicated by the physician. Normally, the first tube is used for chemistry and immunology tests, the second tube for microbiology studies, and the third tube for cell counts.
Review: Yes ☐ No ☐

71. Answer: b
Why: Collection of a buccal (cheek) swab is a less invasive and painless alternative to blood collection for obtaining cells for DNA analysis. The phlebotomist collects the sample by gently massaging the mouth on the inside of the cheek with a special swab. DNA is later extracted from cells on the swab.
Review: Yes ☐ No ☐

72. Answer: b
Why: Semen (seminal fluid) is the sperm-containing thick, yellowish white fluid discharged during male ejaculation. It is analyzed to assess fertility or to determine the effectiveness of sterilization following vasectomy.
Review: Yes ☐ No ☐

73. Answer: c
Why: Use of hair samples is advantageous for drug testing because it is easy to obtain and cannot be as easily tampered with as a urine sample. In addition, hair can show evidence

of chronic drug abuse. Hair samples can also be used for trace and heavy metal analysis. Bone marrow is not easily obtained and is typically used to identify blood disorders, not drug abuse. Buccal swabs are most commonly used for DNA analysis.

Review: Yes ☐ No ☐

74. Answer: d

Why: An ova and parasite (O & P) test is typically performed on a stool (feces) specimen to detect intestinal parasites and their eggs (ova). Ova and parasite testing typically requires small amounts of feces from a fresh stool specimen that are placed in special vials containing preservative (Fig. 13-4). A culture and sensitivity test detects the presence of microorganisms and determines appropriate antibiotics to use against them. A fecal occult blood test (FOBT) detects hidden, tiny amounts of blood in feces. An HCG test detects human chorionic gonadotropin (HCG) in urine to confirm pregnancy.

Review: Yes ☐ No ☐

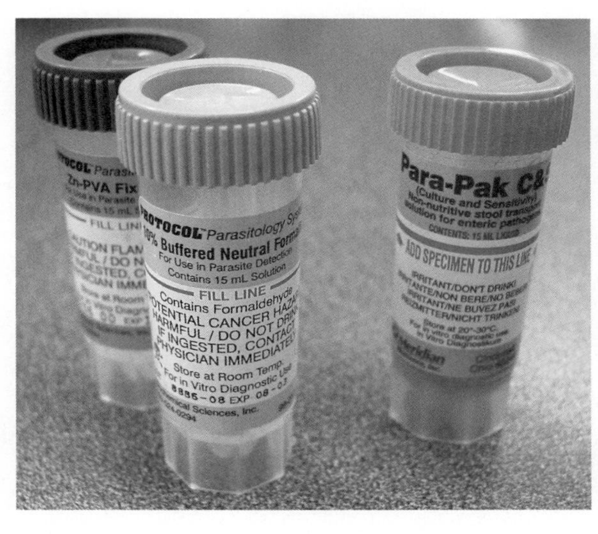

FIGURE 13-4 Ova and parasite specimen containers.

75. Answer: b

Why: The hydrogen breath test is used to evaluate lactose tolerance and is thought to be the most accurate lactose tolerance test.

Review: Yes ☐ No ☐

CHAPTER 14

COMPUTERS AND SPECIMEN HANDLING AND PROCESSING

study tip

Questions in this chapter test knowledge of general computer skills, including the ability to describe components of a computer, define associated computer terminology, and trace the flow of specimens through a laboratory information management system. Questions also test knowledge of routine and special specimen handling and processing procedures, including OSHA-required PPE, the steps involved in processing different types of specimens, time constraints for specimen delivery and processing, and the criteria for specimen rejection.

overview

Today many aspects of patient care are connected through computerized networking, even in the smallest clinic or physician's office. The phlebotomist is involved in certain aspects of the laboratory computer information system as it tracks patient specimens from the time they are collected until the results are reported. This chapter assesses knowledge of computer components, general computer skills, and associated terminology. This chapter also assesses knowledge of proper specimen handling and processing, including the ability to recognize sources of preanalytical error. A thorough understanding of handling and processing helps the phlebotomist avoid preanalytical errors that can render the most skillfully obtained specimen useless and helps ensure that results obtained on a specimen accurately reflect the status of the patient.

REVIEW QUESTIONS

Choose the BEST answer.

1. A mnemonic is a:
   a. memory aid.
   b. number code.
   c. program icon.
   d. secret phrase.

2. A barcode is a:
   a. coded instruction needed to control computer hardware.
   b. confidential computer code that is required by the HIPAA.
   c. series of bars and spaces representing numbers or letters.
   d. unique number given to each test request for ID purposes.

3. A pneumatic tube is a:
   a. pressurized air transportation system.
   b. temporary computer data storage unit.
   c. tube connection between two computers.
   d. type of collection tube for blood gases.

4. This is permanent computer memory that instructs the computer to carry out user-requested operations.
   a. CPU
   b. LIS
   c. RAM
   d. ROM

5. What is output?
   a. coded instruction used in computer processing
   b. information collected for analysis or computation
   c. processed information generated by the computer
   d. storage units for sharing information and resources

6. All of the following can be done to prevent exposure to aerosol generated when the stopper is removed from a specimen tube EXCEPT:
   a. cover the stopper with a 4 × 4-inch gauze while removing it.
   b. remove the stopper with the tube held behind a shield.
   c. use a specially designed safety stopper removal device.
   d. withdraw the specimen through the stopper by syringe.

7. All of the following describes proper aliquot preparation EXCEPT:
   a. do not label tubes until after pipetting the sample into the aliquot tube.
   b. immediately cap or cover aliquot tubes after transferring the specimen.
   c. never pour plasma from different additive tubes into one aliquot tube.
   d. use transfer pipettes instead of pouring specimens into aliquot tubes.

8. This organization develops standards for specimen handling and processing.
   a. CDC
   b. CLIA
   c. CLSI
   d. FDA

9. Interface means:
   a. checking quality control results on instrumentation.
   b. entering data into a laboratory information system.
   c. interacting through the connection of computers.
   d. standardizing all laboratory ordering and testing.

10. ESR determinations on specimens held at room temperature must be made within:
    a. 1 hour.
    b. 4 hours.
    c. 12 hours.
    d. 24 hours.

11. Which of the following is the best way to prepare routine blood specimen tubes for transportation to the lab?
    a. Place the tubes in ice slurry.
    b. Seal the tubes in plastic bags.
    c. Wipe each tube with alcohol.
    d. Wrap them in the requisitions.

12. All of the following are examples of specimens that require special handling EXCEPT:
    a. bilirubin and serum folate.
    b. cholesterol and uric acid.
    c. gastrin and lactic acid.
    d. homocysteine and renin.

13. This is an example of a preanalytical error made at the time of collection.
    a. delay in transporting
    b. failing to mix tubes
    c. incomplete requisition
    d. waiting to centrifuge

14. Transferring specimens into aliquot tubes has inherent risks for all of the following reasons EXCEPT:
    a. aliquot tubes are not prelabeled.
    b. serum and plasma look alike.
    c. specimens can be biohazardous.
    d. transferring can create aerosols.

15. This is a source of preanalytical error that occurs before specimen collection.
    a. dehydrated patient
    b. misidentified patient
    c. mislabeled ETS tube
    d. wrong collection time

16. HIPAA was enacted to do all of the following EXCEPT:
    a. examine all patient healthcare records.
    b. protect privacy of patient information.
    c. provide guidelines for sharing of PHI.
    d. standardize electronic transfer of data.

17. HPC systems are capable of all of the following EXCEPT:
    a. displaying what tubes to collect.
    b. generating labels for specimens.
    c. reading barcodes on ID bracelets.
    d. selecting the site for venipuncture.

18. Critical values (test values that are considered life threatening) are also called:
    a. alarm values.
    b. at-risk values.
    c. panic values.
    d. unstable values.

19. Which of the following would be a preanalytical error related to specimen storage?
    a. exposure to light
    b. faulty technique
    c. inadequate fast
    d. underfilled tube

20. Which of the following would be a preanalytical error related to specimen transport?
    a. agitation-induced hemolysis
    b. contamination caused by dust
    c. incorrect collection tube
    d. strenuous, recent exercise

21. A USB drive is a:
    a. network connection device.
    b. secondary storage device.
    c. terminal linking device.
    d. word processing device.

22. Cellular metabolism in specimens that have not been separated from the cells will affect all of the following analytes EXCEPT:
    a. aldosterone.
    b. calcitonin.
    c. hemoglobin.
    d. phosphorus.

23. Glycolysis by the cells in blood specimens can falsely lower glucose values at a rate of up to:
    a. 50 mg/L per hour.
    b. 100 mg/L per hour.
    c. 200 mg/L per hour.
    d. 250 mg/L per hour.

24. All of the following samples are time sensitive EXCEPT:
    a. blood smears to be made from EDTA specimens.
    b. calcium collected in sodium heparin tubes.
    c. ESR determinations collected in EDTA tubes.
    d. PTTs that are stored at room temperature.

25. Which of the following temperatures would *not* negatively affect the specimen if transportation and handling at room temperature is required?
    a. –20°C
    b. 8°C
    c. 25°C
    d. 37°C

26. Some blood specimens require cooling to:
    a. avoid hemolysis of RBCs.
    b. prevent premature clotting.
    c. promote serum separation.
    d. slow metabolic processes.

27. All of the following activities take place in central processing or triage, EXCEPT specimen:
    a. accessioning or logging.
    b. analysis and reporting.
    c. evaluation for suitability.
    d. sorting by department.

28. Removing the stopper from a specimen can cause all of the following EXCEPT:
    a. contamination.
    b. evaporation.
    c. increase in pH.
    d. loss of iCa^{++}.

29. If a specimen has inadequate identification, the specimen processor may:
    a. add the missing information to the label.
    b. ask the phlebotomist to get a new sample.
    c. contact the patient for correct information.
    d. refer the tube to the laboratory supervisor.

30. Use of one of the newest technologies, RFID, is emerging in healthcare. RFID is a:
    a. method of specimen identification.
    b. mnemonic for a strong disinfectant.
    c. secret code for AIDS patient serum.
    d. test code for chemistry analyzers.

31. An example of a preanalytical error happening during specimen processing is:
    a. faulty collection technique.
    b. inadequate centrifugation.
    c. insufficient specimen.
    d. patient stress and anxiety.

32. To be considered computer literate, an individual must be able to do all of the following EXCEPT:
    a. adapt to changes brought about by computer technology.
    b. design programs for job-specific problems in your area.
    c. perform basic operations to complete required job tasks.
    d. understand the computer and the functions it performs.

33. This is a term for a group of computers linked together for the purpose of sharing information.
    a. junction
    b. network
    c. node unit
    d. terminal

34. Computer input can come from all of the following EXCEPT:
    a. applications.
    b. keyboards.
    c. light pens.
    d. scanners.

35. Computer memory bytes are:
    a. handheld PC assistants.
    b. individual data characters.
    c. local area network systems.
    d. secondary storage drives.

36. Which of the following is *not* a function of a computer CPU?
    a. instruct the computer to carry out user-requested operations
    b. manage the processing and completion of user-required tasks
    c. perform mathematical processes and comparisons of data
    d. provide visible display of all the information being processed

37. Random access memory (RAM):
    a. can be lost when the computer program is closed.
    b. includes data, software, hardware, and peripherals.
    c. instructs the computer to carry out user operations.
    d. is permanent memory installed by manufacturers.

38. Computer peripherals include all of the following EXCEPT:
    a. keyboard.
    b. modem.
    c. programs.
    d. scanner.

39. Systems software includes:
    a. coded instructions that control processing of data.
    b. programs from software companies sold as a unit.
    c. the central processing unit and all hardware additions.
    d. word processing, spreadsheet, and graphic programs.

40. The laboratory has a computerized laboratory information system (LIS). Once an inpatient specimen has been collected by a phlebotomist and returned to the laboratory, what occurs next?
    a. A collection list is generated.
    b. All lab test orders are retrieved.
    c. Collection labels are printed.
    d. Specimen collection is verified.

41. A computer terminal is a:
    a. keyboard and computer screen workstation.
    b. last computer in a series of matching terminals.
    c. printer where information can be displayed.
    d. screen that visually displays data to the user.

42. A computer networking system created to share resources within a facility or organization is also called a:
    a. CPU.
    b. LAN.
    c. RAM.
    d. ROM.

43. Which of the following would be described as logging on?
    a. accessing the Internet from a computer.
    b. entering a password to access the LIS.
    c. turning the computer terminal to "on."
    d. using menus to navigate the program.

44. To process input data, a computer user must:
    a. log off of the Web.
    b. move the cursor.
    c. press the enter key.
    d. select an icon.

45. Computer verification of test orders is *best* described as a process that allows a user to:
    a. access the system to view the patient's diagnosis.
    b. confirm that the test was ordered by a physician.
    c. establish that the appropriate test was ordered.
    d. modify, delete, or accept them after review of data.

46. The "order inquiry" function allows the user to:
a. check the physician's diagnosis.
b. edit or delete duplicate test orders.
c. find errors in patient identification.
d. retrieve all test orders on a patient.

47. Which of the following is confidential and unique to a single computer user?
a. entry icon
b. ID code
c. LIS menu
d. password

48. Typical functions of an LIS can perform include all of the following EXCEPT:
a. acquiring correct samples.
b. entering lab test results.
c. ordering laboratory tests.
d. printing specimen labels.

49. What does the laboratory use to identify a specimen throughout the testing process?
a. accession number
b. hospital number
c. LIS menu icon
d. mnemonic code

50. Using the information from the computer requisition in Fig. 14-1, identify the number that points to the time the specimen is to be collected.
a. 1
b. 6
c. 7
d. 9

51. Using the information from the computer requisition in Fig. 14-1, identify the number that points to the color of tube required.
a. 4
b. 5
c. 7
d. 10

52. Using the information from the computer requisition in Fig. 14-1, identify the number that points to the specimen accession number.
a. 1
b. 3
c. 6
d. 9

53. When using computer-generated specimen labels, what information must be added to the label after a specimen is collected?
a. medical record number
b. patient's complete name
c. patient's date of birth
d. phlebotomist's initials

54. A bidirectional computer interface allows:
a. computer RAM storage capacity to double in size.
b. data to upload or download between two systems.
c. information to go from two analyzers to the LIS.
d. two persons to use a computer at the same time.

55. Which of the following is a characteristic of an intranet?
a. accumulates lab statistics for network workload
b. connects computer networks within a company
c. connects types of lab systems and multiple vendors
d. links lab systems with networks outside the company

56. In computer language, "hard copy" is:
a. data stored on disks or USB drives.
b. information displayed on the CRT.
c. lab results stored on the hard drive.
d. processed data printed on paper.

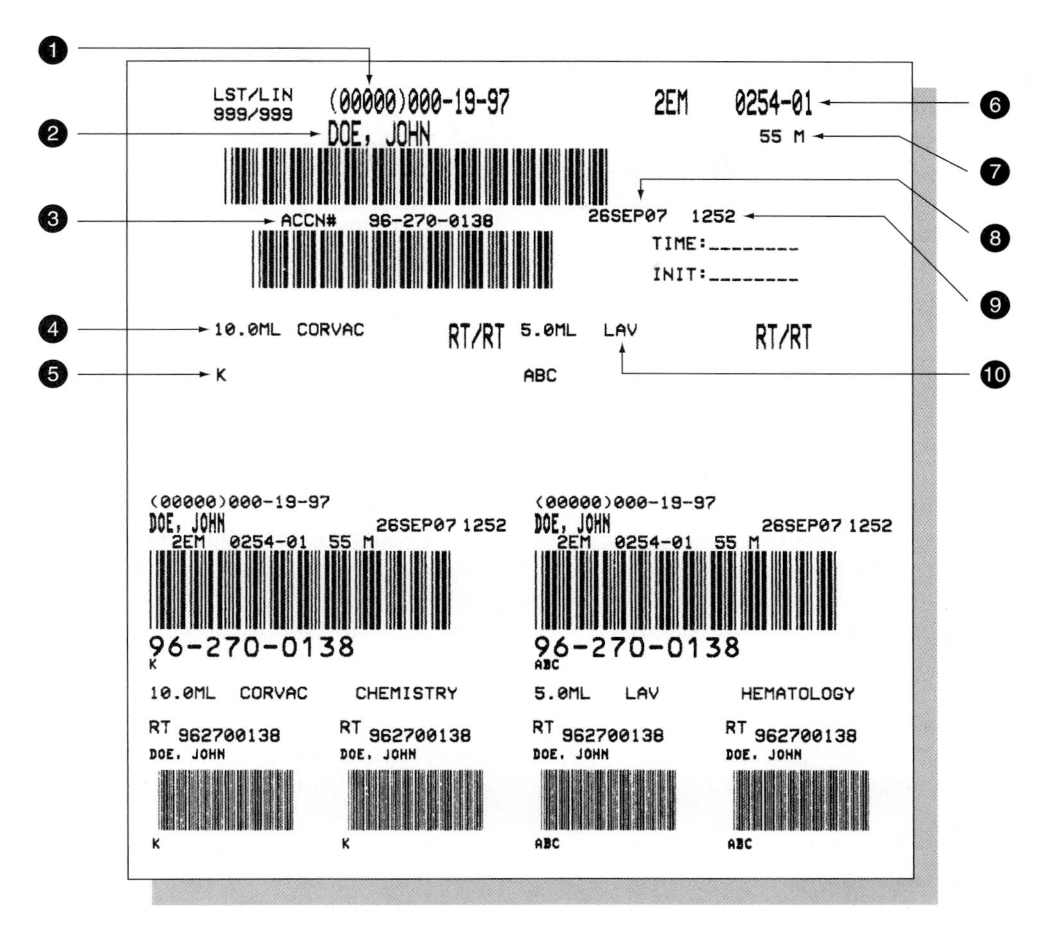

FIGURE 14-1 Computer requisition with bar code.

57. All of the following describe a current trend in laboratory testing EXCEPT:
    a. microchip laboratory technology is increasing.
    b. POCT is replacing most of laboratory testing.
    c. remote reference laboratory testing is increasing.
    d. use of barcode labeling systems is increasing.

58. All of the following are reasons why specimen handling is very important EXCEPT:
    a. effects of mishandling are not always obvious.
    b. improper handling can affect quality of results.
    c. many lab errors occur in the preanalytical phase.
    d. mishandling effects can be corrected if identified.

59. Proper specimen handling begins:
    a. as soon as the specimen is collected.
    b. during specimen collection procedures.
    c. in the course of patient identification.
    d. when the physician orders the test.

60. You are the only phlebotomist in an outpatient drawing station. A physician orders a test that you are not familiar with. What is the appropriate action to take?
   a. Call the physician's office for assistance.
   b. Draw both a serum and a plasma specimen.
   c. Refer to the user manual for instructions.
   d. Send the patient to another drawing station.

61. The number of tube inversions required during specimen collection depends on all of the following EXCEPT:
   a. absence of an additive in the tube.
   b. how difficult it was to get the blood.
   c. manufacturer-suggested inversions.
   d. presence of an additive in the tube.

62. Inadequate mixing of an anticoagulant tube can lead to:
   a. hemolysis of the specimen.
   b. lipemia of the specimen.
   c. microclots in the specimen.
   d. the sample clotting too fast.

63. Which tube does not require mixing?
   a. clot activator
   b. gel separator
   c. liquid EDTA
   d. plain red top

64. Tubes should be transported with the stopper up for all of the following reasons EXCEPT that it:
   a. encourages complete clot formation.
   b. maintains the sterility of the sample.
   c. minimizes stopper-caused aerosols.
   d. reduces agitation-caused hemolysis.

65. Clinical and Laboratory Standards Institute (CLSI) and Occupational Safety and Health Administration (OSHA) guidelines do *not* require specimen transport bags to have:
   a. a visible biohazard logo.
   b. liquid-tight closure top.
   c. shock resistance features.
   d. slip pockets for paperwork.

66. Specimens transported by courier or other air or ground mail systems must follow guidelines defined by all of the following EXCEPT:
   a. DOT.
   b. FAA.
   c. FDA.
   d. OSHA.

67. Which of the following actions will compromise the quality of the specimen?
   a. drawing a BUN in an amber serum tube
   b. mixing an SST by inverting it five times
   c. only partially filling a liquid EDTA tube
   d. transporting a cryofibrinogen at 37°C

68. All of the following analytes require protection from light EXCEPT:
   a. ammonia.
   b. bilirubin.
   c. vitamin B_{12}.
   d. vitamin C.

69. When transporting specimens, rough handling and agitation can do all of the following EXCEPT:
   a. activate the platelets.
   b. affect coagulation tests.
   c. elevate WBC counts.
   d. hemolyze specimens.

70. Which specimen needs to be transported on ice?
   a. ammonia
   b. bilirubin
   c. carotene
   d. potassium

71. The best way to chill a specimen is to:
   a. immerse it in a slurry of ice and water.
   b. put it in a small container of ice cubes.
   c. rubber band it to a large piece of ice.
   d. set it in a chilled metal carrying case.

72. Chilling can cause erroneous results for this analyte.
   a. ammonia
   b. glucagon
   c. lactic acid
   d. potassium

73. How should a cryofibrinogen specimen be transported?
   a. at room temperature
   b. immersed in ice slurry
   c. in a 37°C heat block
   d. protected from light

74. The most probable reason a phlebotomist would wrap a specimen in aluminum foil (Fig. 14-2) would be to:
   a. cool down the specimen.
   b. cover a contaminated tube.
   c. maintain 37°C temperature.
   d. protect it from room light.

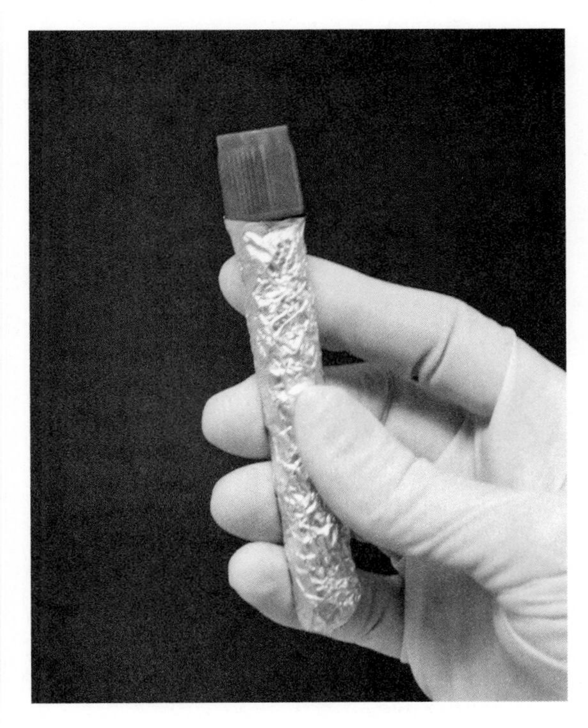

FIGURE 14-2 Specimen wrapped in aluminum foil to protect it from light.

75. A specimen must be transported at or near normal body temperature. Which of the following temperatures meets this requirement?
   a. 25°C
   b. 37°C
   c. 50°C
   d. 98°C

76. According to CLSI, the maximum time limit for separating serum or plasma from cells is:
   a. 15 minutes from the time of collection.
   b. 30 minutes from the time of collection.
   c. 1.0 hour from the time of collection.
   d. 2.0 hours from the time of collection.

77. A separator gel prevents glycolysis:
   a. after the specimen has been centrifuged.
   b. as soon as the specimen is collected.
   c. in tubes used for serum samples only.
   d. when the specimen is thoroughly mixed.

78. A glucose specimen collected in a sodium fluoride tube is generally stable at room temperature for:
   a. 6 hours.
   b. 12 hours.
   c. 24 hours.
   d. 48 hours.

79. Which specimen has priority over all other specimens during processing and testing?
   a. ASAP
   b. fasting
   c. STAT
   d. timed

80. Which of the following specimens does not need to be centrifuged?
   a. BUN in a red/gray SST
   b. CBC in a lavender tube
   c. potassium in a green tube
   d. PTT in a light blue tube

81. Slides made from EDTA specimens must be prepared within 1 hour of specimen collection for all of the following reasons EXCEPT to:
    a. ensure they are made before clots appear.
    b. minimize RBC distortion on the smear.
    c. preserve the integrity of the blood cells.
    d. prevent artifact formation from additive.

82. Examples of protective equipment required when processing specimens include EXCEPT:
    a. booties to cover shoes.
    b. fluid-resistant apron.
    c. protective glasses only.
    d. puncture-proof gloves.

83. All of the following conditions would be reasons to reject a specimen for analysis EXCEPT:
    a. expired evacuated tube.
    b. incomplete identification.
    c. not initialed by collector.
    d. quantity is not sufficient.

84. Which of the following specimens is *least* likely to be rejected for analysis? A specimen for:
    a. electrolytes that is hemolyzed.
    b. fasting glucose that is lipemic.
    c. platelet count with microclots.
    d. total bilirubin that is icteric.

85. A delay in processing longer than 2 hours can lead to erroneously decreased results for all EXCEPT:
    a. carbon dioxide.
    b. fasting glucose.
    c. ionized calcium.
    d. pregnancy test.

86. An aliquot is a:
    a. filter for separating serum from cells.
    b. portion of a specimen being tested.
    c. specimen being prepared for testing.
    d. tube used to balance the centrifuge.

87. Which specimen will be automatically rejected if the tube is not filled until the normal vacuum is exhausted?
    a. complete blood count
    b. plasma electrolytes
    c. postprandial glucose
    d. prothrombin time

88. Vigorous tube mixing can cause hemolysis, which affects test results of all of the following EXCEPT:
    a. amylase.
    b. hemoglobin.
    c. magnesium.
    d. potassium.

89. Tests performed on plasma samples are:
    a. collected in green top tubes.
    b. drawn in anticoagulant tubes.
    c. hematology or serology tests.
    d. obtained from clotted blood.

90. Chemistry tests are often collected in heparin tubes to:
    a. ensure adequate coagulation.
    b. maximize diagnosis potential.
    c. minimize effects of hemolysis.
    d. reduce the turnaround time.

91. It is important to note the type of heparin in a collection tube because:
    a. a few types of heparin do not require tube inversions.
    b. not all types of heparin prevent complete coagulation.
    c. some types of heparin can affect results of certain tests.
    d. some types of heparin make centrifugation unnecessary.

92. To avoid airborne infection while processing specimens:
    a. apply the brake when stopping the centrifuge.
    b. cover tube stoppers with gauze to remove them.

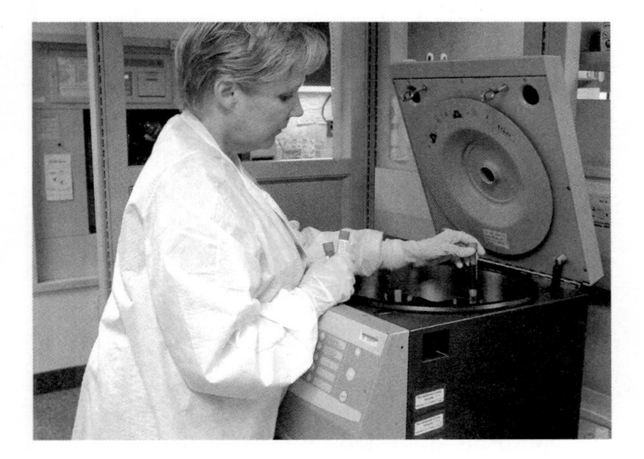

FIGURE 14-3 Specimen processor loading a centrifuge.

c. "pop" tube stoppers when opening serum tubes.
d. pour specimens directly into labeled aliquot tubes.

93. When a non-additive specimen is spun in a centrifuge (Fig. 14-3), the substance that comes to the top is:
a. buffy coat.
b. plasma.
c. red cells.
d. serum.

94. If a serum specimen is not completely clotted before it is centrifuged, the:
a. buffy coat may not form properly.
b. red blood cells in it may hemolyze.
c. separator gel may come to the top.
d. serum may have a fibrin clot in it.

95. A serum specimen may take longer than normal to clot completely for all of the following reasons EXCEPT the:
a. collection was difficult, hemolyzing red cells.
b. patient has an elevated white blood cell count.
c. patient is taking an anticoagulant medication.
d. specimen is chilled soon after being collected.

96. Which of the following tests would be most affected if contaminated with a drop of perspiration?
a. BUN
b. creat
c. lytes
d. SGOT

97. Gloves containing powder are:
a. a potential specimen contamination source.
b. ideal when collecting capillary specimens.
c. not allowed in any laboratory departments.
d. required for use when specimen processing.

98. Minimum precentrifugation time for specimens drawn in serum separator tubes is:
a. 10 minutes.
b. 15 minutes.
c. 20 minutes.
d. 30 minutes.

99. Repeated centrifugation of a specimen can do all of the following EXCEPT:
a. alter test results.
b. cause hemolysis.
c. decrease the volume.
d. deteriorate analytes.

100. Which statement describes proper centrifuge operation?
a. Balance specimens by placing tubes of equal volume and size opposite one another.
b. Centrifuge serum specimens before they start to form clots on the sides of the tubes.
c. Never centrifuge serum specimens and plasma specimens in the same centrifuge.
d. Remove the stoppers from evacuated tubes before placing them in the centrifuge.

ANSWERS AND EXPLANATIONS

1. Answer: a
   Why: A mnemonic is a memory-aiding code or abbreviation, such as 5.0 mL LAV, which tells the phlebotomist the tube type to choose (lavender) and the amount of blood to draw (5 mL).
   Review: Yes ☐ No ☐

2. Answer: c
   Why: A barcode is a parallel array of alternately spaced black bars and white spaces representing a code. The code may represent numbers or letters.
   Review: Yes ☐ No ☐

3. Answer: a
   Why: Pneumatic tube systems (often referred to simply as pneumatic tubes) use pressurized air to transport cylinders that contain items such as patient records, specimens, medications, and test results to and from various locations in a facility.
   Review: Yes ☐ No ☐

4. Answer: d
   Why: Read-only memory (ROM) is computer memory installed by the manufacturer. It is permanently stored and instructs the computer to carry out operations requested by the user.
   Review: Yes ☐ No ☐

5. Answer: c
   Why: Output is the processed information or data generated by a computer and received by the user or someone in another location. Examples of output devices are the computer screen and printer.
   Review: Yes ☐ No ☐

6. Answer: d
   Why: To prevent exposure to aerosol formation when one is opening a tube, the stopper should be covered with a 4 × 4-inch gauze square during removal, removed while the specimen is held behind a safety shield, or removed using a safety stopper removal device. Never withdraw a sample from a tube using a syringe because it is against Occupational Safety and Health Administration (OSHA) regulations and can hemolyze the specimen.
   Review: Yes ☐ No ☐

7. Answer: a
   Why: Proper aliquot preparation involves using transfer pipets (Fig. 14-4) instead of pouring specimens into aliquot tubes, capping or covering tubes after aliquot preparation, and making separate aliquot tubes for serum or plasma specimens from different additive tubes. Always place the aliquot in a labeled tube that matches the original tube.
   Review: Yes ☐ No ☐

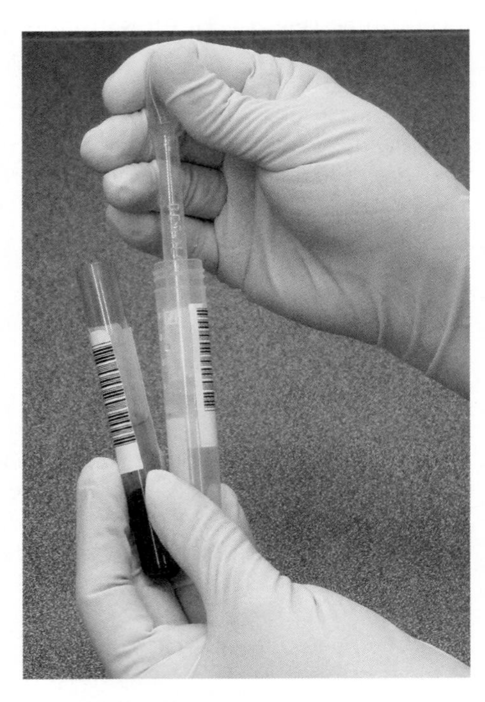

FIGURE 14-4 Transferring a sample from collection tube to aliquot tube.

8. Answer: c
Why: The Clinical and Laboratory Standards Institute (CLSI) develops and publishes standards for handling and processing blood specimens and many other laboratory procedures. The U.S. Food and Drug Administration (FDA), Centers for Disease Control and Prevention (CDC), and the Clinical Laboratory Improvement Amendments (CLIA) have regulations that affect laboratories, but they do not develop standards for handling or processing blood specimens.
Review: Yes ☐ No ☐

9. Answer: c
Why: Many laboratory analyzers have sophisticated computer systems that manage patient data and interface (connect for the purpose of interaction) with the main hospital intranet and through phone lines back to the manufacturer's headquarters.
Review: Yes ☐ No ☐

10. Answer: b
Why: When an erythrocyte sedimentation rate (ESR) is ordered on an EDTA specimen that is held at room temperature, the test must be performed within 4 hours. If the specimen is refrigerated, the time to perform the test is extended up to 12 hours.
Review: Yes ☐ No ☐

11. Answer: b
Why: Blood specimen tubes are typically placed in plastic bags for transportation to the laboratory. Clinical and Laboratory Standards Institute (CLSI) and Occupational Safety and Health Administration (OSHA) guidelines require specimen transport bags to have a biohazard logo with a liquid-tight closure.
Review: Yes ☐ No ☐

12. Answer: b
Why: Bilirubin and serum folate specimens must be protected from light. Gastrin, lactic acid, homocysteine, and renin specimens should be chilled in crushed ice slurry. Cholesterol and uric acid specimens do not require special handling.
Review: Yes ☐ No ☐

13. Answer: b
Why: Failure to mix tubes using the required number of inversions at the time of collection is a preanalytical error that can lead to microclot formation or insufficient clotting.
Review: Yes ☐ No ☐

14. Answer: a
Why: Aliquot tubes are supposed to be prelabeled to help avoid transfer errors. Great care must still be taken to match each specimen with the corresponding labeled aliquot tube to avoid the risk of misidentified samples. Different types of specimens like serum and plasma are virtually indistinguishable once they have been transferred into aliquot tubes, so to avoid errors it is important to match the specimen with the aliquot tube of the requested test as well as the patient. In addition, there is risk of exposure to biohazardous material from spills, splashes, and aerosols if specimens are not handled and transferred carefully.
Review: Yes ☐ No ☐

15. Answer: a
Why: Dehydration of a patient can affect test results and is a source of error that occurs before specimen collection. A misidentified patient, mislabeled tube, and wrong collection time are also sources of preanalytical error; however, they occur at the time of collection (Box 14-1).
Review: Yes ☐ No ☐

16. Answer: a
Why: Computer technology makes sharing of information so simple that patient confidentiality can be easily violated. The Health Insurance Portability and Accountability Act (HIPAA) is designed to protect the privacy

and security of patient information by standardizing the electronic transfer of data and providing guidelines for sharing protected health information (PHI). It was not enacted to have patient healthcare records examined.

Review: Yes ☐ No ☐

17. Answer: d

Why: Handheld personal computers (HPCs) are ideal for patient identification using barcode systems and paperless collection of data because they can go anywhere the patient may be. Today HPCs are being used to read barcodes on patient ID bands and generate the labels used for specimen collection at the patient's bedside. One system from Becton Dickinson (BD) can also display the required collection tubes and the order of draw and identify the person who is performing the phlebotomy. HPCs cannot select the venipuncture site, however.

Review: Yes ☐ No ☐

18. Answer: c

Why: A critical laboratory value, also called a panic value, is a test result that represents such a variance from normal values as to be a threat to the patient's life and requires the immediate attention of the physician. The Clinical and Laboratory Standards Institute (CLIA) requires critical values to be reported to the physician as soon as possible.

Review: Yes ☐ No ☐

19. Answer: a

Why: Proper handling from the time a specimen is collected until the test is performed helps ensure that results obtained on the specimen accurately reflect the status of the patient. Exposure to light during the time a specimen is being stored while awaiting testing can affect test results on several specimens, including bilirubin, carotene, and serum folate.

Review: Yes ☐ No ☐

20. Answer: a

Why: It is important to handle and transport blood specimens carefully. Rough handling and agitation can hemolyze specimens.

Review: Yes ☐ No ☐

21. Answer: b

Why: Secondary storage is storage outside of a computer central processing unit (CPU). A Universal Serial Bus (USB) drive is one type of permanent secondary storage device. Other types include floppy disks, external hard drives, zip drives, CDs, and DVDs.

Review: Yes ☐ No ☐

22. Answer: c

Why: Prompt delivery and separation minimizes the effects of metabolic processes such as glycolysis. Cellular metabolism will affect analytes such as aldosterone, calcitonin, enzymes, and phosphorus. Hemoglobin levels are not affected by cellular metabolism.

Review: Yes ☐ No ☐

23. Answer: c

Why: Glycolysis, breaking down of glucose, by erythrocytes and leukocytes in blood specimens can falsely lower glucose values by up to 200 mg/L per hour. For this reason, glucose specimens must be separated from the cells within 2 hours of collection or collected in tubes containing an antiglycolytic agent such as sodium fluoride. Glucose specimens collected in sodium fluoride tubes are generally stable for 24 hours at room temperature and up to 48 hours when refrigerated at 2° to 8°C.

Review: Yes ☐ No ☐

24. Answer: b

Why: Blood smears made from EDTA specimens must be prepared within 1 hour of collection to preserve the integrity of the blood cells and prevent artifact formation resulting from prolonged contact with the anticoagulant. Specimens for erythrocyte sedimentation rate (ESR) determinations must be tested within 4 hours at room temperature or within 12 hours if refrigerated. Partial thromboplastin time (PTT) test specimens require analysis within 4 hours of collection regardless of storage conditions. Specimens for calcium testing collected in heparin are not time sensitive.

Review: Yes ☐ No ☐

25. Answer: c

Why: A temperature of 25°C is considered normal room temperature and would not hurt the specimen. A temperature of –20°C is below freezing and could damage the specimen. A temperature of 8°C, which is around 45°F, is above freezing but well below room temperature. A temperature of 37°C is body temperature and well above the required temperature.

Review: Yes ☐ No ☐

26. Answer: d

Why: Metabolic processes can continue in a blood specimen after collection and negatively affect some analytes. Cooling slows down metabolic processes. Some analytes are more affected by metabolic processes than others and must be cooled immediately after collection and during transportation. Cooling can delay clotting but is not a desired effect. Cooling does not promote serum separation, nor does it help to avoid hemolysis.

Review: Yes ☐ No ☐

27. Answer: b

Why: Most large laboratories have a specific area, called central processing, where specimens are triaged or screened and prioritized in preparation for testing. Here the specimens are identified, logged/accessioned, sorted by department, and evaluated for suitability for testing. Analysis of specimens and reporting of test results is performed in respective test areas by technicians or technologists after the specimen has been properly processed.

Review: Yes ☐ No ☐

28. Answer: d

Why: Stoppers should remain on tubes awaiting centrifugation. Removing the stopper from a specimen can cause loss of CO_2 and increase the pH, leading to inaccurate results for tests such as pH, CO_2, and acid phosphatase. In addition, leaving the stopper off exposes the specimen to evaporation and contamination.

Review: Yes ☐ No ☐

29. Answer: b

Why: Suitable specimens are required for accurate laboratory results. Unsuitable specimens must be rejected for testing and new specimens obtained. A properly identified specimen is essential because it links the test results to the patient. Consequently, inadequate patient information on a specimen is reason for rejection by the specimen processor and a request for a new specimen.

Review: Yes ☐ No ☐

30. Answer: a

Why: Radio frequency identification (RFID) is a form of identification that is rapidly emerging in healthcare for identifying and tracking records, equipment and supplies, specimens, and patients. RFID tags are tiny silicon chips that transmit data to a wireless receiver. With this technique, it is possible to identify or track many items simultaneously.

Review: Yes ☐ No ☐

31. Answer: b

Why: A preanalytical error that could happen during specimen processing is inadequate centrifugation. This would cause incomplete separation of the sample and contamination of the serum with cells and fibrin.

Review: Yes ☐ No ☐

32. Answer: b

Why: Computer literacy involves the ability to understand a computer and how it functions, perform basic computer operations, and be willing to adapt to changes that computers are making on quality of life.

Review: Yes ☐ No ☐

33. Answer: b

Why: When a number of computers are linked together for the purpose of sharing information, it is called a computer network.

Review: Yes ☐ No ☐

34. Answer: a

Why: "Input" is the term for data entered into a computer. Data can be entered in several different ways, such as by using keyboards, scanners, and light pens. Applications are software programs prepared by software companies or in-house programmers to perform specific tasks required by users.

Review: Yes ☐ No ☐

35. Answer: b

Why: Computer memory bytes are individual characters of data that have been assigned a unique location in random access memory (RAM).

Review: Yes ☐ No ☐

36. Answer: d

Why: The central processing unit (CPU) is made up of many electrical components and microchips and has three elements: hardware, software, and storage. It is the thinking part of the computer that does comparisons, manages tasks, and instructs the computer to carry out user requests. Visible display of data is a function of the computer monitor or display screen, not the CPU.

Review: Yes ☐ No ☐

37. Answer: a

Why: Random access memory (RAM) is temporary storage of data that can be lost if it is not saved to permanent storage before the computer program is closed. Read-only memory (ROM) is permanent memory installed by the manufacturer that instructs the computer to carry out user-requested operations. ROM has characteristics of both hardware and software.

Review: Yes ☐ No ☐

38. Answer: c

Why: The central processing unit (CPU) is the command center of the computer. Things that attach to the CPU such as keyboards, scanners, and modems are referred to as peripherals. Programs or software are coded instructions required to control the hardware in processing data or performing specific tasks are not considered peripherals.

Review: Yes ☐ No ☐

39. Answer: a

Why: Software is the programming, or coded instructions that control computer hardware in the processing of data. There are two types of software, systems software and applications software. Systems software controls normal operation of the computer. Applications software refers to programs developed by software companies or computer programmers to perform specific tasks and includes graphics, spreadsheet, and word processing programs. The central processing unit is hardware.

Review: Yes ☐ No ☐

40. Answer: d

Why: On returning to the lab with a specimen, the first thing a phlebotomist must do is verify collection so that nursing personnel will know the specimen has been collected and no one else will attempt to collect it. Patient information is entered into the system and labels and collection lists are generated before the specimen is collected. Verification of a specimen does not involve retrieval of all test orders.

Review: Yes ☐ No ☐

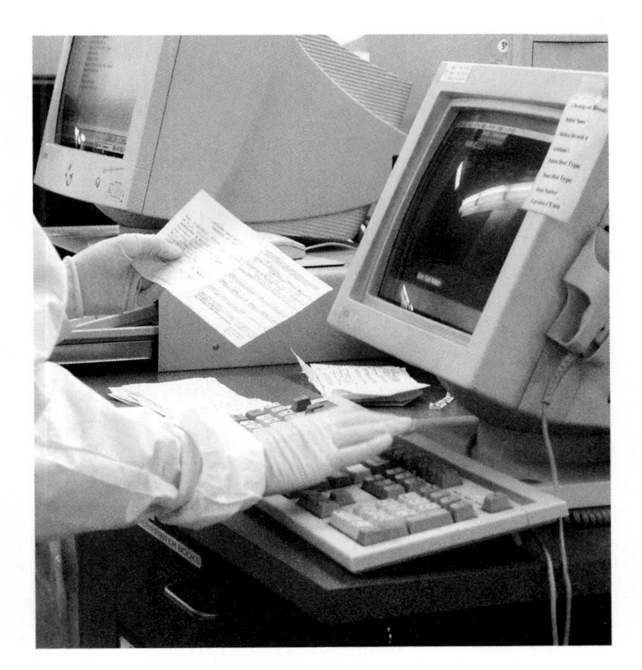

FIGURE 14-5 A computer terminal in the specimen-processing area of the laboratory.

41. Answer: a
    Why: As a minimum, a computer terminal (Fig. 14-5) consists of a monitor or computer screen and a keyboard.
    Review: Yes ☐ No ☐

42. Answer: b
    Why: healthcare organizations can coordinate data by linking a group of computers for the purpose of sharing resources. This is called networking and each individual computer station is called a node. The network interconnection allows all the computers to have access to each other's information or to a large database on a mainframe at a remote site through a special node called a server. The computers can be connected by coaxial cables, fiber optics, standard telephone lines, the Ethernet, or wireless radiowave connections. These networking systems are known as local area networks (LANs).
    Review: Yes ☐ No ☐

43. Answer: b
    Why: Entering a password to gain access to a computer or computer system is called logging on.
    Review: Yes ☐ No ☐

44. Answer: c
    Why: After necessary information has been input into the computer, the enter key must be pressed for information to be processed. When entering patient information in a laboratory information system (LIS), the cursor will automatically reset itself at the correct point for data input after the enter key is pressed.
    Review: Yes ☐ No ☐

45. Answer: d
    Why: The process of verifying an order allows the user to review the information and choose at that point to modify, delete, or accept it before entering. It is not a phlebotomist's duty to determine the appropriateness of a physician's order. Confirmation of the test order takes place before the specimen is collected.
    Review: Yes ☐ No ☐

46. Answer: d
    Why: Selecting the "order inquiry" function allows the user to retrieve any or all test orders associated with a particular patient.
    Review: Yes ☐ No ☐

47. Answer: d
    Why: A password uniquely identifies a person and allows that person to gain entrance into a computer system as a user. ID codes are not always confidential. An icon is an image that represents a document or software program. The LIS menu is a listing of icons or mnemonic codes for selecting a computer function or program to use to enter data into the computer system.
    Review: Yes ☐ No ☐

48. Answer: a
Why: Although specific tasks that LIS performs are defined by and customized for each facility, typical tasks include ordering tests, printing specimen labels, and entering test results. Acquiring the correct sample is still the duty of the phlebotomist.
Review: Yes ☐ No ☐

49. Answer: a
Why: An accession number is a unique number given to a test order. The number is used throughout the collection, handling, processing, and testing process to identify the specimen with its test order. Each new test order will have a different accession number. A hospital or medical record number is unique to the patient and remains the same throughout the patient's hospital stay. A mnemonic code is a memory-aiding code or abbreviation. The LIS menu icon can be found on a list used to select the necessary program in which to enter data into a computer system.
Review: Yes ☐ No ☐

50. Answer: d
Why: Military, or 24-hour time, is used on computer-generated labels to eliminate confusion between AM and PM. The specimen in the requisition example (Fig. 14-3) should be collected at 1252, which is 12:52 PM.
Review: Yes ☐ No ☐

51. Answer: d
Why: The code on the requisition (Fig. 14-1) indicated by number 10 is LAV, which indicates that a lavender top tube should be collected. The size of the lavender tube is indicated as 5.0 mL.
Review: Yes ☐ No ☐

52. Answer: b
Why: An accession number is a unique number generated when the test request is entered. The accession number on the requisition example (Fig. 14-1) is 96-270-0138, and is easily spotted because of the preceding abbreviation "ACCN#."
Review: Yes ☐ No ☐

53. Answer: d
Why: A computer-generated label typically contains the patient's name, medical record number, and date of birth or age. The time of collection and the phlebotomist's initials are added to the label that is placed on the collection tube immediately after the specimen is collected.
Review: Yes ☐ No ☐

54. Answer: b
Why: A bidirectional computer interface allows data to upload (transfer from analyzer to LIS) or download (transfer from LIS to analyzer) between two systems.
Review: Yes ☐ No ☐

55. Answer: b
Why: An intranet is a network of computers within a company. An intranet can be connected to the internet to connect it with outside companies.
Review: Yes ☐ No ☐

56. Answer: d
Why: In computer language, "hard copy" is data printed on paper.
Review: Yes ☐ No ☐

57. Answer: b
Why: Current trends in laboratory testing include the increasing use of microchip technology in testing, more and more tests being performed by off-site reference laboratories, and increased use of barcode labeling systems to increase efficiency and minimize errors. Even though POCT is very popular and cost-effective, it is not expected to replace standard laboratory testing in the near future.
Review: Yes ☐ No ☐

58. Answer: d
Why: Proper handling of specimens is important for quality results. It has been estimated that 46% to 68% of all lab errors occur in the preanalytical phase. Proper handling is important because personnel may not be aware that the integrity of a specimen is compromised; effects of mishandling are not always obvious. Most effects of mishandling *cannot* be corrected.
Review: Yes ☐ No ☐

59. Answer: d
Why: Proper specimen handling begins when a test is ordered and continues throughout the testing process.
Review: Yes ☐ No ☐

60. Answer: c
Why: Procedures and policies concerning specimen collection can be found in the laboratory user manual. A phlebotomist who is unfamiliar with a requested test should consult the user manual for instructions.
Review: Yes ☐ No ☐

61. Answer: b
Why: The number of times a specimen tube should be inverted (Fig. 14-6) depends on whether or not the tube contains an additive and on manufacturer instructions. Non-additive tubes do not require inverting. Additive tubes typically require from 3 to 8 inversions, depending on manufacturer instructions, to adequately mix the additive with the blood in the tube. The difficulty of the draw has no relationship to the number of tube inversions required.
Review: Yes ☐ No ☐

62. Answer: c
Why: Inadequate mixing of an anticoagulant tube can lead to microclots in the specimen. Hemolysis can occur if the specimen is mixed too vigorously. Lipemia is a patient condition that is unrelated to mixing the

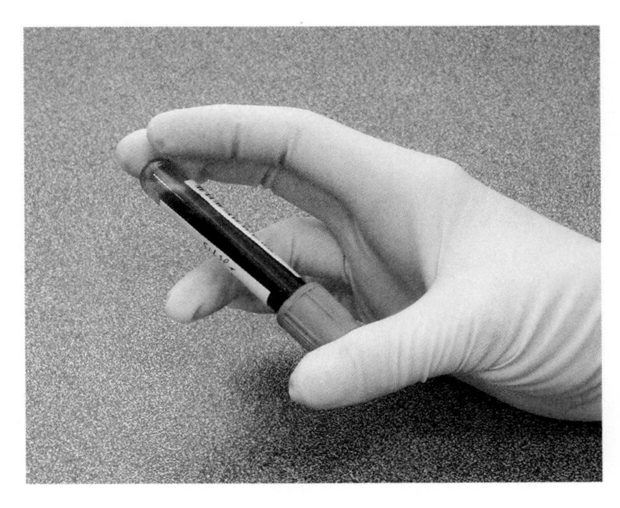

FIGURE 14-6 Mixing of anticoagulated tube.

specimen. An anticoagulant specimen is not supposed to clot.
Review: Yes ☐ No ☐

63. Answer: d
Why: Additive tubes require tube inversions to adequately mix the additive with the blood; non-additive tubes do not. A red top is referred to as a plain red top when it does not contain an additive such as a clot activator. Consequently, it does not require mixing. Glass red top tubes do not contain a clot activator. Plastic red top tubes, however, typically contain a clot activator such as ground glass or silica and do require mixing. A serum separator tube (SST), also called a gel separator, requires mixing because it contains a clot activator. An EDTA tube needs to be mixed regardless of whether or not the anticoagulant EDTA is in liquid or dry form.
Review: Yes ☐ No ☐

64. Answer: b
Why: Transporting tubes with the stopper up aids clotting of serum tubes, allows fluids to drain away from the stopper to minimize aerosol generation when the stopper is removed, and reduces the chance of hemolysis

caused by agitation of the tube contents during transportation. If the tube contents are sterile, they will remain that way until the tube is opened, regardless of tube position during transport.

Review: Yes ☐ No ☐

65. Answer: c

Why: CLSI and OSHA guidelines require a specimen transport bag to have a biohazard logo, a liquid-tight closure, and a slip pocket for paperwork. Pneumatic tube system specimen carriers, as in Fig. 14-7, need to have shock-resistant features to prevent breakage of specimens, but regular transport bags do not need this feature.

Review: Yes ☐ No ☐

66. Answer: c

Why: The Food and Drug Administration (FDA) does not issue guidelines for transporting specimens. Specimens transported by courier or other air or ground mail systems must follow guidelines defined by the Department of Transportation (DOT), the Federal Aviation Administration (FAA), and OSHA guidelines.

Review: Yes ☐ No ☐

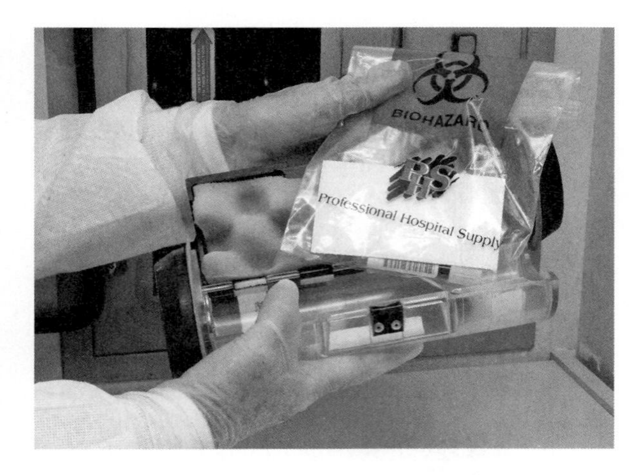

FIGURE 14-7 Specimen prepared for transport through pneumatic tube system.

67. Answer: c

Why: The additive in a tube is designed to work most effectively with an amount of blood that fills the tube until the normal vacuum is exhausted. Results on a specimen from a partially filled liquid EDTA tube may be compromised. Although a blood urea nitrogen (BUN) level does not need to be protected from light, it would not hurt to draw it in an amber serum tube. Serum separator tubes *should* be mixed 5 times. A cryofibrinogen specimen *should* be transported at 37°C.

Review: Yes ☐ No ☐

68. Answer: a

Why: Bilirubin and vitamins C and B_{12} are all analytes that can be broken down in the presence of light. Ammonia requires ASAP transportation in ice slurry but is not affected by light exposure.

Review: Yes ☐ No ☐

69. Answer: c

Why: It is important to handle and transport blood specimens carefully. Rough handling and agitation can activate platelets and affect coagulation tests, hemolyze specimens, and even crack or break tubes. Rough handling does not elevate WBC counts, however.

Review: Yes ☐ No ☐

70. Answer: a

Why: Ammonia specimens are extremely volatile and must be transported ASAP on ice. The expression "on ice" means in an ice slurry (Fig. 14-8). Bilirubin and carotene specimens require protection from light. A potassium specimen should be collected and transported at room temperature.

Review: Yes ☐ No ☐

71. Answer: a

Why: The best way to chill a specimen is to immerse it in an ice and water slurry (Fig. 14-8). Ice cubes without added water may prevent

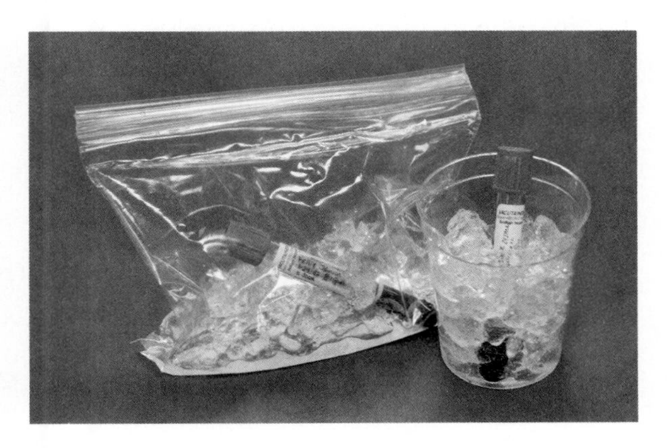

FIGURE 14-8 Specimen immersed in crushed ice and water slurry.

adequate cooling of the specimen. Specimens in contact with a solid piece of ice may freeze, resulting in hemolysis and possible breakdown of the analyte. A metal carrying case may warm back up before the specimen is adequately cooled or delivered to the laboratory.

Review: Yes ☐ No ☐

72. Answer: d

Why: The energy needed to pump potassium into the cells is provided by glycolysis. Cold inhibits glycolysis, causing potassium to leak from the cells, falsely elevating test results. Cooling can also cause hemolysis, which also elevates test results. If a potassium test is ordered along with other tests that require cooling, it must be collected in a separate tube that is not cooled. Ammonia, glucagon, and lactic acid all require cooling for accurate test results.

Review: Yes ☐ No ☐

73. Answer: c

Why: A cryofibrinogen specimen should be transported at body temperature, which is normally 37°C. Small portable heat blocks that hold a 37°C temperature for approximately 15 minutes are available.

Review: Yes ☐ No ☐

74. Answer: d

Why: Wrapping a specimen in aluminum foil (Fig 14-2) is an easy way to protect it from light. A specimen that needs to be cooled quickly should be placed in ice slurry (Fig. 14-8). Heat blocks or special warmers are used to keep specimens warm. A contaminated tube should be wiped with disinfectant and placed in a secondary bag or container.

Review: Yes ☐ No ☐

75. Answer: b

Why: Normal body temperature is approximately 37°C (98.6°F).

Review: Yes ☐ No ☐

76. Answer: d

Why: All specimens should be transported to the laboratory promptly. According to Clinical and Laboratory Standards Institute (CLSI) guidelines, unless conclusive evidence indicates that longer times do not affect the accuracy of test results, specimens should be separated from the cells as soon as possible, with a maximum time limit of 2 hours.

Review: Yes ☐ No ☐

77. Answer: a

Why: Separator gel has a density between that of serum or plasma and cells. During centrifugation it undergoes a change in viscosity and ends up between the liquid portion of the specimen and the cells becoming a physical barrier between the serum or plasma and the cells, that prevents glycolysis. Fig. 14-9 shows two SST tubes, one before centrifugation and the other after.

Review: Yes ☐ No ☐

78. Answer: c

Why: Sodium fluoride can prevent changes in glucose concentration for up to 24 hours at room temperature and up to 48 hours if the tube is refrigerated.

Review: Yes ☐ No ☐

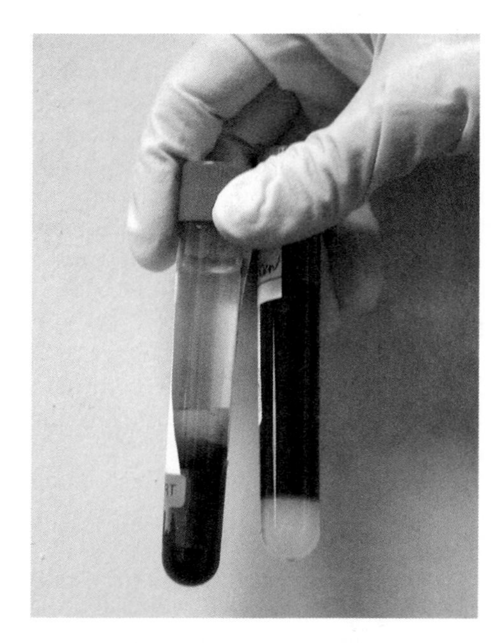

FIGURE 14-9 Hemogard SSTs: *Right*, before being centrifuged; *Left*, after being centrifuged. (Becton Dickinson, Franklin Lakes, NJ.)

79. Answer: c
Why: STAT, or medical emergency specimens, require immediate collection, processing, and testing and have priority over all other specimens.
Review: Yes ☐ No ☐

80. Answer: b
Why: A complete blood count (CBC) is performed on whole blood, and the specimen should never be centrifuged.
Review: Yes ☐ No ☐

81. Answer: a
Why: Prolonged contact with EDTA can distort blood cells, change their staining characteristics, and result in artifact formation. To preserve the integrity of the blood cells and prevent artifact formation, slides made from EDTA specimens must be prepared within 1 hour of specimen collection. If microclots appear on a slide made from an EDTA specimen, it is usually because the specimen was not properly mixed after collection.
Review: Yes ☐ No ☐

82. Answer: a
Why: Occupational Safety and Health Administration (OSHA) regulations require the wearing of protective equipment when processing specimens. Protective equipment includes gloves, fully closed fluid-resistant lab coats or aprons, and protective face gear such as masks and goggles with side shields or chin-length face shields. Shoe covering is not required.
Review: Yes ☐ No ☐

83. Answer: c
Why: Reasons for rejecting a specimen for analysis include missing or incomplete identification, collection in an expired tube, and an insufficient quantity of specimen (referred to as QNS, or quantity not sufficient) to perform the test. If the collector's initials do not appear on the specimen, the specimen is still analyzed even though the collector is unknown.
Review: Yes ☐ No ☐

84. Answer: d
Why: Specimens with high bilirubin levels typically have an abnormal yellow color described as icterus, and the specimen is said to be icteric. Icterus can be expected in some bilirubin specimens and would not be a reason to reject them for testing. A specimen for a platelet count with clots in it would be rejected because clots cause false low results for cell counts, platelets counts in particular. Hemolysis invalidates electrolyte results, potassium results in particular. A lipemic specimen is a clue that the patient may not have been fasting. A non-fasting specimen might be rejected if a fasting specimen was specifically requested.
Review: Yes ☐ No ☐

85. Answer: d
Why: A delay in processing beyond 2 hours can lead to erroneously decreased results for carbon dioxide, glucose, and calcium. A pregnancy testing specimen is not affected by a delay in processing.
Review: Yes ☐ No ☐

86. Answer: b
Why: An aliquot is a portion of a specimen being tested. When several tests are to be performed on the same specimen, portions of the specimen are transferred into separate tubes so that each test has its own tube of specimen. Each portion is called an aliquot, and the tubes containing each portion are called aliquot tubes. Each aliquot tube is labeled with the same identifying information as the original tube.
Review: Yes ☐ No ☐

87. Answer: d
Why: A prothrombin time (PT) is a coagulation test collected in a light blue sodium citrate tube. Coagulation tests require a critical 9-to-1 ratio of blood to anticoagulant for test results to be valid. Therefore, an underfilled light blue top for a PT test would not be accepted for testing. All anticoagulant tubes should be filled until the vacuum is exhausted for best results; however, with the exception of sodium citrate tubes, slightly underfilled anticoagulant tubes are usually accepted for testing. Underfilled serum tubes are almost always accepted for testing provided there is sufficient specimen to perform the test.
Review: Yes ☐ No ☐

88. Answer: b
Why: Hemolysis, regardless of the cause, affects amylase, magnesium, and potassium levels. Hemolysis should not affect hemoglobin levels because the cells are lysed in the testing process in order to measure hemoglobin. Other hematology tests, however, are affected by hemolysis and should not be performed on a hemolyzed specimen.
Review: Yes ☐ No ☐

89. Answer: b
Why: Plasma samples are obtained from blood collected in anticoagulant tubes. A tube containing an anticoagulant must be spun in a centrifuge to obtain plasma for testing. Green top tubes contain the anticoagulant heparin, but not all tests requiring plasma samples are collected in heparin. Most coagulation tests, for example, are performed on plasma obtained from light blue top sodium citrate tubes. Hematology specimens are collected in lavender top tubes containing the anticoagulant EDTA, but the tests are performed on whole blood, not plasma. Serology tests are usually performed on serum. Clotted blood yields serum, not plasma.
Review: Yes ☐ No ☐

90. Answer: d
Why: The ideal specimen for many chemistry tests is serum. However, to obtain serum, the blood must first be allowed to clot completely before it can be centrifuged and separated. Complete clotting takes anywhere from 30 to 60 minutes at room temperature and even longer if the patient is on a blood thinner or has a high white blood cell (WBC) count. Heparin is an anticoagulant. Anticoagulant specimens do not clot and can be spun in a centrifuge immediately to obtain plasma for testing. Collecting chemistry specimens in heparin reduces turnaround time (TAT), which is especially important for STAT tests.
Review: Yes ☐ No ☐

91. Answer: c
Why: There are three types of heparin: ammonium, lithium, and sodium heparin. Ammonium heparin is primarily found in capillary tubes for hematocrit determinations;

however, sodium heparin and lithium heparin are commonly found in evacuated tubes. It is important to note the type of heparin in a collection tube to prevent interference in test results. For example, sodium heparin must not be used for electrolytes, because sodium is one of the electrolytes measured. Lithium heparin must not be used for lithium levels. All heparin tubes prevent coagulation regardless of the type of heparin they contain provided they are mixed properly, and all heparin tubes require mixing. All types of heparin require centrifugation if plasma is needed for testing.

Review: Yes ☐ No ☐

92. Answer: b

Why: Tube stoppers should be removed using commercially available stopper removal devices, by use of robotics, or after being covered with a 4 × 4-inch gauze or tissue to catch any aerosol that may be released. In addition, the tube should be held behind a "splash shield" while the stopper is removed. Applying the brake to stop a centrifuge, "popping" stoppers when opening tubes, and pouring specimens directly into aliquot tubes instead of using transfer pipets are all activities that should be avoided because they can generate infectious aerosols.

Review: Yes ☐ No ☐

93. Answer: d

Why: Blood in a non-additive tube will eventually clot. When a clotted specimen is centrifuged, the clear liquid that separates from the cells and comes to the top of the specimen is called serum. Blood in an anticoagulant tube does not clot. When an anticoagulant tube is centrifuged or allowed to settle, the clear liquid that separates from the cells is called plasma. The red blood cells (RBCs) are heaviest and are at the bottom. The white blood cells and platelets are lighter and form a thin layer on top of the red blood cells called the buffy coat.

Review: Yes ☐ No ☐

94. Answer: d

Why: If a serum specimen is not completely clotted before it is centrifuged, latent fibrin formation may cause the serum to clot. Incomplete clotting does not affect the action of the separator gel or cause hemolysis of the red blood cells. Buffy coat forms when a whole blood specimen is centrifuged. Clotted specimens do not form a buffy coat.

Review: Yes ☐ No ☐

95. Answer: a

Why: A serum specimen may take longer than normal to clot completely if the patient has a high white blood cell count or is on anticoagulant medication. Chilling also delays clot formation. A difficult collection or hemolysis does not normally delay clotting.

Review: Yes ☐ No ☐

96. Answer: c

Why: Sweat contains sodium chloride. Sodium and chloride are two of the four electrolytes measured when a set of electrolytes is ordered. The other two electrolytes are potassium and bicarbonate.

Review: Yes ☐ No ☐

97. Answer: a

Why: Although it does make gloves easier to put on, glove powder is a common source of specimen contamination, especially when collecting capillary specimens or processing specimens. Laboratories may choose not to use powdered gloves, but there are no regulations that either require or disallow their use.

Review: Yes ☐ No ☐

98. Answer: d
Why: Specimens drawn in serum separator tubes (SSTs) generally clot within 30 minutes. Consequently, to prevent latent fibrin formation in the serum, the minimum precentrifugation time for an SST is 30 minutes.
Review: Yes ☐ No ☐

99. Answer: c
Why: A specimen should be centrifuged only once. Repeated centrifugation can cause hemolysis or otherwise deteriorate analytes and lead to erroneous test results. The volume should not be decreased if there is a cap on the specimen.
Review: Yes ☐ No ☐

100. Answer: a
Why: Proper centrifuge operation involves balancing the centrifuge by placing tubes of equal volume and size opposite one another. Specimens should never be centrifuged before they are completely clotted. Specimens should always be centrifuged with the stoppers on to prevent evaporation of the specimen and generation of aerosols. Plasma and serum specimens can be centrifuged at the same time in the same centrifuge.
Review: Yes ☐ No ☐

LABORATORY TESTS

APPENDIX

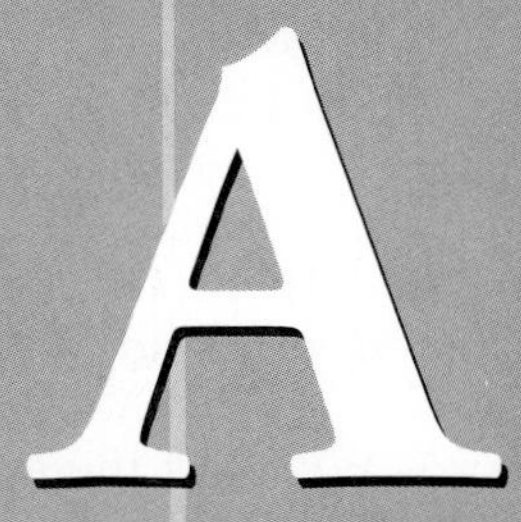

REVIEW QUESTIONS

Choose the BEST answer.

1. The abbreviation for another name for alanine transferase (ALT) is:
   a. ALP.
   b. AST.
   c. SGOT.
   d. SGPT.

2. A chemistry test that may require the patient to be in an upright position for a minimum of 30 minutes before specimen collection is:
   a. aldosterone.
   b. catecholamine.
   c. plasma renin
   d. Stypven time.

3. A royal blue top tube is the best tube for all of the following specimens EXCEPT:
   a. aluminum.
   b. chromium.
   c. copper.
   d. magnesium.

4. A specimen for hemoglobin A1c goes to:
   a. chemistry.
   b. coagulation.
   c. hematology.
   d. microbiology.

5. This is the abbreviation for a chemistry test that is collected in a lavender top tube.
   a. BUN
   b. CO
   c. ESR
   d. GC

6. Which of the following is an abbreviation for a type of antibody?
   a. AFB
   b. CEA
   c. IgM
   d. PSA

7. Most coagulation tests require a plasma specimen collected in a:
   a. gray top tube.
   b. lavender top tube.
   c. light blue top tube.
   d. plasma separator tube.

8. Which of the following is a drug used in the treatment of epilepsy?
   a. carbamazepine
   b. lithium
   c. phenytoin
   d. theophylline

9. Which of the following is a hematology test?
   a. A/G ratio
   b. acid-p'tase
   c. differential
   d. Hgb A1c

10. Which test requires a minimum 12-hour fast before specimen collection?
   a. ADH
   b. CK-MB
   c. HDL/LDL
   d. uric acid

11. Which of the following tests is collected in a red top tube or SST?
   a. ammonia
   b. DIC panel
   c. ETOH
   d. SPEP

12. Gel-barrier tubes are *not* recommended for collection of a specimen for this test.
   a. acid phosphatase
   b. alpha-fetoprotein
   c. salicylate level
   d. thyroid profile

13. Which test is used in the detection of allergies?
   a. CEA
   b. D-dimer
   c. ferritin
   d. RAST

14. Which of the following is a chemistry test performed on either whole blood or serum?
   a. AFB
   b. ANA
   c. cyclosporine
   d. plasminogen

15. Which test requires a whole blood specimen?
   a. CBC
   b. CMV
   c. CRP
   d. EBV

16. Immunology tests are most often performed on:
   a. plasma.
   b. serum.
   c. whole blood.
   d. urine.

17. All of the following tube types can be used for blood bank tests EXCEPT:
   a. lavender top.
   b. non-additive red top.
   c. pink top EDTA.
   d. serum separator tube.

18. This test is used as a tumor marker.
   a. AT-III
   b. BMP
   c. CA 125
   d. HLA

19. Which tests are used in the diagnosis of pancreatitis?
   a. amylase, lipase
   b. BUN, creatinine
   c. HCT, indices
   d. RPR, FTA

20. Name the type of specimen required and the department that performs the CMV test.
   a. plasma, chemistry
   b. serum, immunology
   c. urine, microbiology
   d. whole blood, hematology

21. This test requires whole blood collected from a stasis-free vein.
   a. calcitonin
   b. fibrinogen
   c. lactic acid
   d. zinc RBC

22. Identify the type of tube required and the department that performs the plasminogen test.
   a. green top or PST, chemistry
   b. light blue top, coagulation
   c. red top or SST, chemistry
   d. yellow top, microbiology

23. The microbiology department performs C & S tests on all of the following types of specimens EXCEPT:
    a. blood.
    b. capillary.
    c. sputum.
    d. urine.

24. Which of the following tubes is usually required for hematology tests?
    a. green top
    b. lavender top
    c. light blue top
    d. white top

25. Which of the following is actually a panel of several tests?
    a. BMP
    b. ESR
    c. PTT
    d. TSH

26. An HLA specimen is collected in a tube containing:
    a. ACD.
    b. EDTA.
    c. silica.
    d. thrombin.

27. Which department performs ETOH tests?
    a. chemistry
    b. coagulation
    c. immunology
    d. microbiology

28. Carbamazepine levels are determined in this department.
    a. blood bank
    b. chemistry
    c. hematology
    d. immunology

29. A specimen to be tested for glucose-6-phosphate dehydrogenase deficiency is typically collected in a tube containing:
    a. citrate.
    b. EDTA.
    c. heparin.
    d. oxalate.

30. Which of the following is a blood bank test?
    a. AFP
    b. DAT
    c. NH_4
    d. retic

ANSWERS AND EXPLANATIONS

1. Answer: d
   Why: An older name and abbreviation for alanine transferase (ALT) is serum glutamic-pyruvic transaminase (SGPT). ALP is the abbreviation for alkaline phosphatase. Serum glutamic-oxaloacetic transaminase (SGOT) is an older name for aspartate aminotransferase (AST).
   Review: Yes ☐ No ☐

2. Answer: a
   Why: Aldosterone is an adrenal hormone that plays a role in the absorption of sodium and water in the renal distal tubules. The test is performed in the chemistry department and typically requires the patient to be in an upright position for a minimum of 30 minutes before specimen collection. Catecholamines are a group of organic compounds that include dopamine, epinephrine, and norepinephrine. Catecholamine plasma specimens are ideally collected after the patient has rested quietly in a recumbent (lying down) position for 30 minutes following insertion of a venous catheter. Renin is an enzyme that plays a role in hypertension. Renin levels are best collected after the patient has been resting quietly in a supine position for 2 hours. The specimen is typically collected in EDTA and chilled during transportation and centrifugation. The Stypven time test is a coagulation test collected in a light blue top sodium citrate tube. It is also called a Russell viper venom time (RVVT) or lupus anticoagulant test.
   Review: Yes ☐ No ☐

3. Answer: d
   Why: Aluminum, chromium, and copper are all metals that can be toxic to humans in elevated amounts. They all require collection in trace-element–free royal blue top tubes. A magnesium (Mg) is collected in a gel-barrier tube such as a serum separator tube (SST).
   Review: Yes ☐ No ☐

4. Answer: a
   Why: Hemoglobin A1c (Hgb A1c) is also called glycohemoglobin, glycosylated hemoglobin, and glycated hemoglobin. Glycation is a process in which glucose is bound to hemoglobin. Formation of glycated hemoglobin is irreversible, and the rate of formation is directly proportional to the concentration of glucose in the blood. Hgb A1c concentration therefore reflects the blood glucose concentration over the preceding 6 to 8 weeks. The test is performed in the chemistry department and is ordered to assess long-term glucose control in diabetic patients.
   Review: Yes ☐ No ☐

5. Answer: b
   Why: Carbon monoxide (CO) is a chemistry test collected in a lavender top tube. CO more readily binds to hemoglobin than oxygen and can lead to CO poisoning, which can be fatal. CO bound to hemoglobin is called carboxyhemoglobin (HbCO). Blood urea nitrogen (BUN) is a chemistry test typically performed on serum. The erythrocyte sedimentation rate (ESR) is collected in a lavender top tube, but it is a hematology test. GC stands for gonococcus, a microorganism from the species *Neisseria gonorrhoeae* that causes gonorrhea. A test that screens for GC is performed in microbiology.
   Review: Yes ☐ No ☐

6. Answer: c
   Why: An antibody is a type of protein molecule called an immunoglobulin (Ig). There are five classes of immunoglobulins: IgA, IgD, IgM, IgG, and IgE. AFB is the abbreviation for acid-fast bacillus, a type of bacteria. CEA and PSA are antigens; carcinoembryonic antigen and prostate-specific antigen, respectively.
   Review: Yes ☐ No ☐

7. Answer: c
   Why: Most coagulation tests require plasma specimens collected in light blue top tubes containing the anticoagulant sodium citrate.
   Review: Yes ☐ No ☐

8. Answer: c
   Why: Phenytoin (Dilantin) is a drug used in the treatment of epilepsy. Lithium is a drug used to treat manic depression. Carbamazepine (Tegretol) is a drug used to treat bipolar affective disorder. Theophylline is an asthma drug.
   Review: Yes ☐ No ☐

9. Answer: c
   Why: A differential (diff) is a hematology test that classifies types of leukocytes, describes erythrocyte morphology, and estimates the platelet count. It can be performed automatically by machine or manually by looking at a stained blood smear under a microscope. Albumin/globulin (A/G) ratio, acid phosphatase (acid-p'tase) and glycosylated hemoglobin (also called hemoglobin A1c [Hgb-A1c]) are chemistry tests.
   Review: Yes ☐ No ☐

10. Answer: c
    Why: Lipids are fats such as cholesterol. Cholesterol is transported throughout the body in complexes with protein called lipoprotein. High-density lipoprotein (HDL) is referred to as *good* cholesterol because it plays a role in removing cholesterol from the arteries and transporting it to the liver, where it is removed from the body. Low-density lipoprotein (LDL) is called *bad* cholesterol because it moves cholesterol into the arteries. Accurate measurement of HDL and LDL levels require a 12-hour fast. Antidiuretic hormone (ADH), creatine kinase MB (CK-MB), and uric acid tests do not require fasting specimens.
    Review: Yes ☐ No ☐

11. Answer: d
    Why: Serum protein electrophoresis (SPEP or PEP) requires a serum specimen collected in a red top or serum separator tube (SST). An ammonia test requires a plasma specimen collected in a green top heparin tube. A disseminated intravascular coagulation (DIC) panel consists of several coagulation tests performed on plasma collected in a light blue top sodium citrate tube. Ethanol (ETOH) or blood alcohol is best collected in a gray top sodium fluoride tube.
    Review: Yes ☐ No ☐

12. Answer: c
    Why: It is recommended that salicylate (aspirin) levels *not* be collected in gel-barrier tubes. It is acceptable to collect acid phosphatase, alpha-fetoprotein, and thyroid profile specimens in gel-barrier tubes.
    Review: Yes ☐ No ☐

13. Answer: d
    Why: The radioallergosorbent test (RAST) is used in the detection of allergies. Carcinoembryonic antigen (CEA) is used in diagnosing and monitoring malignancies. D-dimer is a coagulation test. D-dimers are fragments produced by the action of plasmin on fibrin. Ferritin is a reliable indicator of iron stores and is measured in the diagnosis of iron-deficiency anemia and hemochromatosis.
    Review: Yes ☐ No ☐

14. Answer: c
    Why: Cyclosporine is an immunosuppressive drug used to suppress organ rejection in transplant recipients. The test can be performed on whole blood or serum. An acid-fast bacillus (AFB) culture is a microbiology test used to diagnose tuberculosis. The antinuclear antibody (ANA) test is a serology/immunology test used in the diagnosis of systemic lupus erythematosus (SLE) and other autoimmune disorders. Plasminogen is a

coagulation test performed on patients with disseminated intravascular coagulation (DIC) or thrombosis.

Review: Yes ☐ No ☐

15. Answer: a
Why: A complete blood count (CBC) is a hematology test performed on a whole blood specimen. Cytomegalovirus (CMV) is a herpesvirus that can cause devastating effects in a congenitally infected infant and fatal pneumonia in immunocompromised individuals. C-reactive protein (CRP) is an abnormal protein that appears in the blood during inflammatory illnesses, such as rheumatic fever, rheumatoid arthritis, and acute bacterial or viral infections, and as a response to injurious stimuli, such as myocardial infarction and malignancy. Epstein-Barr virus (EBV) is a herpesvirus that is the most common cause of infectious mononucleosis (IM). CMV, CRP, and EBV are serology/immunology tests most commonly performed on serum.
Review: Yes ☐ No ☐

16. Answer: b
Why: Immunology tests are most often performed on serum specimens.
Review: Yes ☐ No ☐

17. Answer: d
Why: Although most blood bank tests have been traditionally performed on serum and cells from clotted blood specimens, tests are increasingly being performed on plasma and cells from EDTA anticoagulated specimens obtained in lavender top tubes or special pink top tubes. Gel-barrier tubes such as serum separator tubes (SSTs) cannot be used for blood bank tests.
Review: Yes ☐ No ☐

18. Answer: c
Why: A tumor marker is a substance found in blood, other body fluids, and tissues that may indicate the existence of malignancy or cancer. Cancer antigen 125 (CA 125) is an antigen that appears in the blood in increased amounts in the presence of ovarian and endometrial tumors. It is detected using an antibody called OC 125. Antithrombin III (AT-III) is the main physiologic inhibitor of thrombin and is measured in the identification of clotting factor deficiencies. A basic metabolic panel (BMP) is a designated number of tests covering a certain body system. Antigens that can be detected on white blood cells are called human leukocyte antigens (HLAs). HLA typing is used in tissue typing for parentage determination and transplant compatibility between donor and recipient.
Review: Yes ☐ No ☐

19. Answer: a
Why: Amylase and lipase are enzymes found in greatest concentrations in the pancreas. They are measured in the diagnosis and treatment of pancreatic disease as well as in differentiating pancreatitis from other abdominal disorders. Urea is an end-product of protein metabolism. In the past it was indirectly measured as blood urea nitrogen (BUN). Most analyzers now measure urea directly, but the term “BUN” may still be used. Creatinine is a product of creatine metabolism in the muscles. Its formation is related to muscle mass, and values vary according to age and gender. BUN and creatinine are excreted by the kidneys and measured in the assessment of kidney function. Hematocrit (HCT) and red blood cell indices are hematology tests used to detect abnormal bleeding and anemia. Rapid plasma reagin (RPR) is a nonspecific test used to screen for syphilis antibodies. The fluorescent treponemal antibody (FTA) test specifically detects antibodies to *Treponema pallidum*, the microorganism that causes syphilis, and is used to confirm positive RPR results.
Review: Yes ☐ No ☐

20. Answer: b
Why: Cytomegalovirus (CMV) is a herpesvirus that can cause devastating effects in

a congenitally infected infant and fatal pneumonia in immunocompromised individuals. It is a serology/immunology test most commonly performed on serum.

Review: Yes ☐ No ☐

21. Answer: c

Why: Lactic acid is a product of carbohydrate metabolism. Excess amounts are produced during hypoxic (oxygen deficiency) states such as shock, hypovolemia (diminished blood volume), and left ventricular failure, and certain metabolic disease states such as diabetes mellitus and drug toxicity. Excess lactic acid in the blood is called lactic acidosis. Strict patient preparation and sample collection and handling procedures must be followed to ensure accurate testing. Patients should be fasting and at rest for 2 hours before testing. Patients should be instructed not to make a fist before or during specimen collection, and specimens should be obtained without the use of a tourniquet because blood levels are affected by stasis (stoppage of blood flow) and hemoconcentration.

Review: Yes ☐ No ☐

22. Answer: b

Why: Plasminogen is a coagulation test collected in a light blue top tube. Plasminogen is a precursor of plasmin, an enzyme that dissolves fibrin and fibrinogen. It circulates in the blood until activated and is converted to plasmin during fibrin clot formation. Its normal function is to dissolve the fibrin clot when healing has occurred and the clot is no longer needed. Substances called antiplasmins destroy any plasmin released into the blood. When pathologic processes such as thrombosis or disseminated intravascular coagulation (DIC) occur, excess amounts of plasmin are released into the blood and begin destroying other coagulation factors, including fibrinogen.

Review: Yes ☐ No ☐

23. Answer: b

Why: The most common type of testing performed in microbiology is culture and sensitivity (C & S) testing of blood and other body fluids and substances such as urine and sputum. C & S testing cannot be performed on capillary specimens because the open collection system exposes the specimen to contamination.

Review: Yes ☐ No ☐

24. Answer: b

Why: Most hematology tests are performed on whole blood specimens collected in lavender or purple top tubes containing the anticoagulant ethylenediaminetetraacetate (EDTA). The most common use of heparin-containing green top tubes is to provide plasma for chemistry tests. Light blue top tubes containing sodium citrate are used for coagulation tests. A white top tube is a plasma preparation tube (PPT) and is used to provide EDTA plasma for molecular diagnostic tests.

Review: Yes ☐ No ☐

25. Answer: a

Why: A basic metabolic panel (BMP) includes a designated number of body system chemistry tests. Erythrocyte sedimentation rate (ESR), partial thromboplastin time (PTT), and thyroid-stimulating hormone (TSH) are individual tests.

Review: Yes ☐ No ☐

26. Answer: a

Why: Human leukocyte antigen (HLA) specimens are typically collected in tubes containing acid citrate dextrose (ACD), although they are sometimes collected in heparin tubes.

Review: Yes ☐ No ☐

27. Answer: a

Why: Blood alcohol (ethanol or ETOH) tests are performed in the toxicology area of the chemistry department. Specimens are typically collected in gray top sodium fluoride tubes. Alcohol is volatile, and specimens must be kept capped during handling and processing to prevent evaporation of the analyte.

Review: Yes ☐ No ☐

28. Answer: b

Why: Carbamazepine (trade name, Tegretol) is a drug used to treat seizure disorders. Drug levels are measured in the toxicology area of the chemistry department.

Review: Yes ☐ No ☐

29. Answer: b

Why: Glucose-6-phosphate dehydrogenase (G-6-PD) is an enzyme that plays a role in glucose metabolism and ultimately in protecting hemoglobin from oxidation. A deficiency of G-6-PD is an inherited sex-linked disorder that can lead to hemolytic anemia. The test for G-6-PD deficiency is commonly performed on a solution of hemolyzed red blood cells obtained from an EDTA specimen. Testing for elevated levels of G-6-PD is performed on serum.

Review: Yes ☐ No ☐

30. Answer: b

Why: The direct antiglobulin test (DAT) is a blood bank or immunohematology test that detects antigen-antibody complexes on the red blood cells, and red blood cell sensitization. It is useful in evaluating hemolytic disease of the newborn (HDN), acquired hemolytic anemias, transfusion reactions, and drug-induced red blood cell sensitization. The alpha-fetoprotein test (AFP) and ammonia test (NH_4) are chemistry tests. A reticulocyte (retic) count is a hematology test.

Review: Yes ☐ No ☐

LABORATORY MATHEMATICS

APPENDIX B

REVIEW QUESTIONS

1. 10 cc of blood equals approximately:
   a. 1.0 mL of blood.
   b. 5.0 mL of blood.
   c. 10 mL of blood.
   d. 20 mL of blood

2. 200 µL is equal to:
   a. 2 mL.
   b. 0.2 mL.
   c. 0.02 mL.
   d. 0.002 mL.

3. Your requisition says that a specimen is to be drawn at 1530. What time would that be in 12-hour time?
   a. 1:30 AM
   b. 3:30 PM
   c. 5:30 AM
   d. 7:30 PM

4. 1:00 PM in 24-hour time is:
   a. 100.
   b. 0100.
   c. 1300.
   d. 01300.

5. Body temperature in centigrade degrees is:
   a. 98.6.
   b. 37.0.
   c. 25.0.
   d. 32.0.

6. If room temperature is 77°F, what is the temperature in centigrade?
   a. 20
   b. 25
   c. 32
   d. 37

7. A specimen must be transported at body temperature, plus or minus 5° Fahrenheit. Which of the following temperature readings is within that range?
   a. 25°C
   b. 35°C
   c. 37°F
   d. 90°F

8. Your text says that factor VIII is the antihemophilic factor. What common Arabic number is this factor?
   a. 4
   b. 8
   c. 13
   d. 23

9. How is the number 12 written in Roman numerals?
   a. IIV
   b. VII
   c. IIX
   d. XII

10. Your paper says that you got 45 of 50 questions correct. What is your grade expressed as a percentage?
    a. 45%
    b. 75%
    c. 90%
    d. 95%

11. If a red blood cell is 8 μm in diameter, what is its size in millimeters?
    a. 0.8
    b. 0.08
    c. 0.008
    d. 0.0008

12. One teaspoon is approximately:
    a. 1 mL.
    b. 5 mL.
    c. 10 mL.
    d. 15 mL.

13. A blood culture bottle containing 45 mL of media requires a 1:10 dilution of specimen. How much blood should be added?
    a. 4 mL
    b. 5 mL
    c. 8 mL
    d. 10 mL

14. Normal infant blood volume is approximately 100 mL/kg. Calculate the approximate blood volume of a baby who weighs 6 lb.
    a. 1.2 L
    b. 2.7 L
    c. 270 mL
    d. 600 mL

15. Normal adult blood volume is approximately 70 mL per kilogram. A patient weighs 130 lb. What is the patient's blood volume?
    a. 1300 mL
    b. 1.3 L
    c. 59 kg
    d. 4.1 L

16. To prepare 100 mL of a 1:10 dilution of bleach, add:
    a. 1 mL water to 100 mL bleach.
    b. 1 mL bleach to 99 mL water.
    c. 10 mL bleach to 90 mL water.
    d. 10 mL water to 100 mL bleach.

17. The basic unit of volume in the metric system is the:
    a. gram.
    b. liter.
    c. meter.
    d. ounce.

18. In the metric system, a millimeter (mm) is:
    a. 1/10 meter.
    b. 1/100 meter.
    c. 1/1000 meter.
    d. 1/10,000 meter.

19. 1.2 kg is equal to how many grams?
    a. 12
    b. 120
    c. 1200
    d. 12,000

20. What does 2.2 pounds (lb) equal in the metric system?
    a. 1 kg
    b. 44 g
    c. 100 g
    d. 454 kg

21. The basic unit of weight in the metric system is the:
    a. gram.
    b. liter.
    c. meter.
    d. ounce.

22. In the metric system the prefix for 1000 is:
    a. centi-.
    b. deci-.
    c. kilo-.
    d. milli-.

23. In the metric system a meter is a measure of:
    a. mass.
    b. density.
    c. distance.
    d. volume.

24. A patient voids 1200 mL of urine for a creatinine clearance test. How much urine is this?
    a. less than a liter
    b. less than a quart
    c. more than a liter
    d. more than 2 liters

25. A test requires 3 mL serum. The laboratory requires that the amount of blood collected be 250% of the volume of specimen required to perform the test. Which size tube should you use to collect the specimen?
    a. 4 mL
    b. 5 mL
    c. 10 mL
    d. 15 mL

ANSWERS AND EXPLANATIONS

1. Answer: c
   Why: For practical purposes, *mL* and *cc* are equivalent and the terms are often used interchangeably in a laboratory setting. Both are approximately equal to one-thousandth of a liter. The term *milliliter* (ml) is used when referring to liquid volume; *cubic centimeter* (cc) is used when referring to volume of gas. However, syringes that are used to extract liquid volume are often calibrated in cc rather than in mL.
   Review: Yes ☐ No ☐

2. Answer: b
   Why: When converting small units to larger units, the decimal point moves to the left the number of spaces determined by subtracting the exponent of the smaller unit from the exponent of the larger unit. A milliliter (mL) is one-thousandth of a liter (L), or 10^{-3} liters. A microliter (µL) is one-millionth of a liter, or 10^{-6} liters. Microliters are smaller than milliliters. Therefore, subtract −6 (µL exponent) from −3 (mL exponent). The result is 3, which means the decimal point moves three places to the left.
   Solution: $-3 - (-6) = -3 + 6 = 3$
   200.0 = 0.2 mL
   Review: Yes ☐ No ☐

3. Answer: b
   Why: To change 24-hour time to 12-hour time, subtract 1200 from any time after 1300. 1530 in 24-hour time less 1200 is 330, which written in 12-hour time format with the colon is 3:30 PM. A clock showing standard and 24-hour (military) time is shown in Fig. AppB-1.
   Review: Yes ☐ No ☐

4. Answer: c
   Why: To convert 12-hour time to 24-hour time, add 1200 to the time (minus the colon) from 1 PM on. 1:00 without the colon is 100. 100 plus 1200 becomes 1300 (See Fig. AppB-1).
   Review: Yes ☐ No ☐

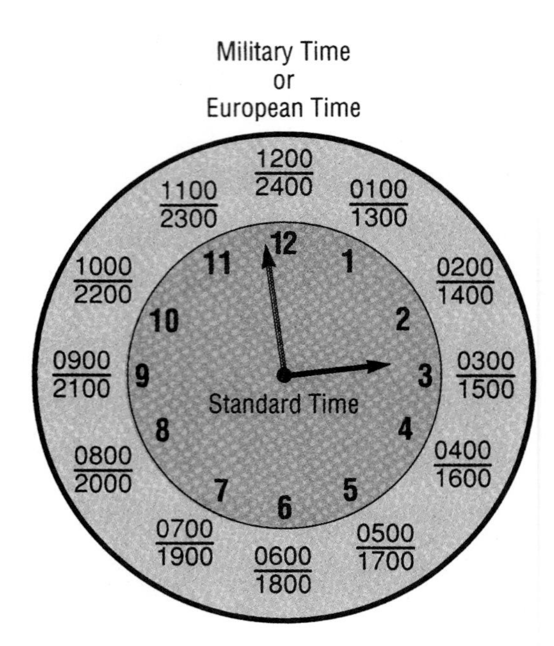

FIGURE APP-B1 Clock showing 24-hour (military) time.

5. Answer: b
   Why: Body temperature in centigrade is 37°. To calculate body temperature in centigrade when given a Fahrenheit reading, subtract 32 from the Fahrenheit temperature and multiply by 5/9. *Note:* A healthcare worker should memorize the centigrade body temperature value along with a few other centigrade temperatures that are common when working in healthcare(Fig. AppB-2).
   Review: Yes ☐ No ☐

6. Answer: b
   Why: Centigrade and Celsius are equal. To convert 77° Fahrenheit (F) temperature to centigrade (C) or Celsius (C), subtract 32 from the Fahrenheit value and multiply the result by 5/9.

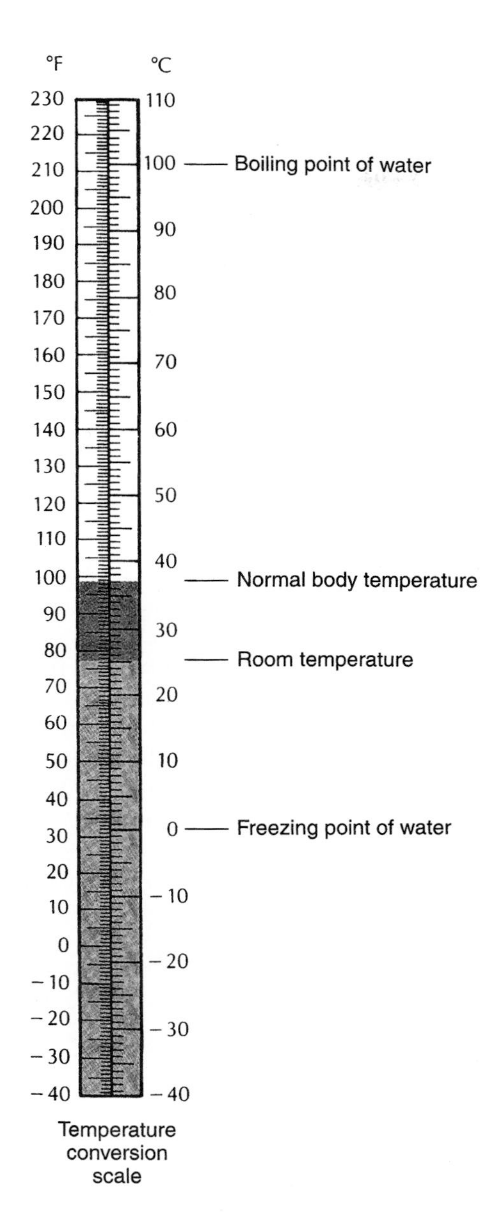

FIGURE APP-B2 Thermometer showing both Fahrenheit and Celsius degrees. (Memmler RL, Cohen BJ, Wood DL.)

Formula: $C = 5/9\ (F - 32)$

Solution: $F - 32 = 77 - 32 = 45$
$5/9\ (45) = 5/9 \times 45/1$
$5/9 \times 45/1 = 225/9$
$225/9 = 25°C$

Room temperature in Celsius or centigrade is 25°C. Healthcare workers should memorize this commonly referenced centigrade temperature (Fig. AppB-2).

Review: Yes ☐ No ☐

7. Answer: b

   Why: Fahrenheit body temperature is 98.6° (Fig. AppB-2). Once we add and subtract 5, we know that we are looking for a temperature that is between 93.6°F and 103.6°F. This eliminates 37°F and 90°F. 25°C (Celsius or centigrade) is the same as 77°F. (See answer 6.) The remaining choice is 35°C. To verify that this is the correct answer, convert 35°C to Fahrenheit temperature:

   Formula: $F = 9/5\ C + 32$

   Solution: $(9/5 \times 35) + 32 = 63 + 32 = 95°F$

   35°C is the correct answer because it is same as 95°F, which meets the transportation temperature requirement.

   Review: Yes ☐ No ☐

8. Answer: b

   Why: Coagulation factors such as the antihemophilic factor are written in Roman numerals. In Roman numerals, letters equal numbers. The Roman numeral V equals 5, and the Roman numeral I equals 1. When numerals of the same value follow in sequence, their values are added. When a numeral is followed by one or more numerals of a lower value, the values are added. Therefore:

   VIII = 5 + 1 + 1 + 1 = 5 + 3 = 8

   Review: Yes ☐ No ☐

9. Answer: d

   Why: Roman numerals are written from left to right in decreasing value (except for numerals that are to be subtracted from subsequent numerals). In addition, there can never be more than three of the same numeral in a sequence. To write a number, you should start with the closest base number and add or subtract other numbers until you reach the desired value. The closest base number to 12 is X, which equals 10. Then add one I for every number 1. Therefore:

12 = X + I + I = XII

Review: Yes ☐ No ☐

10. Answer: c
Why: To calculate a percentage, a number must be converted to parts per 100. First make the number a fraction. Then multiply the numerator of the fraction by 100, divide by the denominator, and add a percent sign.

Solution: 45 of $50 = 45/50$
$45/50 \times 100 = 4500/50$
$4500 \div 50 = 90$

Or reduce the fractions first as follows:

$45/50 \times 100/1 = 45/1 \times 2/1 = 45 \times 2 = 90\%$

Review: Yes ☐ No ☐

11. Answer: c
Why: A micrometer (µm), or micron is equal to one-millionth (10^{-6}) of a meter and a millimeter (mm) is equal to one-thousandth (10^{-3}) of a meter, which means you are converting smaller units to larger units (Table AppB-1). When converting small units to larger units the decimal point moves to the left the number of spaces determined by subtracting the exponent of the smaller unit from the exponent of the larger unit. Therefore, subtract –6 (mL exponent) from –3 (mm exponent). The result is 3, which means the decimal point moves three places to the left.

Solution: $-3 - (-6) = -3 + 6 = 3$
008.0 µm = 0.008 mm

Review: Yes ☐ No ☐

12. Answer: b
Why: By using an English-Metric conversion chart (Table AppB-2), you can find the right answer, or you may choose to memorize certain common conversions, such as 1 tsp = 5 mL.

Review: Yes ☐ No ☐

13. Answer: b
Why: A blood culture dilution of 1:10 means there is 1 mL of blood and 9 mL of media for every 10 mL of blood culture specimen. Forty-five milliliters of media is five times the original proportion of nine milliliters. To maintain the same 1:10 dilution, you must also have five times the original 1 mL proportion of blood. That means you will need to add 5 mL blood to the 45 mL media.

Review: Yes ☐ No ☐

Table App B-1 Commonly Used Metric Measurement Prefixes

Prefix	Multiple	Unit of Measure		
		Meter	Gram	Liter
Kilo- (k)	1000 (10^3)	km	kg	kL
Deci- (d)	1/10 (10^{-1})	dm	dg	dL
Centi- (c)	1/100 (10^{-2})	cm	cg	cL
Milli- (m)	1/1000 (10^{-3})	mm	mg	mL
Micro- (µ)	1/1,000.000 (10^{-6})	µm	µg	µL

Table App B-2 English Metric Equivalents

	English	= Metric
Distance	Yard (yd)	= 0.9 meters (m)
	Inch (in)	= 2.54 centi meters (cm)
Weight	Pound (lb)	= 0.454 kilograms (kg) or 454 grams (g)
	Ounce (oz)	= 28 grams (g)
Volume	Quart (qt)	= 0.95 liters (L)
	Fluid ounce (fl oz)	= 30 milliliters (mL)
	Tablespoon (tbsp)	= 15 milliliters (mL)
	Teaspoon (tsp)	= 5 milliliters (mL)

14. Answer: c
Why: Normal infant blood volume is approximately 100 mL/kg. If a baby's weight is given in pounds, it must be converted to kilograms by multiplying the pounds by the conversion factor 0.454. Once the weight is established in kilograms, multiply that number by 100, because for every kilogram there are 100 mL of blood.
Example:
6 lb × 0.454 = 2.7 kg
(rounded to nearest tenth)
2.7 kg × 100 mL/kg = 270 mL
270 mL/1000 = 0.27 L
Review: Yes ☐ No ☐

15. Answer: d
Why: Normal adult blood volume is approximately 70 mL per kilogram of weight. If the weight is given in pounds, it must be converted to kilograms by multiplying by the conversion factor 0.454 (Table AppB-1). The weight in kilograms is multiplied by 70 because we know that for every kilogram of weight in an adult there is approximately 70 mL of blood. Divide the result by 1000 because adult blood volume is reported in liters and 1 L equals 1000 mL.
Example:
130 lb × 0.454 = 59.02 kg
59 kg × 70 mL/kg = 4130 mL
4130/1000 = 4.13 L
Review: Yes ☐ No ☐

16. Answer: c
Why: A 1:10 dilution of bleach means there is 1 mL of bleach and 9 mL of water for every 10 mL of solution. One hundred milliliters of a 1:10 dilution is 10 times the original 10-mL proportion. That means you will also need 10 times the original amount of bleach and water, or 10 mL bleach and 90 mL water.
Review: Yes ☐ No ☐

17. Answer: b
Why: The basic unit of volume in the metric system is the liter (L), as shown in Table AppB-3 (Metric-English Equivalents). It is easier to remember that the liter is the basic metric unit of volume than to remember other metric measurements, because the soft drink industry in the United States has converted much of their packaging to metric measurements, and we see advertisements for liters of soft drinks all the time.
Review: Yes ☐ No ☐

18. Answer: c
Why: A millimeter (mm) is 1/1000 meter, or 10^{-3}m (Table AppB-2).
Review: Yes ☐ No ☐

19. Answer: c
Why: When converting large units to smaller units, the decimal point moves to the right. To convert large units to basic units, move the decimal point to the right the value of the exponent of the larger unit. A kilogram (k) is 1000 or 10^3 grams (Table AppB-2).

The exponent is 3, so the decimal point moves three places to the right.

Solution: 1.200 kg = 1200 g.

Review: Yes ☐ No ☐

20. Answer: a
Why: One kilogram equals 2.2 lb (Table AppB-3). This is a conversion factor that should be memorized. A helpful hint might be to remember that weight in kilograms is approximately half (divide by 2) the number given in pounds. However, it is important to remember that this number will always be slightly higher than an actual calculation.
Review: Yes ☐ No ☐

21. Answer: a
Why: The basic unit of weight in the metric system is the gram (Table AppB-3).
Review: Yes ☐ No ☐

22. Answer: c
Why: Kilo-, abbreviated "k," means 1000 (Table AppB-1). It can be used with each of the three basic units of measure in the metric system.
Example:
kilogram (kg) = 1000 grams (g)
kiloliter (kL) = 1000 liters (L)
kilometer (km) = 1000 meters (m)
Review: Yes ☐ No ☐

23. Answer: c
Why: Metric-English conversion equivalent for distance (or length) is the meter (m), as shown in Table AppB-3.
Review: Yes ☐ No ☐

Table App B-3 Metric-English Equivalents

	Metric		English
Distance	Meter (m)	=	3.3 fee/ 39.37 inches
	Centimeter (cm)	=	0.4 inches
	Millimeter (mm)	=	0.04 inches
Weight	Gram (g)	=	0.0022 pounds
	Kilogram (kg)	=	2.2 pounds
Volume	Liter (L)	=	1.06 quarts
	Milliliter (mL)[a]	=	0.03 fluid
ounces	Milliliter (mL)[a]	=	0.20 or 1/5 tsp

[a]A milliliter (mL) is approximately equal to a cubic centmeter (cc) and the two terms are often used interchangeably.

24. Answer: c
Why: A liter is equal to 1000 mL and a quart is equal to 950 mL; therefore, 1200 mL is 200 mL more than a liter, 250 mL more than a quart, and 800 mL less than 2 liters (Table AppB-1 and AppB-1).
Review: Yes ☐ No ☐

25. Answer: c
Why: The laboratory needs 250%, or two and one-half times, the 3 mL required for the test. Two times 3 mL is 6 mL. One-half of 3 mL is $1\frac{1}{2}$ mL (or you can multiply 3 times 2.5). Therefore, you need $7\frac{1}{2}$ mL to do the test. The closest tube choice is 10 mL.
Review: Yes ☐ No ☐

Pretest and Written Comprehensive Mock Exam

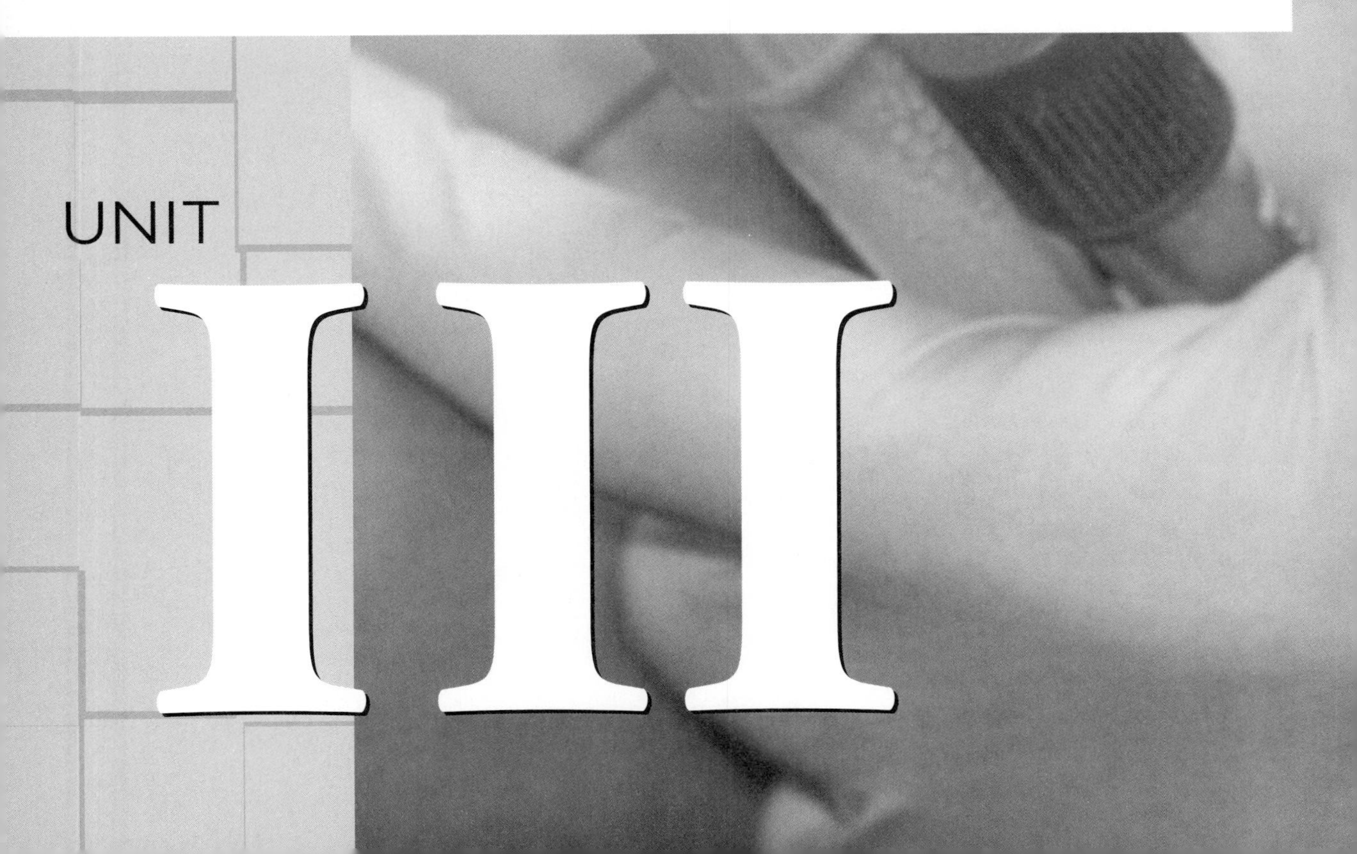

UNIT

III

PRETEST

1. Which of the following infectious disease services is *not* offered through regional Public Health Services agencies?
   a. education
   b. monitoring
   c. screening
   d. treatment

2. Which one of the following should not be an example of a barrier to effective communication with a patient. The patient:
   a. does not speak English.
   b. is a very young child.
   c. is emotionally upset.
   d. is mature male HCW.

3. Which of the following is an example of negative kinesics?
   a. eye contact
   b. frowning
   c. good grooming
   d. smiling

4. Promoting good public relations is a part of the phlebotomist's role for all of the following reasons EXCEPT:
   a. a phlebotomist is a representative of the laboratory.
   b. good public relations promotes harmonious relationships.
   c. patients equate experiences with overall caliber of care received.
   d. skilled public relations can cover up inexperience and insecurity.

5. All of the following are reasons for a phlebotomist to participate in continuing education programs EXCEPT:
   a. eliminate annual evaluations.
   b. learn new skills and techniques.
   c. renew licensure or certification.
   d. stay up-to-date in latest procedures.

6. An individual who has little resistance to an infectious microbe is referred to as a susceptible:
   a. agent.
   b. host.
   c. pathway.
   d. reservoir.

7. MSDS information includes:
   a. general and emergency information.
   b. highly technical chemical formulas.
   c. information on competitor products.
   d. product manufacturing conditions.

8. A person who has recovered from a particular virus and has developed antibodies against that virus is said to be:
   a. a carrier.
   b. immune.
   c. infectious.
   d. susceptible.

9. All pathogens are:
   a. communicable microorganisms.
   b. microbes that can cause disease.
   c. microorganisms that live in soil.
   d. normal flora found on the skin.

10. These are the initials of the two organizations responsible for the latest *Guideline for Isolation Precautions in Hospitals*.
   a. CDC and HICPAC
   b. CLSI and OSHA
   c. HICPAC and NIOSH
   d. NIOSH and OSHA

11. The primary purpose of wearing gloves during phlebotomy procedures is to protect the:
   a. patient from contamination by the phlebotomist.
   b. phlebotomist from exposure to the patient's blood.
   c. specimen from contamination by the phlebotomist.
   d. venipuncture site from contamination by the hands.

12. This equipment is required when collecting a specimen from a patient in airborne isolation.
   a. eye protection
   b. full face shield
   c. mask and goggles
   d. N95 respirator

13. Which of the following is an example of a work practice control that reduces risk of exposure to bloodborne pathogens?
   a. ordering self-sheathing needles
   b. reading the exposure control plan
   c. receiving an HBV vaccination
   d. wearing gloves to draw blood

14. Which of the following statements complies with electrical safety guidelines?
   a. Electrical equipment should be unplugged while being serviced.
   b. Extension cords should be used to conveniently place equipment.
   c. It is safe to use an electrical cord if it is only slightly frayed.
   d. Use electrical equipment carefully if it is starting to malfunction.

15. The "Right to Know" law primarily deals with:
   a. electrical safety issues.
   b. exposure to pathogens.
   c. hazard communication.
   d. labeling of specimens.

16. Blood vessels of the skin are found only in the:
   a. corium and subcutaneous.
   b. dermis and germinativum.
   c. epidermis and adipose layer.
   d. germinativum and corneum.

17. The ability of oxygen to combine with this substance in the red blood cells increases the amount of oxygen that can be carried in the blood by up to 70 times.
   a. carbon dioxide
   b. glucose
   c. hemoglobin
   d. potassium

18. A person's pulse is created by a wave of pressure caused by:
   a. atrial contraction.
   b. atrial relaxation.
   c. ventricular contraction.
   d. ventricular relaxation.

19. The tunica adventitia is the:
   a. external layer of a blood vessel.
   b. inside lining of a blood vessel.
   c. internal layer of a blood vessel.
   d. middle layer of a blood vessel.

20. All of the following are antecubital veins EXCEPT:
   a. accessory cephalic.
   b. median.
   c. median basilic.
   d. subclavian.

21. Which of the following are normally the most numerous of the formed elements?
    a. platelets
    b. red blood cells
    c. reticulocytes
    d. white blood cells

22. This ion is essential to the coagulation process.
    a. calcium.
    b. chloride.
    c. potassium.
    d. sodium.

23. A major cause of respiratory distress in infants and young children is:
    a. airway blockage associated with emphysema.
    b. dyspnea as a consequence of cystic fibrosis.
    c. infection with *Mycobacterium tuberculosis.*
    d. respiratory syncytial virus (RSV) infection.

24. Which of the following are abbreviations for cardiac enzyme tests?
    a. ALP, ALT
    b. BUN, PT
    c. CK, LDH
    d. GTT, ESR

25. What word is used to describe the breakdown of red blood cells?
    a. erythema
    b. erythrocytosis
    c. hemolysis
    d. hemostasis

26. Which of the following word parts are prefixes?
    a. al, lysis, pnea
    b. gastr, lip, onc
    c. ices, ina, nges
    d. iso, neo, tachy

27. A patient who is NPO:
    a. cannot have any food or drink.
    b. cannot have anything but water.
    c. is in critical, but stable condition.
    d. is recovering from minor surgery.

28. There is a sign above the patient's bed that reads, "No blood pressures or venipuncture, right arm". The patient has an IV in the left forearm. You have a request to collect a complete blood count on the patient. How should you proceed?
    a. Ask the patient's nurse to collect the specimen from the IV.
    b. Ask the patient's nurse what to do when the sign is posted.
    c. Collect a CBC from the right arm without using tourniquet.
    d. Collect the specimen from the left hand by finger puncture.

29. Which of the following are all anticoagulants that remove calcium from the specimen by forming insoluble calcium salts, and therefore prevent coagulation?
    a. EDTA, lithium heparin, citrate
    b. NaF, sodium heparin, EDTA
    c. oxalate, SPS, sodium heparin
    d. sodium citrate, EDTA, oxalate

30. All of the following tube stopper colors indicate the presence (or absence) and type of additive in the tube EXCEPT:
    a. green.
    b. lavender.
    c. light blue.
    d. royal blue.

31. What is the purpose of an antiglycolytic agent?
    a. enhance the clotting process
    b. inhibit electrolyte breakdown
    c. preserve glucose
    d. prevent clotting

32. Which one of the following tubes is filled first when multiple tubes are filled from a syringe?
    a. blood culture (SPS) tube
    b. complete blood count tube
    c. nonadditive discard tube
    d. STAT potassium tube

33. The purpose of a tourniquet in the venipuncture procedure is to:
   a. block the flow of arterial blood into the area.
   b. enlarge veins so they are easier to find and enter.
   c. obstruct blood flow to concentrate the analyte.
   d. redirect more blood flow to the venipuncture site.

34. Which type of test is most affected by tissue thromboplastin contamination?
   a. chemistry
   b. coagulation
   c. microbiology
   d. serology

35. Which of the following tests would be most affected by carryover of K_2EDTA?
   a. blood urea nitrogen
   b. glucose
   c. potassium
   d. sodium

36. Symptoms of needle phobia include all of the following EXCEPT:
   a. arrhythmia.
   b. fainting.
   c. lightheadedness.
   d. muscle cramps.

37. Steps taken to unmistakably connect a specimen and the accompanying paperwork to a specific individual are called:
   a. accessioning the specimen.
   b. barcoding specimen labels.
   c. collection verification.
   d. patient identification.

38. Laboratory results can be negatively affected if the phlebotomist:
   a. awakens a sleeping patient and raises the head of the patient's bed.
   b. collects a specimen in dim lighting conditions in the patient's room.
   c. draws a specimen from an unconscious patient without assistance.
   d. startles a patient who is asleep while preparing to collect a specimen.

39. If the tourniquet is too tight, all of the following happens EXCEPT:
   a. arterial flow below it may be stopped.
   b. blood below it may hemoconcentrate.
   c. the pressure can cause the arm to ache.
   d. venous flow increases as veins expand.

40. All of the following will help you avoid inadvertently puncturing an artery during venipuncture EXCEPT:
   a. avoid drawing the basilic vein in the antecubital area.
   b. do not select a site that is near where you feel a pulse.
   c. do not select a vein that overlies or is close to an artery.
   d. stay away from the cephalic vein when the arm is thin.

41. You must collect a light blue top for a special coagulation test from a patient who has an IV in the left wrist area and dermatitis all over the right arm and hand. The veins on the right arm and hand are not readily visible. What is the best way to proceed?
   a. Apply a tourniquet on the right arm over a towel & do the draw.
   b. Ask the patient's nurse to collect the specimen from the IV line.
   c. Collect from the left antecubital area without using a tourniquet.
   d. Collect the specimen by capillary puncture from the left hand.

42. What is the *best* thing to do if the vein can be felt but not seen, even with the tourniquet on?
   a. Insert the needle where you think it is and probe until you find it.
   b. Keep the tourniquet on while cleaning the site and during the draw.

c. Look for visual clues on the skin to remind you where the vein is.
d. Mark the spot using a felt tip pen and clean it off when finished.

43. When is the best time to release the tourniquet during venipuncture?
 a. After the last tube has been filled completely.
 b. After the needle is withdrawn and covered.
 c. As soon as blood begins to flow into the tube.
 d. As soon as the needle penetrates the skin.

44. Proper technique for collecting specimen tubes when using the evacuated tube method includes all of the following EXCEPT:
 a. collect sterile specimens before all other specimens.
 b. draw a "clear" tube before special coagulation tests.
 c. fill each tube until the normal vacuum is exhausted.
 d. position the arm so tubes fill from stopper end first.

45. It is important to fill anticoagulant tubes to the proper level to ensure that:
 a. the specimen yields enough serum for the required tests.
 b there is a proper ratio of blood to anticoagulant additive.
 c. there is an adequate amount of blood to perform the test.
 d. tissue fluid contamination of the specimen is minimized.

46. You have just made two unsuccessful attempts to collect a fasting blood specimen from an outpatient. The patient rotates his arm, and you notice a large vein that you had not seen before. How do you proceed?
 a. Ask another phlebotomist to collect the fasting specimen.
 b. Ask the patient to come back later so that you can try again.
 c. Call the supervisor for permission to make a third attempt.
 d. Make a third attempt on the newly discovered large vein.

47. When drawing blood from an older child the most important consideration is:
 a. assuring the child that it won't be painful.
 b. explaining all of the tests being collected.
 c. explaining the importance of holding still.
 d. offering the child a reward for not crying.

48. Feather is a term used to describe the appearance of:
 a. a newborn screening blood spot.
 b. blood in a thick malaria smear.
 c. lipemia in a bilirubin specimen.
 d. the thinnest area of a blood film.

49. Capillary specimens contain of all of the following EXCEPT:
 a. arterial blood
 b. serous fluids
 c. tissue fluids
 d. venous blood

50. Reference values for this test are higher for capillary specimens:
 a. calcium.
 b. glucose.
 c. phosphorous.
 d. total protein.

51. It is necessary to control the depth of lancet insertion during heel puncture to avoid:
 a. damage to the tendons.
 b. injuring the calcaneus.
 c. puncturing an artery.
 d. unnecessary bleeding.

52. In which of the following areas does capillary specimen collection differ from routine venipuncture when collecting a BUN and CBC?
 a. additives used
 b. antiseptic used

c. ID procedures
d. order of draw

53. A blood smear prepared from an EDTA specimen should be made:
a. after the blood cells settle in the tube.
b. at the time the specimen is collected.
c. before the specimen has been mixed.
d. within 1 hour of specimen collection.

54. An infant may require a blood transfusion if blood levels of this substance exceed 18 mg/dL.
a. bilirubin
b. carnitine
c. galactose
d. thyroxine

55. Phenylketonuria is a:
a. contagious condition caused by lack of phenylalanine.
b. disorder caused by excessive phenylalanine ingestion.
c. genetic disorder involving phenylalanine metabolism.
d. temporary condition caused by lack of phenylalanine.

56. Arteriospasm is defined as:
a. artery contraction due to pain, irritation by a needle, or anxiety.
b. fainting related to hypotension caused by a nervous response.
c. pain that shoots up the side of the arm after needle penetration.
d. tingling feeling in the fingertips when a needle enters an artery.

57. Arterial puncture site selection is based on all of the following EXCEPT:
a. available equipment in the room.
b. presence of collateral circulation.
c. size and accessibility of the artery.
d. type of tissue surrounding the site.

58. Which of the following is a disadvantage of puncturing the radial artery?
a. It is not easy to fully compress.
b. It is small and difficult to feel.
c. The risk of hematoma formation.
d. There is no collateral circulation.

59. In addition to normal patient identification information, an arterial blood gas requisition typically includes all of the following EXCEPT:
a. age at onset of respiratory disease.
b. method of ventilation or delivery.
c. patient activity and body position.
d. temperature and respiration rate.

60. What constitutes a positive modified Allen test? The
a. blood pressure increases in the radial artery.
b. color drains from hand at least 30 seconds.
c. hand color returns to normal in 15 seconds.
d. pulse in the ulnar artery becomes irregular.

61. Some blood specimens require cooling to:
a. avoid hemolysis of RBCs.
b. prevent premature clotting.
c. promote serum separation.
d. slow metabolic processes.

62. All of the following are reasons why specimen handling is very important EXCEPT:
a. effects of mishandling are not always obvious.
b. improper handling can affect quality of results.
c. many lab errors occur in the preanalytical phase.
d. mishandling effects can be corrected if identified.

63. Which of the following actions will compromise the quality of the specimen?
    a. drawing a BUN in an amber serum tube
    b. mixing an SST by inverting it five times
    c. only partially filling a liquid EDTA tube
    d. transporting a cryofibrinogen at 37+C

64. All of the following analytes require protection from light EXCEPT:
    a. ammonia.
    b. bilirubin.
    c. vitamin B_{12}.
    d. vitamin C.

65. Chilling can cause erroneous results for this analyte.
    a. ammonia
    b. glucagon
    c. lactic acid
    d. potassium

66. An example of a QA indicator is:
    a. all phlebotomists will follow universal precautions.
    b. blood culture contamination rates will not exceed 3 percent.
    c. laboratory personnel will not wear lab coats when on break.
    d. no eating, drinking, or smoking is allowed in lab work areas.

67. ESR determinations on specimens held at room temperature must be made within:
    a. 1 hour.
    b. 4 hours.
    c. 12 hours.
    d. 24 hours.

68. All of the following can be done to prevent exposure to aerosol generated when the stopper is removed from a specimen tube EXCEPT:
    a. cover the stopper with a 4 4 gauze while removing it.
    b. remove the stopper with the tube held behind a shield.
    c. use a specially designed safety stopper removal device.
    d. withdraw the specimen through the stopper by syringe.

69. If a specimen has inadequate identification, the specimen processor may:
    a. add the missing information to the label.
    b. ask the phlebotomist to get a new sample.
    c. contact the patient for correct information.
    d. refer the tube to the laboratory supervisor.

70. According to CLSI, the maximum time limit for separating serum or plasma from cells is:
    a. 15 minutes from the time of collection.
    b. 30 minutes from the time of collection.
    c. 1.0 hour from the time of collection.
    d. 2.0 hours from the time of collection.

71. An aliquot is a:
    a. filter for separating serum from cells.
    b. portion of a specimen being tested.
    c. specimen being prepared for testing.
    d. tube used to balance the centrifuge.

72. Which of the following is the best way to prepare routine blood specimen tubes for transportation to the lab?
    a. Place the tubes in ice slurry.
    b. Seal the tubes in plastic bags.
    c. Wipe each tube with alcohol.
    d. Wrap them in the requisitions.

73. Tubes should be transported with the stopper up for all of the following reasons EXCEPT that it:
    a. encourages complete clot formation.
    b. maintains the sterility of the sample.
    c. minimizes stopper caused aerosols.
    d. reduces agitation caused hemolysis.

74. Specimens transported by courier or other air or ground mail systems must follow guidelines defined by all of the following EXCEPT:
    a. DOT.
    b. FAA.

c. FDA.
d. OSHA.

75. Which specimen needs to be transported on ice?
a. ammonia
b. bilirubin
c. carotene
d. potassium

76. A specimen must be transported at or near normal body temperature. Which of the following temperatures meets this requirement?
a. 25°C
b. 37°C
c. 50°C
d. 98°C

77. The liquid portion of a clotted specimen is called:
a. fibrinogen.
b. plasma.
c. saline.
d. serum.

78. A whole blood specimen has an abnormally large buffy coat. This is an indication that the patient has:
a. an elevated leukocyte or platelet count.
b. an increased amount of red blood cells.
c. large numbers of bacteria in the blood.
d. recently eaten a meal with a lot of fat.

79. A urine C & S is typically ordered to:
a. check for glucose in the urine.
b. diagnose urinary tract infection.
c. evaluate function of the kidneys.
d. monitor urinary protein levels.

80. Which of the following tests is sometimes performed on amniotic fluid?
a. alkaline phosphatase
b. alpha-fetoprotein
c. lactic dehydrogenase
d. reticulocyte count

81. This test requires intravenous administration of histamine or pentagastrin.
a. alpha-fetoprotein
b. gastric analysis
c. sweat chloride
d. urine porphyrins

82. A bleeding time (BT) test assesses the functioning of which of the following cellular elements?
a. erythrocytes
b. leukocytes
c. neutrophils
d. thrombocytes

83. The most common reason for glucose monitoring through POCT is to:
a. check for sporadic glucose in the urine.
b. control medication induced mood swings.
c. diagnose glucose metabolism problems.
d. monitor glucose levels for diabetic care.

84. When reading a patient's TB test, there is an area of induration and erythema that measures 7 mm in diameter. The result of the test is:
a. doubtful.
b. negative.
c. positive.
d. unreadable.

85. Point-of-care detection of Group A strep normally requires a:
a. blood sample.
b. nasal collection.
c. throat swab.
d. urine specimen.

86. Which of the following *cannot* be detected in urine on a special reagent strip that is dipped in the urine specimen and then compared visually against color codes on the reagent strip container?
a. bilirubin
b. glucose
c. leukocytes
d. thrombin

87. The AMT, NCA, and ASCP are agencies that:
   a. accredit phlebotomy programs
   b. certify laboratory professionals
   c. license allied health professionals
   d. monitor communicable diseases

88. Which of the following is the name or abbreviation for the federal law that established standards for the electronic exchange of patient information?
   a. CLIA
   b. HIPAA
   c. Medicare
   d. OSHA

89. What is the Clinical and Laboratory Standards Institute (CLSI) recommended way to clean a venipuncture site?
   a. Clean the area thoroughly with disinfectant using concentric circles.
   b. Cleanse with a circular motion from the center to the periphery.
   c. Scrub with an alcohol sponge as vigorously as you can for 1 minute.
   d. Wipe using concentric circles from the outside area to the center.

90. According to CLSI depth of heel puncture should not exceed:
   a. 1.5 mm.
   b. 2.0 mm.
   c. 2.4 mm.
   d. 4.9 mm.

91. The standard of care used in phlebotomy malpractice cases is often based on guidelines from this organization.
   a. CAP
   b. CLIA
   c. CLSI
   d. NAACLS

92. The abbreviation for the federal regulations that established quality standards to ensure the accuracy, reliability, and timeliness of patient test results, regardless of the size, type, or location of the laboratory.
   a. BBP Standard
   b. CLIA '88
   c. JCAHO
   d. OSHA

93. QC protocols prohibit use of outdated evacuated tubes for all of the following reasons except:
   a. additives that prevent clotting may no longer function as required
   b. specimens collected in these tubes may yield erroneous results.
   c. Stoppers may have shrunk causing specimens to leak when inverted
   d. tubes may not fill completely changing the ratio of additive to blood

94. Drawing a patient's blood without his or her permission can result in a charge of:
   a. assault and battery.
   b. breach of confidentiality.
   c. malpractice.
   d. negligence.

95. Civil actions involve:
   a. legal proceedings between private parties.
   b. offenses for which a person may be imprisoned.
   c. regulations established by governments.
   d. violent crimes against the state or nation.

96. Malpractice is a claim of:
   a. breach of confidentiality.
   b. improper treatment.
   c. invasion of privacy.
   d. res ipsa loquitur

97. Diurnal variations associated with some blood components are:
   a. abnormal changes that occur once a day.
   b. changes that follow a monthly cycle.
   c. normal fluctuations throughout the day.
   d. variations that occur on an hourly basis.

98. Which of the following analytes is *most* affected by exercise prior to specimen collection?
    a. bilirubin
    b. calcium
    c. enzymes
    d. uric acid

99. If you have no choice but to collect a specimen from an arm with a hematoma, collect the specimen:
    a. above the hematoma.
    b. beside the hematoma.
    c. distal to the hematoma.
    d. through the hematoma.

100. The ratio of blood to anticoagulant is *most* critical for which of the following tests?
    a. alkaline phosphatase
    b. complete blood count
    c. glycohemoglobin
    d. prothrombin time

PRETEST ANSWERS

1. Answer: d
   Subject: The Healthcare Setting
   Why: Public Health Services, one of the principal units under the Department of Health and Human Services, have agencies at local and state levels. These agencies screen for and monitor infectious diseases, and educate the public about defense against infectious diseases that might spread among the populace. The agencies do not get involved in treatment for infectious diseases.
   Reference: Chapter 1, *Phlebotomy Essentials* 4e.

2. Answer: d
   Subject: Communications
   Why: Language, age and emotions can all be barriers to communication and require special communication techniques for effective exchange of information to occur. In the case of a mature, male healthcare worker (HCW), communication should be without many obstacles since he understands the process and knows what to expect as a practitioner in the healthcare system.
   Reference: Chapter 1, *Phlebotomy Essentials* 4e.

3. Answer: b
   Subject: Communications
   Why: Kinesics is the study of nonverbal communication or body language. Frowning is an example of negative kinesics or body language. Eye contact, good grooming, and smiling are all examples of positive body language.
   Reference: Chapter 1, *Phlebotomy Essentials* 4e.

4. Answer: d
   Subject: Professionalism
   Why: As the "public relations officer" everything the phlebotomist does reflects on the whole facility. The phlebotomist is often the only real contact the patient has with the laboratory. In many cases, the patient equates this encounter with the caliber of care they receive while in the hospital. Positive public relations promotes good will and harmonious relationships with employees and patients. Mastering good public relations does not cover up for inexperience and lack of skills.
   Reference: Chapter 1, *Phlebotomy Essentials* 4e.

5. Answer: a
   Subject: Professionalism
   Why: Continuing education for a health professional is important for maintaining competency in all areas. It is necessary to remain current in the increasingly complex field of healthcare to maintain quality and avoid litigation. By staying current, a phlebotomist can maintain his/her certification through continuing education or by retaking the exam periodically. What continuing education should *not* do is eliminate the need for

annual evaluations. This valuable tool tells the phlebotomist what additional continuing education he or she might need.
Reference: Chapter 1, *Phlebotomy Essentials* 4e.

6. Answer: b
Subject: Infection Control
Why: In healthcare, a susceptible host is someone with decreased ability to resist infection. A microbe responsible for an infection is called the causative or infectious agent. An exit or entry pathway is the way an infectious microbe is able respectively, to leave or to enter a host. A reservoir is a place where an infectious microbe can survive and multiply, and includes humans, animals, food, water, soil, contaminated articles, and equipment.
Reference: Chapter 3, *Phlebotomy Essentials* 4e.

7. Answer: a
Subject: Infection Control
Why: MSDS stands for material safety data sheet, a document that contains general, precautionary, and emergency information for a product with a hazardous warning on the label. The OSHA Hazard Communication (HazCom) Standard requires manufacturers to supply MSDS for their products. Employers are required to obtain the MSDS for every hazardous chemical present in the workplace and have all MSDS readily accessible to employees.
Reference: Chapter 3, *Phlebotomy Essentials* 4e.

8. Answer: b
Subject: Infection Control
Why: Immunity to a particular virus normally exists when a person's blood has antibodies directed against that virus. A person who has recovered from infection with a virus has antibodies directed against it and is considered immune. A person who does not display symptoms of a virus such as hepatitis B, but whose blood contains the virus, is capable of transmitting it to others and is called a carrier. A person who is susceptible to a virus has no antibodies against it.
Reference: Chapter 3, *Phlebotomy Essentials* 4e.

9. Answer: b
Why: Microorganisms (microbes) that are capable of causing disease are called pathogens. Communicable microorganisms are pathogens that can be spread from person to person. Only some pathogenic microbes live in the soil. Normal flora (microorganisms that live on the skin) do not cause disease under normal conditions.
Reference: Chapter 3, *Phlebotomy Essentials* 4e.

10. Answer: a
Subject: Infection Control
Why: The CDC and HICPAC together developed the latest *Guideline for Isolation Precautions in Hospitals.* The guideline identifies two tiers of precautions; standard precautions to be used in the care of all patients, and transmission-based precautions to be used in addition to standard precautions for patients with certain highly transmissible diseases.
Reference: Chapter 3, *Phlebotomy Essentials* 4e.

11. Answer: b
Subject: Infection Control
Why: The OSHA bloodborne pathogen (BBP) standard requires glove use during phlebotomy procedures to protect the phlebotomist from bloodborne pathogen contamination. Gloves do not necessarily protect the patient; in fact, they can be a source of contamination to the patient if the phlebotomist touches contaminated articles before touching the patient's arm. Gloves can also be a source of contamination to capillary puncture specimens. Rather than protecting the

venipuncture site, gloves can contaminate it if the phlebotomist touches the site after it is cleaned.
Reference: Chapter 3, *Phlebotomy Essentials* 4e.

12. Answer: d
Subject: Infection Control
Why: Anyone entering the room of a patient with airborne precautions must wear an N95 respirator, unless the precautions are for rubeola or varicella and the individual entering the room is immune.
Reference: Chapter 3, *Phlebotomy Essentials* 4e.

13. Answer: d
Subject: Infection Control
Why: Work practice controls are routines that alter the manner in which a task is performed to reduce likelihood of exposure to bloodborne pathogens (BBPs). Wearing gloves to draw blood reduces the chance of exposure to BBPs. Ordering self-sheathing needles, reading the exposure control plan, and receiving an HBV vaccination are all important in reducing the risk of exposure to BBPs, but do not in themselves alter the actual performance of a task and are not considered work practice controls.
Reference: Chapter 3, *Phlebotomy Essentials* 4e.

14. Answer: a
Subject: Safety
Why: Electrical equipment should be unplugged before servicing to avoid electrical shock. The use of extension cords should be avoided because they lead to circuit overload, incomplete connections, and potential clutter in the path of workers. Frayed electrical cords are dangerous and should be replaced rather than used. Malfunctioning equipment should be unplugged and not used until fixed.
Reference: Chapter 3, *Phlebotomy Essentials* 4e.

15. Answer: c
Subject: Safety
Why: The OSHA HazCom Standard, which is called the "Right to Know Law", requires manufacturers of hazardous materials to provide MSDS for their products. An MSDS contains general, precautionary, and emergency information about the product.
Reference: Chapter 3, *Phlebotomy Essentials* 4e.

16. Answer: a
Subject: Anatomy and Physiology
Why: Blood vessels are found in the corium (dermis) and subcutaneous layers of the skin. The epidermis is avascular, which means it does not contain blood vessels. The stratum germinativum and stratum corneum are layers of the epidermis. Adipose (fat) cells are found in the subcutaneous.
Reference: Chapter 5, *Phlebotomy Essentials* 4e.

17. Answer: c
Subject: Anatomy and Physiology
Why: The ability of oxygen to combine with a protein in red blood cells called hemoglobin increases the oxygen-carrying capacity of the blood. Hemoglobin combined with oxygen is called oxyhemoglobin.
Reference: Chapter 5, *Phlebotomy Essentials* 4e.

18. Answer: c
Subject: Circulatory System
Why: The wave of pressure created as the ventricles contract and blood is forced out of the heart and through the arteries creates the throbbing beat known as the pulse.
Reference: Chapter 6, *Phlebotomy Essentials* 4e.

19. Answer: a
Subject: Circulatory System
Why: Blood vessels have three main layers. The tunica adventitia (also called tunica

externa) is the term applied to the outer layer of an artery or a vein. It is made up of connective tissue and is thicker in arteries than veins. The tunica intima (also called tunica interna) is the inner layer or lining of a blood vessel and is composed of a single layer of endothelial cells with an underlying basement membrane, connective tissue layer, and elastic membrane. The tunica media is the middle layer, composed of smooth muscle and some elastic fibers. The tunica media is much thicker in arteries than in veins.
Reference: Chapter 6, *Phlebotomy Essentials* 4e.

20. Answer: d
Subject: Circulatory System
Why: The subclavian vein begins in the shoulder area and leads into the chest. The accessory cephalic median basilic, and median veins all have portions that are in the antecubital fossa.
Reference: Chapter 6, *Phlebotomy Essentials* 4e.

21. Answer: b
Subject: Circulatory System
Why: The formed elements are red blood cells, white blood cells, and platelets. The erythrocyte (red blood cell) is normally the most numerous formed element in the blood, averaging 4.5–5.0 million per cubic millimeter of blood.
Reference: Chapter 6, *Phlebotomy Essentials* 4e.

22. Answer: a
Subject: Circulatory System
Why: Ions are particles that carry an electrical charge. The coagulation process requires the presence of calcium ions, which have a positive charge, for proper function. An anticoagulant prevents coagulation by binding or chelating calcium and not allowing it to enter into the coagulation process for which it is essential. Chloride, sodium and potassium are also ions. They function in other body processes, however.
Reference: Chapter 6, *Phlebotomy Essentials* 4e.

23. Answer: d
Subject: Tests and Disorders
Why: Infection with respiratory syncytial virus causes acute respiratory problems in children. Cystic fibrosis, emphysema, and *Mycobacterium tuberculosis* can cause respiratory distress in children but are not nearly as common.
Reference: Chapter 5, *Phlebotomy Essentials* 4e.

24. Answer: c
Subject: Tests and Disorders
Why: Creatine kinase (CK) and lactate dehydrogenase (LDH) are enzymes present in cardiac muscle. They are released during myocardial infarction. Alkaline phosphatase (ALP) and alanine aminotransferase (ALT) are enzymes measured most commonly to determine liver function. Blood urea nitrogen (BUN) is a kidney function test, and prothrombin time (PT) is a coagulation test used to monitor anticoagulant therapy. A glucose tolerance test (GTT) measures glucose metabolism, and erythrocyte sedimentation rate (ESR) is a nonspecific indicator of disease, especially inflammatory conditions such as arthritis.
Reference: Chapter 5, *Phlebotomy Essentials* 4e.

25. Answer: c
Subject: Terminology
Why: Hemolysis is the breakdown of red blood cells. The combining form *hemo* means blood. The suffix *lysis* means breakdown.
Reference: Chapter 4, *Phlebotomy Essentials* 4e.

26. Answer: d
Subject: Terminology
Why: The word parts *iso-*, *neo-*, and *tachy-* are prefixes. The word parts *-al -lysis*, and *-pnea* are suffixes; *gastr*, *lip* and *onc* are word roots; and *ices*, *ina*, and *nges* are plural endings.

Reference: *Chapter 4, Phlebotomy Essentials* 4e.

27. Answer: a
Subject: Patient Considerations
Why: NPO comes from Latin (*non per os*) and means nothing by mouth. Patients who are NPO cannot have food or drink, not even water. Patients are typically NPO before surgery, not after.
Reference: Chapter 8, *Phlebotomy Essentials* 4e.

28. Answer: d
Subject: Tests and Disorders
Why: Because the specimen is a complete blood count (CBC), it can easily be collected by fingerstick from the left hand. The right arm should not be used. Collecting the CBC from the IV is not worth the risk when it can easily be collected by capillary puncture. A competent phlebotomist should be able to decide what to do in this situation without having to ask the nurse.
Reference: Chapter 1, *Phlebotomy Essentials* 4e.

29. Answer: d
Subject: Equipment
Why: Sodium citrate, oxalate and EDTA are all anticoagulants that prevent blood from clotting by chelating (binding) or precipitating calcium so it is not available to the coagulation process. Sodium polyanethol sulfonate (SPS) also binds calcium, however lithium and sodium heparin prevent clotting by inhibiting the formation of thrombin needed to convert fibrinogen to fibrin in the coagulation process. Sodium fluoride is an antiglycolytic agent, not an anticoagulant.
Reference: Chapter 7, *Phlebotomy Essentials* 4e.

30. Answer: d
Subject: Equipment
Why: Most tube stopper colors indicate the presence (or absence) and type of additive in a tube. A green stopper indicates heparin, a lavender stopper indicates EDTA, and light blue normally indicates sodium citrate. A royal blue stopper, however, indicates that the tube and stopper are virtually trace-element–free. A royal blue top can contain no additive, potassium EDTA, or sodium heparin. Additive color-coding of a royal blue top tube is typically indicated on the label.
Reference: Chapter 7, *Phlebotomy Essentials* 4e.

31. Answer: c
Subject: Equipment
Why: An antiglycolytic agent is a substance that inhibits or prevents glycolysis (metabolism of glucose) by the cells of the blood. The most common glycolytic inhibitors are sodium fluoride and lithium iodoacetate.
Reference: Chapter 7, *Phlebotomy Essentials* 4e.

32. Answer: a
Subject: Equipment
Why: Tubes or containers for specimens such as blood cultures that must be collected in a sterile manner are always collected first in both the syringe and ETS system of venipuncture.
Reference: Chapter 7, *Phlebotomy Essentials* 4e.

33. Answer: b
Subject: Equipment
Why: The purpose of a tourniquet in the venipuncture procedure is to block the venous flow, not the arterial flow, so that blood flows freely into the area but not out. This causes the veins to enlarge, making them easier to find and penetrate with a needle. The tourniquet does not redirect blood flow, but does change the volume of the flow. The tourniquet must not be left on for longer than 1 minute because obstruction of blood flow changes the concentration of some analytes, leading to erroneous test results.
Reference: Chapter 7, *Phlebotomy Essentials* 4e.

34. Answer: b
Subject: Equipment
Why: Tissue thromboplastin affects coagulation tests the most because it is a substance found in tissue that activates the extrinsic coagulation pathway. Tissue thromboplastin is picked up by the needle as it penetrates the skin during venipuncture and is flushed into the first tube filled during ETS collection, or mixed with blood collected in a syringe. Although it is no longer considered a significant problem for prothrombin time (PT) and partial thromboplastin time (PTT) tests unless the draw is difficult or involves a lot of needle manipulation, it may compromise results of other coagulation tests. Therefore, any time a coagulation test other than PT or PTT is the first or only tube collected, a few milliliters of blood should be drawn into a "discard" tube.
Reference: Chapter 7, *Phlebotomy Essentials* 4e.

35. Answer: c
Subject: Equipment
Why: K_2EDTA contains potassium. (K is the chemical symbol for potassium, and K_2EDTA is an abbreviation for dipotassium EDTA.) Carryover of potassium EDTA formulations into tubes for potassium testing have been known to significantly increase potassium levels in the specimen, causing erroneously elevated test results.
Reference: Chapter 7, *Phlebotomy Essentials* 4e.

36. Answer: d
Subject: Venipuncture
Why: Symptoms of needle phobia include pallor (paleness), profuse sweating, lightheadedness, nausea, and fainting. In severe cases, patients have been known to suffer arrhythmia and even cardiac arrest, but not muscle cramps.
Reference: Chapter 8, *Phlebotomy Essentials* 4e.

37. Answer: a
Subject: Venipuncture
Why: The steps taken to unmistakably connect a specimen and the accompanying paperwork to a specific individual is called accessioning the specimen. The accession number is automatically assigned when the request is entered into the computer.
Reference: Chapter 8, *Phlebotomy Essentials* 4e.

38. Answer: d
Subject: Venipuncture
Why: A startle reflex can affect test results and should be avoided. Collecting the specimen in dim lighting or collecting a specimen from an unconscious patient should not affect test results, provided the specimen is collected properly. When a phlebotomist awakens a patient and elevates the head of the patient's bed before collecting the specimen, there should be no negative effect to the specimen.
Reference: Chapter 8, *Phlebotomy Essentials* 4e.

39. Answer: d
Subject: Venipuncture
Why: A tourniquet that is too tight may prevent arterial blood flow into the area, resulting in failure to obtain blood. A tourniquet that is too tight increases the effects of hemoconcentration and contributes to erroneous results on the sample. A tourniquet that is too tight will pinch and hurt the patient and cause the arm to turn red or purple. A tight tourniquet will not allow for an increase in venous blood flow.
Reference: Chapter 8, *Phlebotomy Essentials* 4e.

40. Answer: d
Subject: Venipuncture
Why: To avoid inadvertently puncturing an artery never select a vein that overlies or is close to an artery or near where you feel a pulse. Avoid drawing from the basilic vein as it is in the area of the brachial artery.

Reference: Chapter 8, *Phlebotomy Essentials* 4e.

41. Answer: a
Subject: Venipuncture
Why: When a person has dermatitis and there is no other site available, it is acceptable to apply the tourniquet over a towel or washcloth placed over the patient's arm. A coagulation test should not be collected from an IV and a coagulation tube cannot be collected by fingerstick. The area above an IV must not be used regardless of whether or not you use a tourniquet.
Reference: Chapter 8, *Phlebotomy Essentials* 4e.

42. Answer: c
Subject: Venipuncture
Why: If the vein can be felt, but not seen, try to mentally visualize its location. It often helps to note the position of the vein in reference to a mole, hair, or skin crease. Never insert the needle blindly or probe to find a vein as damage to nerves and tissue may result. Never leave the tourniquet on for more than 1 minute as hemoconcentration of the specimen may result. Marking the site with a felt tip pen could contaminate the specimen or transfer disease from patient to patient.
Reference: Chapter 8, *Phlebotomy Essentials* 4e.

43. Answer: a
Subject: Venipuncture
Why: According to CLSI guidelines, the best time to release the tourniquet is as soon as blood begins to flow into the first tube. Releasing the tourniquet as well as having the patient release the fist minimizes the effects of stasis and hemoconcentration on the specimen. A tourniquet should not remain in place longer than 1 minute.
Reference: Chapter 8, *Phlebotomy Essentials* 4e.

44. Answer: d
Subject: Venipuncture
Why: The arm should be in a downward position during venipuncture so that tubes fill from the bottom up and *not* from the stopper end first. This keeps blood in the tube from coming in contact with the needle, preventing reflux of tube contents into the patient's vein, and minimizing the chance of additive carryover between tubes. Collecting sterile specimens before filling tubes for other specimens, clearing for special coagulation tests, and filling tubes until the normal vacuum is exhausted are all part of proper venipuncture technique.
Reference: Chapter 8, *Phlebotomy Essentials* 4e.

45. Answer: b
Subject: Venipuncture
Why: It is important to fill additive tubes to the proper fill level to ensure a proper ratio of additive to blood. The proper fill level is attained by allowing the tube to fill until the normal vacuum is exhausted and blood ceases to flow into the tube. Tubes will not fill completely as there is always dead space at the top. Blood in an anticoagulant tube does not clot. A partially filled tube would likely yield enough specimen to perform the test; however, the results would be inaccurate. Tissue thromboplastin is a problem for some tests, particularly special coagulation tests collected in light blue tops. However, contamination can be minimized by first collecting a discard tube to flush the tissue thromboplastin out of the needle.
Reference: Chapter 8, *Phlebotomy Essentials* 4e.

46. Answer: a
Subject: Venipuncture
Why: After two unsuccessful attempts at blood collection, *do not* try a third time. Ask another phlebotomist to take over. Unsuccessful venipuncture attempts are frustrating

to the patient and the phlebotomist. With the exception of STAT and other priority specimens, if the second phlebotomist is also unsuccessful, it is a good idea to give the patient a rest and come back at a later time. An outpatient may be given the option of returning another day after consultation with his or her physician.
Reference: Chapter 8, *Phlebotomy Essentials* 4e.

47. Answer: c
Subject: Venipuncture
Why: Older children appreciate honesty and will be more cooperative if you explain what you are going to do and stress the importance of holding still. *Never* tell the child it won't hurt, because chances are it will, even if just a little. It is all right to offer the child a reward for being brave, but *do not* put conditions on receiving the reward such as, "You can only have the reward if you don't cry." Some crying is to be anticipated, and it is important to let the child know that it is all right to cry.
Reference: Chapter 8, *Phlebotomy Essentials* 4e.

48. Answer: d
Subject: Capillary
Why: A properly made blood film or smear shows a smooth transition from thick to thin. The thinnest area of the film is only one cell thick and is called the feather because of its appearance when held up to the light. The feather is the area where a manual differential is performed.
Reference: Chapter 10, *Phlebotomy Essentials* 4e.

49. Answer: b
Subject: Capillary
Why: Capillary specimens are a mixture of arterial and venous blood, and tissue fluids that include interstitial fluid from the tissue spaces between the cells, and intracellular fluid from within the cells. Serous fluids are pale yellow watery fluids similar to serum that are found between double-layered membranes that line the pleural, pericardial, and peritoneal cavities.
Reference: Chapter 10, *Phlebotomy Essentials* 4e.

50. Answer: b
Subject: Capillary
Why: Reference values for glucose tests are higher for capillary puncture specimens. They are lower for calcium, phosphorous, and total protein.
Reference: Chapter 10, *Phlebotomy Essentials* 4e.

51. Answer: b
Subject: Capillary
Why: The depth of lancet insertion must be controlled to avoid injuring the heel bone. The medical term for the heel bone is calcaneus. Puncturing an artery or damaging tendons is avoided by puncturing in a recommended area. A deep puncture does not necessarily produce more bleeding.
Reference: Chapter 10, *Phlebotomy Essentials* 4e.

52. Answer: d
Subject: Capillary
Why: Capillary puncture releases tissue thromboplastin, which activates the coagulation process and leads to platelet clumping and microclot formation in specimens that are not collected quickly. This affects hematology specimens the most, consequently they are collected first. Serum specimens are collected last because they are supposed to clot. In the order of draw for venipuncture, which was designed to minimize problems caused by additive carryover between tubes, serum specimens are collected before hematology specimens. Carryover is not an issue with capillary collection. Isopropyl alcohol is the recommended antiseptic for capillary puncture and routine venipuncture.

Patient identification is the same regardless of specimen collection method. Additives in microcollection tubes and stopper colors correspond to those of evacuated tubes.
Reference: Chapter 10, *Phlebotomy Essentials* 4e.

53. Answer: d
Subject: Capillary
Why: A blood smear prepared from an EDTA specimen should be made within 1 hour of collection to prevent cell distortion caused by prolonged contact with the anticoagulant.
Reference: Chapter 10, *Phlebotomy Essentials* 4e.

54. Answer: a
Subject: Capillary
Why: Bilirubin can cross the blood–brain barrier in infants, accumulating to toxic levels that can cause permanent brain damage or even death. A transfusion may be needed if levels increase at a rate equal to or greater than 5 mg/dL per hour or when levels exceed 18 mg/dL.
Reference: Chapter 10, *Phlebotomy Essentials* 4e.

55. Answer: c
Subject: Capillary
Why: Phenylketonuria (PKU) is a hereditary disorder caused by an inability to metabolize the amino acid phenylalanine. Patient's with PKU lack the enzyme necessary to convert phenylalanine to tyrosine. Phenylalanine accumulates in the blood and can rise to toxic levels. PKU cannot be cured but it can normally be treated with a diet low in phenylalanine. If left untreated or not treated early on, PKU can lead to brain damage and mental retardation.
Reference: Chapter 10, *Phlebotomy Essentials* 4e.

56. Answer: a
Subject: Arterial Blood Gases
Why: Pain or irritation caused by needle penetration of the artery muscle and even patient anxiety can cause a reflex (involuntary) contraction of the artery referred to as an arteriospasm. The condition is transitory but can make it difficult to obtain a specimen.
Reference: Chapter 12, *Phlebotomy Essentials* 4e.

57. Answer: a
Subject: Arterial Blood Gases
Why: Several different sites can be used for arterial puncture, and the choice of site is never based on what equipment is available in the room or on the phlebotomist's tray. The criteria for site selection include the presence of collateral circulation, how large and accessible the artery is, and the type of tissue surrounding the puncture site.
Reference: Chapter 12, *Phlebotomy Essentials* 4e.

58. Answer: b
Subject: Arterial Blood Gases
Why: One disadvantage of puncturing the radial artery is it requires considerable skill to successfully puncture because it is so small. The presence of ligaments and bone in the area to aid in compression decrease the chance of hematoma formation, which is an advantage. The presence of collateral circulation via the ulnar artery is also an advantage.
Reference: Chapter 12, *Phlebotomy Essentials* 4e.

59. Answer: a
Subject: Arterial Blood Gases
Why: An ABG requisition typically includes the patient's body temperature and respiratory rate, method of ventilation or delivery, patient activity and body position in addition to normal patient identification information. The patient's age at onset of respiratory disease is not found on the requisition.
Reference: Chapter 12, *Phlebotomy Essentials* 4e.

60. Answer: c
Subject: Arterial Blood Gases
Why: When performing the modified Allen test, both the ulnar and radial arteries are compressed to stop arterial flow to the hand.

With both arteries compressed the hand should appear blanched or drained of color. If the patient has collateral circulation, the hand will flush pink or normal color when the ulnar artery is released even though the radial artery is still compressed. The presence of collateral circulation constitutes a positive modified Allen test.
Reference: Chapter 12, *Phlebotomy Essentials* 4e.

61. Answer: d
Subject: Handling
Why: Metabolic processes can continue in a blood specimen after collection and negatively affect some analytes. Cooling slows down metabolic processes. Some analytes are more affected by metabolic processes than others and must be cooled immediately after collection and during transportation. Cooling can delay clotting, but is not a desired effect. Cooling does not promote serum separation, nor does it help to avoid hemolysis.
Reference: Chapter 14 , *Phlebotomy Essentials* 4e.

62. Answer: d
Subject: Handling
Why: Proper handling of specimens is important for quality results. It has been estimated that 46 to 68% of all lab errors occur in the preanalytical phase. Proper handling is important because personnel may not be aware that the integrity of a specimen is compromised because effects of mishandling are not always obvious. Most effects of mishandling *cannot* be corrected.
Reference: Chapter 14, *Phlebotomy Essentials* 4e.

63. Answer: c
Subject: Handling
Why: The additive in a tube is designed to work most effectively with an amount of blood that fills the tube until the normal vacuum is exhausted. Results on a specimen from a partially filled liquid EDTA tube may be compromised. Although a blood urea nitrogen (BUN) level does not need to be protected from light, it would not hurt to draw it in an amber serum tube. Serum separator tubes *should* be mixed. A cryofibrinogen specimen *should* be transported at 37°C.
Reference: Chapter 14, *Phlebotomy Essentials* 4e.

64. Answer: a
Subject: Handling
Why: Bilirubin, and vitamins C and B_{12} are all analytes that can be broken down in the presence of light. Ammonia requires ASAP transportation in ice slurry, but is not affected by light exposure.
Reference: Chapter 4, *Phlebotomy Essentials* 4e.

65. Answer: d
Subject: Handling
Why: The energy needed to pump potassium into the cells is provided by glycolysis. Cold inhibits glycolysis, causing potassium to leak from the cells, falsely elevating test results. Cooling can also cause hemolysis, which also elevates test results. If a potassium test is ordered along with other tests that require cooling, it must be collected in a separate tube that is not cooled. Ammonia, glucagon, and lactic acid all require cooling for accurate test results.
Reference: Chapter 14, *Phlebotomy Essentials* 4e.

66. Answer: b
Subject: Regulatory Agencies
Why: Following standard precautions guidelines, not wearing lab coats outside of work areas, and not eating, drinking or smoking in lab work areas are all safety rules. QA indicators are not considered rules but are statements that serve as monitors of patient care. By setting a limit or threshold value, the QA indicators serve as initiators of action plans.
Reference: Chapter 2, *Phlebotomy Essentials* 4e.

67. Answer: b
Subject: Processing
Why: When an erythrocyte sedimentation rate (ESR) is ordered on an EDTA specimen that is held at room temperature, the test must be performed within 4 hours. If the specimen is refrigerated, the time to perform the test is extended up to 12 hours.
Reference: Chapter 14, *Phlebotomy Essentials* 4e.

68. Answer: d
Subject: Processing
Why: To prevent exposure to aerosol formation when opening a tube, the stopper should be covered with a 4 × 4 gauze square during removal, removed while the specimen is held behind a safety shield, or removed using a safety stopper removal device. Never withdraw a sample from a tube using a syringe because it is against OSHA regulations and can hemolyze the specimen.
Reference: Chapter 14, *Phlebotomy Essentials* 4e.

69. Answer: b
Subject: Processing
Why: Suitable specimens are required for accurate laboratory results. Unsuitable specimens must be rejected for testing and new specimens obtained. A properly identified specimen is essential because it links the test results to the patient. Consequently, inadequate patient information on a specimen is reason for rejection by the specimen processor and a request for a new specimen.
Reference: Chapter 14, *Phlebotomy Essentials* 4e.

70. Answer: d
Subject: Processing
Why: All specimens should be transported to the laboratory promptly. According to Clinical and Laboratory Standards Institute (CLSI) guidelines, unless conclusive evidence indicates that longer times do not affect the accuracy of test results, specimens should be separated from the cells as soon as possible with a maximum time limit of two hours.
Reference: Chapter 14, *Phlebotomy Essentials* 4e.

71. Answer: b
Subject: Processing
Why: An aliquot is a portion of a specimen being tested. When several tests are to be performed on the same specimen, portions of the specimen are transferred into separate tubes so that each test has its own tube of specimen. Each portion is called an aliquot, and the tubes containing each portion are called aliquot tubes. Each aliquot tube is labeled with the same identifying information as the original tube.
Reference: Chapter 14, *Phlebotomy Essentials* 4e.

72. Answer: b
Subject: Processing
Why: Blood specimen tubes are typically placed in plastic bags for transportation to the laboratory. CLSI and OSHA guidelines require specimen transport bags to have a bio-hazard logo and a liquid-tight closure.
Reference: Chapter 14, *Phlebotomy Essentials* 4e.

73. Answer: b
Subject: Transporting
Why: Transporting tubes with the stopper up aids clotting of serum tubes, allows fluids to drain away from the stopper to minimize aerosol generation when the stopper is removed, and reduces the chance of hemolysis caused by agitation of the tube contents during transportation. If the tube contents are sterile they will remain that way until the tube is opened regardless of tube position during transport.
Reference: Chapter 14, *Phlebotomy Essentials* 4e.

74. Answer: c
Subject: Transporting
Why: The Food and Drug Administration (FDA) does not issue guidelines for

transporting specimens. Specimens transported by courier or other air or ground mail systems must follow guidelines defined by the Department of Transportation (DOT), the Federal Aviation Administration (FAA), OSHA.
Reference: Chapter 14, *Phlebotomy Essentials* 4e.

75. Answer: a
Subject: Transporting
Why: Ammonia specimens are extremely volatile and must be transported ASAP on ice. The expression "on ice" means in an ice slurry. Bilirubin and carotene specimens require protection from light. A potassium specimen should be collected and transported at room temperature.
Reference: Chapter 14, *Phlebotomy Essentials* 4e.

76. Answer: b
Subject: Transporting
Why: Normal body temperature is approximately 37 ° C (98.6 F).
Reference: Chapter 14, *Phlebotomy Essentials* 4e.

77. Answer: d
Subject: Circulatory System
Why: A clotted blood specimen is actually made up of two parts, a clotted portion containing cells enmeshed in fibrin, and a liquid portion called serum. The liquid portion is called serum because it does not contain fibrinogen. The fibrinogen was used up in the process of clot formation.
Reference: Chapter 6, *Phlebotomy Essentials* 4e.

78. Answer: a
Subject: Specimen Types
Why: The buffy coat of a whole blood specimen is made up of white blood cells and platelets. Therefore a specimen with an abnormally large buffy coat has either a high white blood cell count or a high platelet count.
Reference: Chapter 6, *Phlebotomy Essentials* 4e.

79. Answer: b
Subject: Specimen Types
Why: The most common reason for ordering a culture and sensitivity (C&S) on a urine specimen is to diagnose urinary tract infection (UTI). Urine C&S testing can detect the presence of UTI by culturing (growing) and identifying microorganisms present in the urine. When microorganisms are identified, an antibiotic susceptibility test is performed to determine which antibiotics are effective against the microorganism.
Reference: Chapter 13, *Phlebotomy Essentials* 4e.

80. Answer: b
Subject: Specimen Types
Why: Alpha-fetoprotein (AFP) is an antigen normally present in the human fetus that is also found in amniotic fluid and maternal serum. Abnormal AFP levels may indicate problems in fetal development such as neural tube defects. AFP testing is initially performed on maternal serum, and abnormal results are confirmed by AFP testing on amniotic fluid.
Reference: Chapter 13, *Phlebotomy Essentials* 4e.

81. Answer: b
Subject: Specimen Types
Why: A typical gastric analysis called a basal gastric analysis, involves aspirating a sample of gastric secretions by means of a tube passed through the mouth and throat (oropharynx) or nose and throat (nasopharynx) into the stomach following a period of fasting. This sample is tested to determine acidity. After the basal sample has been collected, a gastric stimulant, most commonly histamine or pentagastrin, is administered intravenously and several more samples are collected at timed intervals. Serum gastrin levels may also be collected.
Reference: Chapter 13, *Phlebotomy Essentials* 4e.

82. Answer: d
Subject: POCT
Why: Thrombocyte is the medical term for platelet. A bleeding time (BT) test evaluates platelet plug formation in the capillaries to detect platelet function disorders and capillary integrity problems. Platelet plug formation at the site of a standardized incision is evaluated. Blood is wicked away from the site to determine the endpoint. The "wicking" technique is critical in getting the correct endpoint of the test.
Reference: Chapter 1, *Phlebotomy Essentials* 4e.

83. Answer: d
Subject: POCT
Why: Glucose monitoring in diabetics (people with diabetes mellitus) is the most common reason for performing glucose testing through point-of-care testing (POCT).
Reference: Chapter 11, *Phlebotomy Essentials* 4e.

84. Answer: a
Subject: POCT
Why: Skin test reactions often produce erythema (redness) or induration (hardness), or both, around the injection site. Interpretation of a TB skin test is based upon the presence or absence of induration, or firm raised area of swelling around the injection site. A positive test results when the area of induration measures 10 mm or greater in diameter. An area between 5 to 9 mm is considered doubtful. An area less than 5 mm is considered negative.
Reference: Chapter 11, *Phlebotomy Essentials* 4e.

85. Answer: c
Subject: POCT
Why: Point-of-care detection of Group A strep normally requires a throat swab specimen. Secretions from the swab are tested for the presence of strep A antigen. A number of different companies make special test kits, for rapid detection of strep A.
Reference: Chapter 11, *Phlebotomy Essentials* 4e.

86. Answer: d
Subject: POCT
Why: Bilirubin, glucose, and leukocytes are all commonly detected in urine by reagent strip methods. Reagent strips also typically detect bacteria, blood, pH, protein, specific gravity, and urobilinogen. A chemical reaction resulting in color changes to the strip take place when the strip is dipped in a urine specimen. Results are determined visually by comparing color changes on the strip with the chart of color codes on the reagent strip container.
Reference: Chapter 11, *Phlebotomy Essentials* 4e.

87. Answer: b
Subject: Regulatory Agencies
Why: American Medical Technologists (AMT), National Credentialing Agency (NCA) and American Society for Clinical Pathology (ASCP) are among the agencies that offer certification for all levels of laboratory professionals. These agencies do not license healthcare allied health professionals because that is the responsibility of the states that have passed licensure laws. They do not accredit phlebotomy programs because that is the role of NAACLS. Public Health Services (PHS) at the state and local level monitor communicable diseases.
Reference: Chapter 1, *Phlebotomy Essentials* 4e.

88. Answer: b
Subject: Regulatory Agencies
Why: To more closely secure protected health information (PHI) and regulate patient privacy, a federal law was enacted and went into effect in 2003. The law, HIPAA, established national standards for the electronic exchange of PHI. The law, CLIA '88 mandates

that all laboratories must be regulated using the same standard measurement regardless of the location, type or size
Reference: Chapter 1, *Phlebotomy Essentials* 4e.

89. Answer: b
Subject: CLSI Guidelines
Why: CLSI venipuncture guidelines recommend cleaning the site with a circular motion from the center to the periphery. In other words, start at the center and wipe outward in ever increasing circles.
Reference: Chapter 8, *Phlebotomy Essentials* 4e.

90. Answer: b
Subject: CLSI Guidelines
Why: Studies have shown that heel punctures deeper than 2.0 mm risk injuring the calcaneus or heel bone. For this reason, the latest CLSI capillary puncture standard states that heel puncture depth should not exceed 2.0 mm.
Reference: Chapter 10, *Phlebotomy Essentials* 4e.

91. Answer: c
Subject: Professional Standards
Why: Clinical and Laboratory Standards Institute (CLSI) publishes standards for phlebotomy procedures. These national standards are recognized as the legal standard of care for phlebotomy procedures. CLIA and College of American Pathologists (CAP) set standards for healthcare organizations and laboratories, respectively, but not specifically for phlebotomy procedures. NAACLS approves phlebotomy programs.
Reference: Chapter 2, *Phlebotomy Essentials* 4e.

92. Answer: b
Subject: Regulatory Agencies
Why: The Clinical Laboratory Improvement Amendments of 1988 (CLIA '88) are federal regulations whose aim is to ensure the accuracy, reliability, and timeliness of patient test results no matter what the type, size, or location of the laboratory. The Occupational Safety and Health Act and also the Occupational Safety and Health Administration (OSHA) were designed to safely protect employees. The Bloodborne Pathogen (BBP) Standard was instituted to protect healthcare employees from bloodborne pathogens.
Reference: Chapter 1, *Phlebotomy Essentials* 4e.

93. Answer: c
Subject: Preanalytical Considerations
Why: Outdated tubes should never be used. The tube vacuum and the integrity of any additive that might be in the tube are guaranteed by the manufacturer, but only if the tube is used before the expiration date. After that date, the additive may break down and no longer function as intended. In addition, outdated tubes may lose some of the vacuum and no longer fill completely. In either situation, the results may be incorrect or erroneous. It has not been shown that the tube stoppers shrink when held past the expiration date.
Reference: Chapter 9, *Phlebotomy Essentials* 4e.

94. Answer: c
Subject: The Law and Ethics
Why: Drawing a person's blood without permission can be perceived as assault, the act or threat of intentionally causing a person to be in fear of harm to his or her person. If the act or threat is actually committed than it can be perceived as battery also. Battery is defined as the intentional harmful or offensive touching of a person without consent or legal justification. Breach of confidentiality involves failure to keep medical information private or confidential. Negligence requires doing something that a reasonable person would not do, or not doing something a reasonable person would do. Malpractice is negligence by a professional.
Reference: Chapter 2, *Phlebotomy Essentials* 4e.

95. Answer: a
Subject: The Law and Ethics
Why: Civil actions involve actions between private parties. The most common civil actions involve tort. For example, a claim of malpractice because of harm or injury to a patient by a phlebotomist is a civil wrong or tort. Crimes against the state or that violate laws established by governments are criminal actions for which a guilty individual may be imprisoned.
Reference: Chapter 2, *Phlebotomy Essentials* 4e.

96. Answer: b
Subject: The Law and Ethics
Why: Malpractice can be described as improper or negligent treatment resulting in injury, loss, or damage. Breach of confidentiality involves failure to keep medical information private or confidential as opposed to invasion of privacy. This tort involves physical intrusion or the unauthorized publishing or releasing of private information.
Reference: Chapter 2, *Phlebotomy Essentials* 4e.

97. Answer: c
Subject: Preanalytical Considerations
Why: Diurnal means "happening daily". The levels of many blood components normally exhibit diurnal variations or normal fluctuations throughout the day.
Reference: Chapter 9, *Phlebotomy Essentials* 4e.

98. Answer: c
Subject: Preanalytical Considerations
Why: Muscular activity elevates blood levels of a number of components, including enzymes. Some enzymes, such as creatine kinase and lactate dehydrogenase, may stay elevated for 24 hours or more.
Reference: Chapter 9, *Phlebotomy Essentials* 4e.

99. Answer: c
Subject: Preanalytical Considerations
Why: If you have no other choice, it is acceptable to collect a blood specimen distal, or below a hematoma, where blood flow is least affected by it. A venipuncture in the area of a hematoma, including above, beside, or through it, is painful to the patient, and can yield erroneous results related to the obstruction of blood flow by the hematoma. It can also result in collection of contaminated and possibly hemolyzed blood from the hematoma, instead of blood from the vein.
Reference: Chapter 9, *Phlebotomy Essentials* 4e.

100. Answer: d
Subject: Preanalytical Considerations
Why: A prothrombin time is a coagulation test. The ratio of blood to anticoagulant is *most* critical for coagulation tests because a ratio of nine parts blood to one part anticoagulant must be maintained for accurate test results. The excess anticoagulant in a short draw dilutes the plasma portion of the specimen used for testing, causing falsely prolonged test results.
Reference: Chapter 9, *Phlebotomy Essentials* 4e.

Exam Topics and Study Hours by Topic

General Knowledge 26%	**Specimen Collection 60%**	**Quality Assurance 14%**
Healthcare System ☐ Recommended study time__ hr.	Patient Considerations ☐ Recommended study time__ hr.	Regulatory Agencies ☐ Recommended study time__ hr.
Communication ☐ Recommended study time__ hr.	Equipment ☐ Recommended study time__ hr.	Preanalytical Considerations ☐ Recommended study time__ hr.
Professionalism ☐ Recommended study time__ hr.	Venipuncture ☐ Recommended study time__ hr.	The Law and Ethics ☐ Recommended study time__ hr.
Infection Control ☐ Recommended study time__ hr.	Capillary ☐ Recommended study time__ hr.	Professional Standards ☐ Recommended study time__ hr.
Safety ☐ Recommended study time__ hr.	Arterial ☐ Recommended study time__ hr.	
Anatomy & Physiology ☐ Recommended study time__ hr.	Handling ☐ Recommended study time__ hr.	
Circulatory System ☐ Recommended study time__ hr.	Processing ☐ Recommended study time__ hr.	
Terminology ☐ Recommended study time__ hr.	Transporting ☐ Recommended study time__ hr.	
Tests & Disorders ☐ Recommended study time__ hr.	Specimen Types ☐ Recommended study time__ hr.	
	POCT ☐ Recommended study time__ hr.	

Summary of Study Hours

Study Item	**Hours**
Pretest Suggested Study Hours	
Additional study hours added for Specimen Collection and Handling which is >50% of the test questions on all exams	4
Timed mock exam (computer or written) and final prep hours	4
Total suggested minimum study hours	

WRITTEN COMPREHENSIVE MOCK EXAM

Choose the BEST answer.

1. The hematology department performs tests that:
   a. concern the ability of the blood to form and dissolve clots.
   b. deal with the antigen-antibody responses of the body.
   c. identify abnormalities of the blood and blood-forming tissues.
   d. involve culturing fluids to identify infectious microorganisms.

2. A phlebotomist who collects a specimen from an inpatient with this disease would be required to wear an N-95 respirator while in the patient's room.
   a. diabetes mellitus
   b. infectious hepatitis
   c. pulmonary tuberculosis
   d. respiratory syncytial virus

3. Red blood cells are also called:
   a. erythrocytes.
   b. leukocytes.
   c. lymphocytes.
   d. thrombocytes.

4. While organizing your phlebotomy tray, you notice that your vinyl tourniquet is soiled with blood. What should you do?
   a. Autoclave it before reuse.
   b. Throw it in biohazard waste.
   c. Wash it with a bleach solution.
   d. Wipe it three times with alcohol.

5. You have a STAT request to collect an H & H on a post-op patient. Which of the following scenarios best describes the proper response?
   a. During the next sweep, collect that specimen first, and send it down to the lab in the tube system before proceeding with the rest.
   b. Go immediately to the surgical recovery room, collect a lavender top tube on the patient, and deliver it immediately to the laboratory.
   c. Proceed to post-op as soon as possible, collect one red top tube on the patient, and return it to the laboratory as soon as possible.
   d. Proceed to surgery, collect a red top and a lavender top tube on the patient, and call someone from the lab to come get the specimens.

6. You asrrive to collect a specimen on a patient named John Doe in 302B. How do you verify that the patient in 302B is indeed John Doe?
   a. Ask him, "Are you John Doe?"; if he says yes, collect the specimen.
   b. Ask him to state his name and date of birth and match it to the requisition.

c. Check the patient's ID band; if it matches the requisition, draw the specimen.
d. Have the nurse verify the patient's name after you check his ID band.

7. A delay in processing longer than 2 hours can lead to erroneously decreased results for:
a. blood glucose.
b. carbon dioxide.
c. ionized calcium.
d. occult blood.

8. Which mode of infection transmission occurs from touching contaminated bed linens?
a. direct contact
b. droplet contact
c. indirect contact
d. vehicle contact

9. Oncology is the medical specialty that treats patients who have:
a. benign and malignant tumors.
b. kidney malfunction and disorders.
c. problems associated with aging.
d. vision problems or eye diseases.

10. The abbreviation for the virus that causes acquired immune deficiency syndrome (AIDS) is:
a. HAV.
b. HBV.
c. HCV.
d. HIV.

11. All of the following could be a cause of hematoma formation during venipuncture EXCEPT:
a. inadequate site pressure is applied after needle removal.
b. the needle bevel is centered in the lumen of the vein.
c. the needle bevel is only partially inserted in the vein.
d. the needle has penetrated through the back of the vein.

12. Which of the following is a proper laboratory safety procedure?
a. Keep food on a different shelf than lab reagents.
b. Keep your mouth closed when you chew gum.
c. Tie back hair that is longer than shoulder length.
d. Wear your protective laboratory coat at all times.

13. Antiseptics are:
a. corrosive liquid chemical compounds.
b. designed to kill pathogenic microbes.
c. safe and effective to use on human skin.
d. used to disinfect contaminated surfaces.

14. A laboratory procedure that requires the use of goggles to prevent exposure from sprays or splashes also requires this protective attire.
a. earplugs
b. face mask
c. respirator
d. sterile gown

15. The respiratory therapy department is responsible for:
a. administering needed oxygen treatments.
b. performing magnetic resonance imaging.
c. performing therapeutic drug monitoring.
d. providing therapy to restore mobility.

16. Standard precautions should be followed:
a. if a patient is in airborne isolation.
b. when a patient is known to be HIV-positive.
c. when a patient is known to have HBV.
d. with all of the patients, at all times.

17. The composition of capillary puncture blood more closely resembles:
a. arterial blood.
b. lymph fluid.
c. tissue fluid.
d. venous blood.

18. You accidentally splash a bleach solution into your eyes while preparing it for cleaning purposes. What is the first thing to do?
   a. Blot your eyes with a wet paper towel several times.
   b. Flush your eyes with water for a minimum of 15 minutes.
   c. Proceed to the emergency room as quickly as possible.
   d. Put 10–20 drops of saline in your eyes and repeat twice.

19. All of the following specimens have conditions that could cause them to be rejected for testing EXCEPT a:
   a. bilirubin specimen that is icteric.
   b. CBC specimen that has clots in it.
   c. fasting glucose specimen that is lipemic.
   d. potassium specimen that is hemolyzed.

20. At what interval is the blood blotted during a bleeding time test?
   a. 10 seconds
   b. 20 seconds
   c. 30 seconds
   d. 60 seconds

21. What is the *best* means of preventing nosocomial infection?
   a. proper immunizations
   b. hand decontamination
   c. isolation procedures
   d. wearing disposable gloves

22. The suffix of the term "hepatitis" means:
   a. condition.
   b. deficiency.
   c. infection.
   d. inflammation.

23. Symptoms of shock include:
   a. decreased breathing.
   b. expressionless face.
   c. rapid, strong pulse.
   d. warm, moist skin.

24. You are unfamiliar with a test that has been ordered. The procedure manual says it requires a serum specimen. Which of the following tubes will yield a serum specimen?
   a. green top
   b. lavender top
   c. light blue top
   d. plain red top

25. Exposure time, distance, and shielding are the main principles involved in:
   a. biohazard safety.
   b. chemical safety.
   c. electrical safety.
   d. radiation safety.

26. When the threshold value of a QA indicator is exceeded and a problem is identified:
   a. a corrective action plan is implemented.
   b. an incident report is written and filed.
   c. patient specimens must be drawn again.
   d. patients' physicians must be notified.

27. A phlebotomist arrives to collect a 2-hour postprandial glucose specimen on an inpatient and discovers that 2 hours have not elapsed since the patient's meal. What should the phlebotomist do?
   a. Ask the patient's nurse to verify the correct time to draw the specimen.
   b. Come back 2 hours from the time the patient says he finished his meal.
   c. Draw the specimen and write the time collected on the specimen label.
   d. Fill out an incident report form and give it to the phlebotomy supervisor.

28. Which of the following is referred to as a delivering chamber of the heart?
   a. aortic arch
   b. left ventricle
   c. right atrium
   d. vena cava

29. Which of the following is an example of a work practice control that reduces risk of exposure to bloodborne pathogens?
    a. a red biohazard sticker
    b. an exposure control plan
    c. frequent hand washing
    d. hepatitis B vaccination

30. An inpatient refused to let a phlebotomist collect blood from him one afternoon. Early the next morning, another phlebotomist who had been advised of the situation arrived to collect a specimen on the same patient. The phlebotomist drew the specimen without waking him. The phlebotomist could be charged with:
    a. assault and battery.
    b. invasion of privacy.
    c. res ipsa loquitur.
    d. vicarious liability.

31. A phlebotomist is accidentally punctured on the thumb by a needle that was used to collect a blood specimen from a patient. The first thing he or she should do is:
    a. decontaminate the site and fill out an incident report.
    b. find the patient's chart and check the medical records.
    c. go to the employee health service and get a tetanus booster.
    d. leave the area so that the patient does not see the injury.

32. What should a phlebotomist do if a patient feels faint during a blood draw?
    a. Have the patient lower his or her head and continue the blood draw.
    b. Immediately discontinue the draw and lower the patient's head.
    c. Remove the needle and shake the patient to revive him or her.
    d. Use one hand to hold the patient upright and continue the draw.

33. Which of the following is an example of a nosocomial infection? A:
    a. catheter site of a patient in intensive care becomes infected.
    b. child breaks out with measles a day after hospital admission.
    c. drug addict contracts hepatitis from a contaminated needle.
    d. patient is admitted with symptoms suggestive of Hantavirus.

34. All of the following are reasons to eliminate a potential venipuncture site EXCEPT:
    a. petechiae appear with tourniquet application.
    b. the arm is noticeably edematous from an IV.
    c. there is a massive scar in the antecubital area.
    d. the only palpable vein feels hard and cordlike.

35. These are the initials of the two organizations responsible for the latest *Guideline for Isolation Precautions in Hospitals*.
    a. CDC and HICPAC
    b. CLSI and OSHA
    c. HICPAC and NIOSH
    d. NIOSH and OSHA

36. According to laboratory policy, you are required to collect a specimen that will yield 2.5 times the amount of specimen needed to perform the test. If a chemistry test requires 0.5 mL of serum, which of the following tubes is the smallest that can be used?
    a. plain bullet
    b. 3 mL red top
    c. 5 mL SST
    d. 7 mL PST

37. A short in the wiring of a centrifuge causes a fire. Which type of extinguisher is best for putting it out?
    a. Class A
    b. Class B
    c. Class C
    d. Class D

38. To minimize effects of hemoconcentration caused by blockage of blood flow during venipuncture, the tourniquet should never be left in place longer than:
 a. 30 seconds.
 b. 60 seconds.
 c. 2 minutes.
 d. 4 minutes.

39. Which of the following is an acceptable chemical safety procedure?
 a. Familiarize oneself with the MSDS for any new reagent.
 b. If mixing acid and water together, add the water to the acid.
 c. Mix bleach with other cleaners for extra disinfecting power.
 d. Store chemicals at eye level so the labels are easy to see.

40. The minimum education level of a clinical laboratory scientist (CLS) is a(n):
 a. advanced degree.
 b. associate's degree.
 c. bachelor's degree.
 d. high school diploma.

41. You have just been hired as a phlebotomist but have not been vaccinated against hepatitis B. You are immediately assigned to phlebotomy duties. According to federal law, your employer must offer you hepatitis B vaccination free of charge:
 a. after any probationary period is over.
 b. immediately upon being hired.
 c. within 1 month of employment.
 d. within 10 working days of assignment.

42. While staying in a healthcare facility, one of the patient expectations as listed in *The Patient Care Partnership* brochure is the right to:
 a. a 1:1 patient to nurse ratio.
 b. a quiet, private room.
 c. help with billing claims.
 d. information on roommates.

43. CLSI and OSHA guidelines do *not* require specimen transport bags to have:
 a. a visible biohazard logo.
 b. liquid-tight closure tops.
 c. shock-resistance features.
 d. slip pockets for paperwork.

44. Which of the following needles has the largest diameter?
 a. 18-gauge hypodermic needle
 b. 21-gauge multisample needle
 c. 22-gauge multisample needle
 d. 23-gauge butterfly needle

45. A phlebotomist explains to a patient that a blood specimen is going to be collected. The patient extends his arm and pushes up his sleeve. This is an example of:
 a. expressed consent.
 b. implied consent.
 c. informed consent.
 d. refusal of consent.

46. The main difference between serum and plasma is:
 a. plasma has fibrinogen; serum does not.
 b. plasma is obtained from clotted blood.
 c. serum is usually clear; plasma is cloudy.
 d. serum is pale yellow; plasma is colorless.

47. While processing blood specimens, you accidentally spill blood on the countertop. What is the best way to clean it up?
 a. Absorb it with a damp cloth and wash the area with soapy water.
 b. Absorb it with a paper towel and wipe the area with disinfectant.
 c. Wait for it to dry and then scrape it into a biohazard bag.
 d. Wipe it up immediately with an alcohol pad and let it dry.

48. Which statement concerning human anatomy is true?
    a. A patient who is supine is lying down on his or her back.
    b. Phalanges is the medical term for the curved heel bone.
    c. Sagittal planes divide the body into upper and lower portions.
    d. The elbow is distal to the wrist and proximal to the shoulder.

49. Identify the tubes that can be used to collect a WBC, PT, and STAT calcium by color and in the proper order of collection for a multi-tube draw.
    a. gold top, yellow top, light blue top
    b. lavender top, SST, royal blue top
    c. light blue top, green top, lavender top
    d. red top, gray top, light blue top

50. Which type of test is most affected by tissue thromboplastin contamination?
    a. chemistry
    b. coagulation
    c. microbiology
    d. serology

51. The silica particles in an SST:
    a. enhance the process of coagulation.
    b. keep RBCs from sticking to the tube.
    c. minimize hemolysis of blood cells.
    d. stop glycolysis by enhancing clotting.

52. The best choice of equipment for drawing difficult veins is:
    a. butterfly and evacuated tube holder.
    b. lancet and microcollection container.
    c. needle and evacuated tube holder.
    d. small gauge needle and 5cc syringe.

53. A blood smear made from blood collected in EDTA must be prepared within:
    a. a few minutes of collection.
    b. 30 minutes of collection.
    c. 1.0 hour of collection.
    d. 4.0 hours of collection.

54. Anaerobic conditions must be maintained when collecting and handling this specimen.
    a. bilirubin
    b. blood gases
    c. glucose
    d. plasma renin

55. Some specimens require cooling to:
    a. avoid cold agglutinin activation.
    b. prevent the blood from clotting.
    c. separate serum more completely.
    d. slow down metabolic processes.

56. Proper collection and handling of anticoagulant tubes includes all of the following EXCEPT:
    a. collecting them in the proper order of draw to prevent additive carryover between tubes.
    b. filling them until the vacuum is exhausted to maintain correct ratio of blood to additive.
    c. inverting them the recommended number of times to prevent microclots from forming.
    d. transporting them in a horizontal position so they continue to mix during transportation.

57. HIPAA was enacted to do all of the following EXCEPT:
    a. examine all patient healthcare records.
    b. protect privacy of patient information.
    c. provide guidelines for sharing of PHI.
    d. standardize electronic transfer of data.

58. The patient asks if the test you are about to draw is for diabetes. How do you answer?
    a. Explain that it is best to discuss the test with the physician.
    b. If the test is for glucose say, "Yes, it is," but do not elaborate.
    c. Say, "HIPAA confidentiality rules won't let me tell you."
    d. Tell the patient that it is not for a glucose test even if it is.

59. Which of the following is a safe area for infant heel puncture? The:
    a. area of the arch.
    b. central plantar area.
    c. medial plantar surface.
    d. posterior curvature.

60. Which of the following is a function of the muscular system?
    a. eliminate waste
    b. produce heat
    c. regulate fluids
    d. secrete hormones

61. The major structural difference between arteries and veins is:
    a. arteries are larger in diameter.
    b. arteries have more tissue layers.
    c. veins have a thicker muscle layer.
    d. veins have valves that direct flow.

62. You arrive to draw a fasting specimen. The patient is eating breakfast. What do you do?
    a. Ask his nurse if it should be collected and document it as a "non-fasting" specimen if drawn.
    b. Collect the specimen anyway, because the patient had not finished eating all of his breakfast.
    c. Do not collect the specimen; fill out an incident report, and ask the nurse to re-order the test.
    d. Draw the specimen anyway, but write "non-fasting" on the test order and the specimen label.

63. The additive and color code associated with coagulation tests is:
    a. lithium heparin, green.
    b. potassium EDTA, lavender.
    c. sodium citrate, light blue.
    d. thixotropic gel, red/gray.

64. What is the CLSI-recommended blood culture site disinfectant for infants 2 months and older?
    a. chlorhexidine gluconate
    b. benzalkonium chloride
    c. Betadine swabsticks
    d. isopropyl alcohol swab

65. All of the following statements concerning an employee bloodborne pathogen exposure incident are true EXCEPT:
    a. all exposure incidents should be reported to the immediate supervisor.
    b. an exposed employee has access to a free confidential medical evaluation.
    c. the exposure should be documented on a standard incident report form.
    d. the source patient must submit to HIV and HBV testing within 48 hours.

66. Which additive prevents coagulation by binding calcium?
    a. lithium heparin
    b. potassium EDTA
    c. sodium fluoride
    d. thixotropic gel

67. Which of the following statements complies with electrical safety guidelines?
    a. electrical equipment should be unplugged while being serviced
    b. extension cords should be used to conveniently place equipment
    c. it is fairly safe to use an electrical cord that is only slightly frayed
    d. use electrical equipment carefully if it is starting to malfunction

68. You must collect an ETOH specimen on a patient for forensic purposes. Which of the following tubes would be the best choice to collect the specimen?
    a. gray top sodium fluoride tube
    b. green top plasma separator tube
    c. plain red top clot activator tube
    d. royal blue with a green-coded label

69. You are the only phlebotomist on the night shift. You receive orders for all of the following tests within minutes of one another. Which test has the greatest collection priority?
    a. ASAP electrolytes in CCU
    b. STAT CBC in labor and delivery
    c. STAT electrolytes in the ER
    d. timed blood cultures in ICU

70. It is necessary to control the depth of lancet insertion during capillary puncture to avoid:
   a. excessive bleeding.
   b. injury to the calcaneus.
   c. puncture of an artery.
   d. specimen contamination.

71. Which of the following is the best way to tell if a specimen is arterial? As the specimen is collected, the blood:
   a. appears bright cherry red.
   b. exhibits some air bubbles.
   c. looks thick and dark blue.
   d. pumps into the syringe.

72. You must collect a specimen on a 6-year-old. The child is a little fearful. Which of the following is the best thing to do?
   a. Explain what is going to happen in simple terms and ask the child to cooperate.
   b. Have someone restrain the child and draw the specimen without any explanation.
   c. Tell the child to remain very still and not to worry because then it will not hurt.
   d. Tell the child that you will give him a special treat if he is still and does not cry.

73. You must collect a prothrombin specimen from a patient with IVs in both arms. The best place to collect the specimen is:
   a. above one of the IVs.
   b. below one of the IVs.
   c. from an ankle vein.
   d. from one of the IVs.

74. What is the meaning of the following symbol?
   a. biological hazard
   b. chemical hazard
   c. microbial hazard
   d. radiation hazard

75. A patient complains of significant pain when you insert the needle. The pain does not subside and radiates down the patient's arm. What should you do?
   a. Ask the patient if it is all right to continue the draw.
   b. Collect the necessary amount as quickly as possible.
   c. Remove the needle and discontinue the draw immediately.
   d. Tell the patient there will be another stick if you stop now.

76. Which of the following microcollection containers should be filled first if collected by capillary puncture?
   a. gray top
   b. green top
   c. lavender top
   d. red top

77. Quality assurance (QA) procedures include all of the following EXCEPT:
   a. checking needles for blunt tips and barbs before use.
   b. following strict requirements for labeling specimens.
   c. keeping track of and logging employee absenteeism.
   d. recording results of refrigerator temperature checks.

78. If the phlebotomist makes a blood smear that is too short, he or she should try again and:
   a. decrease the angle of the spreader slide.
   b. exert more pressure on the spreader slide.
   c. increase the angle of the spreader slide.
   d. place a smaller drop of blood on the slide.

79. The bleeding time (BT) test assesses:
   a. effectiveness of heparin therapy.
   b. functioning of the red blood cells.
   c. platelet plug formation in capillaries.
   d. therapeutic action of a blood thinner.

80. Which of the following diseases can be transmitted through blood and body fluids?
   a. anemia
   b. leukemia
   c. rubella
   d. syphilis

81. The most common reason for glucose monitoring through POCT is to:
   a. check for sporadic glucose in the urine.
   b. control medication-induced mood swings.
   c. diagnose glucose metabolism problems.
   d. monitor glucose levels for diabetic care.

82. All of the following are examples of possible "parenteral" means of transmission EXCEPT:
   a. drinking water from a glass that is contaminated.
   b. getting stuck by a needle used on a patient with AIDS.
   c. rubbing the eyes without first washing the hands.
   d. touching infectious material with chapped hands.

83. Which of the following pieces of information is typically required on an inpatient specimen label?
   a. diagnosis or CPT code
   b. medical record number
   c. name of the physician
   d. room and bed number

84. Which additional identification information is typically required on a nonblood specimen label?
   a. accession number
   b. patient diagnosis
   c. physician's name
   d. specimen source

85. All of the following analytes require protection from light EXCEPT:
   a. ammonia.
   b. bilirubin.
   c. vitamin B_{12}.
   d. vitamin C.

86. A technologist asks you to collect 5 cc of whole blood for a special test. What volume tube should you use?
   a. 3.0 mL
   b. 5.0 mL
   c. 10 mL
   d. 15 mL

87. Your hospital uses computer-generated specimen labels. What information is typically added to the label manually when the specimen is collected?
   a. medical record number
   b. patient's date of birth
   c. patient's full name
   d. phlebotomist's initials

88. You are the only phlebotomist in an outpatient drawing station. A physician orders a test with which you are unfamiliar. What is the appropriate action to take?
   a. call the physician's office for assistance
   b. draw both a serum and a plasma specimen
   c. refer to the specimen collection manual
   d. send the patient to another drawing station

89. Promoting good public relations is a part of the phlebotomist's role for all of the following reasons EXCEPT:
   a. a phlebotomist is a representative of the laboratory.
   b. good public relations promotes harmonious relationships.
   c. patients equate experiences with overall caliber of care received.
   d. skilled public relations can cover up inexperience and insecurity.

90. Tubes should be transported with the stopper up for all of the following reasons EXCEPT that it:
   a. encourages complete clot formation.
   b. maintains the sterility of the sample.
   c. minimizes stopper-caused aerosols.
   d. reduces agitation-caused hemolysis.

91. You are performing a sweat chloride test on a toddler. What infection control precautions apply to the sweat specimen that is collected?
   a. contact precautions
   b. droplet precautions
   c. no special precautions
   d. standard precautions

92. Specimens transported by courier or other air or ground mail systems must follow guidelines defined by all of the following EXCEPT:
   a. DOT.
   b. FAA.
   c. FDA.
   d. OSHA.

93. Which of the following is *not* a required characteristic of a sharps container?
   a. leak-proof
   b. lid that locks
   c. puncture-resistant
   d. red in color

94. Which statement describes proper centrifuge operation?
   a. Avoid centrifuging serum specimens in the same centrifuge as plasma specimens.
   b. Balance specimens by placing tubes of equal volume and size opposite one another.
   c. Centrifuge serum specimens as soon as possible to stimulate the clotting process.
   d. Remove stoppers from the tubes before balancing specimen tubes in the centrifuge.

95. The manufacturer must supply an MSDS for:
   a. certain prescribed medications.
   b. fluid-resistant laboratory coats.
   c. isopropyl and methyl alcohol.
   d. isotonic sodium chloride solution.

96. Which type of specimen has processing and testing priority over all other specimens?
   a. ASAP
   b. fasting
   c. STAT
   d. timed

97. What is the recommended procedure for collecting a 24-hour urine specimen?
   a. Collect the first morning specimen and all other urine for 24 hours except the first specimen the following morning.
   b. Collect the first morning specimen and all other urine for 24 hours including the first specimen the next morning.
   c. Discard the first morning specimen; collect all the following specimens including the next morning's specimen.
   d. Drink 500 cc of water before starting the timing; collect all urine for a 24-hour period including the first and last.

98. The abbreviation for the federal agency that instituted and enforces regulations requiring the labeling of hazardous materials is:
   a. CDC.
   b. CLSI.
   c. NFPA.
   d. OSHA.

99. Continuing education units (CEUs) are:
   a. certificates awarded for participating in skills courses.
   b. college credits for taking related healthcare courses.
   c. documentation of passing a national certification exam.
   d. proof of participation in workshops to upgrade knowledge.

100. The most common nosocomial infection in the United States is:
   a. hepatitis infection.
   b. respiratory infection.
   c. surgical site infection.
   d. urinary tract infection.

ANSWERS TO THE WRITTEN COMPREHENSIVE MOCK EXAM

Answers to the Written Comprehensive Mock Exam Topics and chapters from Phlebotomy Essentials 4th edition.

1. Ans: c
   Cognitive level: Recall
   Topic: Laboratory Departments
   Chapter: 1

2. Ans: c
   Cognitive level: Application
   Topic: Infection Control
   Chapter: 3

3. Ans: a
   Cognitive level: Recall
   Topic: Circulatory System
   Chapter: 6

4. Ans: b
   Cognitive level: Recall
   Topic: Blood Collection Equipment
   Chapter: 7

5. Ans: b
   Cognitive level: Application
   Topic: Test Priority
   Chapter: 8

6. Ans: b
   Cognitive level: Application
   Topic: Patient Identification
   Chapter: 8

7. Ans: a
   Cognitive level: Recall
   Topic: Specimen Handling
   Chapter: 14

8. Ans: c
   Cognitive level: Recall
   Topic: Infection Control
   Chapter: 3

9. Ans: a
   Cognitive level: Recall
   Topic: Medical Specialties
   Chapter: 1

10. Ans: d
    Cognitive level: Recall
    Topic: Infection Control
    Chapter: 3

11. Ans: b
    Cognitive level: Analysis
    Topic: Procedural Error Risks
    Chapter: 9

12. Ans: c
    Cognitive level: Application
    Topic: Safety
    Chapter: 3

13. Ans: c
    Cognitive level: Analysis
    Topic: Blood Collection Equipment
    Chapter: 7

14. Ans: b
    Cognitive level: Recall
    Topic: Infection Control Methods
    Chapter: 3

15. Ans: a
    Cognitive level: Recall
    Topic: Hospital Service Areas
    Chapter: 1

16. Ans: d
    Cognitive level: Recall
    Topic: Infection Control
    Chapter: 3

17. Ans: a
    Cognitive level: Recall
    Topic: Capillary Puncture Principles
    Chapter: 10

18. Ans: b
    Cognitive level: Application
    Topic: Chemical Safety
    Chapter: 3

19. Ans: a
    Cognitive level: Analysis
    Topic: Specimen Processing
    Chapter: 14

20. Ans: c
    Cognitive level: Recall
    Topic: Point-of-Care Testing
    Chapter: 11

21. Ans: b
    Cognitive level: Recall
    Topic: Infection Control
    Chapter: 3

22. Ans: d
    Cognitive level: Recall
    Topic: Medical Terminology
    Chapter: 4

23. Ans: b
    Cognitive level: Analysis
    Topic: First Aid
    Chapter: 3

24. Ans: d
    Cognitive level: Application
    Topic: Evacuated Tubes
    Chapter: 7

25. Ans: d
    Cognitive level: Recall
    Topic: Radiation Safety
    Chapter: 3

26. Ans: a
    Cognitive level: Application
    Topic: Quality Assurance
    Chapter: 2

27. Ans: a
    Cognitive level: Application
    Topic: Special Collections
    Chapter: 11

28. Ans: b
    Cognitive level: Recall
    Topic: Heart Structure
    Chapter: 6

29. Ans: c
    Cognitive level: Application
    Topic: Biosafety
    Chapter: 3

30. Ans: a
    Cognitive level: Analysis
    Topic: Legal Issues
    Chapter: 2

31. Ans: a
    Cognitive level: Application
    Topic: Biosafety
    Chapter: 3

32. Ans: b
    Cognitive level: Application
    Topic: Patient Complications and Conditions
    Chapter: 9

33. Ans: a
    Cognitive level: Recall
    Topic: Infection Control
    Chapter: 3

34. Ans: a
    Cognitive level: Application
    Topic 1: Problem Sites
    Topic 2: Patient Complications and Conditions
    Chapter: 9

35. Ans: a
    Cognitive level: Recall
    Topic: Infection Control
    Chapter: 3

36. Ans: b
    Cognitive level: Application
    Topic: Blood Composition
    Chapter: 6

37. Ans: c
    Cognitive level: Application
    Topic: Electrical Safety
    Chapter: 3

38. Ans: b
    Cognitive level: Recall
    Topic 1: Routine ETS Venipuncture
    Topic 2: Specimen Quality Concerns
    Chapters: 8, 9

39. Ans: a
    Cognitive level: Analysis
    Topic: Chemical Safety
    Chapter: 3

40. Ans: c
    Cognitive level: Recall
    Topic: Clinical Laboratory Personnel
    Chapter: 1

41. Ans: d
    Cognitive level: Recall
    Topic: Biosafety
    Chapter: 3

42. Ans: c
    Cognitive level: Recall
    Topic: Patients' Rights
    Chapter: 1

43. Ans: c
    Cognitive level: Recall
    Topic: Specimen Handling
    Chapter: 14

44. Ans: a
    Cognitive level: Recall
    Topic: Venipuncture Equipment
    Chapter: 7

45. Ans: b
    Cognitive level: Application
    Topic: Legal Issues
    Chapter: 2

46. Ans: a
    Cognitive level: Analysis
    Topic: Blood Composition
    Chapter: 6

47. Ans: b
    Cognitive level: Application
    Topic: Biosafety
    Chapter: 3

48. Ans: a
    Cognitive level: Analysis
    Topic: Anatomy and Physiology
    Chapter: 5

49. Ans: c
    Cognitive level: Application
    Topic 1: Venipuncture Equipment
    Topic 2: Order of Draw
    Chapter: 7

50. Ans: b
    Cognitive level: Recall
    Topic: Special Collections
    Chapter: 11

51. Ans: a
    Cognitive level: Recall
    Topic: Venipuncture Equipment
    Chapter: 7

52. Ans: a
    Cognitive level: Recall
    Topic 1: Venipuncture Equipment
    Topic 2: Butterfly procedures
    Chapter: 7,8

53. Ans: c
    Cognitive level: Recall
    Topic: Routine Blood Film Preparation
    Chapter: 10

54. Ans: b
    Cognitive level: Recall
    Topic: Arterial Puncture Procedures
    Chapter: 12

55. Ans: d
    Cognitive level: Recall
    Topic: Specimen Handling
    Chapter: 14

56. Ans: d
    Cognitive level: Analysis
    Topic: Anticoagulants
    Chapter: 7

57. Ans: a
    Cognitive level: Recall
    Topic: Confidentiality
    Chapter: 1

58. Ans: a
    Cognitive level: Application
    Topic: Addressing Patient Inquiries
    Chapter: 8

59. Ans: c
    Cognitive level: Recall
    Topic: Capillary Puncture
    Chapter: 10

60. Ans: b
    Cognitive level: Recall
    Topic: Anatomy and Physiology
    Chapter: 5

61. Ans: d
    Cognitive level: Analysis
    Topic: Blood Vessel Structure
    Chapter: 6

62. Ans: c
    Cognitive level: Analysis
    Topic: Diet Restrictions
    Chapter: 8

63. Ans: c
    Cognitive level: Recall
    Topic: Blood Collection Additives
    Chapter: 7

64. Ans: b
    Cognitive level: Recall
    Topic: Special Collections
    Chapter: 11

65. Ans: d
    Cognitive level: Analysis
    Topic: Biosafety
    Chapter: 3

66. Ans: b
    Cognitive level: Recall
    Topic: Blood Collection Additives
    Chapter: 7

67. Ans: a
Cognitive level: Application
Topic: Electrical Safety
Chapter: 3

68. Ans: a
Cognitive level: Recall
Topic 1: Blood Collection Additives
Topic 2: Toxicology Specimens
Chapters: 7, 11

69. Ans: c
Cognitive level: Analysis
Topic: Test Status and Collection Priority
Chapter: 8

70. Ans: b
Cognitive level: Recall
Topic: Capillary Puncture Procedures
Chapter: 10

71. Ans: d
Cognitive level: Recall
Topic: Arterial Puncture Procedures
Chapter: 12

72. Ans: a
Cognitive level: Analysis
Topic: Pediatric Venipuncture
Chapter: 8

73. Ans: b
Cognitive level: Application
Topic: Vascular Access Devices (VADs) and Sites
Chapter: 9

74. Ans: a
Cognitive level: Recall
Topic: Safety
Chapter: 3

75. Ans: c
Cognitive level: Application
Topic 1: Patient Complications Conditions
Topic 2: Procedural Error risks
Chapter: 9

76. Ans: c
Cognitive level: Recall
Topic: Capillary Puncture Order of draw
Chapter: 10

77. Ans: c
Cognitive level: Application
Topic: Quality Assurance
Chapter: 2

78. Ans: a
Cognitive level: Analysis
Topic: Routine Blood Film Preparation
Chapter: 10

79. Ans: c
Cognitive level: Analysis
Topic: Point-of-Care Testing
Chapter: 11

80. Ans: d
Cognitive level: Recall
Topic: Infection Control
Chapter: 3

81. Ans: d
Cognitive level: Application
Topic: Point-of-Care Testing
Chapter: 11

82. Ans: a
Cognitive level: Application
Topic: Biosafety
Chapter: 3

83. Ans: b
Cognitive level: Recall
Topic: Tube Labeling
Chapter: 8

84. Ans: d
Cognitive level: Recall
Topic: Nonblood Specimens and Tests
Chapter: 13

85. Ans: a
Cognitive level: Recall
Topic: Specimen Handling
Chapter: 14

86. Ans: b
Cognitive level: Recall
Topic: Blood Composition
Chapter: 6

87. Ans: d
Cognitive level: Recall
Topic: Requisitions
Chapter: 8

88. Ans: c
Cognitive level: Application
Topic: Quality Assurance
Chapter: 2

89. Ans: d
Cognitive level: Application
Topic: Public Relations and Client Interaction
Chapter: 1

90. Ans: b
Cognitive level: Application
Topic: Specimen Handling
Chapter: 14

91. Ans: c
Cognitive level: Application
Topic: Infection Control
Chapter: 3

92. Ans: c
Cognitive level: Recall
Topic: Specimen Handling
Chapter: 14

93. Ans: d
Cognitive level: Recall
Topic: Blood Collection Equipment
Chapter: 7

94. Ans: b
Cognitive level: Application
Topic: Specimen Processing
Chapter: 14

95. Ans: c
Cognitive level: Application
Topic: Chemical Safety
Chapter: 3

96. Ans: c
Cognitive level: Recall
Topic: Collection Priority
Chapter: 8

97. Ans: c
Cognitive level: Application
Topic: Nonblood Specimens and Tests
Chapter: 13

98. Ans: d
Cognitive level: Recall
Topic: Safety
Chapter: 3

99. Ans: d
Cognitive level: Recall
Topic: Official Recognition
Chapter: 1

100. Ans: d
Cognitive level: Recall
Topic: Infection Control
Chapter: 3

INDEX

Page numbers followed by *f* indiacte figures. Page numbers followed by *t* indicate tables.